THEORETICAL FOUNDATIONS OF ELECTRON SPIN RESONANCE

This is Volume 37 of
PHYSICAL CHEMISTRY
A Series of Monographs

Editor: ERNEST M. LOEBL, *Polytechnic Institute of New York*

A complete list of titles in this series appears at the end of this volume.

THEORETICAL FOUNDATIONS OF ELECTRON SPIN RESONANCE

JOHN E. HARRIMAN

Department of Chemistry and
Theoretical Chemistry Institute
University of Wisconsin
Madison, Wisconsin

ACADEMIC PRESS New York San Francisco London 1978

A Subsidiary of Harcourt Brace Jovanovich, Publishers

ACADEMIC PRESS, INC.
111 Fifth Avenue, New York, New York 10003

United Kingdom Edition published by
ACADEMIC PRESS, INC. (LONDON) LTD.
24/28 Oval Road, London NW1 7DX

Library of Congress Cataloging in Publication Data

Harriman, John E.
Theoretical foundations of electron spin resonance.

(Physical chemistry, a series of monographs ;)
Bibliography: p.
Includes index.
1. Electron paramagnetic resonance spectroscopy. I. Title. II. Series.
QC763.H37 538'.3 77-75573
ISBN 0-12-326350-6

PRINTED IN THE UNITED STATES OF AMERICA

CONTENTS

APPENDICES

PREFACE

When I was in high school and college, one activity I enjoyed was formal competitive debate. The first speaker in such a debate always began by defining terms so everyone would be in agreement as to just what was the subject. I will begin this introduction by giving my "definitions" of the terms which appear in the title. In doing so I hope to establish part of the context in which the book was written.

Theoretical. It is clear that this book is theoretical in its approach. Only a few references to experimental results are made, although the nature of experimental work in the field has influenced the selection of material to be treated. More important, perhaps, is that the organization of the book is on a theoretical basis. I have tried to exhibit some of the unity present in this branch of theoretical chemistry; it is a unity that is sometimes obscured when results are developed on the basis of need in a particular experimental context.

Foundations. This book is not elementary. I have in fact assumed reasonable prior knowledge on the part of the reader of both the fundamentals of ESR and ordinary quantum chemistry. Foundations are referred to by way of distinction from applications. I have tried to establish the foundations firmly; I have not attempted to build upon them applications to other branches of chemistry or physics.

Electron Spin Resonance. If the assumption that the reader already has some knowledge of the subject is correct, the only word requiring comment is "spin." Objection might be made that the term electron *spin* resonance is inappropriate in certain cases and thus that the more general term electron *paramagnetic* resonance is preferable. It is precisely because of this implied limitation that I have chosen "spin." In selecting the topics to be discussed I had in mind applications to polyatomic, probably organic, free radicals in condensed phases. Questions of orbital angular momentum in first order, applicable to transition metal complexes, and of rotational angular momentum, applicable to small radicals in the gas phase, have not been addressed.[†] Electron paramagnetic resonance in nonmolecular solids has also been excluded from explicit consideration. Many of the results obtained here are, of course, applicable to these systems, but problems, methods, and approximations specifically addressed to them have been avoided.

Another major restriction on the subjects addressed is not inherent in the title. This book confines itself to essentially static phenomena: the description and determination of stationary-state energy levels. Dynamic aspects other than the ESR transition itself have not been considered. When the book was first planned, I expected that topics such as relaxation, hindered rotation, inter- and intramolecular electron transfers, etc. would be discussed. I have since abandoned these topics for a number of reasons.

One is just the fact that I have done little work in these areas and thus feel less comfortable with them. A related consideration is the time that would have been required to develop a careful treatment. Another reason is the recent appearance of several books in this area [145, 159]. The decisive factor, however, is my feeling that the theory of relaxation and related processes is still in a state of rapid development. While present treatments are entirely satisfactory in some cases and at least useful in others, they do not as yet present an essentially unified, firmly grounded, a priori theory such as is possible (at least very nearly) for the static phenomena. I came to suspect that I would be unsatisfied with anything I did in this area, so I did nothing. Besides, the book was getting rather long anyway.

As I have indicated, I have assumed the reader to have some familiarity with elementary ESR. To provide some background and possibly an indication of motivation to those readers with very limited previous experience, a brief review has been provided in Chapter 0. I have also assumed some familiarity with elementary quantum chemistry, I hope comparable to that provided in a typical graduate course. The necessary aspects of relativistic quantum mechanics are developed as needed. More advanced techniques such as second quantization and diagrammatic perturbation theory have been avoided. Relevant features of classical mechanics and electromagnetic theory, as well as of the quantum theory of angular momentum and rotations, are reviewed in appendices.

Where appropriate, atomic units have been used. In the early sections I have chosen not to use atomic or natural units because constants with dimensions make it easier to keep track of terms. Gaussian rather than SI units have been chosen. I believe they will be more familiar to more readers

[†] These topics are treated by, for example, Abgragam and Bleany [2] and by Carrington, [31], respectively.

and, in addition, despite the clear advantages offered by the International System, I prefer Coulomb's law to have the simplest possible form for this work, where Coulomb forces dominate. A comparison of systems of units is presented at the end of Appendix A.

A few words next about the organization of the book. The fundamental unit is the section, although sections vary considerably in length. These sections are grouped into chapters, the titles of which I believe to be self-explanatory. The progression is one of logical development rather than historical or in terms of practical interest. This is one aspect of the assumption of some prior knowledge of ESR. Motivation—why something is of interest—is in the early stages to be supplied by the reader if required. When significance is not apparent, I request a suspension of judgment. I hope it will eventually be recognizable.

References have been presented primarily on the basis of two criteria: when my treatment was explicitly based on another work, appropriate credit is given; when another point of view or further development is likely to be useful, references are provided. In both cases my primary concern was utility rather than historical precedence. I have therefore cited review papers or books in preference to the original literature in many cases. With the exception of a very few topics, I have not attempted to completely survey the literature in the field. To the many workers who might have been cited, and to the hopefully few who clearly should have been but were not, I offer my apologies.

ACKNOWLEDGMENTS

I would like to express my appreciation to the friends and colleagues, past and present, who contributed to this work. I was introduced to ESR by A. H. Maki when we were both at Harvard, and to modern theoretical chemistry by P. O. Löwdin in Uppsala. J. O. Hirschfelder is responsible, more than anyone else, for the existence of and favorable environment within the Theoretical Chemistry Institute where this book was written. I thank them especially.

Among those who read portions of the manuscript and provided helpful comments were C. F. Curtiss, J. M. Dietrich, S. T. Epstein, E. M. Loebl, J. M. Norbeck, B. T. Sutcliffe, and F. A. Weinhold. Suggestions and corrections were also received from graduate students with whom the manuscript was reviewed. They were Melodye Block, David Fish, Nancy Piltch, Charles Szmanda, and James Tortorelli. A truly superb job of technical typing, which I greatly appreciate, was done by Patty Spires.

Financial support that contributed directly or indirectly to the development of the book was received from the National Science Foundation and the Alfred P. Sloan Foundation.

I would like to express my sincere thanks to my wife and son for putting up with me during this project and for not asking too frequently, "How is the book coming?" To my colleagues on faculty committees where I spent many hours that might have been used to hasten completion of this work, my forgiveness; it was my choice.

CHAPTER 0

REVIEW OF ELEMENTARY ELECTRON SPIN RESONANCE

Systems Studied by Electron Spin Resonance

In magnetic resonance spectroscopy, transitions are observed between energy levels which depend on the strength of a magnetic field.‡ Electron spin resonance (ESR) is a branch of magnetic resonance spectroscopy dealing with molecules (or occasionally atoms, or "centers" in nonmolecular solids) in which the total spin quantum number S is different from zero. This statement implies that the quantum mechanical states of the system are, at least to a good approximation, eigenfunctions of $\mathscr{S}^2$. When this is not the case a somewhat more involved description is necessary. For now, we will assume each molecular state can be characterized by, among other things, spin quantum numbers S and M_S.

Many of the spin-dependent properties of such a molecule are determined by its spin density distribution. The spin density at any point in the molecule is the probability of finding an electron there with spin "up" minus the probability of finding one there with spin "down." The entire spin density distribution is proportional to M_S. When $M_S = 0$, including the case of a singlet state with $S = M_S = 0$, the spin density is everywhere zero. Most of the nondynamic information obtainable from an ESR observation is information about the spin density distribution. This in turn gives information about the structure of the molecule being observed.

The overwhelming majority of molecules exist in singlet states and are, therefore, unobservable by ESR. We can use the term "molecule" in a very general sense in considering systems which are of interest to ESR. Many atoms have ground states or accessible excited states in which $S \neq 0$. They can be observed by ESR in the gas phase or trapped in relatively inert matrices. Equivalent information may also be available from high-resolution optical spectroscopy. Transition metal and lanthanide ions form many

‡ There are very many books on magnetic resonance, among them Refs. [32, 192], which include both nuclear magnetic resonance (NMR) and electron paramagnetic resonance (EPR).

complexes in which $S \neq 0$. It is often necessary in these cases to consider electronic orbital angular momentum as well as spin, and the term "electron paramagnetic resonance" (EPR) is probably preferable to ESR for such cases. This is also true for a variety of paramagnetic, localized defects or impurities which can be observed in nonmolecular crystals.

Some molecular systems also have stable nonsinglet ground states. The most important now are probably the nitroxides used as spin labels. Less stable molecular radicals may, under appropriate circumstances, have lifetimes long enough that they can be observed by ESR. Small, highly reactive radicals are of interest in interstellar and upper atmosphere chemistry. Irradiation of solid materials often produces radical species via bond rupture or ionization. They are potentially very reactive but are unable to move rapidly enough through their environment to find a reaction partner. Oxidation or reduction reactions in solution under carefully controlled circumstances may produce radical ions with lifetimes ranging from milliseconds to days. It is clear that many samples suitable for study by ESR can be obtained, and that information about them is of interest in a variety of applications.

The Basic Electron Spin Resonance Experiment

We examine now the basic ESR experiment. Consider a molecule with a net electronic spin different from zero. Associated with this spin will be a magnetic moment. If a magnetic field is applied, the moment will interact with it. If the molecule is, for example, in a state with $S = \frac{1}{2}$ but spatially nondegenerate, there are two energy levels which are degenerate in zero field but are split in the field by an amount proportional to the field strength. Any other interaction of the net spin will for now be assumed to be absent or negligible, so we have a two-level system. The basic ESR experiment consists of observing a transition between these two levels.

Transitions between the two levels can be induced by an appropriately oriented, oscillating magnetic field if the resonance condition $h\nu = \Delta E = g\beta B$ is satisfied. In cgs-Gaussian units the Bohr magneton β is 9.27×10^{-21} erg/G and Planck's constant h is 6.63×10^{-27} erg sec. The dimensionless constant g is very nearly 2 for organic free radicals. A typical x-band microwave frequency of 9.5 GHz thus corresponds to a field strength of 3400 G. The oscillating field has the same probability of causing upward and downward transitions, but at equilibrium in the static field the lower level will be more highly populated than the upper so there will be more upward than downward transitions and a net transfer of energy to the sample from the oscillating field. It is this absorption which is observed.

Let n_+ be the number of molecules in the sample with energy $g\beta B/2$ and n_- be the number with energy $-g\beta B/2$. At equilibrium in the static field

$$n_+/n_- = e^{-\Delta E/kT} = e^{-g\beta B/kT}.$$

Boltzmann's constant k is 1.38×10^{-16} erg/K so at room temperature of 298 K, $g\beta B/kT = 1.5 \times 10^{-3}$ for $B = 3400$ G. Then $n_-/n_+ = 1.0015$, and the population difference $\Delta n = n_- - n_+$ as a fraction of the total population $n = n_- + n_+$ is

$$\frac{\Delta n_{\text{eq}}}{n} = \frac{(n_- - n_+)_{\text{eq}}}{n_- + n_+} = \tanh\left(\frac{g\beta B}{2kT}\right) \sim 0.003.$$

Let P be the probability per unit time that a transition in either direction will be induced. Clearly P depends on the strength of the microwave field as well as other factors. The rate of absorption of energy by the sample from the microwave field is $W = h\nu P\,\Delta n$, and unless there is some mechanism tending to reestablish equilibrium, Δn will approach zero.

We assume that there is a relaxation mechanism tending to reestablish equilibrium, and further assume it to be first order:

$$\frac{d\Delta n}{dt} = \frac{\Delta n_{\text{eq}} - \Delta n}{T_1}.$$

The first-order rate constant is written as $1/T_1$ and T_1 is known as the spin–lattice or longitudinal relaxation time. This combines with the changes produced by the microwave field to give

$$\left(\frac{d\Delta n}{dt}\right)_{\text{total}} = -2P\,\Delta n + \frac{\Delta n_{\text{eq}} - \Delta n}{T_1}.$$

For steady-state conditions we assume this rate of change to be zero and get

$$\Delta n_{\text{steady state}} = \frac{\Delta n_{\text{eq}}}{1 + 2PT_1}.$$

The steady-state absorption of power by the system due to ESR transitions is

$$w_{\text{steady state}} = h\nu \frac{P}{1 + 2PT_1}.$$

Before treating other interactions of the electron spin which give structure to the spectrum, we will briefly consider other aspects of relaxation, obtaining a simple description of the resonance lineshape. A detailed treatment is beyond the scope of this chapter, and will in fact not be considered at all in this book. At this point we continue with a macroscopic, phenomenological point of view.

Relaxation and Lineshape

The magnetic moment associated with the net electronic spin in a single molecule is described in quantum mechanics by an operator proportional to the spin operator $\mathcal{S}$. Since the operators for the different components of $\mathcal{S}$ do not commute, it is not meaningful to talk about precise values for each component simultaneously, or about the "direction" of the vector $\mathcal{S}$. This quantum mechanical restriction does not apply to a macroscopic observable, however. Consider a volume of the sample which is large enough to contain very many molecules and yet small enough that, e.g., external fields can be considered uniform over the volume. We let **M** be the net magnetic moment in this sample volume due to the magnetic moments of all the individual molecules. This is a macroscopic vector quantity and can be assigned definite direction as well as magnitude.

The equation of motion governing the behavior of **M** turns out to be the same in classical and quantum treatments. If **M** has any component perpendicular to the magnetic field **B**, there will be a torque proportional to $\mathbf{M} \times \mathbf{B}$ causing **M** to precess about **B**. Consider, e.g., the quantum mechanical description in the Heisenberg formulation. The operator for the magnetic moment of one molecule is

$$\boldsymbol{\mu} = -g\beta\mathcal{s}.$$

(The minus sign enters explicitly because the electronic charge is negative but we are taking β to be positive.) The Hamiltonian giving the energy of interaction of the moment with the field is

$$\mathcal{H} = -\boldsymbol{\mu} \cdot \mathbf{B} = g\beta\mathcal{s} \cdot \mathbf{B}$$

and the Heisenberg equation of motion gives

$$i\hbar \frac{d\boldsymbol{\mu}}{dt} = [\boldsymbol{\mu}, \mathcal{H}] = -g^2\beta^2[\mathcal{s}, \mathcal{s} \cdot \mathbf{B}] = i\hbar g^2\beta^2\mathcal{s} \times \mathbf{B}$$

from the commutation properties of the spin operators. The magnetization **M** is a sum of contributions, $\mathbf{M} = \sum \boldsymbol{\mu}$, and spin operators associated with different molecules commute so this equation becomes

$$\frac{d\mathbf{M}}{dt} = -g\beta\mathbf{M} \times \mathbf{B}.$$

At equilibrium, in a static field **B**, **M** will be parallel to **B**. We use M_0 to denote the equilibrium magnitude and take **B** to define the z direction of a laboratory-fixed set of coordinates. If the system is not at equilibrium, we assume it will seek to return to equilibrium by a first-order process. For the z component of **M**

$$\frac{dM_z}{dt} = \frac{M_0 - M_z}{T_1}$$

corresponding to our previous assumption about Δn. The x and y components have equilibrium values zero, so

$$\frac{dM_x}{dt} = -\frac{M_x}{T_2}, \qquad \frac{dM_y}{dt} = -\frac{M_y}{T_2}.$$

The rate constant is written as $1/T_2$, where T_2 is known as the spin–spin or transverse relaxation time. For reasons that we will not go into here, T_1 and T_2 are in general different. They can be directly observed by appropriate pulse experiments, which are more readily done in NMR than ESR.

We next consider what will happen if, in addition to the static field, there is an oscillating field in the laboratory x direction, $B_1(t) = B_1 \cos \omega t$. An oscillating field is the normal experimental situation, but to simplify the analysis we write it as the sum of two fields rotating in opposite directions. The total field is then written

$$\mathbf{B} = (0, 0, B_0) + \kappa\left(\frac{B_1}{2}\cos \omega t, \frac{B_1}{2}\sin \omega t, 0\right) + \lambda\left(\frac{B_1}{2}\cos \omega t, -\frac{B_1}{2}\sin \omega t, 0\right).$$

The parameters κ and λ are inserted as labels to let us keep track of the contributions due to the various field terms, and the magnitude of the static field is now B_0.

We combine the precessional and relaxational contributions to the time dependence of $\mathbf{M}$ to obtain the Bloch equations

$$\frac{d\mathbf{M}}{dt} = -g\beta(\mathbf{M} \times \mathbf{B}) - \mathbf{k} \cdot (\mathbf{M} - \mathbf{M}_0),$$

where $\mathbf{k} = (1/T_2, 1/T_2, 1/T_1)$ and $\mathbf{M} = (0, 0, M_0)$. We now choose to write the components of $\mathbf{M}$ not in terms of the laboratory-fixed coordinate system x, y, z, but in terms of a coordinate system rotating with the applied field. In particular, M_x and M_y are replaced by

$$u = \cos \omega t\, M_x + \sin \omega t\, M_y, \qquad v = -\sin \omega t\, M_x + \cos \omega t\, M_y.$$

In terms of these components the equations governing $\mathbf{M}$ can be written

$$\frac{du}{dt} = -\frac{1}{T_2}u + (\omega - \omega_0)v + \frac{\lambda B_1}{2}\sin 2\omega t\, M_z,$$

$$\frac{dv}{dt} = -(\omega - \omega_0)u - \frac{1}{T_2}v + \frac{\kappa B_1}{2}M_z + \frac{\lambda B_1}{2}\cos 2\omega t\, M_z,$$

$$\frac{dM_z}{dt} = \frac{\kappa B_1}{2}v - \frac{(M_z - M_0)}{T_1} + \frac{\lambda B_1}{2}[\sin 2\omega t\, u + \cos 2\omega t\, v],$$

where $\omega_0 = g\beta B_0$. In the typical situation ω is fixed and B_0 is a slowly changing function of time, and we are interested in that part of $\mathbf{M}$ which is (in the rotating frame of reference) essentially static. The high-frequency terms (multiplied by λ) coming from the counter-rotating component of the field will have little effect on the static part of **M**, so we discard them. We can then set $\kappa = 1$. The part of **M** which is static in the rotating frame is then obtained by setting $du/dt = dv/dt = dM_z/dt = 0$ and solving the resultant algebraic equations. We obtain

$$u \simeq \frac{B_1 M_0}{2} \frac{\omega - \omega_0}{[(1/T_2^2) + (B_1^2 T_1/4T_2) + (\omega_0 - \omega)^2]},$$

$$v \simeq \frac{B_1^2 M_0}{4} \frac{1}{[(1/T_2^2) + (B_1^2 T_1/4T_2) + (\omega_0 - \omega)^2]}.$$

The out-of-phase component v shows a Lorentzian absorption lineshape while the in-phase component u is a dispersion. Most ESR spectrometers can be adjusted to detect either component, but the absorption mode is commonly chosen in free radical ESR. The presence of a time-dependent modulation field in the z direction complicates the analysis but the principal effect is usually to result in an observed signal that is approximately a first derivative of absorption.‡ It should also be noted that in solids there are usually unresolved interactions with neighboring molecules such that a Gaussian lineshape function describes what is observed more accurately than does the Lorentzian.

The assumption of a first-order relaxation process has led us to a Lorentzian lineshape. We have not considered the nature of the relaxation mechanisms, or whether a simple first-order characterization is adequate. Comparison with experimental results indicated that it is certainly quite good. A more detailed treatment of relaxation and its consequences will not be given here.

The Spin Hamiltonian

An important intermediate in the interpretation of most ESR experiments is the spin Hamiltonian. It is essentially a model which allows experimental data to be summarized in terms of a small number of parameters. These parameters are at least in principle susceptible to theoretical evaluation as well. Frequently it is possible to establish empirical correlations relating spin Hamiltonian parameter values to structural or other chemically interesting information.

A spin Hamiltonian contains operators for an effective electronic spin and for nuclear spins, the external magnetic field, and parameters. Its eigen-

‡ For an extensive discussion, see R. Ernst [50]; a simpler treatment of lineshapes is given by Wahlquist [204].

functions determine the allowed energy levels of the system, or at least those aspects of interest for an ESR experiment.

The parameters occur in sets or arrays commonly called tensors, although some of them may not actually transform properly as tensors.‡ In solution ESR only the isotropic average of each tensor is relevant because radical tumbling is random and rapid on the appropriate time scale. In single crystal ESR, the various tensor components can be separately obtained. Spectra obtained from glassy or polycrystalline samples are superpositions of many single-crystal-like spectra for radicals in all orientations. Their analysis requires use of anisotropic parameters but less information is available than from a single crystal study.

We now return to the question of energy levels and the positions of spectral lines, associating the various interactions with appropriate spin Hamiltonian terms.

The Electronic Zeeman Interaction

In a spectrum without structure (a single line), not considering possible dynamic information given by the linewidth or shape, there is only one piece of information. From the spectrometer frequency ν and field strength B at the center of the line we can obtain $g = h\nu/\beta B$. For a free electron g_e is found to have the value 2.0023191... . Free radicals are found to have somewhat different g values.

In another relatively simple case, we could consider an atom or atomic ion in a field sufficiently weak that the spin–orbit interaction completely dominates the Zeeman interaction. In such a case states will be characterized by quantum numbers J, M_J, as well as (at least approximately) L and S. The energy is $g_J/\beta BM_J$ and the g factor is given by the Landé formula

$$g_J = 1 + \frac{J(J+1) + S(S+1) - L(L+1)}{2J(J+1)}$$

with the approximation that the magnetic moment associated with the spin is $2\beta\mathscr{S}$. At the other extreme, if the field is strong enough that spin–orbit coupling is negligible compared with the Zeeman splittings, states will be characterized by M_L and M_S values with magnetic energies $(M_L + g_e M_S)\beta B$. At intermediate field strenghts the energy is not linear in the field strength.

When the atom or ion is incorporated into a molecule or complex, the Born–Oppenheimer electronic potential is no longer spherically symmetric; $\mathscr{L}^2$ does not commute with the Hamiltonian and L is not a good quantum

‡ This is particularly significant when the effective spin of the spin Hamiltonian differs from the true spin of the system. Compare Abragam and Bleaney [2].

number. In a complex dominated by a single, heavy atom there may be states enough like those of the free atom or ion that the latter provide a good starting point for a perturbation treatment of the complex. One may then wish to speak of the orbital angular momentum as being partially "quenched" in the complex. If the interaction with the ligands is not too strong, states corresponding to degenerate states of the free ion will remain relatively closely spaced in energy. If the symmetry of the complex is high enough, exact degeneracies may persist, at least in the orbital energies of a molecular orbital (thus approximate) description of the system. The methods used to determine g in these cases are essentially those of degenerate perturbation theory. It should be noted that g is defined as a proportionality factor relating magnetic field strength and frequency or energy level differences. In a spin Hamiltonian, the operator with which g is associated may involve an effective spin, not simply related to a true spin operator when degeneracies other than true M_S degeneracies are involved.

In a nonlinear molecule not dominated by one atom, electronic orbital angular momentum operators do not commute even approximately with the Hamiltonian and there is no closely related system in which total electronic orbital angular momentum quantum numbers are defined. They thus cease to be useful even as labels. In the typical case where molecular rotations are not considered (because the sample is in a condensed phase), the net electronic spin is the only angular momentum, in lowest order (other than nuclear spins which do not affect the electronic Zeeman energy). Not surprisingly, then, the g value is found to be close to g_e. Small relativistic corrections within the ground state and contributions from excited states mixed in by spin–orbit or other operators result in a small shift of g from g_e. For typical, organic free radicals made up of first row atoms, g is in the range 2.003–2.005. Very precise measurements are thus necessary if interesting information is to be obtained.

Because of the role played by the spin–orbit interaction in the shift of g away from g_e, and because of the strong dependence of this interaction on nuclear charge, the g shift is quite sensitive to the Z values of atoms in the molecular radical. The inclusion of oxygen in a carbon framework may make a noticeable difference. Inclusion of a second-row atom like Si or S can increase the g shift by an order of magnitude. Comparisons in series of radicals show that the g shift can be approximately related to the spin density centered on the heavier (higher Z) atoms in many cases.

The g value depends on the orientation of the radical relative to the magnetic field. The term in the spin Hamiltonian describing the interaction of spin and field can be written $\beta \mathscr{S} \cdot \mathbf{g} \cdot \mathbf{B}$, and various components of $\mathbf{g}$ can be determined from measurements on oriented radicals in single crystals. In solution ESR, only the isotropic average of $\mathbf{g}$ is observed.

Magnetic Hyperfine Interactions

Luckily for the preservation of interest in the subject, most ESR spectra do not consist of a single line; they have structure. We consider first what is known as hyperfine structure, due to interactions between the electronic spin density and nuclear spins in the radical. Among the more common nuclei with nonzero spin and magnetic moments are ^{1}H, ^{14}N, ^{19}F and the other halogens, ^{31}P, etc. Even in natural abundance there is enough ^{13}C that its effects are sometimes observed. It and other isotopic species can also be artificially enriched. We need not be concerned here with the detailed mechanisms of interaction which cause energy levels to depend on nuclear spin state. Splittings are closely connected with the spin density at or near the nucleus causing them and can thus be used to map the spin density distribution in the radical. Splittings are small, typically a few percent to a fraction of a percent of the electronic Zeeman interaction.

It is an excellent approximation for a mobile radical and a useful first approximation for a radical in a fixed orientation to consider the nuclear spin state to be unchanged in the course of the ESR transition. The macroscopic system can thus be thought of as consisting of a number of subsystems, each containing radicals with a particular nuclear spin state. The number of energy levels available to the radicals in any subsystem is just $2S + 1$ ($= 2$ for a doublet). The multi-line spectrum then consists of a superposition of one-line spectra, one arising from the radicals in each subsystem.

In order for this to be a valid description, the radicals must be far enough apart that they do not interact with one another. If intermolecular electron spin magnetic dipole interactions—or Heisenberg exchange pseudo-spin interactions—are not negligible, hyperfine contributions from many radicals are averaged. All nuclear spin states are essentially equally likely, and the average over all states of the hyperfine interaction energy is zero, so in concentrated samples the hyperfine structure collapses.

For a radical in dilute solution the hyperfine interaction adds to the spin Hamiltonian a term $A\mathbf{S}\cdot\mathbf{I}$ for each nucleus with which the electron spin interacts. If $g\beta B \gg A$, the treatment can be simplified and an excellent approximate description obtained by replacing this term by AS_zI_z. In this approximation the energy of the radical is given by

$$E(M_S, m_{I1}, m_{I2}, \ldots) = g\beta BM_S + \sum_{\nu} A_\nu m_{I\nu} M_S.$$

The sum extends over nuclei, labeled by ν, for which $I \neq 0$ and A is large enough to be significant.

The nuclear moments also interact with the external field. The resultant nuclear Zeeman energy is the same for both states involved in an ESR transition for solution ESR, so it cancels out. The nuclear Zeeman interaction can then be omitted entirely.

Suppose, for example, that in the system of interest $S = \frac{1}{2}$, and there is a single magnetic nucleus with $I = \frac{1}{2}$. The energy levels are shown in Fig. 0-1. In practice the spectrometer frequency is fixed and the field strength is varied. Energy will be absorbed by the sample when the resonance condition $\Delta E(B) = h\nu$ is satisfied.

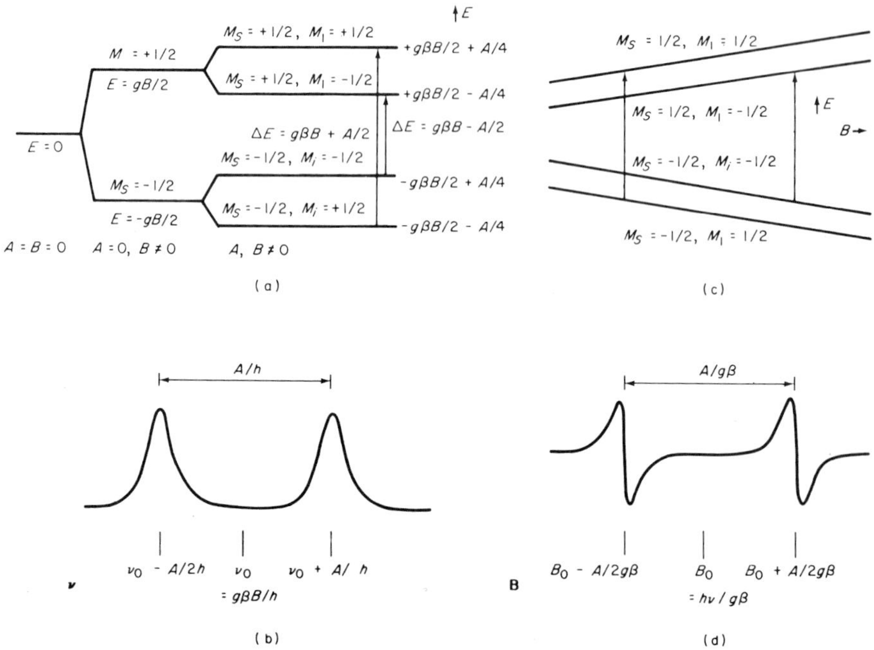

FIG. 0-1. Magnetic energy levels and transitions in a system with $S = \frac{1}{2}$ and one nucleus with $I = \frac{1}{2}$. (a) Energy levels and allowed transitions. (The magnitude of A relative to $g\beta B$ is exaggerated.) (b) Transitions as a function of frequency at fixed field strength (absorption). (c) Energy levels as a function of field strength. (d) Transitions as a function of field strength at fixed frequency (first derivative of absorption).

Equivalent Nuclei and Intensity Patterns

Nuclei which are equivalent because of molecular symmetry will have the same hyperfine coupling constants. It is the average interaction on the ESR time scale which is significant and thus, e.g., methyl protons are equivalent (except possibly at very low temperature) because of the rapid internal rotation. When there are equivalent nuclei, several nuclear spin states will have the same hyperfine interaction energy and lines of higher relative

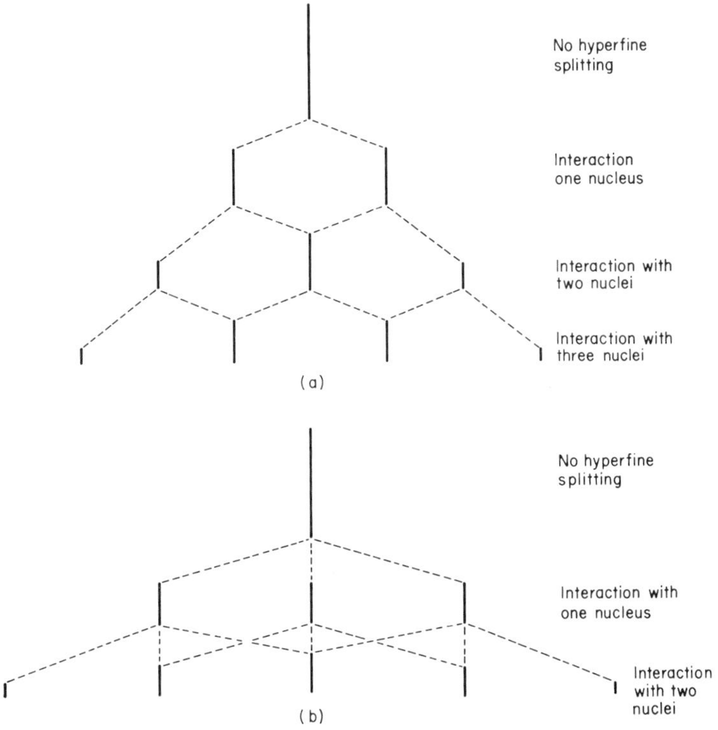

FIG. 0-2. Hyperfine splitting patterns due to equivalent nuclei. (a) Equivalent nuclei of spin $\frac{1}{2}$. The intensity pattern follows a binomial distribution. (b) Equivalent nuclei of spin 1.

intensity will occur in the spectrum. This phenomenon is illustrated in Fig. 0-2. In a "stick diagram" such as this the line height is proportional to intensity (strength of absorption). Hyperfine interactions do not increase the total intensity, but divide it among several lines. Each line is thus less intense.

The intensity patterns characteristic of equivalent nuclei provide assistance in identifying radicals and in assigning hyperfine coupling constants to particular nuclei. As an example, Fig. 0-3 shows the experimental spectrum and its stick diagram reconstruction for the *p*-nitrobenzoate dianion radical. The large splitting, A_N, producing a triplet of intensity ratio 1 : 1 : 1 must correspond to interaction with the spin-1 ^{14}N nucleus. The other two splittings, each producing a triplet with intensity ratio 1 : 2 : 1, must correspond to interactions with the two sets of two equivalent ring protons. There is no way on the basis of this spectrum alone that one can decide which splitting corresponds to which set of protons. A comparison with calculated results and with spectra of similar radicals for which deuterium substituted

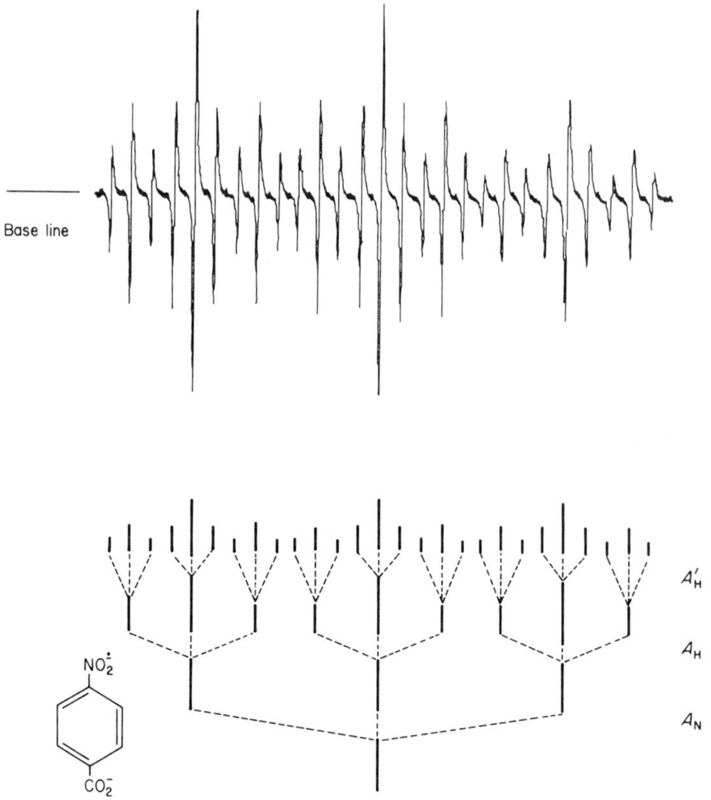

FIG. 0-3. Electron spin resonance spectrum of the *p*-nitrobenzoate dianion radical. (Room temperature, $\sim 10^{-3}$ *M*, in dimethylsulfoxide, generated electrolytically with 0.1 *M* tetra-n-propylammonium perchlorate as supporting electrolyte. From K. M. Brubaker [26].

radicals have been studied indicates that the smallest splitting, A'_H, is associated with the protons closer to the CO_2 while the intermediate splitting, A_H, is associated with the protons closer to the NO_2.

This spectrum also illustrates the phenomenon of linewidth variation. Consider just the three strongest lines. If the center line is assigned a width of 1.00, the line at low field (left) has a width 1.06 and the high field (right) line has a width 1.48 on the same scale [26]. Since the integrated intensities of the three are the same, an increase in width results in a decrease in peak-to-peak amplitude. Theories of relaxation more sophisticated than the simple Bloch equations considered here can explain the dependence of linewidth on nuclear spin state. The linewidths provide useful additional information about radical dynamics.

For oriented radicals the hyperfine interaction must be treated in the form $\mathbf{S} \cdot \mathbf{A} \cdot \mathbf{I}$, and the various components of $\mathbf{A}$ determined. If nuclear Zeeman energies are not negligible compared with hyperfine interactions, they must also be considered. In such a case, if more than one nucleus is involved, a single nuclear spin state cannot be readily assigned.

There are also circumstances in which changes in nuclear spin state must be considered, because of interstate relaxation, in a multiple-resonance experiment, etc. We will not be concerned here with such situations.

Other Interactions

Other interactions may also be important. A nucleus with $I \geq 1$ may have an electric quadrupole moment which will interact with the molecular electronic charge distribution. The resultant splitting produces an additional dependence of energy levels on nuclear spin state which may have directly observable effects in single crystal ESR. The interaction averages to zero in solution but may be indirectly observed because of its contribution to nuclear spin relaxation.

When $S \geq 1$ energy differences associated with the direct or indirect interactions of the spin moments of different electrons may occur. If they are significant, M_S is no longer a good quantum number and states within the spin multiplet will have different energies in the absence of an external field and hyperfine interactions. The resultant "fine structure" in the ESR spectrum arises from this effect, known as zero field splitting.

In a triplet state, for example, the appropriate spin Hamiltonian term can be written $\mathbf{S} \cdot \mathbf{D} \cdot \mathrm{S}$. Observations on single crystals can determine the elements of $\mathbf{D}$. In amorphous solid phases the ESR spectrum is often so broad as to be unobservable, but the breakdown in selection rules associated with the fact that M_S is no longer a good quantum number allows the observation of a somewhat sharper transition at about half the usual field strength.

The rest of this book will be concerned with the detailed development of the theory of energy levels of interest to ESR and of the resultant spectra.

CHAPTER I

THE ORIGIN OF MAGNETIC ENERGY LEVELS

1. The Dirac Electron

The Dirac theory of the electron [46, 47] resulted from an attempt to reconcile the fundamental requirements of quantum mechanics with those of the special theory of relativity. It can be elegantly formulated, and its predictions are experimentally verified, subject only to small corrections due to quantum field effects. In this theory the electron spin and magnetic moment arise naturally. It thus provides a reasonable starting point for a discussion of magnetic interactions. In discussing the Pauli treatment of spin, Dirac said "The question remains as to why Nature should have chosen this particular model for the electron instead of being satisfied with the point-charge. One would like to find some incompleteness in the previous methods of applying quantum mechanics to the point-charge electron such that, when removed, the whole of the duplexity phenomena [spin effects] follow without arbitrary assumptions" [46]. This goal was achieved.

The Dirac equation can be solved exactly for a number of cases, including an electron in a uniform magnetic field or a Coulomb field. Other problems can be treated by perturbation theory. The properties of the Dirac equation and some of its solutions will be discussed in this section. The relationship of Dirac theory to nonrelativistic quantum mechanics, field theories, and the use of approximate methods will be discussed in later sections.

Origin of the Dirac Equation

The general principles of quantum mechanics as it is now usually formulated include these:

1. *The state of a system is represented by a state vector*, which in the Schrödinger picture is the wave function Ψ, a function of the positions of the particles in the system, any variables associated with internal degrees of freedom such as spin, and the time. This function is to be interpreted as a probability amplitude so that $|\Psi|^2\, d\tau$ gives the probability of finding the system in a volume element $d\tau$ about the specified point in configuration space at the specified time. As a consequence of this interpretation, $\int |\Psi|^2\, d\tau$, the integral over all space of the probability density, must be finite and independent of time. (An equivalent Lorentz-invariant condition exists in the form of an equation of continuity.)

2. *An equation of motion exists which determines the state vector for all times if it is given for one time.*

3. *A linear combination of state vectors is itself a possible state vector.* This principle of superposition requires that the equation of motion be linear and homogeneous in the state vector.

It can be shown [47] that these conditions imply that the equation of motion must be the form

$$\mathscr{H}\Psi = i\hbar\, \partial\Psi/\partial t, \tag{1-1}$$

where $\mathscr{H}$ is a linear, Hermitian operator. (The constants are chosen for convenience.) The operator $\mathscr{H}$ corresponds to the energy of the system and can be identified with an operator form of the Hamiltonian function of classical physics.

In the nonrelativistic case this is just

$$\mathscr{H} = p^2/2m \tag{1-2}$$

for a free particle of mass m. Appropriate additions are made if the particle is charged and there are fields present.

For the coordinate representation in this Schrödinger picture, $p_x = (\hbar/i)\, \partial/\partial x$, and Eq. (1-1) is second order in the space derivatives. Since it involves only a first derivative with respect to time, it is clearly not Lorentz invariant and is thus not acceptable in a relativistic theory. The relativistic expression for the classical Hamiltonian of a free particle is (Appendix A)

$$\mathscr{H} = (m^2c^4 + p^2c^2)^{1/2}. \tag{1-3}$$

It is not clear how a corresponding operator involving the square root would be interpreted. A quadratic form of the equation can be written as

$$\mathscr{H}^2\Psi = (p^2c^2 + m^2c^4)\Psi = -\hbar^2\, \partial^2/\partial t^2 \Psi, \tag{1-4}$$

but because the second derivative with respect to time is involved, the resultant wave function does not conserve probability; i.e., the integral of $|\Psi|^2$

over all space varies with time. (A different definition of the probability density could be used.)

A possible alternative to the quadratic approach is to try to find linear factors for the square root by letting

$$\mathscr{H} = \boldsymbol{\alpha} \cdot \mathbf{p}c + \beta mc^2, \tag{1-5}$$

where the constants c and mc^2 are chosen for convenience and the Hermitian operators $\boldsymbol{\alpha} = (\alpha_x, \alpha_y, \alpha_z)$ and β are to be chosen so that

$$\mathscr{H}^2 = (\boldsymbol{\alpha} \cdot \mathbf{p}c + \beta mc^2)(\boldsymbol{\alpha} \cdot \mathbf{p}c + \beta mc^2) = p^2c^2 + m^2c^4. \tag{1-6}$$

This requires that

$$\alpha_j\alpha_k + \alpha_k\alpha_j = 0, \quad j \neq k; \quad \alpha_j\beta + \beta\alpha_j = 0; \quad \alpha_j^2 = \beta^2 = 1. \tag{1-7}$$

Since we are discussing a free particle in isotropic space, the α_j's and β must be independent of position or momentum. They thus act on some new degree of freedom of the wave function Ψ. Their properties will be further discussed below.

If Eq. (1-1) with $\mathscr{H}$ given by Eq. (1-5) is multiplied by β, and new operators are defined by

$$\gamma_k = -i\beta\alpha_k, \quad k = 1,2,3; \quad \gamma_4 = \beta, \tag{1-8}$$

the resultant equation can be written in the highly symmetric form

$$\left(\sum_{\mu=1}^{4} \gamma_\mu \frac{\partial}{\partial x_\mu} + \frac{mc}{\hbar}\right)\Psi = 0. \tag{1-9}$$

The 4-vector x_μ has components $(\mathbf{r}, ict)$ (Appendix A). It can be verified that this equation is Lorentz invariant (see, e.g., Rose [172, Section 14].)

In order to obtain the equation in the presence of an electromagnetic field, we make the usual change to the gauge-invariant momentum

$$p_\mu \to \Pi_\mu = p_\mu + eA_\mu/c \tag{1-10}$$

for a particle of charge $-e$, where A_μ is the 4-vector potential $(\mathbf{A} - i\phi)$ (Appendix A). If we again separate the fourth component from the first three we can obtain the following useful form of the Dirac equation:

$$[c\boldsymbol{\alpha} \cdot (\mathbf{p} + e\mathbf{A}/c) - e\phi + \beta mc^2]\Psi = i\hbar\, \partial\Psi/\partial t. \tag{1-11}$$

It can be verified that gauge transformations of the electromagnetic potentials simply introduce a phase change into the wave function as they do in non-relativistic quantum mechanics (Appendix B).

A brief summary has been given above indicating how the Dirac equation arises in a natural way from the principles of quantum mechanics and the requirements of the special theory of relativity. Of course, this does not constitute a "derivation" of the equation. We will instead at this point assert Eq. (1-11) as a postulate from which we will derive our results. The operators $\boldsymbol{\alpha}$ and β are defined by their commutation properties, Eq. (1-7), and the other operators are interpreted as in nonrelativistic quantum mechanics with unit operators on the $\boldsymbol{\alpha}$, β-space inserted where necessary.

General properties of the Dirac equation are discussed extensively in books on relativistic quantum mechanics. We will concentrate on certain aspects of particular interest to ESR.

Some Properties of the Dirac Equation and Dirac Operators

The Hermitian operators γ_k or $\boldsymbol{\alpha}$ and β occurring in the Dirac equation are seen from Eqs. (1-7) and (1-8) to anticommute and to be idempotent:

$$\gamma_\mu \gamma_\nu + \gamma_\nu \gamma_\mu = 2\delta_{\mu\nu}. \tag{1-12}$$

Since $\gamma_\mu^2 = 1$, the eigenvalues of γ_μ are ± 1. It also follows that

$$\operatorname{tr} \gamma_\mu = \operatorname{tr} \gamma_\nu^2 \gamma_\mu = \operatorname{tr} \gamma_\nu \gamma_\mu \gamma_\nu,$$

since the trace of a product is unaffected by cyclic permuations of factors. However, since $\gamma_\mu \gamma_\nu = -\gamma_\nu \gamma \mu$,

$$\operatorname{tr} \gamma_\nu \gamma_\mu \gamma_\nu = -\operatorname{tr} \gamma_\nu^2 \gamma_\mu = -\operatorname{tr} \ \gamma_\mu,$$

and thus

$$\operatorname{tr} \gamma_\mu = 0. \tag{1-13}$$

The set of eigenvalues of γ_μ must thus contain the same number of $+1$'s and -1's, and if a matrix representation is used it must of even dimension.

It can in fact be shown (see, e.g., Rose [172, Section 11]) that 16 distinct operators can be formed: 1 (the unit operator), the four γ_μ, the six products $i\gamma_\mu\gamma_\nu$, four products $i\gamma_\mu\gamma_\nu\gamma_\lambda$, and the product $\gamma_1\gamma_2\gamma_3\gamma_4$. These 16 are linearly independent, but no other combination of the γ_μ can be formed which is linearly independent of all of them. Further, any operator which commutes with all 16 of these must be a multiple of the unit operator in the γ space. It seems plausible, then, to take a 4×4 matrix representation of the γ_μ, and any other representation can be shown to be at most a trivial extension of the 4×4 matrix representation.

This representation is of course not necessary, and results can be obtained without reference to any particular representation of the γ's. It is more convenient to work in one particular representation, however. There is still freedom as to which 4×4 representation to use, i.e., which matrices to take as diagonal. The most useful representation for our purposes, as well as the most common choice, is expressible as

$$\alpha_k = \begin{pmatrix} 0 & \sigma_k \\ \sigma_k & 0 \end{pmatrix}, \qquad \beta = \begin{pmatrix} 1 & 0 \\ 0 & -1 \end{pmatrix}, \tag{1-14}$$

where 0 and 1 are the 2×2 zero and unit matrices and the σ_k are the 2×2 Pauli spin matrices

$$\sigma_x = \begin{pmatrix} 0 & 1 \\ 1 & 0 \end{pmatrix}, \qquad \sigma_y = \begin{pmatrix} 0 & -\mathrm{i} \\ \mathrm{i} & 0 \end{pmatrix}, \qquad \sigma_z = \begin{pmatrix} 1 & 0 \\ 0 & -1 \end{pmatrix}. \tag{1-15}$$

We will also have occasion to use 4×4 σ matrices

$$\sigma_k = \begin{pmatrix} \sigma_k & 0 \\ 0 & \sigma_k \end{pmatrix} \tag{1-16}$$

and will depend on context to make it clear whether the Dirac or Pauli σ is intended in specific cases.

The use of 4×4 matrices for the operators requires that the wave function have four components. It is convenient to follow the partitioning suggested by Eq. (1-14) and divide Ψ into two "upper" and two "lower" components.

$$\Psi = \begin{pmatrix} \psi_\mathrm{u} \\ \psi_l \end{pmatrix} \tag{1-17}$$

with

$$\psi_\mathrm{u} = \begin{pmatrix} \psi_1 \\ \psi_2 \end{pmatrix}, \qquad \psi_l = \begin{pmatrix} \psi_3 \\ \psi_4 \end{pmatrix}. \tag{1-18}$$

Transformation properties of the matrices and the components of the wave function have been extensively examined, but we will introduce only the properties we require, at the time we need them.

It is convenient to distinguish between even and odd Dirac operators. An operator is said to be even if it is of the form

$$\Omega_\mathrm{e} = \begin{pmatrix} a & 0 \\ 0 & b \end{pmatrix} \tag{1-19a}$$

and odd if it is of the form

$$\Omega_\mathrm{o} = \begin{pmatrix} 0 & c \\ d & 0 \end{pmatrix}. \tag{1-19b}$$

The operator β commutes with an even operator and anticommutes with an odd operator. Clearly any operator can be separated into odd and even parts.

We will occasionally have to deal with commutators involving matrix operators. Two useful results can be summarized as

$$
\begin{aligned}
\left[\begin{pmatrix} p & q \\ r & s \end{pmatrix}, \begin{pmatrix} a & 0 \\ 0 & b \end{pmatrix}\right] &= \begin{pmatrix} pa - ap & qb - aq \\ ra - br & sb - bs \end{pmatrix} \\
\left[\begin{pmatrix} p & q \\ r & s \end{pmatrix}, \begin{pmatrix} 0 & c \\ d & 0 \end{pmatrix}\right] &= \begin{pmatrix} qd - cr & pc - cs \\ sd - dp & rc - dq \end{pmatrix}
\end{aligned}
\tag{1-20}
$$

These may be thought of as involving 2×2 matrices of simple operators or as 4×4 matrices made up of 2×2 operator matrices.

Solutions of the Dirac equation exist for both positive and negative energies. By "negative energies" we do not mean the usual negative energies of bound states, but rather $E \sim -mc^2$. Such negative energy solutions occur in the Dirac case even for free particles. They are properly interpreted as describing the behavior of positrons (with positive energy) rather than of electrons with negative energy. For electron solutions, $E \sim mc^2$ and $\|\psi_u\| \gg \|\psi_l\|$, while for the positron solutions $\|\psi_l\| \gg \|\psi_u\|$. When E is substantially different in magnitude from mc^2, the distinction is not as clear in these terms. If sufficient energy is available ($2mc^2$ or more), electron–positron pairs can be produced. The Dirac theory is thus inescapably a many-particle theory, and should properly be dealt with by field-theoretic techniques. For $E \sim mc^2$, however, only solutions corresponding to a single electron need be considered.

Solutions of the Dirac Equation

The Dirac equation can be solved exactly or constants of motion simply obtained in a number of cases, some of which are of interest to ESR. We will consider first the case of a Dirac electron in a uniform magnetic field and then the hydrogen atom or Coulomb field problem.

Uniform Magnetic Field [85,90]

For a constant magnetic field the scalar potential can be taken to be zero

$$\phi \equiv 0. \tag{1-21}$$

The stationary state Dirac equation, in terms of upper and lower components, is then

$$\begin{pmatrix} mc^2 & c\boldsymbol{\sigma} \cdot \boldsymbol{\pi} \\ c\boldsymbol{\sigma} \cdot \boldsymbol{\pi} & -mc^2 \end{pmatrix} \begin{pmatrix} \psi_u \\ \psi_l \end{pmatrix} = E \begin{pmatrix} \psi_u \\ \psi_l \end{pmatrix}. \tag{1-22}$$

Since $E \pm mc^2$ is just a constant, we can easily solve for one pair of components in terms of the other

$$\psi_l = \frac{c\boldsymbol{\sigma} \cdot \boldsymbol{\pi}}{E + mc^2} \psi_{\mathrm{u}} \tag{1-23}$$

and thus obtain an equation involving the upper component only

$$\left[mc^2 + \frac{c^2(\boldsymbol{\sigma} \cdot \boldsymbol{\pi})^2}{E + mc^2}\right]\psi_{\mathrm{u}} = E\psi_{\mathrm{u}} \tag{1-24}$$

or, by an appropriate transfer of constants,

$$\frac{1}{2m}(\boldsymbol{\sigma} \cdot \boldsymbol{\pi})^2\psi_{\mathrm{u}} = \varepsilon\psi_{\mathrm{u}}, \tag{1-25}$$

where $\varepsilon = \frac{1}{2}(1 + (E/mc^2))(E - mc^2)$ is approximately the energy in excess of the rest mass energy.

Since

$$(\boldsymbol{\sigma} \cdot \boldsymbol{\pi})^2 = \pi^2 + i\boldsymbol{\sigma} \cdot \boldsymbol{\pi} \times \boldsymbol{\pi} \tag{1-26}$$

and for j, k, l any cyclic permutation of x, y, z

$$\begin{aligned}(\boldsymbol{\pi} \times \boldsymbol{\pi})_j &= (p_k + eA_k/c)(p_l + eA_l/c) - (p_l + eA_l/c)(p_k + eA_k/c) \\ &= \frac{e\hbar}{ic}\left(\frac{\partial A_l}{\partial x_k} - \frac{\partial A_k}{\partial x_l}\right) = -i\frac{e\hbar}{c}B_j,\end{aligned} \tag{1-27}$$

we have

$$(\boldsymbol{\sigma} \cdot \boldsymbol{\pi})^2 = \pi^2 + \frac{e\hbar}{c}\boldsymbol{\sigma} \cdot \mathbf{B} \tag{1-28}$$

and

$$[\pi^2/2m + \beta_{\mathrm{e}}\boldsymbol{\sigma} \cdot \mathbf{B}]\psi_{\mathrm{u}} = \varepsilon\psi_{\mathrm{u}} \tag{1-29}$$

with $\beta_{\mathrm{e}} = e\hbar/(2mc)$. The first term is simply that which appears in the nonrelativistic quantum mechanical treatment of a (spinless) charged particle in a magnetic field. The second term describes the interaction of the electron spin magnetic moment with the field. Thus far the only assumption we have made about the field is that it does not vary with time. If we further restrict it to be uniform in space, then the second term above will be independent of both position and momentum. The first term contains only the implicit unit Dirac operator, so the two terms commute and can be considered separately.

Before further consideration of the relativistic problem, let us treat the nonrelativistic (spinless) case. We will treat this case at some length because it provides a basis for understanding much of what follows. As noted above, the Hamiltonian is

$$\mathscr{H}_{\mathrm{nr}} = \pi^2/2m. \tag{1-30}$$

For a uniform field taken to be in the z direction, $\mathbf{B} = (0, 0, B)$, we can take

$$\mathbf{A} = \tfrac{1}{2}(\mathbf{B} \times \mathbf{r}) = (-\tfrac{1}{2}By, \tfrac{1}{2}Bx, 0), \tag{1-31}$$

and

$$\mathscr{H}_{\mathrm{nr}} = \mathscr{H}_{\perp} + \mathscr{H}_z \tag{1-32}$$

with

$$\mathscr{H}_{\perp} = (\pi_x^2 + \pi_y^2)/2m, \qquad \mathscr{H}_z = p_z^2/2m. \tag{1-33}$$

It follows that the z behavior is separable and is just that of a free particle with p_z, which commutes with $\mathscr{H}_{\mathrm{nr}}$, a constant of the motion. We further note that [cf. Eq. (1-27)]

$$[\pi_x, \pi_y] = (\boldsymbol{\pi} \times \boldsymbol{\pi})_z = -i\frac{e\hbar B}{c}, \tag{1-34}$$

and thus, apart from constants, $\mathscr{H}$ behaves like a one-dimensional harmonic oscillator Hamiltonian. Because an operator treatment of the harmonic oscillator problem is well known (see, e.g., Messiah [138, Chapter XII]), it will only be sketched here.

We begin by defining

$$\pi_{\pm} = \pi_x \pm i\pi_y \tag{1-35}$$

and note that

$$\mathscr{H}_{\perp} = (\pi_+\pi_-/2m) + \beta_e B \tag{1-36}$$

It follows from Eqs. (1-34) and (1-35) that

$$[\pi_+, \pi_-] = -i[\pi_x, \pi_y] + i[\pi_y, \pi_x] = -2(e\hbar/c)B, \tag{1-37}$$

and thus that

$$[\pi_{\pm}, \mathscr{H}_{\perp}] = [\pi_{\pm}, \pi_+\pi_-]/2m = \mp 2\beta_e B\pi_{\pm}. \tag{1-38}$$

Suppose that $|n\rangle$ is an eigenstate of $\mathscr{H}_{\perp}$ with eigenvalue $E_{\perp,n}$:

$$\mathscr{H}_{\perp}|n\rangle = E_{\perp,n}|n\rangle. \tag{1-39}$$

Then

$$\pi_{\pm}\mathscr{H}_{\perp}|n\rangle = \mathscr{H}_{\perp}\pi_{\pm}|n\rangle + [\pi_{\pm}, \mathscr{H}_{\perp}]|n\rangle = (\mathscr{H}_{\perp} \mp 2\beta_e B)\pi_{\pm}|n\rangle \tag{1-40}$$

or

$$\mathscr{H}_\perp(\pi_\pm|n\rangle) = (E_{\perp,n} \pm 2\beta_e B)(\pi_\pm|n\rangle). \tag{1-41}$$

The operators $\pi_\pm$ thus act as raising and lowering operators for the eigenvalues of $\mathscr{H}_\perp$. In the usual way it can be shown that since $\pi_+^\dagger = \pi_-$, $\langle\mathscr{H}_\perp\rangle \geq \beta_e B$, and thus there is a lowest state with

$$\pi_-|0\rangle = 0, \qquad \mathscr{H}_\perp|0\rangle = \beta_e B|0\rangle. \tag{1-42}$$

It follows that

$$|n\rangle \propto (\pi_+)^n|0\rangle, \qquad E_{\perp,n} = (2n+1)\beta_e B, \qquad n \geq 0. \tag{1-43}$$

The change in normalization on applying π_+ is readily found. We have not yet considered degeneracy and constants of motion other than the energy. Since the system is in two dimensions after the separation of z, we expect two quantum numbers to be necessary to specify the state.

It is possible to write $\mathscr{H}_\perp$ as

$$\mathscr{H}_\perp = \frac{1}{2m}(p_x^2 + p_y^2) + \frac{e^2B^2}{8mc^2}(x^2 + y^2) + \frac{eB}{2mc}(xp_y - yp_x). \tag{1-44}$$

We recognize the first two terms as being equivalent to a two-dimensional harmonic oscillator with a force constant, $e^2B^2/4mc^2$, dependent on the magnetic field strength. The last term involves the operator $L_z = xp_y - yp_x$ coupled to the field. Transforming to cylindrical coordinates

$$x = \rho\cos\phi, \qquad y = \rho\sin\phi, \tag{1-45}$$

we find

$$\mathscr{H}_\perp = -\frac{\hbar^2}{2m}\left(\frac{\partial^2}{\partial\rho^2} + \frac{1}{\rho}\frac{\partial}{\partial\rho}\right) + \frac{L_z^2}{2m\rho^2} + \frac{e^2B^2}{8mc^2}\rho^2 + \frac{eB}{2mc}L_z. \tag{1-46}$$

It is clear that

$$L_z = xp_y - yp_x = \frac{\hbar}{i}\frac{\partial}{\partial\phi} \tag{1-47}$$

commutes with $\mathscr{H}_\perp$ and in fact with $\mathscr{H}_{\mathrm{nr}}$. Note, however, that L_z does not commute with $\pi_\pm$:

$$[L_z, \pi_\pm] = \pm\hbar\pi_\pm, \tag{1-48}$$

so that $\pi_\pm$ raise or lower the eigenvalues of L_z by $\hbar$ at the same time they change the eigenvalues of $\mathscr{H}_\perp$ by $\pm 2\beta_e B$.

The $\mathscr{H}_\perp$ eigenvalue equation is separable in cylindrical coordinates

$$|n\rangle \leftrightarrow \psi(\rho, \phi) = P(\rho)\Phi(\phi) \tag{1-49}$$

and since we are free to use eigenfunctions of L_z we take

$$\Phi_{m_l}(\phi) = (1/\sqrt{2\pi})e^{im_l\phi}. \tag{1-50}$$

Suppose we have a ψ with eigenvalue $m_l\hbar$ of L_z, but with

$$\pi_- \psi_{0,m_l} = 0. \tag{1-51}$$

In cylindrical coordinates

$$\pi_\pm = e^{\pm i\phi}\left[\frac{\hbar}{i}\frac{\partial}{\partial\rho} \pm \frac{\hbar}{\rho}\frac{\partial}{\partial\phi} \pm i\frac{eB}{2c}\rho\right], \tag{1-52}$$

so the equation we obtain for P in this case is

$$e^{i(m_l-1)\phi}\left[\frac{\hbar}{i}\left(P' + \frac{m_l}{\rho}P\right) - i\frac{eB}{2c}\rho P\right] = 0 \tag{1-53}$$

or

$$P' + [(m_l/\rho) + \gamma\rho]P = 0, \tag{1-54}$$

where $\gamma = eB/(2\hbar c)$. A solution of this equation is

$$P(\rho) = A\rho^{-m_l}e^{-(\gamma/2)\rho^2}. \tag{1-55}$$

In order for the function to be quadratically integrable, $-m_l$ must be non-negative, so $m_l \leq 0$.

Eigenfunctions with higher energies can be obtained by applying π_+. Alternatively, one can solve the P eigenvalue equation

$$P'' + (1/\rho)P' - [(m_l^2/\rho^2) + \gamma^2\rho^2 + 2\gamma m_l - \lambda]P = 0, \tag{1-56}$$

where $\lambda = 2mE_\perp/\hbar^2$. It is found that for each integer $n' \geq 0$, there is a solution

$$P_{n',|m_l|} = g_{n'}(\rho)\rho^{|m_l|}e^{-\gamma\rho^2/2}, \tag{1-57}$$

where the coefficients in the power series

$$g_{n'}(\rho) = \sum_{j=0}^{n'} a_{2j}\rho^{2j} \tag{1-58}$$

satisfy a recursion relation

$$a_{2j+2} = \frac{(j-n')}{(j+1)(j+|m_l|+1)}\gamma a_{2j}. \tag{1-59}$$

The constant term a_0 is nonzero and can be determined from the normalization condition. The corresponding eigenvalue is

$$\lambda = 2\gamma(2n' + |m_l| + m_l + 1), \qquad E_\perp = \beta_e B(2n' + |m_l| + m_l + 1). \quad (1\text{-}60)$$

We can identify n with $n' + \frac{1}{2}(|m_l| + m_l)$ and note now that each energy level is in fact infinitely degenerate. As a consequence of this degeneracy, our particular choice for the form of the eigenfunctions is not unique.

The energy of the two-dimensional harmonic oscillator problem, as defined by the first two terms in Eq. (1-44) is $E_{\text{HO}} = \beta_e B(2n' + |m_l| + 1)$. The potential energy in this case is a diamagnetic-like term. The additional m_l contribution to $E_\perp$ arises from the L_z term in $\mathscr{H}_\perp$ and corresponds to the interaction of the magnetic field and the magnetic moment associated with the orbital motion of the electron.

To complete the treatment of the nonrelativistic problem, we need only combine these results with the solutions to the equation governing the z behavior.

$$Z(z) = e^{ikz}, \qquad E_Z = \hbar^2 k^2/2m, \quad (1\text{-}61)$$

where k is any real number. The z component of linear momentum is $k\hbar$. The complete solutions of the problem are thus

$$|n, k, m_l\rangle = C_1 e^{i(kz + m_l\phi)} P_{n', |m_l|}(\rho) \quad (1\text{-}62)$$

with $n' = n - \frac{1}{2}(|m_l| + m_l)$ and $P_{n'|m_l|}$ as given by Eq. (1-51), or

$$|n, k, m_l\rangle = C_2 e^{ikz}(\pi_+)^n \rho^{n - m_l} e^{-\gamma\rho^2/2 + i(m_l - n)\phi}. \quad (1\text{-}63)$$

These solutions are eigenfunctions of $\mathscr{H}_{\text{nr}}$, p_z, and L_z with eigenvalues of $\hbar^2 k^2/2m + (2n + 1)\beta_e B$, $k\hbar$, and $m_l\hbar$, respectively, and m_l must be less than or equal to n. This picture is consistent with the classical picture of the charged particle moving in a helix with axis parallel to the field. The contributions to the energy are those associated with the axial and transverse components of motion and the interaction energy of the external field with the field resulting from the motion of the charged particle. The normalization constants C_1 or C_2 depend on the choice of normalization for the free-particle-like z behavior as well as on the quantum numbers for the state involved.

We can now return to the two-component Dirac ψ_u. With this uniform magnetic field, $\boldsymbol{\sigma} \cdot \mathbf{B} = \sigma_z B$, and Eq. (1-29) becomes

$$\begin{pmatrix} \dfrac{\pi^2}{2m} + \beta_e B & 0 \\ 0 & \dfrac{\pi^2}{2m} - \beta_e B \end{pmatrix} \begin{pmatrix} \psi_1 \\ \psi_2 \end{pmatrix} = \varepsilon \begin{pmatrix} \psi_1 \\ \psi_2 \end{pmatrix}. \quad (1\text{-}64)$$

There are clearly two possibilities:

$$\psi_1 \propto |n, k, m_l\rangle, \qquad \psi_2 \equiv 0 \tag{1-65a}$$

with

$$\varepsilon = (2n + 2)\beta_e B + \frac{k^2\hbar^2}{2m}, \tag{1-65b}$$

or

$$\psi_1 \equiv 0, \qquad \psi_2 \propto |n, k, m_l\rangle \tag{1-66a}$$

with

$$\varepsilon = 2n\beta_e B + \frac{k^2\hbar^2}{2m}. \tag{1-66b}$$

We note that ψ_u is an eigenfunction of $\mathscr{H}_\perp$, p_z, and L_z, as is $|n, k, m_l\rangle$, and ψ_u is also an eigenfunction of σ_z. In anticipation of what is to follow, we call the σ_z eigenvalue $2m_s$. It can be ± 1. One term in ε will be $2m_s\beta H$.

The lower components of the four-component Dirac function are given by Eq. (1-23) in terms of the upper components. The four-component functions are eigenfunctions of the Dirac Hamiltonian $\mathscr{H}$ with eigenvalues

$$E = \pm mc^2[1 - 2\varepsilon/(mc^2)]^{1/2} = \pm[mc^2 + \varepsilon - \tfrac{1}{2}\varepsilon^2/(mc^2) + \cdots]. \tag{1-67}$$

The linear momentum operator p_z commutes with $\mathscr{H}$ as well as with $\mathscr{H}_{nr}$, and the four-component functions are still eigenfunctions of p_z with eigenvalues $k\hbar$. The operator L_z does not commute with $\mathscr{H}$, however, and different components of ψ are associated with different m_l values. It can be directly shown that the operator

$$J_z = L_z + (\hbar/2)\sigma_z \tag{1-68}$$

does commute with $\mathscr{H}$ and with p_z. This suggests that $s_z = (\hbar/2)\sigma_z$ is the z component of an operator $\mathbf{s} = (\hbar/2)\boldsymbol{\sigma}$ corresponding to an internal or spin angular momentum. The energy term involving m_s describes the interaction of the field with the magnetic moment associated with this internal angular momentum. We note that the proportionality constant is greater than that associated with m_l by a factor of 2. (The magnetic moment is antiparallel to the angular momentum because the electron is negatively charged.)

The relativistic states are characterized by quantum numbers n, k, and m_j. States exist for each nonnegative integer n. For any $n > 0$ we can, in accord with the discussion above, write two functions which are eigenfunctions of

$\mathscr{H}$, p_z, and J_z with eigenvalues E_n, $k\hbar$, and $m_j\hbar$, respectively. The energy E_n will be given by Eq. (1-67) with $\varepsilon = 2n\beta_e B$. The functions are

$$\psi^{+}_{n,k,m_j} = C_+ \begin{pmatrix} |n-1, k, m_j - \frac{1}{2}\rangle \\ 0 \\ \dfrac{k\hbar c}{E_n + mc^2}|n-1, k, m_j - \frac{1}{2}\rangle \\ \dfrac{2\hbar c(\gamma n)^{1/2}}{E_n + mc^2}|n, k, m_j + \frac{1}{2}\rangle \end{pmatrix},$$

$$\psi^{-}_{n,k,m_j} = C_- \begin{pmatrix} 0 \\ |n, k, m_j + \frac{1}{2}\rangle \\ \dfrac{2\hbar c(\gamma n)^{1/2}}{E_n + mc^2}|n-1, k, m_j - \frac{1}{2}\rangle \\ -\dfrac{k\hbar c}{E_n + mc^2}|n, k, m_j + \frac{1}{2}\rangle \end{pmatrix}. \qquad (1\text{-}69)$$

The angular momentum quantum number m_j can have any half-integer value $\leq n - \frac{1}{2}$, and k can have any value. When $n = 0$, only the second function is defined.

When there are two states with the same set of eigenvalues, it is usually desirable to introduce an additional operator, commuting with all three of the previous operators, but having different eigenvalues for ψ^+ and ψ^-. One possible choice for such an operator is

$$\Lambda = \frac{1}{E}\begin{pmatrix} mc^2\sigma_z & c\sigma_z\boldsymbol{\sigma}\cdot\boldsymbol{\pi} \\ c\boldsymbol{\sigma}\cdot\boldsymbol{\pi}\sigma_z & -mc^2\sigma_z \end{pmatrix}, \qquad (1\text{-}70)$$

which has the property that

$$\Lambda\psi^{\pm} = \lambda^{\pm}\psi^{\pm}, \qquad \lambda^{\pm} = \pm 1. \qquad (1\text{-}71)$$

It is not defined when $E = 0$‡, but in that case $n = 0$ so that ψ^+ does not exist and there is no need for an operator to distinguish between ψ^+ and ψ^-. The nonrelativistic quantum numbers m_l and m_s are not defined for the full relativistic functions, but they are for the large components. They can be obtained from m_j and λ as

$$m_l = m_j - (\lambda/2), \qquad m_s = m_j - m_l. \qquad (1\text{-}72)$$

‡ Note that $E\Lambda$ has eigenvalues $\pm E$. If $E = 0$ there is only one possibility, otherwise there are two.

Another quantum number n', which characterizes the ρ behavior of the large component can be defined by

$$n' = n - \tfrac{1}{2}(|m_l| + m_l), \tag{1-73}$$

and the energy can then be expressed in terms of

$$\varepsilon = (k^2\hbar^2/2m) + [(2n' + |m_l|) + m_l + 2m_s]\beta_e B \tag{1-74}$$

in which the contributions of the dipole–field interactions are made explicit.

Coulomb Field [47,172]

A second case in which the Dirac equation can be solved is the Coulomb field, or the hydrogenlike atom or ion with atomic number Z in the limit of infinite nuclear mass. The natural choice of potentials in this case is

$$\phi = Ze/r, \qquad \mathbf{A} \equiv 0. \tag{1-75}$$

The Dirac equation thus assumes the form

$$\begin{pmatrix} mc^2 - \dfrac{Ze^2}{r} & c\boldsymbol{\sigma}\cdot\mathbf{p} \\ c\boldsymbol{\sigma}\cdot\mathbf{p} & -mc^2 - \dfrac{Ze^2}{r} \end{pmatrix} \begin{pmatrix} \psi_u \\ \psi_l \end{pmatrix} = E\begin{pmatrix} \psi_u \\ \psi_l \end{pmatrix}. \tag{1-76}$$

Although the potential is spherically symmetric, L^2 and the components of $\mathbf{L}$ do not commute with the Hamiltonian as they do in the nonrelativistic case. If L_k is any component of $\mathbf{L}$,

$$[\mathscr{H}, L_k] = c\begin{pmatrix} 0 & [\boldsymbol{\sigma}\cdot\mathbf{p}, L_k] \\ [\boldsymbol{\sigma}\cdot\mathbf{p}, L_k] & 0 \end{pmatrix} \neq 0, \tag{1-77}$$

since the components of $\mathbf{p}$ and $\mathbf{L}$ do not in general commute: $[p_x, L_y] = i\hbar p_z$, etc. On the other hand, the square of the spin angular momentum

$$s^2 = \frac{\hbar^2}{4}\boldsymbol{\sigma}\cdot\boldsymbol{\sigma} = \frac{3\hbar^2}{4}\,1 \tag{1-78}$$

is just a multiple of the unit operator and does commute with $\mathscr{H}$. Its z component does not, as in the previous case of the magnetic field. Again it is possible to construct the total angular momentum operator $\mathbf{J} = \mathbf{L} + \mathbf{S}$. Both J^2 and J_z do commute with the Hamiltonian, with s^2, and with each other. An additional operator commuting with J^2, J_z, and $\mathscr{H}$ can be defined:

$$K = \beta[\boldsymbol{\sigma}\cdot\mathbf{L} + 1]. \tag{1-79}$$

A consideration of these operators will allow us to determine the angular behavior of the components of ψ.

The total angular momentum operators J^2 and J_z are even [in the sense of Eq. (1-19)] and in fact just apply the same J^2 and J_z to ψ_u and ψ_l. Both ψ_u and ψ_l must thus be eigenfunctions of J^2 and J_z with the same eigenvalues. The method of coupling the spin eigenfunctions, which in this representation are the two unit vectors $\binom{1}{0}$ and $\binom{0}{1}$, with the Y_l^m eigenfunctions of L^2 and L_z to obtain J^2, J_z eigenfunctions is well known. Both ψ_u and ψ_l must be of the form

$$\psi = \phi(r)[C_1 Y_l^{m-1/2}(\theta, \phi)\tbinom{1}{0} + C_2 Y_l^{m+1/2}(\theta, \phi)\tbinom{0}{1}]. \tag{1-80}$$

The constants C_1 and C_2 are appropriate Clebsch–Gordan coefficients. Two values of l, either $j + \frac{1}{2}$ or $j - \frac{1}{2}$, are possible and since the four-component function is not an eigenfunction of L^2, different l's must occur in ψ_u and ψ_l.

The operator K is also even but because of the β it is $(\boldsymbol{\sigma} \cdot \mathbf{L} + 1)$ on ψ_u but $-(\boldsymbol{\sigma} \cdot \mathbf{L} + 1)$ on ψ_l. The two components are individually eigenfunctions of L^2, and thus $(\boldsymbol{\sigma} \cdot \mathbf{L} + 1) = J^2 - L^2 - s^2 + 1 = J^2 - L^2 + \frac{1}{4}$ will have eigenvalue $l + 1$ if $j = +\frac{1}{2}$ and $-l$ if $j = -\frac{1}{2}$. The eigenvalue of K is customarily denoted by κ,

$$\kappa = \begin{cases} l = j + \frac{1}{2}, & \text{if} \quad j = l - \frac{1}{2}, \\ -l - 1 = -(j + \frac{1}{2}), & \text{if} \quad j = l + \frac{1}{2}. \end{cases} \tag{1-81}$$

It should be noted that the case $j = l - \frac{1}{2}$ is not possible when $l = 0$. Thus $\kappa = \pm 1, \pm 2, \ldots$ and both j and l can be determined from κ. Although L^2 does not commute with the Hamiltonian, l is of rigorous significance because it fixes the parity of the eigenfunction. (It also gives the L^2 behavior of the large component of the wave function.)

In order to have this correct angular momentum behavior, the two components of ψ_u must have a common radial factor, as indicated in Eq. (1-80). Similarly, the two components of ψ_l must have a common radial factor, but this need not be the same as that occurring in ψ_u. Combining these results, inserting the appropriate Clebsch–Gordan coefficients, and assigning customary phases, we find if $j = l + \frac{1}{2}$,

$$\psi_u = \begin{pmatrix} g(r)\left(\dfrac{l + m_j + \frac{1}{2}}{2l + 1}\right)^{1/2} Y_l^{m_j - 1/2}(\theta, \phi) \\[2ex] -g(r)\left(\dfrac{l - m_j + \frac{1}{2}}{2l + 1}\right)^{1/2} Y_l^{m_j + 1/2}(\theta, \phi) \end{pmatrix}$$

$$\psi_l = \begin{pmatrix} -if(r)\left(\dfrac{l - m_j + \frac{3}{2}}{2l + 3}\right)^{1/2} Y_{l+1}^{m_j - 1/2}(\theta, \phi) \\[2ex] -if(r)\left(\dfrac{l + m_j + \frac{3}{2}}{2l + 3}\right)^{1/2} Y_{l+1}^{m_j + 1/2}(\theta, \phi) \end{pmatrix}, \tag{1-82}$$

and if $j = l - \frac{1}{2}$,

$$\psi_u = \begin{pmatrix} g(r)\left(\dfrac{l - m_j + \frac{1}{2}}{2l + 1}\right)^{1/2} Y_l^{m_j - 1/2}(\theta, \phi) \\ g(r)\left(\dfrac{l + m_j + \frac{1}{2}}{2l + 1}\right)^{1/2} Y_l^{m_j + 1/2}(\theta, \phi) \end{pmatrix},$$

$$\psi_l = \begin{pmatrix} -if(r)\left(\dfrac{l + m_j - \frac{1}{2}}{2l - 1}\right)^{1/2} Y_{l-1}^{m_j - 1/2}(\theta, \phi) \\ -if(r)\left(\dfrac{l - m_j - \frac{1}{2}}{2l - 1}\right)^{1/2} Y_{l-1}^{m_j + 1/2}(\theta, \phi) \end{pmatrix}. \tag{1-83}$$

Substitution into the Dirac equation then leads to coupled equations for the radial functions f and g

$$\left(E + \frac{Ze^2}{r} + mc^2\right)f - \hbar c\left(\frac{dg}{dr} + [1 + \kappa]\frac{g}{r}\right) = 0,$$
$$\hbar c\left(\frac{df}{dr} + [1 - \kappa]\frac{f}{r}\right) + \left(E + \frac{Ze^2}{r} - mc^2\right)g = 0. \tag{1-84}$$

These equations can be solved by conventional techniques, with which we will not be concerned here. As usual, it is found that quadratically integrable solutions result only for certain values of E. It is convenient to define

$$\zeta = Ze^2/\hbar c = Z\alpha,$$

where $\alpha = e^2/\hbar c \sim \frac{1}{137}$ is the fine structure constant.‡ Then

$$E = mc^2\left[1 + \frac{\zeta^2}{(n' + \sqrt{\kappa^2 - \zeta^2})^2}\right]^{-1/2}. \tag{1-85}$$

Noting that $|\kappa| = j + \frac{1}{2}$, we see that E depends on $n' = 0, 1, 2, \ldots$ and on j, but not on l. The radial functions can be expressed as

$$f(r) = C_f \rho^{\gamma - 1} e^{-\rho/2}[n'F(-n' + 1, 2\gamma + 1, \rho) - (\kappa - \zeta/\lambda)F(-n', 2\gamma + 1, \rho)],$$
$$g(r) = C_g \rho^{\gamma - 1} e^{-\rho/2}[-n'F(-n' + 1, 2\gamma + 1, \rho) - (\kappa - \zeta/\lambda)F(-n', 2\gamma + 1, \rho)], \tag{1-86}$$

where F is the confluent hypergeometric function

$$F(a, c, x) = 1 + \frac{a}{c}x + \frac{a(a + 1)}{c(c + 1)}\frac{x^2}{2!} + \cdots, \tag{1-87}$$

‡ If $Z > 137$, ζ will be greater than 1, and since κ^2 can be 1, solutions of the form considered here will not exist. This is not a problem for "light" atoms, or for any as-yet-known atom.

$\gamma = (\kappa^2 - \zeta^2)^{1/2}$ and $\rho = 2\lambda r$ with

$$\lambda = \left[1 + \left(\frac{n' + \gamma}{\zeta}\right)^2\right]^{-1/2}. \tag{1-88}$$

The normalization constants C_f and C_g are complicated functions of the quantum numbers and need not concern us here. A few explicit solutions for low quantum numbers are given in Table 1-1. They are presented in a way which indicates the relationship with the nonrelativistic, Schrödinger radial functions.

For very small values of ρ, f and g behave like $\rho^{\gamma-1}$. When $|\kappa| = 1$, γ is slightly less than 1, and the solutions exhibit a singularity at the origin. Since $\delta = 1 - \gamma$ is small, this singularity is mild and the solutions are quadratically integrable. The Dirac radial functions also differ slightly from the Schrödinger functions in other ways. These differences become more significant as the atomic number Z increases.

TABLE 1-1

Some Dirac Hydrogenic Radial Functions[a]

State	$g(r)$	$f(r)$
$1s_{1/2}$	$r^{-\delta}e^{-Zr}$	$\mu r^{-\delta}e^{-Zr}$
$2s_{1/2}$	$r^{-\delta}[2(1-\eta) - Zr]e^{-(1+\xi)(Zr/2)}$	$\mu' r^{-\delta}[4(1-\eta') - Zr]e^{-(1+\xi)(Zr/2)}$
$2p_{1/2}$	$r^{-\delta}(Zr + \nu)e^{-(1+\xi)(Zr/2)}$	$\mu' r^{-\delta}[Zr - 6(1-\nu')]e^{-(1+\xi)(Zr/2)}$
$2p_{1/2}$	$r^{1-\delta'}e^{-Zr/2}$	$\mu' r^{1-\delta'}e^{-Zr/2}$

Parameter	Parameter values[b] $Z = 1$	$Z = 7$	$Z = 55$
δ	2.66×10^{-5}	1.31×10^{-3}	8.41×10^{-2}
μ	3.65×10^{-3}	2.55×10^{-2}	2.09×10^{-1}
ξ	6.66×10^{-6}	3.27×10^{-4}	2.17×10^{-2}
η	2.66×10^{-5}	1.31×10^{-3}	8.27×10^{-2}
η'	2.33×10^{-5}	1.14×10^{-3}	7.28×10^{-2}
μ'	1.82×10^{-3}	1.28×10^{-2}	1.04×10^{-1}
ν	3.99×10^{-5}	1.96×10^{-3}	1.23×10^{-1}
ν'	1.77×10^{-5}	8.70×10^{-4}	5.56×10^{-2}
δ'	1.33×10^{-5}	6.52×10^{-4}	4.07×10^{-2}

[a] These functions are not normalized, but the relative normalization of large and small components is given by μ or μ'. The variable r is in units of the Bohr radius a_0.

[b] The nonrelativistic solutions have all these parameters set to 0.

To relate the energy given by Eq. (1-85) to the nonrelativistic result, we can make an expansion in powers of ζ, which will be a small parameter unless Z becomes very large.

$$(n' + \sqrt{\kappa^2 - \zeta^2})^{-2} = (n' + |\kappa|\sqrt{1 - (\zeta/\kappa)^2})^{-2} = \frac{1}{n^2}\left(1 + \frac{\zeta^2}{|\kappa| n} + \cdots\right) \tag{1-89}$$

in which we have defined $n = n' + |\kappa|$, and

$$\begin{aligned} E &= mc^2[1 - \tfrac{1}{2}\zeta^2(n' + \sqrt{\kappa^2 - \zeta^2})^{-2} + \tfrac{3}{8}\zeta^4(n' + \sqrt{\kappa^2 - \zeta^2})^{-4} + \cdots] \\ &= mc^2 - \frac{mZ^2e^4}{2\hbar^2 n^2} + \frac{mZ^4e^8}{\hbar^4 c^2}\left(\frac{3}{8}\frac{1}{n^4} - \frac{1}{2}\frac{1}{n^3|\kappa|}\right) + \cdots . \end{aligned} \tag{1-90}$$

The first term is the rest mass energy and the second is just the Schrödinger result for a nonrelativistic, one-electron atom. The next term is the lowest order relativistic correction. It represents a sum of several contributions which can best be examined when we consider the relationship between relativistic and nonrelativistic results in the next section. One of the contributions corresponds to spin–orbit coupling, another to variation of mass with velocity, etc.

Conclusions Suggested by Exact Solutions

As a result of the behavior of a Dirac electron in a uniform magnetic field or in a Coulomb field, we find that it has associated with it an intrinsic angular momentum and magnetic moment. The gyromagnetic ratio associated with this intrinsic angular momentum is twice that associated with the orbital angular momentum. Both moments interact with a magnetic field and they interact with each other. The nature of these properties will become more clear in the next section when we consider the relationship of Dirac theory to nonrelativistic quantum mechanics.

Perturbations of the Dirac Hydrogen Atom

The four-component solutions for hydrogenlike atoms can be used as the zero-order solutions of some perturbation problems of interest in magnetic resonance: a uniform magnetic field or a nuclear magnetic moment. Conventional methods of perturbation theory can be applied in this relativistic formulation, and the results may shed some light on the conclusions to be drawn later in the more commonly treated nonrelativistic case. We will not go into the details of the calculation here, but will summarize the results. For further information the reader is referred to the book by Rose [172].

In the presence of a magnetic field as well as the Coulomb field, the Hamiltonian becomes

$$\mathscr{H} = c\boldsymbol{\alpha}\cdot\boldsymbol{\pi} - (Ze^2/r) + \beta mc^2 = \mathscr{H}_0 + \mathscr{H}', \tag{1-91}$$

where

$$\mathscr{H}_0 = c\boldsymbol{\alpha}\cdot\mathbf{p} - (Ze^2/r) + \beta mc^2 \tag{1-92}$$

is the H-atom Hamiltonian dealt with above and

$$\mathscr{H}' = c\boldsymbol{\alpha}\cdot(\boldsymbol{\pi} - \mathbf{p}) = e\boldsymbol{\alpha}\cdot\mathbf{A} \tag{1-93}$$

is the perturbation due to the field.

For the Zeeman interaction with a uniform external field in the z direction [cf. Eq. (1-31)]

$$\mathscr{H}' = (eB/2)(x\alpha_y - y\alpha_x) = (eB/2)r\cos\theta(\cos\phi\,\alpha_y - \sin\phi\,\alpha_x). \tag{1-94}$$

It is readily verified that J_z commutes with $\mathscr{H}'$ and thus with $\mathscr{H}$, but J^2 does not. The perturbation operator will have nonzero matrix elements between states of different j but not between states with different m_j. In a first-order treatment, matrix elements between states of different principal quantum number can be neglected, but among the degenerate or nearly degenerate states with a given n, off-diagonal as well as diagonal matrix elements must be included.

The radial and angular parts of the integrals can be separated to give

$$\langle n\kappa m|\mathscr{H}'|n\kappa' m\rangle = -(ieB/2)R_{\kappa\kappa'}^{(n)}A_{\kappa\kappa'}^{(m_j)}. \tag{1-95}$$

Although matrix elements between states of different n are being neglected and those between states of different m_j are zero, the integrals do depend on these quantum numbers. The radial integral is

$$R_{\kappa\kappa'}^{(n)} = \int_0^\infty r^3(g_{n\kappa}f_{n\kappa'} + g_{n\kappa'}f_{n\kappa})\,dr, \tag{1-96}$$

while the angular integral is given by

$$A_{\kappa\kappa'}^{(m_j)} = i\left[\frac{2(2\bar{l}'+1)}{2l+1}\right]^{1/2} C(\bar{l}'1l;00)\sum_\tau C(l\tfrac{1}{2}j;m_j-\tau,\tau)$$
$$\times\, C(\bar{l}'\tfrac{1}{2}j';m_j+\tau,-\tau)C(\bar{l}'1l;m_j+\tau,-2\tau), \tag{1-97}$$

where the C's are the Clebsch–Gordan coefficients $C(j_1j_2j;m_1,m-m_1)$ and

$$l = \kappa, \qquad \bar{l} = \kappa - 1, \qquad \text{for} \quad \kappa > 0;$$
$$l = -\kappa - 1, \qquad \bar{l} = -\kappa, \qquad \text{for} \quad \kappa < 0.$$

It follows from the triangle condition for nonvanishing Clebsch–Gordan coefficients that $l - \bar{l} = 0, \pm 2$.

In the particular cases $n = 1$ and 2, l values greater than 1 are not available and the nonzero $A_{\kappa\kappa'}$ are

$$A_{\kappa\kappa} = i\frac{4\kappa m_j}{4\kappa^2 - 1}, \qquad A_{\pm|\kappa|, \mp(|\kappa|+1)} = \pm i\frac{[(|\kappa| + \frac{1}{2})^2 - m_j^2]^{1/2}}{2|\kappa| + 1}. \tag{1-98}$$

The radial integrals in this case are readily evaluated and are given by Rose. Some of the results for low lying states are given in Table 1-2.

TABLE 1-2

Some Zeeman Energies for the Dirac H Atom[a]

State	g_j	$E^{(1)} = g_j\beta B m_j(1 + \xi)$ (atomic units)		
		$\xi: Z = 1$	$\xi: Z = 7$	$\xi: Z = 55$
$1s_{1/2}$	2	1.78×10^{-5}	8.70×10^{-4}	5.61×10^{-2}
$2s_{1/2}$	2	4.44×10^{-6}	2.18×10^{-4}	1.42×10^{-2}
$2p_{3/2}$ $(m_j = \pm\frac{3}{2})$[b]	$\frac{4}{3}$	5.33×10^{-6}	2.61×10^{-4}	1.63×10^{-2}

[a] $g_j = 1 + \dfrac{j(j+1) + s(s+1) - l(l+1)}{2j(j+1)}$ is the Landé g factor.

ξ gives the result of relativistic effects. It would be zero in nonrelativistic theory including spin in the Pauli sense.

[b] The $2p_{1/2}$ and $2p_{3/2}$, $m_j = \pm\frac{1}{2}$ states are mixed, so explicit results will not be reported here. The calculation is reported by Rose [172].

The hyperfine interaction can be treated in a very similar way. The perturbation in Eq. (1-94) is replaced by that due to the magnetic field of a dipole $\boldsymbol{\mu} = g_N\beta_N\mathbf{I}$ at the nucleus. In this expression g_N is the nuclear gyromagnetic ratio and $\beta_N = e\hbar/(2cM_{\text{proton}})$ is the nuclear magneton. The vector potential is

$$\mathbf{A} = \boldsymbol{\mu} \times \mathbf{r}/r^3 \tag{1-99}$$

for a magnetic dipole at the origin, and thus

$$\mathscr{H}' = e\boldsymbol{\alpha}\cdot(\boldsymbol{\mu} \times \mathbf{r}/r^3) = e\boldsymbol{\mu}\cdot(\mathbf{r} \times \boldsymbol{\alpha}/r^3). \tag{1-100}$$

The first-order energy which results is most readily expressed for states in which the electronic angular momentum $\mathbf{J}\hbar$ and the nuclear spin angular momentum $\mathbf{I}\hbar$ have been combined to yield a total angular momentum $\mathbf{F}\hbar$. The angular momentum coupling is readily done in closed form and the result is

$$E^{(1)} = [2\kappa/(4\kappa^2 - 1)]2\beta_e g_N\beta_N[F(F+1) - I(I+1) - j(j+1)]R_\kappa \tag{1-101}$$

with

$$R_\kappa = 2\int_0^\infty g_\kappa f_\kappa \, dr. \tag{1-102}$$

Some particular results are given in Table 1-3.

TABLE 1-3

Some Hyperfine Energies for the Dirac H Atom[a]

			$E^{(1)}/\Delta = \rho Z^3(1+\xi)$		
State	F[b]	ρ	$\xi : Z = 1$	$\xi : Z = 7$	$\xi : Z = 55$
$1s_{1/2}$	0	$-\frac{3}{4}$	7.99×10^{-5}	3.93×10^{-3}	3.12×10^{-1}
	1	$\frac{1}{4}$			
$2s_{1/2}$	0	$-\frac{3}{32}$	1.13×10^{-4}	5.57×10^{-3}	4.62×10^{-1}
	1	$\frac{1}{32}$			
$2p_{1/2}$	0	$-\frac{1}{32}$	1.04×10^{-4}	5.13×10^{-3}	4.20×10^{-1}
	1	$\frac{1}{96}$			
$2p_{3/2}$	1	$-\frac{1}{96}$	1.55×10^{-5}	7.26×10^{-4}	4.92×10^{-2}
	2	$\frac{1}{160}$			

[a] $\Delta = [E^{(1)}(1s_{1/2}, F = 1) - E^{(1)}(1s_{1/2}, F = 0)]_{\rm nr}^{Z=1}$; ρ = the nonrelativistic ratio for $Z = 1$: ξ = the relativistic correction.

[b] All values of F assume $I = \frac{1}{2}$.

Other Calculations with Four-Component Functions

The hydrogen molecule ion is the prototype for molecular calculations, and the nonrelativistic Schrödinger equation can be solved exactly for this problem, in the fixed nucleus approximation. It would thus clearly be of interest to obtain solutions of the Dirac equation with a double Coulomb potential, $\phi = e(Z_a/r_a + Z_b/r_b)$. This has not been done, however. The Schrödinger equation for fixed-nuclei H_2^+ can be separated in confocal elliptic coordinates and the resultant three ordinary differential equations can be solved analytically [13]. The results are presented in many standard texts [154]. The Dirac equation, on the other hand, is not completely separable [87, 175]. The coordinate corresponding to rotation about the internuclear axis is separable, and the resultant equation can be trivially solved, but the remaining coordinates do not separate.

Although this problem is not solvable exactly, it has been treated by variation and perturbation methods [112,156]. These are more readily discussed in terms of approximate relativistic equations, however, and will not be considered at present.

We have been able to treat interaction with a uniform magnetic field exactly for the case of an otherwise free electron, and as a perturbation of the H-like atom. We have also considered a point magnetic dipole at the origin of the Coulomb field in this perturbation sense to first order. We will see in the next section that terms involving higher than the first order of the magnetic point dipole cause trouble in a nonrelativistic-plus-perturbations treatment. It would be of interest to have an exact solution for the magnetic dipole only, to shed additional light on the nature of the hyperfine interaction. Unfortunately, two of the three coordinates in this problem are also inseparable, and any approximate treatment is further complicated by the fact that there are no bound states in the problem.

When Z becomes sufficiently large, relativistic effects in atoms can become appreciable, even in comparison with nonrelativistic energies. Spin–orbit coupling and the variation of electronic mass with velocity are usually the most important effects. Variational calculations for many-electron systems in the self-consistent field (SCF) approximation can include relativistic effects. These are usually done by adding correction terms to the nonrelativistic Hamiltonian, rather than by dealing with Dirac operators. We will see that there are difficulties associated with a completely relativistic many-electron theory. In the case of light atoms and the free radicals of primary interest to us, it has thus far been impossible to deal effectively with relativistic effects except by perturbation theory.

Summary of Section 1

In this section we have examined some solutions of the Dirac equation. This equation combines the requirements of special relativity with those of quantum mechanics. From the solutions in a uniform magnetic field and in a Coulomb field we find that the electron has an intrinsic angular momentum (with quantum number $s = \frac{1}{2}$*) and a magnetic moment proportional to that angular momentum. The proportionality constant is twice that associated with the orbital-angular-momentum magnetic moment. These properties arise naturally and need not be separately postulated as in the Pauli treatment of spin.*

Zeeman and magnetic hyperfine interactions in Dirac hydrogenlike ions can be treated by perturbation theory, but solutions of the Dirac equation for even such simple molecular problems as H_2^+ *have not been attained. A more generally hopeful approach thus will be found in expressing Dirac results in terms of nonrelativistic quantum mechanics and corrections which can be treated by perturbation theory.*

2. The Relationship between Relativistic and Nonrelativistic Theories

In the previous section, the Dirac theory of the electron was discussed. In many cases, however, one may not wish to deal with a fully relativistic theory even when it is possible; often it is impossible. The relationships between relativistic and nonrelativistic formulations, which will be discussed in this section, facilitate both understanding and practical utility of results arising from the Dirac theory.‡ Consideration will continue in this section to be restricted to one electron moving in classical fields.

The relativistic theory referred to here is the Dirac theory in which a four-component wave function describes the electron's behavior. (In a more general but equivalent formulation there is a four-valued variable associated with the electron's "internal coordinates.") By a nonrelativistic theory is meant one in which the wave function has two components and spin is treated in the Pauli sense. The nonrelativistic wave function can equivalently be expressed in terms of purely spatial functions and the two spin eigenfunctions α and β.

Reasons for wishing to establish a connection between these two theories fall into two categories. Understanding of a theory often depends to a significant extent on establishing a physical picture or model in terms of which the predictions of the theory can be interpreted. Such a model is, of course, not "real" and must be used with caution. There is a natural tendency to base new models on revisions of those existing previously, and thus to relate relativistic quantum mechanics to nonrelativistic quantum mechanics, which is in turn related to classical mechanics. The second reason for establishing the connection is a practical one. Most of the "relativistic" effects are quite small compared in magnitude to the total quantities involved. This is particularly true in magnetic resonance, in which one is usually interested in very fine details of the energy level structure of states which are degenerate if relativistic and spin effects are neglected. In the hydrogen atom ground state, for example, the ratio of the hyperfine interaction energy to the electronic binding energy is 4.3×10^{-7}. In molecular radicals the total energy is larger and the hyperfine energy smaller by several orders of magnitude. Further, the experimentalist may be interested in effects appearing in the second or third figure

‡ The presentation here is based on earlier, unpublished work of the author [74].

of the hyperfine energy. The precise determination of nonrelativistic energies in systems of more than one electron is itself a major undertaking. In any system for which approximate calculations must be made, therefore, it will clearly be impossible to obtain total energies with sufficient accuracy to get the small differences by subtraction. Rather the quantities of interest, like Zeeman and hyperfine splittings, should be obtained directly to a level of approximation which will hopefully approach the *relative* accuracy obtainable for the total energy. This can best be attempted by perturbation theory, provided the Hamiltonian is expressed as the ordinary spin-free, nonrelativistic Schrödinger Hamiltonian, plus spin-dependent perturbation terms arising from the relativistic treatment. Titchmarsh has shown that, at least for the H atom, a convergent perturbation series exists [201].

Since for practical work one will be dealing with a nonrelativistic Hamiltonian plus perturbations, the question immediately arises: Why not just start from there? The ordinary, spin-free Hamiltonian is well known, and magnetic interaction terms can be easily added by analogy with classical theory once the electron's spin and magnetic moment are postulated. Two objections to this procedure can be raised. One is the difficulty in obtaining all the relevant terms. It is probably impossible to be certain that everything has been included, and indeed there are some terms for which classical analogs are remote, being recognized only after the terms were known. The correspondence principle which provides the usual bridge between classical and quantum theories cannot help us here, because spin itself does not exist in the classical limit. In contrast, a careful reduction of a relativistic theory to nonrelativistic form will provide all of the terms inherent in the original theory. (There may still be some terms missing, but in that case the basic theory needs revision.) The second objection is more subjectively based and is essentially aesthetic in character. A piecemeal or patch-up theory is inherently less satisfactory than one obtained from a simply formulated and elegant starting point.

The first step in considering transformations from a relativistic to a nonrelativistic theory will be for us to formulate criteria by which various transformations can be judged. Several methods will be compared in terms of these criteria, and finally various results will be summarized. The goal is to obtain from the Dirac equation an equation which is in some sense approximately equivalent to it, but which also more closely resembles the nonrelativistic Schrödinger equation.

Characteristics of and Criteria for Transformations

In order to discuss the relative advantages of various methods of reducing the Dirac equation to two-component form, we must have in mind a clear idea of the purpose for which this reduction is intended. Such purposes have been discussed above. It cannot be expected that one method will necessarily lead to the result best suited for all purposes. The question will arise as to the sense in which a two-component equation is to be approximately equivalent to the Dirac equation.

It may be well to review some of the information given by the Dirac equation in a particular Lorentz frame. It can be written

$$D\Psi = i\hbar\,(\partial\Psi/\partial t) \tag{2-1}$$

with

$$D = c\boldsymbol{\alpha}\cdot[\mathbf{p} + (e\mathbf{A}/c)] - e\phi + \beta mc^2. \tag{2-2}$$

All of the information defining the particular system under consideration is in the potentials ϕ and $\mathbf{A}$ contained in the Hamiltonian operator D. The equation is invariant under a gauge transformation, although D itself is not always so. Changes in D with a transformation from one gauge to another are offset by changes in the phase of the wave function, just as in the nonrelativistic case (Appendix B). The eigenfunctions of D are state vectors for possible stationary states of the system; the eigenvalues are the energies (including the rest-mass energy) of these states. The time-dependent equation determines the behavior in time of a state vector: It determines $\Psi(t)$ when an initial state $\Psi(t_0)$ is known. Finally, the expectation value for any observable, F, is predictable when the state vector is known as $\langle\Psi|F|\Psi\rangle/\langle\Psi|\Psi\rangle$ with the usual corresponding formula for transition moments between states.

It is not possible for a two-component equation to duplicate all of these properties exactly. The Dirac equation has solutions corresponding to both negatron (electron) and positron states. A two-component equation is restricted to one or the other of these. Attention will be concentrated on equations approximately describing negatron behavior. The object of reducing the Dirac equation to two-component form is then to obtain an operator $\mathscr{H}$, acting on two-component functions Φ, with as many as possible of the following properties:

1. The low energy eigenvalues of $\mathscr{H}$ should agree, apart possibly from a constant displacement by mc^2, to within any desired degree of accuracy specified in advance, with the low-energy (i.e., close to mc^2) negatron-state eigenvalues of D.
2. If some initial state of the system is well described by a linear combination of low-energy stationary states, and its evolution in time is such that high-energy states do not become involved, then the time-dependent two-component equation should accurately give the evolution of the two-component function, maintaining the proper correspondence between it and the four-component function.

3. It should be possible to calculate, with any desired prespecified accuracy, the expectation values (and transition moments) of observables when the two-component functions are known. Expressions other than the simple expectation values or transition moments with respect to the two-component functions may be involved, however.

4. The two-component equation should be gauge invariant. It would also be desirable that $\mathscr{H}$ be Hermitian, but if the expression for conservation of probability in terms of the two-component function Φ is not the usual one this may be unnecessary or impossible.

The Foldy–Wouthuysen Transformation

One method of obtaining a two-component equation from the Dirac equation is to transform to a representation in which D is an even operator. The four-component equation then consists of a pair of uncoupled two-component equations. Methods for making such a transformation have been developed by Foldy and Wouthuysen [57] and their successors [10,56]. (See also Rose [172, Section 22].) In the case of a free electron or an electron in a uniform magnetic field, the transformation can be made completely and in closed form. When electric fields are present, as in the H atom, a series of transformations can be defined making the separation to as high an order as desired, but some difficulties may arise.

Naturally, when the transformation is made on D it is also made on other operators, and a corresponding transformation made on the wave functions. The transformation of operators supplies a possible interpretation of several relativistic effects and thus provides one of the advantages of the Foldy–Wouthuysen (FW) method.

A Hermitian operator S is to be chosen so that

$$\mathscr{H} = e^{iS}De^{-iS} - i\hbar e^{iS}\,(\partial e^{-iS}/\partial t) \tag{2-3}$$

is even, or if this is not possible, so that the odd component of $\mathscr{H}$ is sufficiently small to have a negligible effect at the desired level of approximation. The corresponding change in the wave function is

$$\Phi = e^{iS}\Psi \tag{2-4}$$

and thus, $D\Psi = i\hbar(\partial\Psi/\partial t)$ implies that $\mathscr{H}\Phi = i\hbar(\partial\Phi/\partial t)$.

As an example, we will consider an electron moving in a stationary magnetic field. The FW transformation in this situation was considered by Case [33]. We will expand somewhat on his treatment. The transformation for a free electron, first considered by Foldy and Wouthuysen, is closely related. In the absence of an electric field, with gauge chosen so that $\phi \equiv 0$, the Dirac Hamiltonian is

$$D = \beta mc^2 + c\boldsymbol{\alpha}\cdot\boldsymbol{\pi}. \tag{2-5}$$

Let

$$S = -(i/2mc)\beta\boldsymbol{\alpha}\cdot\boldsymbol{\pi}f \tag{2-6}$$

where f is a function of $\boldsymbol{\sigma}\cdot\boldsymbol{\pi}$ to be defined by its series expansion. Since $\boldsymbol{\sigma}\cdot\boldsymbol{\pi}$ commutes with $\beta\boldsymbol{\alpha}\cdot\boldsymbol{\pi}$ and with D in this case, no complications will arise. We also note that β anticommutes with the components of $\boldsymbol{\alpha}$ so that $\beta\boldsymbol{\alpha}\cdot\boldsymbol{\pi}$ is anti-Hermitian and S will be Hermitian provided that f is real. This S is not explicitly time-dependent so

$$\mathscr{H} = e^{iS}De^{-iS} = e^{2iS}D. \tag{2-7}$$

The second equality follows from the readily verified fact that S anticommutes with D so that in the series expansion of the exponential $DS^k = (-S)^kD$. We also note that

$$\begin{aligned} e^{2iS} &= \sum_{n=0}^{\infty}\frac{1}{n!}\left[\frac{1}{mc}\beta\boldsymbol{\alpha}\cdot\boldsymbol{\pi}f\right]^n = \sum_{k=0}^{\infty}\frac{1}{(2k)!}\left[\left(\frac{1}{mc}\beta\boldsymbol{\alpha}\cdot\boldsymbol{\pi}f\right)^2\right]^k \\ &\quad + \sum_{k=0}^{\infty}\frac{1}{(2k+1)!}\frac{\beta\boldsymbol{\alpha}\cdot\boldsymbol{\pi}f}{mc}\left[\left(\frac{1}{mc}\beta\boldsymbol{\alpha}\cdot\boldsymbol{\pi}f\right)^2\right]^k. \end{aligned} \tag{2-8}$$

But

$$\left(\frac{1}{mc}\beta\boldsymbol{\alpha}\cdot\boldsymbol{\pi}f\right)^2 = \left(\frac{f}{mc}\right)^2\beta\boldsymbol{\alpha}\cdot\boldsymbol{\pi}\beta\boldsymbol{\alpha}\cdot\boldsymbol{\pi} = -\left(\frac{f}{mc}\right)^2(\boldsymbol{\sigma}\cdot\boldsymbol{\pi})^2, \tag{2-9}$$

so

$$\begin{aligned} e^{2iS} &= \sum_{k=0}^{\infty}\frac{(-1)^k}{(2k)!}\left[\frac{f}{mc}\boldsymbol{\sigma}\cdot\boldsymbol{\pi}\right]^{2k} + \beta\rho_1\sum_{k=0}^{\infty}\frac{(-1)^k}{(2k+1)!}\left[\frac{f}{mc}\boldsymbol{\sigma}\cdot\boldsymbol{\pi}\right]^{2k+1} \\ &= \cos\left(\frac{f}{mc}\boldsymbol{\sigma}\cdot\boldsymbol{\pi}\right) + \beta\rho_1\sin\left(\frac{f}{mc}\boldsymbol{\sigma}\cdot\boldsymbol{\pi}\right), \end{aligned} \tag{2-10}$$

use having been made of the Dirac matrix

$$\rho_1 = \begin{pmatrix} 0 & 1 \\ 1 & 0 \end{pmatrix}$$

with the property $\rho_1\boldsymbol{\sigma} = \boldsymbol{\alpha}$. It follows that

$$\mathscr{H} = e^{2iS}D = \left[\cos\left(\frac{f}{mc}\boldsymbol{\sigma}\cdot\boldsymbol{\pi}\right) + \beta\rho_1\sin\left(\frac{f}{mc}\boldsymbol{\sigma}\cdot\boldsymbol{\pi}\right)\right][\beta mc^2 + c\boldsymbol{\alpha}\cdot\boldsymbol{\pi}],$$

and if we use the relationships

$$[\rho_1, \boldsymbol{\sigma}] = [\rho_1, \beta]_+ = 0, \qquad \rho_1^2 = 1,$$

we see that

$$\begin{aligned}\mathscr{H} &= [\beta mc^2 + c\rho_1 \boldsymbol{\sigma}\cdot\boldsymbol{\pi}]\cos\left(\frac{f}{mc}\boldsymbol{\sigma}\cdot\boldsymbol{\pi}\right) - [mc^2\rho_1 - c\beta\boldsymbol{\sigma}\cdot\boldsymbol{\pi}]\sin\left(\frac{f}{mc}\boldsymbol{\sigma}\cdot\boldsymbol{\pi}\right)\\ &= \beta c\left[mc\cos\left(\frac{f}{mc}\boldsymbol{\sigma}\cdot\boldsymbol{\pi}\right) + \boldsymbol{\sigma}\cdot\boldsymbol{\pi}\sin\left(\frac{1}{mc}\boldsymbol{\sigma}\cdot\boldsymbol{\pi}\right)\right]\\ &\quad + \rho_1 c\left[\boldsymbol{\sigma}\cdot\boldsymbol{\pi}\cos\left(\frac{f}{mc}\boldsymbol{\sigma}\cdot\boldsymbol{\pi}\right) - mc\sin\left(\frac{f}{mc}\boldsymbol{\sigma}\cdot\boldsymbol{\pi}\right)\right].\end{aligned} \tag{2-11}$$

Since β and $\boldsymbol{\sigma}\cdot\boldsymbol{\pi}$ are even operators, $\mathscr{H}$ will be even if the coefficient of the odd operator ρ_1 vanishes. This will be the case provided

$$\boldsymbol{\sigma}\cdot\boldsymbol{\pi}\cos\left(\frac{f}{mc}\boldsymbol{\sigma}\cdot\boldsymbol{\pi}\right) = mc\sin\left(\frac{f}{mc}\boldsymbol{\sigma}\cdot\boldsymbol{\pi}\right)$$

or

$$f = \left(\frac{\boldsymbol{\sigma}\cdot\boldsymbol{\pi}}{mc}\right)^{-1}\arctan\left(\frac{\boldsymbol{\sigma}\cdot\boldsymbol{\pi}}{mc}\right). \tag{2-12}$$

This leads to

$$\begin{aligned}\sin\left(\frac{f}{mc}\boldsymbol{\sigma}\cdot\boldsymbol{\pi}\right) &= \frac{\boldsymbol{\sigma}\cdot\boldsymbol{\pi}}{[(mc)^2 + (\boldsymbol{\sigma}\cdot\boldsymbol{\pi})^2]^{1/2}},\\ \cos\left(\frac{f}{mc}\boldsymbol{\sigma}\cdot\boldsymbol{\pi}\right) &= \frac{mc}{[(mc)^2 + (\boldsymbol{\sigma}\cdot\boldsymbol{\pi})^2]^{1/2}}\end{aligned} \tag{2-13}$$

and thus

$$\mathscr{H} = \beta c\frac{(mc)^2 + (\boldsymbol{\sigma}\cdot\boldsymbol{\pi})^2}{[(mc)^2 + (\boldsymbol{\sigma}\cdot\boldsymbol{\pi})^2]^{1/2}} = \beta c[(mc)^2 + (\boldsymbol{\sigma}\cdot\boldsymbol{\pi})^2]^{1/2}. \tag{2-14}$$

This Hamiltonian provides separate equations for upper and lower components and is consistent with the previously found eigenvalues $E = \pm mc^2[1 + 2\varepsilon/(mc^2)]^{1/2}$ with ε the eigenvalue of $(\boldsymbol{\sigma}\cdot\boldsymbol{\pi})^2/2m$ [Eqs. (1-25) and (1-69)]. Results for the more commonly treated case of the free-electron are obtained by replacing $\boldsymbol{\pi}$ by $\mathbf{p}$.

The transformation operators $e^{\pm iS}$ can conveniently be defined in terms of E. We find, by a transformation like that leading to Eq. (2-10), that

$$e^{\pm iS} = \cos\left[\frac{1}{2}\left(\frac{f}{mc}\boldsymbol{\sigma}\cdot\boldsymbol{\pi}\right)\right] \pm \beta\rho_1\sin\left[\frac{1}{2}\left(\frac{f}{mc}\boldsymbol{\sigma}\cdot\boldsymbol{\pi}\right)\right]. \tag{2-15}$$

Using Eqs. (2-13), with $[(mc^2)^2 + c^2(\boldsymbol{\sigma}\cdot\boldsymbol{\pi})^2]^{1/2} = E$, and trigonometric identities which are valid for the operators involved in this case, we obtain

$$\begin{aligned} e^{\pm iS} &= \left[\frac{E + mc^2}{2E}\right]^{1/2} \pm \beta\rho_1\left[\frac{E - mc^2}{2E}\right]^{1/2} \\ &= \frac{E + mc^2 \pm \beta\rho_1[E^2 - (mc^2)^2]^{1/2}}{[2E(E + mc^2)]^{1/2}} \\ &= \frac{E + mc^2 \pm c\beta\boldsymbol{\alpha}\cdot\boldsymbol{\pi}}{[2E(E + mc^2)]^{1/2}}. \end{aligned} \tag{2-16}$$

It is straightforward to verify that in fact these expressions lead to $e^{iS}De^{-iS} = \beta E$.

Any operator other than the Hamiltonian must be transformed in the same way. In the field-free case the linear momentum operator is unchanged by the transformation. This is not surprising since the momentum of a free particle is a constant of motion in both relativistic and nonrelativistic quantum mechanics. However, even such simple operators as position and spin assume quite a complicated form in the new representation. Alternatively, one can look for operators which become simple position, spin or orbital angular momentum operators in the new representation and consider them to be the appropriate relativistic analogs of the ordinary nonrelativistic operators [57]. They have a complex form in the original, untransformed representation, where they are sometimes called the mean position, mean spin, and mean orbital angular momentum. Among their interesting properties are the fact that the mean spin and mean orbital angular momentum are separately constants of the motion in the relativistic case.

The mean position operator can be analyzed in a way which shows that it corresponds to an averaging of the electron's position over a small region of space. Similarly, the wave function in the new representation is related that in the original representation by an integral transformation: The transformed function at a point depends on the original function in a small region about that point. We will not consider explicitly the operators or the integral transformation. They are available in the paper of Foldy and Wouthuysen [57] and elsewhere. Rather, we will seek some understanding of the nonlocal character of position by reexamining Dirac theory itself, with particular emphasis on position [47].

We will consider a free electron or, equivalently, concentrate on the z component of motion of an electron in a uniform magnetic field in the z direction. It is more instructive to work in the Heisenberg picture in this case. The Heisenberg equation of motion for z is

$$i\hbar\dot{z} = [z, D] = [z, \beta mc^2 + c\boldsymbol{\alpha}\cdot\boldsymbol{\pi}] = c\alpha_z[z, p_z] = i\hbar c\alpha_z \tag{2-17}$$

or

$$\dot{z} = c\dot{\alpha}_z. \tag{2-18}$$

Since the eigenvalues of α_z are ± 1, any measurements of v_z for the electron will give c, the velocity of light! As Dirac points out, however, this should not be surprising in view of the uncertainty principle [47]. Measurement of *velocity* (as opposed to momentum) requires the very precise measurement of the position of the electron at two closely spaced times. The uncertainty in momentum will thus be large, infinite in the limit corresponding to $v = c$, the maximum possible velocity in a relativistic theory.

Further understanding is facilitated by an examination of the time dependence of α_z itself. Again in the Heisenberg picture,

$$i\hbar\dot{\alpha}_z = [\alpha_z, D] = 2\alpha_z D - 2cp_z, \tag{2-19}$$

since $\alpha_z^2 = 1$. We note that of course $\dot{D} = 0$ and $\dot{p}_z = 0$ in this case also, so by a second differentiation

$$\ddot{\alpha}_z = -(2i/\hbar)\dot{\alpha}_z D \tag{2-20}$$

or

$$\dot{\alpha}_z(t) = \dot{\alpha}_z(0)e^{-2iDt/\hbar}, \tag{2-21}$$

where $\dot{\alpha}_z(0)$ is some initial value of $\dot{\alpha}_z$ (constant). Thus

$$2\alpha_z D - 2cp_z = i\hbar\dot{\alpha}_z(0)e^{-2iDt/\hbar}$$

or

$$\alpha_z(t) = \frac{i\hbar}{2}\dot{\alpha}_z(0)e^{-2iDt/\hbar}D^{-1} + cp_z. \tag{2-22}$$

For a stationary state in which the eigenvalue of D is E,

$$\dot{z} = \frac{i\hbar c}{E}\dot{\alpha}_z(0)e^{-2iEt/\hbar} + \frac{c^2 p_z}{E}. \tag{2-23}$$

The second term is just the classical (relativistic) velocity. The first term describes a very rapidly oscillating component of motion which averages to zero but accounts for the instantaneous values of $\pm c$ for $\dot{z}$. This rapid motion of the electron is known as *zitterbewegung*. Some of the interactions of the electron with its surroundings which arise in relativistic theory can be interpreted in terms of the *zitterbewegung* or the effective smearing out of the electron.

Foldy–Wouthuysen Transformation with Electric Fields Present

When electric fields are present there is no closed-form expression of Foldy–Wouthuysen type which will produce a Hamiltonian free of odd operators. A series of transformations can be defined, however, to reduce the remaining odd operators to as small an order as desired. Unfortunately, other problems may arise for higher orders.

A series of Hamiltonians is defined by

$$\mathscr{H}_{n+1} = e^{iS_n}\mathscr{H}_n e^{-iS_n} - i\hbar e^{iS_n}(\partial e^{-iS_n}/\partial t) \tag{2-24}$$

in which

$$S_n = -i(\lambda/2)\beta\mathcal{O}_n^{(n)} \tag{2-25}$$

with $\lambda = (mc^2)^{-1}$ being the parameter determining orders of smallness and $\mathcal{O}_n^{(n)}$ being the odd term of lowest order in $\mathscr{H}_n$ (as the notation implies, it will be of order n). The series starts with

$$\begin{aligned} \mathscr{H}_0 &= D = \lambda^{-1}\beta + \mathscr{E} + \mathcal{O}, \qquad \mathscr{E} = -e\phi, \qquad \mathcal{O} = c\boldsymbol{\alpha}\cdot\boldsymbol{\pi}, \\ S_0 &= -(i\lambda/2)\beta\mathcal{O}. \end{aligned} \tag{2-26}$$

The effect of the transformation can be seen by keeping only the lowest-order terms in

$$e^{\pm iS_0} = 1 \pm iS_0 - \cdots$$

and making use of the facts that β anticommutes with odd operators and $\beta^2 = 1$. Neglecting possible time dependence of S_0, we find

$$\begin{aligned} \mathscr{H}_1 &= (1 + (\lambda/2)\beta\mathcal{O} + \cdots)(\lambda^{-1}\beta + \mathscr{E} + \mathcal{O})(1 - (\lambda/2)\beta\mathcal{O} - \cdots) \\ &= \lambda^{-1}\beta + \mathscr{E} + \mathcal{O} + \tfrac{1}{2}(\beta\mathcal{O}\beta - \beta^2\mathcal{O}) + \text{terms of order } \lambda \text{ or higher} \\ &= \lambda^{-1}\beta + \mathscr{E} + \text{terms of order } \lambda \text{ or higher} \end{aligned} \tag{2-27}$$

Any remaining odd operators must thus be of at least first order in λ.

When the sequence of transformations is made it is convenient to use the operator identities (Appendix E)

$$\begin{aligned} e^A B e^{-A} &= B + [A, B] + \frac{1}{2!}[A, [A, B]] + \frac{1}{3!}[A, [A, [A, B]]] + \cdots \\ e^A \frac{\partial e^{-A}}{\partial t} &= -\frac{\partial A}{\partial t} - \frac{1}{2!}\left[A, \frac{\partial A}{\partial t}\right] - \frac{1}{3!}\left[A, \left[A, \frac{\partial A}{\partial t}\right]\right] - \cdots. \end{aligned} \tag{2-28}$$

The algebra will not be reproduced here, but the result is of the form

$$\mathscr{H} = \lambda^{-1}\beta + \sum_{k=1}^{N} \lambda^k \mathscr{E}^{(k)} + R_N, \tag{2-29}$$

TABLE 2-1

Results of the Foldy–Wouthuysen Transformation[a,b]

k	$\mathcal{E}^{(k)}$	$\lambda^k \mathcal{E}^{(k)}$
0	$\mathcal{E}$	$-e\phi$
1	$\frac{1}{8}[\beta\mathcal{O}, \beta]^{(2)} + \frac{1}{2}[\beta\mathcal{O}, \mathcal{O}]$	$\frac{1}{2m}\beta(\boldsymbol{\sigma}\cdot\boldsymbol{\pi})^2$
2	$\frac{1}{8}[\beta\mathcal{O}, \mathcal{E}]^{(2)} + \frac{i\hbar}{8}\left[\beta\mathcal{O}, \frac{\partial\mathcal{O}}{\partial t}\right]$	$\frac{e\hbar^2}{8m^2c^2}\operatorname{div}\mathbf{E} + \frac{e\hbar}{8m^2c^2}\boldsymbol{\sigma}\cdot(\mathbf{E}\times\boldsymbol{\pi} - \boldsymbol{\pi}\times\mathbf{E})$
3	$\frac{1}{384}[\beta\mathcal{O}, \beta]^{(4)} + \frac{1}{48}[\beta\mathcal{O}, \mathcal{O}]^{(3)}$	$-\frac{1}{8m^3c^2}\beta(\boldsymbol{\sigma}\cdot\boldsymbol{\pi})^4 + \frac{e^2\hbar^2}{8m^3c^4}E^2$
	$+\frac{1}{2}\beta\left(\frac{1}{2}[\beta\mathcal{O}, E] + \frac{i\hbar}{2}\beta\frac{\partial\mathcal{O}}{\partial t}\right)^2$	
⋮	⋮	⋮

[a] $\mathcal{E} = -e\phi$, $\mathcal{O} = c\boldsymbol{\alpha}\cdot\boldsymbol{\pi}$, and $[A, B]^{(n)} \equiv \underbrace{[A, \ldots [A,}_{n\ \text{brackets}} B] \ldots]$.

[b] For the two-component equation for electrons, β may be replaced by 1 and $\boldsymbol{\sigma}$ interpreted as the 2×2 Pauli operator.

where R_N includes odd (and even) terms of order $N + 1$ and higher. The first few terms in the expansion are given in Table 2-1 in the form in which they first appear and in an expanded form. The significance of these terms will be discussed after they are compared with those obtained by the partitioning technique.

It is of course possible to continue the treatment to obtain terms of higher order. Certain difficulties arise, however, and can already be seen in the last term in Table 2-1, proportional to E^2. It has arisen here after odd terms of second order have been eliminated and since it involved c^{-4} it should make a very small contribution. Suppose, however, that $\mathbf{E}$ is a Coulomb field:

$$\mathbf{E} \propto \mathbf{r}/r^3.$$

The $E^2 \propto r^{-4}$ and many of the integrals arising from the use of this term in a perturbation treatment will be divergent.

We know that the Coulomb field does not lead to difficulties in the Dirac equation; the problem can be solved exactly. It is also true that if the corresponding transformation is also made on the exact wave function and the higher-order terms are retained, factors will appear which exactly cancel the effect of the transformation of D and problems will be avoided. This does not alter the fact that we have clearly failed to reach our stated goal of obtaining operators which can be used for a perturbation treatment starting with (exact or approximate) Schrödinger wave functions. Additional terms leading to still more strongly divergent integrals continue to arise as the transformation is carried to higher order.

The origin of these difficulties is immediately clear when we consider that the treatment is based on a power series expansion of $\exp(\pm iS_n)$. Although S_0 does not contain ϕ, the potential will occur in higher-order S's, and thus if $\phi \propto 1/r$, we are employing an expansion of $\exp(1/r)$; we must expect to encounter difficulties for small r. Our conclusion is that although the Foldy–Wouthuysen transformation is valid and very useful for slowly varying fields, it cannot be satisfactorily employed when point sources are present.

In an attempt to avoid this difficulty as well as to obtain a further understanding of the relationship between relativistic and nonrelativistic formulations we will consider another method of converting the Dirac equation to two-component form.

Partitioning of the Dirac Equation

The traditional "method of the large component" (see, e.g., Bethe and Salpeter [17, Section 12]) for the reduction of the Dirac equation to two-component form, particularly as presented by Breit [22], is essentially a partitioning method. It has been so formulated by Löwdin [111] and by Blinder [19]. This method has been anticipated in Section 1 in our treatment of an electron in a uniform magnetic field.

If we write the 4×4 Dirac matrices in terms of 2×2 submatrices, the general Dirac equation is

$$\begin{pmatrix} mc^2 - e\phi - \hat{E} & c\boldsymbol{\sigma}\cdot\boldsymbol{\pi} \\ c\boldsymbol{\sigma}\cdot\boldsymbol{\pi} & -mc^2 - e\phi - \hat{E} \end{pmatrix} \begin{pmatrix} \psi_{\mathrm{u}} \\ \psi_l \end{pmatrix} = 0, \tag{2-30}$$

where $\hat{E}$ can be thought of either as the eigenvalue of D or as the operator $i\hbar(\partial/\partial t)$. It is convenient to substitute for $\hat{E}$

$$\hat{E} = W + mc^2, \tag{2-31}$$

where W is the energy in excess of that associated with the rest mass. If in a time-dependent case W is now assumed to correspond to $i\hbar(\partial/\partial t)$, the effect will merely be to introduce an unobservable phase shift. For a stationary state, for example,

$$\psi(t) = e^{i\hat{E}t/\hbar}\psi(0) = e^{imc^2t/\hbar}(e^{iWt/\hbar}\psi(0)). \tag{2-32}$$

The second of Eqs. (2-30) can be solved formally to give

$$\psi_l = (W + e\phi + 2mc^2)^{-1} c\boldsymbol{\sigma}\cdot\boldsymbol{\pi}\psi_{\mathrm{u}}. \tag{2-33}$$

If we define an operator $\hat{k}$ by

$$\hat{k} = 2mc^2(W + e\phi + 2mc^2)^{-1} = [1 + (\lambda/2)(W + e\phi)]^{-1}, \tag{2-34}$$

where again $\lambda = (mc^2)^{-1} \ll 1$, then

$$\psi_l = \frac{1}{2mc}\hat{k}\boldsymbol{\sigma}\cdot\boldsymbol{\pi}\psi_{\mathrm{u}} \tag{2-35}$$

and thus, from the first of Eqs. (2-30)

$$[(1/2m)\boldsymbol{\sigma}\cdot\boldsymbol{\pi}\hat{k}\boldsymbol{\sigma}\cdot\boldsymbol{\pi} - e\phi - W]\psi_{\mathrm{u}} = 0. \tag{2-36}$$

In a stationary state with $\phi \equiv 0$, $\hat{k}$ is just a number $k = (1 + \lambda W/2)^{-1}$, and the result is equivalent to that obtained previously [Eq. (1-25)]. For more general cases, additional properties of $\hat{k}$ must be considered. Löwdin [111] has shown that for any operator F,

$$[\hat{k}, F] = (\lambda/2)\hat{k}[F, \hat{E} + e\phi]\hat{k} \tag{2-37}$$

and further, that if ψ_{u} is the upper component of a solution of the Dirac equation for the given potentials,

$$\hat{k}\psi_{\mathrm{u}} = (1 - (\lambda/4m)\hat{k}\boldsymbol{\sigma}\cdot\boldsymbol{\pi}\hat{k}\boldsymbol{\sigma}\cdot\boldsymbol{\pi})\psi_{\mathrm{u}}. \tag{2-38}$$

These expressions can be used to provide what is essentially an expansion of $\hat{k}$ in powers of λ.

In Eq. (2-36), $\hat{k}$ can be moved to the right and a correction added as specified by Eq. (2-37). If ψ_{u} is assumed to be a solution of the equation, Eq. (2-38) can be used to give the effect of $\hat{k}$. This process can clearly be repeated as many times as desired to remove $\hat{k}$ from lower-order terms; only terms of higher than some specified order in λ will retain $\hat{k}$. The results of such a transformation are indicated in Table 2-2. The lower-order results are seen to agree with those provided by the Foldy–Wouthuysen transformation (Table 2-1). Problems again arise because of the occurrence of large negative powers of r in the higher-order terms when ϕ is a Coulomb potential.

These results can be put in more familiar form if we make use of some relationships among the operators involved. Recall that $\hat{E} = W + mc^2$, but in a commutator mc^2 does not matter so that either $\hat{E}$ or W can be associated with $i\hbar(\partial/\partial t)$. Then, for example,

$$\begin{aligned}[\sigma_x\pi_x, \hat{E} + e\phi] &= \sigma_x\left[p_x + \frac{e}{c}A_x, i\hbar\frac{\partial}{\partial t} + e\phi\right] \\ &= \sigma_x\left(\frac{e\hbar}{i}\frac{\partial\phi}{\partial x} - i\frac{e\hbar}{c}\frac{\partial A_x}{\partial t}\right) = ie\hbar\sigma_x E_x,\end{aligned} \tag{2-39}$$

and we see that

$$[(\boldsymbol{\sigma}\cdot\boldsymbol{\pi}), \hat{E} + e\phi] = ie\hbar\boldsymbol{\sigma}\cdot\mathbf{E}. \tag{2-40}$$

TABLE 2-2

Results of Partitioning with $\hat{k}$ Transferred to Higher Order

n	$\mathscr{H}^{(n)} \quad [\mathscr{H} = \sum_n \lambda^n \mathscr{H}^{(n)}]$
0	$-e\phi + \frac{1}{2m}(\boldsymbol{\sigma}\cdot\boldsymbol{\pi})^2$
1	$-\frac{1}{8m^2}(\boldsymbol{\sigma}\cdot\boldsymbol{\pi})^4 + \frac{1}{4m}(\boldsymbol{\sigma}\cdot\boldsymbol{\pi})[(\boldsymbol{\sigma}\cdot\boldsymbol{\pi}), \hat{E} + e\phi]$
2	$-\frac{1}{16m^3}(\boldsymbol{\sigma}\cdot\boldsymbol{\pi})^6 + \frac{1}{8m}(\boldsymbol{\sigma}\cdot\boldsymbol{\pi})[[(\boldsymbol{\sigma}\cdot\boldsymbol{\pi}), \hat{E} + e\phi], \hat{E} + e\phi]$
	$-\frac{1}{16m^2}\{2(\boldsymbol{\sigma}\cdot\boldsymbol{\pi})^3[(\boldsymbol{\sigma}\cdot\boldsymbol{\pi}), \hat{E} + e\phi] + (\boldsymbol{\sigma}\cdot\boldsymbol{\pi})^2[(\boldsymbol{\sigma}\cdot\boldsymbol{\pi}), \hat{E} + e\phi](\boldsymbol{\sigma}\cdot\boldsymbol{\pi})$
	$+ 2(\boldsymbol{\sigma}\cdot\boldsymbol{\pi})[(\boldsymbol{\sigma}\cdot\boldsymbol{\pi}), \hat{E} + e\phi](\boldsymbol{\sigma}\cdot\boldsymbol{\pi})^2\}$
⋮	⋮

Products involving two or more $\boldsymbol{\sigma}$'s can be simplified by use of the identity

$$(\boldsymbol{\sigma}\cdot\mathbf{a})(\boldsymbol{\sigma}\cdot\mathbf{b}) = \mathbf{a}\cdot\mathbf{b} + i\boldsymbol{\sigma}\cdot(\mathbf{a}\times\mathbf{b}), \tag{2-41}$$

where $\mathbf{a}$ and $\mathbf{b}$ are any operators which commute with $\boldsymbol{\sigma}$. When $\mathbf{a} = \mathbf{b} = \boldsymbol{\pi}$, we will need to evaluate $\boldsymbol{\pi}\times\boldsymbol{\pi}$. The x component, for example, is

$$\begin{aligned}(\boldsymbol{\pi}\times\boldsymbol{\pi})_x &= \left[\frac{\hbar}{i}\frac{\partial}{\partial y} + \frac{e}{c}A_y, \frac{\hbar}{i}\frac{\partial}{\partial z} + \frac{e}{c}A_z\right] \\ &= \frac{ie\hbar}{c}\left(\frac{\partial A_z}{\partial y} - \frac{\partial A_y}{\partial z}\right) = -\frac{ie\hbar}{c}B_x,\end{aligned} \tag{2-42}$$

so

$$\boldsymbol{\pi}\times\boldsymbol{\pi} = -\frac{ie\hbar}{c}\mathbf{B}. \tag{2-43}$$

It thus follows that

$$(\boldsymbol{\sigma}\cdot\boldsymbol{\pi})^2 = \pi^2 + (e\hbar/c)\boldsymbol{\sigma}\cdot\mathbf{B}. \tag{2-44}$$

When the higher-order operators in the table are expanded, terms like E^2 appear and for a Coulomb field will lead to divergent integrals. This could have been anticipated because the continued use of Eq. (2-37) will again produce a power series in ϕ (or in $\mathbf{E}$). How then can the Dirac equation be transformed in a way which will be acceptable even for the simple case of the hydrogen atom?

One approach is to leave $\hat{k}$ in place after the first transformation and work with the operator

$$\begin{aligned}\mathscr{H} &= -e\phi + \frac{1}{2m}\boldsymbol{\pi}\cdot k\boldsymbol{\pi} + \frac{i}{2m}\boldsymbol{\sigma}\cdot(\boldsymbol{\pi}\times\hat{k}\boldsymbol{\pi}) \\ &= -e\phi + \frac{1}{2m}\boldsymbol{\pi}\cdot k\boldsymbol{\pi} - \frac{e\hbar}{2mc}\hat{k}\boldsymbol{\sigma}\cdot\left(\mathbf{B} + \frac{\mathbf{E}\times k\boldsymbol{\pi}}{2mc}\right).\end{aligned} \tag{2-45}$$

The higher-order terms are included implicitly in such a way that divergent integrals apparently do not appear. It should be recalled that $\hat{k}$ depends on W, however, and thus

$$\mathscr{H}\psi_{\mathrm{u}} = W\psi_{\mathrm{u}}$$

is not a simple eigenvalue equation for stationary states, and as a time-dependent equation is very complicated.

The stationary-state equation can be dealt with by substituting for W in $\mathscr{H}$ an approximate value W_0 obtained from the solution of the equation in which $\hat{k}$ is replaced by 1. The error which results will be of higher order and can in principle be removed by a series of successive approximations using the W resulting from one cycle as input to $\mathscr{H}$ in the next, following the usual methods of partitioning theory. For higher-order results this method is not amenable to the direct calculation of small energy differences, which we have set as one of our goals. This approach thus also leaves something to be desired.

We have seen that problems of one sort arise from the ϕ dependence of $\hat{k}$ if $\hat{k}$ is removed from the Hamiltonian operator, while problems of another sort arise from the W dependence of $\hat{k}$ if it is not removed. Thus one should obviously remove the W dependence but leave in a modified $\hat{k}$ containing ϕ. Such a separation is possible and can be carried out without great difficulty, but then a new problem appears. The combination $W + e\phi$ which occurs in $\hat{k}$ corresponds to a fourth component, π_4, of the gauge invariant momentum with first three components $\boldsymbol{\pi} = \mathbf{p} + (e/c)\mathbf{A}$. If the parts of π_4 are separated and treated in different ways then the equation will not remain gauge invariant. The effect of a gauge transformation in quantum mechanics is to produce a phase change in the wave function such that when derivatives are taken the shifts in the potentials will be exactly offset. The separation of W from ϕ in $\hat{k}$ followed by an expansion producing powers of one but not the other destroys this possibility.

There does not seem to be any completely satisfactory resolution to this dilemma. A partial solution leading to workable results is possible, however. The gauge transformations which lead to difficulty if W and ϕ are separated are those which are time dependent. On the other hand, the potentials which lead to difficulties if $\hat{k}$ is expanded are those which arise from point sources. Point sources are introduced to approximate the effects of other particles. The other particles ought to be given proper quantum mechanical treatment including relativistic particle–particle interactions, but this is very difficult, as will be discussed in a later section. The additional approximation is usually made of considering nuclei as *fixed* point sources. For a fixed source there is no need for a time-dependent gauge transformation. External fields, for which the possibility of time-dependent gauge transformation may be desirable, do not involve point sources in the region of interest.

It is appropriate at this point to note still one further complication. A nucleus may include not only an electric monopole (charge) but an electric quadrupole, magnetic dipole, etc. These may lead to difficulty in the point source approximation. For example, the vector potential arising from a point magnetic dipole at the origin is $\mathbf{A} = (\boldsymbol{\mu} \times \mathbf{r})/r^3$, where $\boldsymbol{\mu}$ is the magnetic dipole moment. All the methods of reduction of the Dirac equation thus far considered include a term proportional to π^2. Indeed this term occurs in nonrelativistic theory when potentials are added. But π^2 includes a term $(e/c)^2A^2$, which for a point–dipole source is proportional to r^{-4}, and will again lead to divergent integrals in even a first-order perturbation treatment. This term has often been dismissed because the coefficient is small, but a divergent integral remains divergent, no matter how small the finite coefficient multiplying it. Again we are faced with a problem resulting from the inadequate approximation of a nucleus (or another electron) as a static point source. [Some of the problems can be avoided by the use of a finite-dimensional nuclear model (cf. Moore and Moss [143]).] This will be further discussed later.

We can define a partitioning procedure [74] which yields a satisfactory result for a limited class of fields, namely those for which

1. **B** does not arise from point sources
2. **E** can be divided into two parts

$$\mathbf{E} = \mathbf{E}_{\text{int}} + \mathbf{E}_{\text{ext}} \tag{2-46}$$

where $\mathbf{E}_{\text{int}}$ is stationary and $\mathbf{E}_{\text{ext}}$ does not arise from point sources.

For such fields it is possible to choose potentials, without sacrificing any useful freedom of gauge, such that $\phi = \phi_{\text{int}} + \phi_{\text{ext}}$, with $\dot{\phi}_{\text{int}} = 0$ and ϕ_{ext} not coming from point sources.

$$\begin{aligned} \mathbf{E}_{\text{int}} &= -\text{grad}\ \phi_{\text{int}} \\ \mathbf{E}_{\text{ext}} &= -\text{grad}\ \phi_{\text{ext}} - \frac{1}{c}\frac{\partial \mathbf{A}}{\partial t} \\ \mathbf{B} &= \text{curl}\ \mathbf{A}. \end{aligned} \tag{2-47}$$

Only gauge transformations for which these equations remain valid are allowed. This is equivalent to the condition that $\phi_{\rm int}$ is fixed, apart from a possible additive time-independent term of vanishing gradient.

With this restriction on the allowed fields and choice of potentials, we rewrite $\hat{k}$ as

$$\hat{k} = [k_0^{-1} + (\lambda/2)(W + e\phi_{\rm ext})]^{-1}, \tag{2-48}$$

where

$$k_0 = (1 + (\lambda/2)e\phi_{\rm int})^{-1}. \tag{2-49}$$

The operator $\hat{k}$ can then be expanded using the identity (Appendix E)

$$\begin{aligned}(A + B)^{-1} &= A^{-1} - A^{-1}BA^{-1} + A^{-1}BA^{-1}BA^{-1} - \cdots \\ &= A^{-1}\sum_{n=0}^{\infty}(-BA^{-1})^n,\end{aligned}$$

which leads in this case to

$$\begin{aligned}k &= k_0 \sum_{n=0}^{\infty} [-(\lambda/2)(W + e\phi_{\rm ext})k_0]^n \\ &= \sum_{n=0}^{\infty}(-\lambda/2)^n(W + e\phi_{\rm ext})^n k_0^{n+1} = \sum_{n=0}^{\infty}(-\lambda/2)^n k_0^{n+1}(W + e\phi_{\rm ext})^n.\end{aligned} \tag{2-50}$$

The commutation of k_0 and $(W + e\phi_{\rm ext})$ which has been assumed in obtaining these expressions follows from our requirement that $\phi_{\rm int}$ be stationary.

The potential can also be divided into two parts in the partitioned equation, with the result that Eq. (2-36) can be written

$$[(1/2m)\boldsymbol{\sigma}\cdot\boldsymbol{\pi}\hat{k}\boldsymbol{\sigma}\cdot\boldsymbol{\pi} - e\phi_{\rm int}]\psi_{\rm u} = (W + e\phi_{\rm ext})\psi_{\rm u}. \tag{2-51}$$

The expansion of $\hat{k}$ can then be substituted and all factors $(W + e\phi_{\rm ext})$ moved to the right, with appropriate commutator corrections. They can of course equally well be moved to the left.

$$\begin{aligned}\boldsymbol{\sigma}\cdot\boldsymbol{\pi}\hat{k}\boldsymbol{\sigma}\cdot\boldsymbol{\pi} &= \sum_{n=0}^{\infty}(-\lambda/2)^n\boldsymbol{\sigma}\cdot\boldsymbol{\pi}(W + e\phi_{\rm ext})^n k_0^{n+1}\boldsymbol{\sigma}\cdot\boldsymbol{\pi} \\ &= \sum_{n=0}^{\infty}\vec{\Omega}_n(W + e\phi_{\rm ext})^n = \sum_{n=0}^{\infty}(W + e\phi_{\rm ext})^n\overleftarrow{\Omega}_n.\end{aligned} \tag{2-52}$$

The operators $\vec{\Omega}_n$ and $\overleftarrow{\Omega}_n$ are defined implicitly in this way as the coefficients (independent of $W + e\phi_{\rm ext}$) which arise. The index n no longer labels a power of λ, however, since the commutators may introduce additional

TABLE 2-3

Operators $\Omega_n^{(k)}$[a]

k	n	$\vec{\Omega}_n^{(k)}$
0	0	$\boldsymbol{\sigma}\cdot\boldsymbol{\pi}k_0\boldsymbol{\sigma}\cdot\boldsymbol{\pi}$
1	0	$\frac{ie\hbar}{2}\boldsymbol{\sigma}\cdot\boldsymbol{\pi}k_0^2\boldsymbol{\sigma}\cdot\mathbf{E}_{\text{ext}}$
1	1	$-\frac{1}{2}\boldsymbol{\sigma}\cdot\boldsymbol{\pi}k_0^2\boldsymbol{\sigma}\cdot\boldsymbol{\pi}$
2	0	$\frac{e\hbar^2}{4}\boldsymbol{\sigma}\cdot\boldsymbol{\pi}k_0^3\boldsymbol{\sigma}\cdot\dot{\mathbf{E}}_{\text{ext}}$
2	1	$-\frac{ie\hbar}{2}\boldsymbol{\sigma}\cdot\boldsymbol{\pi}k_0^3\boldsymbol{\sigma}\cdot\mathbf{E}_{\text{ext}}$
2	2	$\frac{1}{4}\boldsymbol{\sigma}\cdot\boldsymbol{\pi}k_0^3\boldsymbol{\sigma}\cdot\boldsymbol{\pi}$
⋮	⋮	⋮

[a] Only $\vec{\Omega}_n^{(k)}$ is given. In each case $\overleftarrow{\Omega}_n^{(k)} = [\vec{\Omega}_n^{(k)}]^\dagger$

factors proportional to λ. Each Ω_n is clearly of at least order n and to separate the powers of λ we can define $\Omega_n^{(k)}$ independent of λ and such that

$$\Omega_n = \sum_{k=n}^{\max(n)} \lambda^k \Omega_n^{(k)}. \tag{2-53}$$

Some of the operators $\vec{\Omega}_n^{(k)}$ and $\overleftarrow{\Omega}_n^{(k)}$ are given in Table 2-3. A more symmetric result and one in which Hermiticity is more readily apparent is obtained by combining results of transfers to right and left and working with half the sum at each order.

$$\begin{aligned}(\mathscr{H} + e\phi_{\text{ext}})\psi_{\text{u}} &= \sum_{n=0}^{\infty}\sum_{k=n}^{\max(n)} \frac{\lambda^k}{4m}\{(W + e\phi_{\text{ext}})^n\overleftarrow{\Omega}_n^{(k)} + \vec{\Omega}_n^{(k)}(W + e\phi_{\text{ext}})^n\}\psi_{\text{u}} \\ &= (W + e\phi_{\text{ext}})\psi_{\text{u}}.\end{aligned} \tag{2-54}$$

Successive approximations to $\mathscr{H}$, not containing W, can then be obtained by replacing $W + e\phi_{\text{ext}}$ by an approximate $\mathscr{H} + e\phi_{\text{ext}}$. Thus

$$\mathscr{H}_0 = -e\phi + \tfrac{1}{2}\{\overleftarrow{\Omega}_0^{(0)} + \vec{\Omega}_0^{(0)}\}, \tag{2-55}$$

and through order N

$$\mathscr{H}_N = -e\phi + \frac{1}{4m}\sum_{k=0}^{N}\sum_{n=0}^{k}\{(\mathscr{H}_{N-k})^n|_{N-k}\overleftarrow{\Omega}_n^{(k)} + \vec{\Omega}_n^{(k)}(\mathscr{H}_{N-k})^n|_{N-k}\}. \tag{2-56}$$

The notation $(\mathscr{H}_l)^n|_l$ means that after $(\mathscr{H}_l)^n$ is determined all terms of order higher than the lth are dropped.

A formal separation of $\mathscr{H}$ into orders is possible, with

$$\mathscr{H} = \sum_n \mathscr{H}^{(n)}, \qquad \mathscr{H}^{(n)} = \mathscr{H}_{N=n} - \mathscr{H}_{N-1=n-1}. \tag{2-57}$$

The terms of each order, $\mathscr{H}^{(n)}$, are Hermitian, independent of W, and do not lead to divergent integrals (except possibly for higher-order magnetic dipole terms). The Nth order approximate equation $\mathscr{H}_N\psi \sim W\psi$ is, for each N, invariant under the class of gauge transformations consistent with Eq. (2-47). It should be noted, however, that the "order" of a given term is somewhat artificial and does not necessarily give the magnitude of its contribution accurately in all cases. A term may be effectively of one order over most of space but give a "contact term" of lower order near a point source.

The lower-order contributions to be obtained in this way are

$$\begin{aligned}
\mathscr{H}^{(0)} &= -e\phi + \frac{1}{2m}\boldsymbol{\sigma}\cdot\boldsymbol{\pi}k_0\boldsymbol{\sigma}\cdot\boldsymbol{\pi} \\
\mathscr{H}^{(1)} &= \frac{ie\hbar}{8m^2c^2}[\boldsymbol{\sigma}\cdot\boldsymbol{\pi}k_0^2\boldsymbol{\sigma}\cdot\mathbf{E}_{\text{ext}} - \boldsymbol{\sigma}\cdot\mathbf{E}_{\text{ext}}k_0^2\boldsymbol{\sigma}\cdot\boldsymbol{\pi}] \\
&\quad - \frac{1}{16m^3c^2}[\boldsymbol{\sigma}\cdot\boldsymbol{\pi}k_0(\boldsymbol{\sigma}\cdot\boldsymbol{\pi})^2k_0^2\boldsymbol{\sigma}\cdot\boldsymbol{\pi} + \boldsymbol{\sigma}\cdot\boldsymbol{\pi}k_0^2(\boldsymbol{\sigma}\cdot\boldsymbol{\pi})^2k_0\boldsymbol{\sigma}\cdot\boldsymbol{\pi}] \\
&\quad + \frac{e}{8m^2c^2}[\phi\boldsymbol{\sigma}\cdot\boldsymbol{\pi}k_0^2\boldsymbol{\sigma}\cdot\boldsymbol{\pi} + \boldsymbol{\sigma}\cdot\boldsymbol{\pi}k_0^2\boldsymbol{\sigma}\cdot\boldsymbol{\pi}\phi]
\end{aligned} \tag{2-58}$$

We can use the commutation relation

$$[k_0, \boldsymbol{\sigma}\cdot\boldsymbol{\pi}] = \frac{ie\hbar}{2mc^2}k_0^2\boldsymbol{\sigma}\cdot\mathbf{E}_{\text{int}} \tag{2-59}$$

to transfer all the k_0 factors to the far right or the far left. It is again best to do each and take half the sum of the two results so operators obtained will be explicitly Hermitian. The commutation contribution from the second term in $\mathscr{H}^{(0)}$ combined conveniently with the first term of $\mathscr{H}^{(1)}$ to give a term involving $\mathbf{E}_{\text{ext}} + \mathbf{E}_{\text{int}} = \mathbf{E}$. The commutator contributions from terms in $\mathscr{H}^{(1)}$ will be of order c^{-4} or smaller, and will be neglected.

This method could be carried to higher order by retaining these commutator terms and including contributions from $\mathscr{H}^{(2)}$. The algebra becomes quite involved, however, and is probably not worth the trouble. We will see in later sections that it is not practical to go beyond order c^{-2} for two or more electrons. The lower-order results are summarized in Table 2-4. The subscript index used on the terms in this table is merely a label for convenience in referring to the terms.

TABLE 2-4

Results of Modified Partitioning

n	k	$\mathscr{H}_k^{(n)}$ $[\mathscr{H} = \sum_{n,k} \mathscr{H}_k^{(n)}]$
0	1	$\frac{1}{4m}[k_0(\boldsymbol{\sigma}\cdot\boldsymbol{\pi})^2 + (\boldsymbol{\sigma}\cdot\boldsymbol{\pi})^2 k_0]$
0	2	$-e\phi$
1	1	$-\frac{ie\hbar}{8m^2c^2}[k_0^2(\boldsymbol{\sigma}\cdot\mathbf{E})(\boldsymbol{\sigma}\cdot\boldsymbol{\pi}) - (\boldsymbol{\sigma}\cdot\boldsymbol{\pi})(\boldsymbol{\sigma}\cdot\mathbf{E})k_0^2]$
1	2	$-\frac{1}{16m^3c^2}[k_0^3(\boldsymbol{\sigma}\cdot\boldsymbol{\pi})^4 + (\boldsymbol{\sigma}\cdot\boldsymbol{\pi})^4 k_0^3]$
1	3	$\frac{e}{8m^2c^2}[k_0^2\phi(\boldsymbol{\sigma}\cdot\boldsymbol{\pi})^2 + (\boldsymbol{\sigma}\cdot\boldsymbol{\pi})^2\phi k_0^2]$
⋮	⋮	⋮

Discussion of Terms Occurring in the Hamiltonian

We will consider the various terms occurring in Table 2-4 in succession and compare them with the results of the FW transformation (Table 2-1). To aid in interpreting these terms and to provide expressions that will be useful in the future, we will examine the forms they assume when the fields include a uniform external magnetic field and nuclear Coulomb and magnetic dipolar fields.‡

$$\phi_{\text{int}} = \frac{Z_\nu e}{r_\nu}, \qquad \mathbf{E}_{\text{int}} = \frac{Z_\nu e}{r_\nu^3}\mathbf{r}_\nu. \tag{2-60}$$

$$\mathbf{A}_0 = \frac{1}{2}(\mathbf{B}_0 \times \mathbf{r}), \qquad \mathbf{A}_\nu = \frac{1}{r_\nu^3}(\boldsymbol{\mu}_\nu \times \mathbf{r}_\nu), \qquad \mathbf{B}_\nu = -\frac{\boldsymbol{\mu}_\nu}{r_\nu^3} + 3\frac{(\boldsymbol{\mu}_\nu\cdot\mathbf{r}_\nu)}{r_\nu^5}\mathbf{r}_\nu. \tag{2-61}$$

The subscript ν is added to indicate a nuclear contribution. Nucleus ν is the origin for $\mathbf{r}_\nu$ and $\boldsymbol{\mu}_\nu$ is the nuclear magnetic moment. The subscript 0 identifies contributions from the uniform magnetic field. Contributions from other fields will not be considered explicitly.

‡ We have already noted that the approximation of a point magnetic dipole source will lead to difficulty. It is included, however, as the simplest way of approximating magnetic hyperfine interactions.

Expanding $\boldsymbol{\sigma} \cdot \boldsymbol{\pi}$ with the help of Eqs. (2-44) and (1-10), we can write $\mathscr{H}_1^{(0)}$ as the sum of four contributions:

$$\mathscr{H}_{1a}^{(0)} = \frac{1}{4m} [k_0 p^2 + p^2 k_0],$$

$$\mathscr{H}_{1b}^{(0)} = \frac{e}{4mc} [k_0(\mathbf{p} \cdot \mathbf{A} + \mathbf{A} \cdot \mathbf{p}) + (\mathbf{p} \cdot \mathbf{A} + \mathbf{A} \cdot \mathbf{p})k_0], \tag{2-62}$$

$$\mathscr{H}_{1c}^{(0)} = \frac{e^2}{2mc^2} k_0 A^2, \qquad \mathscr{H}_{1d}^{(0)} = \frac{e\hbar}{2mc} k_0 \boldsymbol{\sigma} \cdot \mathbf{B}.$$

In $\mathscr{H}_{1a}^{(0)}$, k_0 is not needed as a convergence factor so its effect can be transferred to higher order. It follows from the definition of k_0 [Eq. (2-49)] that

$$k_0[1 + (\lambda/2)e\phi_{\text{int}}] = 1,$$

$$k_0 = 1 - (\lambda/2)e\phi_{\text{int}} k_0 = 1 - \frac{e}{2mc^2} \phi_{\text{int}} k_0. \tag{2-63}$$

This expansion corresponds in its effect to the use of Eq. (2-38) in the original partitioning method and can lead to the same difficulties. There will be no problem if it is used here, however.

This subsitution for k_0 leads to

$$\mathscr{H}_{1a}^{(0)} = \frac{p^2}{2m} - \frac{e}{8m^2c^2} (k_0 \phi_{\text{int}} p^2 + p^2 \phi_{\text{int}} k_0). \tag{2-64}$$

The first term is of course the ordinary nonrelativistic *kinetic energy*. It will occur also in the FW expression. We defer discussion of the second term until we consider contributions from $\mathscr{H}_3^{(1)}$.

To treat $\mathscr{H}_{1b}^{(0)}$, we note that

$$\mathbf{p} \cdot \mathbf{A} + \mathbf{A} \cdot \mathbf{p} = 2\mathbf{A} \cdot \mathbf{p} - i\hbar \operatorname{div} \mathbf{A}, \tag{2-65}$$

and that for the vector potentials we are considering explicitly div $\mathbf{A} = 0$. For the uniform field

$$\mathbf{A}_0 \cdot \mathbf{p} = \tfrac{1}{2}(\mathbf{B}_0 \times \mathbf{r}) \cdot \mathbf{p} = \tfrac{1}{2}\mathbf{B}_0 \cdot \mathbf{r} \times \mathbf{p} = (\hbar/2)\mathbf{B}_0 \cdot \mathbf{l}, \tag{2-66}$$

where $\mathbf{l}$ is defined as $\hbar^{-1}(\mathbf{r} \times \mathbf{p})$ and is thus dimensionless. It is computed with respect to the same origin as that used for $\mathbf{r}$ in $\mathbf{A}_0$. If there is only a single nucleus, k_0 is spherically symmetric and commutes with $\mathbf{l}$ if the nucleus is taken to be the origin. In general

$$[\mathbf{l}, k_0] = -\frac{ie\hbar}{2mc^2} k_0^3 \mathbf{r} \times \mathbf{E}_{\text{int}}. \tag{2-67}$$

Alternatively, we note that k_0 is not needed to provide a convergence factor in this term so we can transfer its effect to higher order by using Eq. (2-63). The result is

$$\mathscr{H}^{(0)}_{1b0} = \frac{e\hbar}{2mc}\mathbf{B}_0 \cdot \mathbf{l} - \frac{e^2\hbar}{8m^2c^2}(k_0 \phi_{\text{int}} \mathbf{B}_0 \cdot \mathbf{l} + \mathbf{B}_0 \cdot \mathbf{l}\phi_{\text{int}} k_0). \tag{2-68}$$

The second term is a higher-order correction to the first. The first is the *orbital Zeeman* term describing the interaction of the electrons orbital motion with the magnetic field. An identical term occurs in the FW treatment.

For the dipolar field

$$\mathbf{A}_\nu \cdot \mathbf{p} = (1/r_\nu^3)\boldsymbol{\mu}_\nu \times \mathbf{r}_\nu \cdot \mathbf{p} = (\hbar/r_\nu^3)\boldsymbol{\mu}_\nu \cdot \mathbf{l}_\nu, \tag{2-69}$$

where $\mathbf{l}_\nu = \hbar^{-1}(\mathbf{r}_\nu \times \mathbf{p})$ is the orbital angular momentum about nucleus ν. Terms arising from commutators of k_0 and $\mathbf{l}$ will be negligible since $|\boldsymbol{\mu}_\nu|$ is itself small, but in this case it is convenient to retain k_0 as a convergence factor.

$$\mathscr{H}^{(0)}_{1b\nu} = \frac{e\hbar}{mc} k_0 \frac{\boldsymbol{\mu}_\nu \cdot \mathbf{l}_\nu}{r_\nu^3}. \tag{2-70}$$

In the vicinity of nucleus ν, ϕ_{int} is dominated by the contribution from that nucleus, $\phi_\nu = Z_\nu e/r_\nu$. For sufficiently small r_ν, k_0 is essentially proportional to r_ν, so the operator will behave near the nucleus like r_ν^{-2}, and integrals will present no problems. The same feature will occur in connection with other terms considered below. The term represents an *orbital hyperfine interaction.* In the FW result it occurs without the k_0.

If several contributions to the vector potential are simultaneously present, $\mathscr{H}^{(0)}_{1c}$ will include both squares and cross terms. For a uniform field and several nuclei

$$\begin{aligned} A^2 &= A_0^2 + 2\sum_\nu \mathbf{A}_0 \cdot \mathbf{A}_\nu + \sum_{\nu,\nu'} \mathbf{A}_\nu \cdot \mathbf{A}_{\nu'} \\ &= \frac{1}{4}[B_0^2 r^2 - (\mathbf{B}_0 \cdot \mathbf{r})^2] + \sum_\nu \frac{1}{r_\nu^3}[(\boldsymbol{\mu}_\nu \cdot \mathbf{B}_0)(\mathbf{r} \cdot \mathbf{r}_\nu) - (\mathbf{B} \cdot \mathbf{r}_\nu)(\mathbf{r} \cdot \boldsymbol{\mu}_\nu)] \\ &\quad + \sum_{\nu,\nu'} \frac{1}{r_\nu^3 r_{\nu'}^3}[(\boldsymbol{\mu}_\nu \cdot \boldsymbol{\mu}'_\nu)(\mathbf{r}_\nu \cdot \mathbf{r}_{\nu'}) - (\boldsymbol{\mu}_\nu \cdot \mathbf{r}_{\nu'})(\boldsymbol{\mu}_{\nu'} \cdot \mathbf{r}_\nu)]. \end{aligned}$$

The purely uniform field contributions present no problems. The effect of k_0 can be transferred to higher order, where it is negligible, and

$$\mathscr{H}^{(0)}_{1c00} = \frac{e^2}{8mc^2}[B_0^2 r^2 - (\mathbf{B}_0 \cdot \mathbf{r})^2]. \tag{2-71}$$

In the common case where the direction of $\mathbf{B}_0$ determines the z direction, this is

$$\mathscr{H}^{(0)}_{1c00}(\mathbf{B}_0 \| \hat{z}) = \frac{e^2 B_0^2}{8mc^2}(x^2 + y^2).$$

This is the familiar *diamagnetic* term. The same term is found by the FW method. We note at this point that if the origin with respect to which $\mathbf{A}_0$ is defined is changed, this is a gauge transformation. The same origin must be used for $\mathbf{A}_0$ and for $\mathbf{l}$ in $\mathscr{H}^{(0)}_{1b0}$. The effects of such gauge transformations will be considered in Section 9.

The cross terms between uniform and dipolar fields contribute

$$\mathscr{H}^{(0)}_{1c0\nu} = \frac{e^2}{2mc^2} k_0 \frac{1}{r_\nu^3}[(\boldsymbol{\mu}_\nu \cdot \mathbf{B}_0)(\mathbf{r} \cdot \mathbf{r}_\nu) - (\mathbf{r} \cdot \boldsymbol{\mu}_\nu)(\mathbf{r}_\nu \cdot \mathbf{B}_0)], \tag{2-72}$$

which is a correction to the nuclear Zeeman interaction. The term behaves like k_0/r^2 near the nucleus, so integrals will be convergent.

The contribution from purely dipolar fields is

$$\mathscr{H}^{(0)}_{1c\nu\nu'} = \frac{e^2}{2mc^2} k_0 \frac{1}{r_\nu^3 r_{\nu'}^3}[(\boldsymbol{\mu}_\nu \cdot \boldsymbol{\mu}_{\nu'})(\mathbf{r}_\nu \cdot \mathbf{r}_{\nu'}) - (\boldsymbol{\mu}_\nu \cdot \mathbf{r}_{\nu'})(\boldsymbol{\mu}_{\nu'} \cdot \mathbf{r}_\nu)]. \tag{2-73}$$

If $\nu' \neq \nu$, integrals will be convergent. Near nucleus ν, k_0 behaves like r_ν and near nucleus ν' it behaves like $r_{\nu'}$. When $\nu' = \nu$, however, the overall behavior near the nucleus will be like r_ν^{-3} so integrals will diverge. The divergence is even worse for the FW result where k_0 is absent. This represents a breakdown in the point–dipole approximation for the nuclear magnetic moment.

The remaining term in $\mathscr{H}^{(0)}_1$ describes the interaction of the electron's magnetic moment with a magnetic field. For the uniform field case the effect of k_0 is not significant and can be transferred to higher order. The contribution is thus

$$\mathscr{H}^{(0)}_{1d0} = \frac{e\hbar}{2mc}\boldsymbol{\sigma} \cdot \mathbf{B}_0, \tag{2-74}$$

which is the usual *Zeeman* term and occurs also in the FW approach. The dipolar contribution from this term is

$$\mathscr{H}^{(0)}_{1d\nu} = -\frac{e\hbar}{2mc} k_0 \left(\frac{\boldsymbol{\sigma} \cdot \boldsymbol{\mu}_\nu}{r_\nu^3} - 3\frac{(\boldsymbol{\sigma} \cdot \mathbf{r}_\nu)(\boldsymbol{\mu}_\nu \cdot \mathbf{r}_\nu)}{r_\nu^5} \right). \tag{2-75}$$

The effect of k_0 is negligible except for very small r_ν, where it provides a convergence factor so that no integral difficulties arise. This term describes the interaction between electron and nuclear magnetic moments and is the *dipolar hyperfine interaction* term.

The same term arises in the FW method, except that k_0 is there replaced by 1. Further discussion of the small r behavior is then required. The treatment by Messiah [138, Section 32], for example, begins by noting that $\mathbf{A}_\nu$ can be written as

$$\mathbf{A}_\nu = \text{curl}\, \boldsymbol{\mu}_\nu / r_\nu, \tag{2-76}$$

so that

$$\mathbf{B}_\nu = \text{curl curl}\, \frac{\boldsymbol{\mu}_\nu}{r_\nu} = \text{grad div}\, \frac{\boldsymbol{\mu}_\nu}{r_\nu} - \nabla^2 \frac{\boldsymbol{\mu}_\nu}{r_\nu}, \tag{2-77}$$

and

$$\begin{aligned} \boldsymbol{\sigma} \cdot \mathbf{B}_\nu &= (\boldsymbol{\sigma} \cdot \nabla)(\boldsymbol{\mu}_\nu \cdot \nabla)(1/r_\nu) - (\boldsymbol{\sigma} \cdot \boldsymbol{\mu}_\nu)\nabla^2(1/r_\nu) \\ &= [(\boldsymbol{\sigma} \cdot \nabla)(\boldsymbol{\mu}_\nu \cdot \nabla) - \tfrac{1}{3}(\boldsymbol{\sigma} \cdot \boldsymbol{\mu}_\nu)\nabla^2](1/r_\nu) - \tfrac{2}{3}\boldsymbol{\sigma} \cdot \boldsymbol{\mu}_\nu \nabla^2(1/r_\nu). \end{aligned} \tag{2-78}$$

The final form is selected because each of the two terms is an irreducible tensor operator (Appendix C): The first is of order 2; the second of order 0. Thus,

$$\mathscr{H}^{(0)}_{1\text{d}\nu}(\text{FW}) = \sum_{j,k} \sigma_j \mu_{\nu k} T^{(2)}_{jk} + \sum_{j,k} \sigma_j \mu_{\nu k} T^{(0)}_{jk}, \tag{2-79}$$

where $\mathbf{T}^{(2)}$ and $\mathbf{T}^{(0)}$ contain all the spatial operators. (The derivatives in Eq. (2-78) operate only on the $1/r_\nu$, not on the function the operator is acting on.)

In the evaluation of integrals involving $\mathscr{H}^{(0)}_{1\text{d}}$, the spatial part of the integrand can be expanded about the position of nucleus ν as

$$\sum_{l,m} f_{lm}(r_\nu) Y_l^m(\theta, \phi),$$

where Y_l^m is a spherical harmonic and f_{lm} is a function of the distance r_ν with the property that it will certainly go to zero as r_ν^l for small r_ν. The only terms which will give nonzero contributions are those involving Y_2 with $\mathbf{T}^{(2)}$ and those involving Y_0 with $\mathbf{T}^{(0)}$. The term $\mathbf{T}^{(2)}$ gives the dipolar interaction and behaves like $1/r_\nu^3$. It will survive angular integration only in terms with r_ν^2 behavior for small r_ν, so the radial integrals will converge.

The $\mathbf{T}^{(0)}$ term can be rewritten in terms of a Dirac δ function, since

$$\nabla^2(1/r) = -4\pi\delta(\mathbf{r}). \tag{2-80}$$

Its contribution comes from the spherically symmetric (Y_0) part of the distribution. This is the *Fermi contact interaction*

$$\mathscr{H}^{(0)}_{1\text{d}\nu'}(\text{FW}) = \frac{8\pi}{3} \frac{e\hbar}{2mc} \boldsymbol{\sigma} \cdot \boldsymbol{\mu}_\nu \delta(\mathbf{r}_\nu). \tag{2-81}$$

It would seem that an equivalent term would result if we apply similar arguments to examine the partitioning result. In that case, however, the term is multiplied by k_0, and k_0 is zero at $r_\nu = 0$, so there will be no contribution. As we shall see, the Fermi contact term arises in another way in the partitioning treatment.

The next term in Table 2-4 is $\mathscr{H}_2^{(0)}$. For a Coulomb field it contributes

$$\mathscr{H}_{2\nu}^{(0)} = -Ze^2/r_\nu. \tag{2-82}$$

This is the standard *nuclear attraction* term of the nonrelativistic Hamiltonian. It is included in both the FW and partitioning treatments and requires no further comment.

We now proceed to the terms first order in $\lambda = 1/mc^2$. In $\mathscr{H}_1^{(1)}$ we again expand π and make use of Eq. (2-41) to obtain a sum of five terms:

$$\begin{aligned}
\mathscr{H}_{1a}^{(1)} &= -\frac{ie\hbar}{8m^2c^2}[k_0^2\mathbf{E}\cdot\mathbf{p} - \mathbf{E}\cdot\mathbf{p}k_0^2],\\
\mathscr{H}_{1b}^{(1)} &= \frac{e\hbar^2}{8m^2c^2}k_0^2 \operatorname{div}\mathbf{E},\\
\mathscr{H}_{1c}^{(1)} &= \frac{e\hbar}{8m^2c^2}[k_0^2\boldsymbol{\sigma}\cdot\mathbf{E}\times\mathbf{p} - \boldsymbol{\sigma}\cdot\mathbf{p}\times\mathbf{E}k_0^2],\\
\mathscr{H}_{1d}^{(1)} &= -\frac{ie^2\hbar}{8m^2c^3}[k_0^2\mathbf{E}\cdot\mathbf{A} - \mathbf{E}\cdot\mathbf{A}k_0^2] \equiv 0,\\
\mathscr{H}_{1e}^{(1)} &= \frac{e^2\hbar}{8m^2c^3}[k_0^2\boldsymbol{\sigma}\cdot\mathbf{E}\times\mathbf{A} - \boldsymbol{\sigma}\cdot\mathbf{A}\times\mathbf{E}k_0^2] = \frac{e^2\hbar}{4m^2c^3}k_0^2\boldsymbol{\sigma}\cdot\mathbf{E}\times\mathbf{A}.
\end{aligned} \tag{2-83}$$

In $\mathscr{H}_{1a}^{(1)}$ we note that the terms involved would cancel if k_0 commuted with $\mathbf{E}\cdot\mathbf{p}$, but

$$[\mathbf{E}\cdot\mathbf{p}, k_0] = \frac{ie\hbar}{2mc^2}k_0^2\mathbf{E}\cdot\mathbf{E}_{\text{int}}. \tag{2-84}$$

Since $\mathscr{H}_{1a}^{(1)}$ already contains a factor c^{-2}, this term would seem to be negligibly small. We must be careful, however, because of possible near singularities. The Coulomb contribution to $\mathbf{E}$ and $\mathbf{E}_{\text{int}}$ gives

$$\mathbf{E}\cdot\mathbf{E}_{\text{int}} = \frac{Z_\nu^2e^2}{r_\nu^4}. \tag{2-85}$$

The k_0 provides a convergence factor so that the small r_ν behavior is as $1/r_\nu^2$. If we neglect contributions to k_0 other than that from nucleus ν and let $r_0 = e^2/mc^2$,

$$k_0^2 = [1 + (Z/2)(r_0/r)]^2$$

and

$$\mathscr{H}_{1\mathrm{av}}^{(1)} = \frac{e^2\hbar^2}{16m^3c^4} k_0^2 \mathbf{E} \cdot \mathbf{E}_{\mathrm{int}} = \frac{e^2\hbar^2}{16m^3c^4} \frac{Z_\nu^2 e^2}{r_\nu^4[1 + (Z/2)(r_0/r)]^2} \tag{2-86}$$

will be of order c^{-4} for all values of $r_\nu \gg r_0$. For $r_\nu \ll r_0$, however, $k_0^2 \sim 4r_\nu^2/Z^2r_0^2$ and the term is of order c^0. Since $r_0 \sim 2.8 \times 10^{-13}$ cm is so very small, it is reasonable to suppose that any functions occurring together with $\mathscr{H}_{1\mathrm{av}}^{(1)}$ in an integrand will be essentially constant over the region 0 to r_0 and can be brought outside the integral. (The contribution from the region over which these functions vary will be negligible because of the small coefficient.) Only the spherically symmetric part of the integrand will survive the angular integration, which will introduce a factor of 4π. There remains

$$\int_0^\infty \frac{r^2\,dr}{r^4[1 + (Z/2)(r_0/r)]^2} = \int_0^\infty \frac{dr}{[r + (Zr_0/2)]^2} = \int_{Zr_0/2}^\infty \frac{dx}{x^2} = \frac{2}{Zr_0} = \frac{2mc^2}{Ze^2}. \tag{2-87}$$

It will thus be a good approximation to write

$$\mathscr{H}_{1\mathrm{av}}^{(1)} = \frac{\pi e^2\hbar}{2m^2c^2} Z_\nu \delta(\mathbf{r}_\nu). \tag{2-88}$$

This is usually known as the *Darwin term*. It can be considered a *zitterbewegung* correction. If the electron's charge were spread over a small volume, the first correction to the Coulomb interaction would be of this form [172, p. 129]. Since $k_0 = 1$ in the FW results there is no term there corresponding to $\mathscr{H}_{1\mathrm{a}}^{(1)}$. The Darwin term arises elsewhere in the FW treatment. In fact, we now consider $\mathscr{H}_{1\mathrm{b}}^{(1)}$ and note that for a Coulomb field

$$\operatorname{div} \mathbf{E} = Z_\nu e 4\pi\delta(\mathbf{r}_\nu). \tag{2-89}$$

Since $k_0 = 0$ for $r_\nu = 0$, this term does not contribute at all in the partitioning treatment. In the FW method the term is obtained with k_0 replaced by 1 so that it contributes the same Darwin term obtained above.

We come next to $\mathscr{H}_{1\mathrm{c}}^{(1)}$. A vector cross product changes sign when the factors are reversed, so the two terms would be equal if $\mathbf{p}$ commuted with $\mathbf{E}k_0^2$. Apart from small contributions from terms in k_0 due to other nuclei, we expect this commutator to vanish since it is essentially the curl of a gradient. Consider the x component, for example:

$$\begin{aligned}(\mathbf{p} \times \mathbf{E})_x k_0^2 &= (p_y E_z - p_z E_y)k_0^2 \\ &= k_0^2 E_z p_y - k_0^2 E_y p_z + \frac{\hbar}{i}\left[\frac{\partial}{\partial y}(E_z k_0^2) - \frac{\partial}{\partial z}(E_y k_0^2)\right] \\ &= -k_0^2(\mathbf{E} \times \mathbf{p})_x - i\hbar[\operatorname{curl}(\mathbf{E}k_0^2)]_x.\end{aligned} \tag{2-90}$$

For $\mathbf{E} = \mathbf{r}_\nu/\mathbf{r}_\nu^3$, neglecting the dependence of k_0 on variables other than r_ν, and taking the origin of the coordinate system to be at nucleus ν, we find

$$[\mathrm{curl}(\mathbf{E}k_0^2)]_x = \frac{\partial}{\partial y}\left(z\frac{k_0^2}{r^3}\right) - \frac{\partial}{\partial z}\left(y\frac{k_0^2}{r^3}\right)$$
$$= zyf'(r) - yzf'(r) = 0, \tag{2-91}$$

where $f'(r) = (d/dr)(k_0^2/r^3)$. If there is more than one nucleus present k_0 is not a function of $r\ (= r_\nu)$ only, and other terms will result. They are of higher order and will be negligible, however.

For the Coulomb field, then,

$$\mathscr{H}^{(1)}_{1c\nu} = \frac{e\hbar}{4m^2c^2} k_0^2 \boldsymbol{\sigma}\cdot\mathbf{E}\times\mathbf{p} = \frac{Ze^2\hbar}{4m^2c^2}\frac{k_0^2}{r_\nu^3}\boldsymbol{\sigma}\cdot\mathbf{r}_\nu\times\mathbf{p}$$
$$= Z_\nu \frac{e^2\hbar^2}{4m^2c^2}\frac{k_0^2}{r_\nu^3}\boldsymbol{\sigma}\cdot\mathbf{l}_\nu \tag{2-92}$$

This is the familiar *spin–orbit interaction* term. It occurs in the FW treatment without the k_0^2, which is, however, useful as a convergence factor. If it is absent, an indeterminate result will sometimes occur in which $\langle \mathbf{l}\cdot\boldsymbol{\sigma}\rangle = 0$ but $\langle 1/r^3\rangle = \infty$, and the arguments required to show that the product is in fact zero are not as simple as one might desire. On the other hand, $\langle k_0^2/r^3\rangle$ is always finite.

Since **E**, **A**, and k_0 all commute, $\mathscr{H}^{(1)}_{1d} = 0$ as had already been indicated. This term does not appear in the FW treatment. In $\mathscr{H}^{(1)}_{1e}$ this commutation results in the equivalence of the two contributions. When **E** is a Coulomb field and **A** describes a uniform magnetic field

$$\mathscr{H}^{(1)}_{1e\nu 0} = \frac{Z_\nu e^3\hbar}{8m^2c^3}\frac{k_0^2}{r_\nu^2}\boldsymbol{\sigma}\cdot[\mathbf{r}_\nu\times(\mathbf{B}_0\times\mathbf{r})]$$
$$= \frac{Z_\nu e^3\hbar}{8m^2c^3}\frac{k_0^2}{r_\nu^3}(\mathbf{r}_\nu\cdot\mathbf{r}\,\boldsymbol{\sigma}\cdot\mathbf{B}_0 - \boldsymbol{\sigma}\cdot\mathbf{r}\,\mathbf{r}_\nu\cdot\mathbf{B}_0). \tag{2-93}$$

This term represents a correction to the Zeeman interaction, but is of higher order and no near singularities are involved. An equivalent term with $k_0 = 1$ is implicit in the FW treatment, but is usually not considered.

For Coulomb and magnetic dipolar fields (which may come from different nuclei),‡

$$\mathscr{H}^{(1)}_{1e\nu\nu'} = \frac{Z_{\nu'}e^3\hbar}{m^2c^3}\frac{[k_0(r_{\nu'})]^2}{r_\nu^3 r_{\nu'}^3}\boldsymbol{\sigma}\cdot\mathbf{r}_{\nu'}\times(\boldsymbol{\mu}_\nu\times\mathbf{r}_\nu)$$
$$= \frac{Z_{\nu'}e^3\hbar}{4m^2c^3}\frac{[k_0(r_{\nu'})]^2}{r_\nu^3 r_{\nu'}^3}[(\mathbf{r}_\nu\cdot\mathbf{r}_{\nu'})(\boldsymbol{\sigma}\cdot\boldsymbol{\mu}_\nu) - (\boldsymbol{\sigma}\cdot\mathbf{r}_\nu)(\boldsymbol{\mu}_\nu\cdot\mathbf{r}_{\nu'})] \tag{2-94}$$

‡ We make use of the vector identity $\mathbf{a}\times(\mathbf{b}\times\mathbf{c}) = (\mathbf{a}\cdot\mathbf{c})\mathbf{b} - (\mathbf{a}\cdot\mathbf{b})\mathbf{c}$. Note also that $k_0(r_{\nu'} = 0) = 0$ but $k_0(r_{\nu'} = r_\nu) \simeq 1$ if $\nu \neq \nu'$.

This term is also of higher order, but it cannot be neglected because of its near-singular behavior at $r_\nu = 0$ when $\nu' = \nu$. As in the case of $\mathscr{H}^{(0)}_{1d\nu}$(FW), we consider resolution of this operator into irreducible tensorial components.

$$\boldsymbol{\sigma}\cdot\boldsymbol{\mu}_\nu - \frac{(\boldsymbol{\sigma}\cdot\mathbf{r}_\nu)(\boldsymbol{\mu}_\nu\cdot\mathbf{r}_\nu)}{r_\nu^2} = \left[\frac{1}{3}\boldsymbol{\sigma}\cdot\boldsymbol{\mu}_\nu - \frac{(\boldsymbol{\sigma}\cdot\mathbf{r}_\nu)(\boldsymbol{\mu}_\nu\cdot\mathbf{r}_\nu)}{r_\nu^2}\right] + \frac{2}{3}\boldsymbol{\sigma}\cdot\boldsymbol{\mu}_\nu$$

$$= \sum_{j,k} \sigma_j \mu_{\nu k} T^{(2)}_{jk} + \sum_{jk} \sigma_j \mu_{\nu k} T^{(0)}_{jk}. \qquad (2\text{-}95)$$

The $\mathbf{T}^{(2)}$ term will give a nonzero expectation value on angular integration only for terms with radial parts behaving like r_ν^2 for small r_ν. There are thus no near singularities and the contribution from this term will be negligible because of the small coefficient.

For the spherically symmetric $\mathbf{T}^{(0)}$ term, however, the functions involved do not go to zero as r_ν goes to zero. The operator is proportional to $k_0^2/r_\nu\ \boldsymbol{\sigma}\cdot\boldsymbol{\mu}_\nu$, and we have seen in our examination of $\mathscr{H}^{(1)}_{1a\nu}$ that $k_0^2/r_\nu^4 \sim (2mc^2/Z_\nu e^2)4\pi\delta(\mathbf{r}_\nu)$ and thus

$$\mathscr{H}^{(1)}_{1e\nu\nu} = \frac{e\hbar}{2mc}\frac{8\pi}{3}\delta(\mathbf{r}_\nu)\boldsymbol{\sigma}\cdot\boldsymbol{\mu}_\nu, \qquad (2\text{-}96)$$

which is the *Fermi contact hyperfine* term. A term corresponding in form to $\mathscr{H}^{(1)}_{1e\nu\nu}$ as given in Eq. (2-94) but with $k_0 = 1$ is implicit in the FW treatment. It is not usually considered explicitly. Divergent integrals would clearly result.

The next term to be considered is $\mathscr{H}^{(1)}_2$. It can be expressed as a sum of terms involving $\mathbf{p}$ and $\mathbf{A}$ or $\mathbf{B}$.

$$\mathscr{H}^{(1)}_{2a} = -\frac{1}{16m^3c^2}[k_0^3 p^4 + p^4 k_0^3]$$

$$\mathscr{H}^{(1)}_{2b} = -\frac{e}{16m^3c^3}\{k_0^3[p^2(\mathbf{A}\cdot\mathbf{p} + \mathbf{p}\cdot\mathbf{A}) + (\mathbf{A}\cdot\mathbf{p} + \mathbf{p}\cdot\mathbf{A})p^2]$$
$$+ [p^2(\mathbf{A}\cdot\mathbf{p} + \mathbf{p}\cdot\mathbf{A}) + (\mathbf{A}\cdot\mathbf{p} + \mathbf{p}\cdot\mathbf{A})p^2]k_0^3\} \qquad (2\text{-}97)$$

$$\mathscr{H}^{(1)}_{2c} = -\frac{e\hbar}{16m^3c^3}\{k_0^3[p^2\boldsymbol{\sigma}\cdot\mathbf{B} + \boldsymbol{\sigma}\cdot\mathbf{B}p^2] + [p^2\boldsymbol{\sigma}\cdot\mathbf{B} + \boldsymbol{\sigma}\cdot\mathbf{B}p^2]k_0^3\}$$
$$\vdots$$

The terms involving more than one factor of $\mathbf{A}$ or $\mathbf{B}$ have been omitted. They are of higher order in $1/c$ (but of course will be divergent for a point dipolar magnetic field).

In $\mathscr{H}^{(1)}_{2a}$ the effect of k_0 is not usually essential so it can be transferred to higher order. The remaining term is

$$\mathscr{H}^{(1)}_{2a} = -\frac{1}{8m^3c^2}p^4. \qquad (2\text{-}98)$$

The same term occurs in the FW method. This is the well known *relativistic correction to the kinetic energy*. It occurs in classical relativistic mechanics if the Hamiltonian is expanded as a power series in $1/c^2$.

In $\mathscr{H}_{2b}^{(1)}$ we assume that div $\mathbf{A} = 0$ and ignore commutators of k_0 and $\mathbf{p}$ as being of higher order. Then

$$\mathscr{H}_{2b}^{(1)} \simeq -\frac{e}{2m^3c^3} k_0^3 p^3 \mathbf{A} \cdot \mathbf{p}.$$

For the uniform and nuclear dipole fields this becomes

$$\mathscr{H}_{2b0}^{(1)} \simeq -\frac{e\hbar}{4m^3c^3} k_0^3 p^2 \mathbf{B}_0 \cdot \mathbf{l}, \qquad \mathscr{H}_{2b\nu}^{(1)} \simeq -\frac{e\hbar}{2m^3c^3} k_0^3 p^2 \frac{\boldsymbol{\mu}_I \cdot \mathbf{l}_\nu}{r_\nu^3}. \tag{2-99}$$

Similarly, the uniform field contribution to $\mathscr{H}_{1c}^{(1)}$ leads to

$$\mathscr{H}_{1c0}^{(1)} \simeq -\frac{e\hbar}{2m^3c^3} k_0^3 \boldsymbol{\sigma} \cdot \mathbf{B}_0 p^2. \tag{2-100}$$

A corresponding nuclear dipole contribution will be neglected. None of these terms involves a near singularity and all are of higher order. They are implicit in the FW treatment with $k_0 = 1$, but they are usually ignored.

Finally we come to $\mathscr{H}_3^{(1)}$. It will also be a sum of terms of which the lower-order two are

$$\begin{aligned} \mathscr{H}_{3a}^{(1)} &= \frac{e}{8m^2c^2} [k_0^2 \phi p^2 + p^2 \phi k_0^2], \\ \mathscr{H}_{3b}^{(1)} &= \frac{e^2}{8m^2c^3} [k_0^2 \phi(\mathbf{A} \cdot \mathbf{p} + \mathbf{p} \cdot \mathbf{A}) + (\mathbf{A} \cdot \mathbf{p} + \mathbf{p} \cdot \mathbf{A})\phi k_0^2]. \end{aligned} \tag{2-101}$$

The first can be combined with the term of order c^{-2} that arose in connection with $\mathscr{H}_{1a}^{(0)}$. If we transfer the effect of k_0 to higher order in each case the sum of the two is

$$\mathscr{H}_{3a'}^{(1)} = \frac{e}{8m^2c^2} [(\phi - \phi_{\text{int}})p^2 + p^2(\phi - \phi_{\text{int}})]. \tag{2-102}$$

This term vanishes in the absence of an external scalar potential. If div $\mathbf{A} = 0$ and k_0 is transferred to higher order

$$\mathscr{H}_{3b}^{(1)} \simeq \frac{e^2}{4m^2c^3} (\phi \mathbf{A} \cdot \mathbf{p} + \mathbf{A} \cdot \mathbf{p} \phi), \tag{2-103}$$

and this term will also be neglected.

These results are summarized as the one-electron terms in Appendix F. We have seen that the partitioning and FW treatments give essentially the same results to order $1/c^2$. Interestingly, some of the terms seem to arise in different ways in the two treatments. In a few cases the partitioning method provides useful convergence factors which are absent in the FW method.

Hydrogenic Ion Results

Before leaving the discussion of the reduction of the Dirac equation to nonrelativistic form, let us treat a hydrogenlike ion as a check and an illustration of the magnitudes of the terms involved. To reduce the number of constants required we will work now in atomic units $e = \hbar = m = 1$. The zero-order Hamiltonian is of course

$$\mathscr{H}_0 = \tfrac{1}{2}p^2 - Z/r. \tag{2-104}$$

The zero-order eigenfunctions will be denoted by $|n, l\rangle$ (m_l and m_s have been suppressed), and

$$\mathscr{H}_0|n, l\rangle = -(Z^2/2n^2)|n, l\rangle. \tag{2-105}$$

In the absence of magnetic fields the perturbation we have found is

$$\mathscr{H}' = \alpha^2\left[-\frac{1}{8}p^4 + \frac{Z}{2}\frac{k_0^2}{r^3}\mathbf{l}\cdot\mathbf{s} + \frac{\pi Z}{2}\delta(\mathbf{r})\right]. \tag{2-106}$$

The first-order energy corresponding to this perturbation is readily obtained. The nonrelativistic quantum theory of H-like ions has been thoroughly studied and [154]

$$\left\langle\frac{1}{r}\right\rangle_{nl} = \frac{Z}{n^2}, \qquad \left\langle\frac{1}{r^2}\right\rangle_{nl} = \frac{Z^2}{n^3(l+\frac{1}{2})}, \qquad \left\langle\frac{1}{r^3}\right\rangle_{nl} = \frac{Z^3}{n^3 l(l+\frac{1}{2})(l+1)}. \tag{2-107}$$

From Eqs. (2-105) and (2-106)

$$p^2|n, l\rangle = \left(\frac{2Z}{r} - \frac{Z^2}{n^2}\right)|nl\rangle \tag{2-108}$$

so

$$\langle p^2\rangle_{nl} = Z^2/n^2, \tag{2-109}$$

$$\langle p^4\rangle_{nl} = \||p^2|nl\rangle\|^2 = \frac{Z^4}{n^3}\left[\frac{4}{(l+\frac{1}{2})} - \frac{3}{n}\right]. \tag{2-110}$$

We note also that

$$\mathbf{l}\cdot\mathbf{s} = \tfrac{1}{2}[(\mathbf{l}+\mathbf{s})^2 - l^2 - s^2],$$

so that for a state with $\mathbf{l}$ and $\mathbf{s}$ coupled to $\mathbf{j}$,

$$\langle\mathbf{l}\cdot\mathbf{s}\rangle_{nlj} = \tfrac{1}{2}[j(j+1) - l(l+1) - \tfrac{3}{4}]. \tag{2-111}$$

Finally, to evaluate the δ-function term we note that

$$|nl\rangle = R_{nl}(r)Y_l^m(\theta, \phi) \cdot (\text{spin}), \tag{2-112}$$

where R_{nl} and Y_l^m are separately normalized and

$$R_{nl}(r) = \left[\left(\frac{2Z}{n}\right)^3 \frac{(n-l-1)!}{2n\{(n+l)!\}^3}\right]^{1/2} e^{-\rho/2}\rho^l L_{n+l}^{2l+1}(\rho),$$

$$L_{n+l}^{2l+1}(\rho) = \sum_{k=0}^{n-l-1} (-1)^k \frac{\{(n+l)!\}^2}{(n-l-1-k)!(2l+1+k)!k!}\rho^k, \tag{2-113}$$

$$\rho = \frac{2Z}{n}r.$$

We will require the value

$$[R_{nl}(0)]^2 = \delta_{l0}\left(\frac{2Z}{n}\right)^3 \frac{(n-1)!}{2n(n!)^3}\left[\frac{(n!)^2}{(n-1)!j!0!}\right]^2 = \delta_{l0}\frac{4Z^3}{n^3}. \tag{2-114}$$

The p^4 and δ-function terms are straightforward. The $\mathbf{l} \cdot \mathbf{s}$ term must be more carefully examined, however, because when $l = 0$ the expression given leads to $\langle 1/r^3 \rangle_{n0} = \infty$, $\langle \mathbf{l} \cdot \mathbf{s} \rangle_{n01/2} = 0$, and the product is ambiguous. In general, when $j = l + \frac{1}{2}$, Eq. (2-111) gives

$$\langle \mathbf{l} \cdot \mathbf{s} \rangle = \tfrac{1}{2}[(l + \tfrac{1}{2})(l + \tfrac{3}{2}) - l(l+1) - \tfrac{3}{4}] = \tfrac{1}{2}l.$$

The inclusion of k_0^2 in the $1/r^3$ integral will have negligible effect for $l > 0$, but provides a convergence factor so that $\langle k_0^2/r^3 \rangle$ is finite for $l = 0$. Thus

$$\langle (k_0^2/r^3)\mathbf{l} \cdot \mathbf{s} \rangle_{n,l,j=l+1/2} = \begin{cases} \dfrac{Z^3}{2n^3(l+\frac{1}{2})(l+1)}, & \text{if} \quad l > 0, \\ 0, & \text{if} \quad l = 0. \end{cases} \tag{2-115}$$

Of course the case $j = l - \frac{1}{2}$ does not allow $l = 0$, so we need not consider k_0 and

$$\langle \mathbf{l} \cdot \mathbf{s}/r^3 \rangle_{n,l,j=l-1/2} = -\frac{Z^3}{2n^3 l(l+\frac{1}{2})}. \tag{2-116}$$

Combining these results we find

$$\langle \mathscr{H}' \rangle = \begin{cases} \dfrac{\alpha^2 Z^4}{2n^3}\left(\dfrac{3}{4}\dfrac{1}{n} - \dfrac{1}{l+1}\right), & \text{if} \quad j = l + \frac{1}{2}, \\ \dfrac{\alpha Z^4}{2n^3}\left(\dfrac{3}{4}\dfrac{1}{n} - \dfrac{1}{l}\right), & \text{if} \quad j = l - \frac{1}{2}. \end{cases} \tag{2-117}$$

From Eq. (1-90) a series expansion of the Dirac energy gives

$$E = mc^2 - \frac{Z^2}{2n^2} + \alpha^2 Z^4\left(\frac{3}{8}\frac{1}{n^4} - \frac{1}{2}\frac{1}{n^3|\kappa|}\right) + \cdots,$$

and since Eq. (1-81) tells us

$$\kappa = \begin{cases} l, & \text{if } j = l - \frac{1}{2}, \\ -l - 1, & \text{if } j = l + \frac{1}{2}, \end{cases}$$

we see that the first-order energy corresponds exactly to the term of order α^2 in the series expansion of the Dirac result.

Summary of Section 2

In this section we have considered the relationship between relativistic and nonrelativistic quantum mechanics for one electron. Two techniques, the Foldy–Wouthuysen transformation and the partitioning method, have been used to convert the Dirac equation into a form that looks like a Schrödinger equation with perturbation corrections. The FW approach provides useful insights into the nature of the relativistic corrections, but is not properly applicable when point sources are present. With the partitioning approach, convergence factors appear naturally to avoid many of the divergent-perturbation-operator problems. Divergences still arise in higher order if point magnetic dipole sources are included.

Perturbation correction operators obtained include the usual Zeeman and hyperfine terms, as well as a number of smaller terms and terms which are spin independent. These operators are summarized as the one-electron terms in Appendix F.

As an illustration and check on the results, the perturbations for a hydrogen-like ion in the absence of magnetic fields were evaluated through first order. The result was found to agree completely with the first relativistic term in a series expansion of the exact Dirac result.

3. Radiative Corrections

The Dirac theory provides an elegant description of the properties of an electron. Spin and magnetic moment arise naturally, and the quantitative predictions of the theory are generally in good agreement with experiment. This agreement is not complete, however. For example, the magnetic moment of an electron is predicted by Dirac theory to be exactly two Bohr magnetons and the observed value is about 0.1% larger than this (the anomalous magnetic moment); the $2s_{1/2}$ and $2p_{1/2}$ states of a hydrogen atom are predicted by Dirac theory to be exactly degenerate and a small energy difference (the Lamb shift) is observed. In this section we will consider how these discrepancies between theory and experiment can be removed.

Some potential sources of error such as the neglect of finite nuclear size and mass are not inherent in the Dirac theory. They can often be corrected for in straightforward ways to be discussed in later sections. Two aspects of Dirac theory essential to it but leading to error are the treatment of the electromagnetic field classically rather than quantum mechanically and the neglect of states involving several electrons or positrons. These aspects are more correctly treated in the theory known as quantum electrodynamics, with the result that theoretical predictions and experimental observations are brought into essentially complete agreement.

Quantum Electrodynamics

Standard treatments of quantum electrodynamics make use of the formalisms of second quantization and diagrammatic perturbation theory. It is likely that many of the readers of this book will not be familiar with these formalisms, and an attempt to develop them here would require more space and effort than can be justified. We will thus confine ourselves here to a brief qualitative discussion, hopefully leading to some understanding of the phenomena involved, and to a presentation without proof of the most important results. We will also consider how these results can be incorporated into the systematic, approximate treatment of the previous section.

The Electromagnetic Field

It is well known that electromagnetic radiation occurs in quanta or photons with energy proportional to the frequency of the radiation. Each photon state can be characterized by the frequency and the directions of propagation and polarization. (The frequency and direction of propagation together determine the momentum of the photon. The polarization provides an extra, discrete degree of freedom.) The state of the radiation field can be specified by stating how many photons occupy each possible photon state. Since the photons are bosons, any nonnegative occupation number is possible and it is not meaningful to distinguish different states on the basis of "which" photons are in a given state.

The nonradiative portion of the field, such as a stationary Coulomb field, is more difficult to treat but can be dealt with.

It is quite obvious that the number of photons present is not a constant but is dependent on the state of the field.

The Dirac Field

We are accustomed in nonrelativistic theories to think of the number of particles of each type as constant, part of the characterization of the system under consideration. With the introduction of the relativistic equivalence of mass and energy, however, this ceases to be the case. We are familiar with experiments in which one type of particle is converted into another or particle–antiparticle pairs are created or destroyed, subject to the overall conservation of mass–energy.

Dirac theory applies to both electrons and positrons, and if enough energy is available, electron–positron pairs can be produced. Neglect for the moment interactions between particles. The state of any one particle is then determined by specifying the quantum numbers characterizing the solution of the Dirac equation. This is normally taken to be the free-particle equation but could, e.g., be that for a Coulomb potential. In this approach the state of the Dirac field is given by specifying which of the one-particle states are occupied. Since electrons and positrons are fermions the only possible occupation numbers are 0 and 1, and it is not meaningful to distinguish states of the field on the basis of "which" particle is in a given particle state. In this way of describing things, different numbers of particles correspond not to different systems but to different states of a single system—the Dirac field.

Interactions

The separate treatment of the radiation field and of noninteracting Dirac particles is not realistic. The particles are charged, so they will be subjected to forces if an electromagnetic field is present. In addition, they serve as sources for the electromagnetic field. Provision must be made in the theory to describe the interaction between Dirac and electromagnetic fields. This can be done, but an exact, closed-form solution is no longer possible even in cases where the Dirac equation can be solved analytically. In consequence, the interaction is usually treated by perturbation theory.

We note that in perturbation theory the zero-order state of interest is modified by the admixture of small components of other zero-order states. In a field theory these other states may differ from the state of interest in the number of particles or photons involved. Energies beyond the first order of perturbation also involve contributions from other, "virtual" states.

A Model

As a simple example of this sort of behavior, consider two interacting harmonic oscillators described by a total Hamiltonian

$$\begin{aligned}\mathscr{H} &= \mathscr{H}_1^{(0)} + \mathscr{H}_2^{(0)} + \mathscr{H}',\\ \mathscr{H}_j^{(0)} &= -\frac{\hbar^2}{2m_j}\frac{\partial^2}{\partial x_j^2} + \frac{k_j}{2}x_j^2, \qquad j = 1, 2, \\ \mathscr{H}' &= \lambda x_1 x_2,\end{aligned} \tag{3-1}$$

with the interaction term $\mathscr{H}'$ being described by perturbation theory. (The total problem, including $\mathscr{H}'$, can be solved exactly, since an appropriate change of variables will result in two decoupled oscillator problems. It is more instructive for this example to use perturbation theory, however.)

Zero-order energies are

$$E_{n_1 n_2}^{(0)} = \hbar\omega_1(n_1 + \tfrac{1}{2}) + \hbar\omega_2(n_2 + \tfrac{1}{2}) \tag{3-2}$$

with $\omega_j = (k_j/m_j)^{1/2}$. Zero-order eigenfunctions are

$$\begin{aligned}\psi_{n_1 n_2}^{(0)}(x_1, x_2) &= \psi_{n_1}^{(0)}(x_1)\psi_{n_2}^{(0)}(x_2)\\ &= [C_{n_1} H_{n_1}(\xi_1)e^{-\xi_1^2/2}][C_{n_2} H_{n_2}(\xi_2)e^{-\xi_2^2/2}],\end{aligned} \tag{3-3}$$

where C_n is a normalization constant, H_n a Hermite polynomial, and

$$\xi_j = \left(\frac{m_j k_j}{\hbar}\right)^{1/4} x_j. \tag{3-4}$$

These follow from the separability of the zero-order problem and simple, one-dimensional harmonic oscillator results (to be found in nearly any quantum mechanics text, e.g., Messiah [138, Chapter XII]).

Matrix elements of the perturbation with respect to the zero-order functions will factor into products of integrals involving only x_1 or only x_2, and these integrals are all known. It is found that the first-order energy is zero, but that the second-order energy and first-order wave functions are nonzero.

In particular, for the ground state $n_1 = n_2 = 0$,

$$\lambda^2 E_{00}^{(2)} = -\frac{\lambda^2 \hbar\omega_1\omega_2}{4k_1k_2(\omega_1 + \omega_2)}, \tag{3-5}$$

and the wave function through first order is given by

$$\psi_{0,0} = \psi_{00}^{(0)} - \frac{\lambda}{2}\frac{1}{\omega_1 + \omega_2}\left(\frac{\omega_1\omega_2}{k_1k_2}\right)^{1/2}\psi_{11}^{(0)}. \tag{3-6}$$

We see that states with different values of n are being mixed.

In the zero-order problem we can define operators

$$\mathcal{N}_j = \mathcal{H}_j/h\omega_j - \tfrac{1}{2}. \tag{3-7}$$

These commute with the total zero-order Hamiltonian $\mathcal{H}^{(0)} = \mathcal{H}_1^{(0)} + \mathcal{H}_2^{(0)}$, and their eigenvalues are just the quantum numbers n_j. The operators $\mathcal{N}_j$ do not commute with $\mathcal{H}'$ however, e.g.,

$$[\mathcal{N}_1, \mathcal{H}'] = \frac{\lambda\hbar}{m_1\omega_1} x_2 \frac{\partial}{\partial x_1}, \tag{3-8}$$

and thus we cannot expect the n_j to remain good quantum numbers in the perturbed problem.

This example contains the essential features of the problem we are concerned with. The radiation field is not a harmonic oscillator, although it is formally equivalent to an infinite set of oscillators with different frequencies, and the Dirac field is not an oscillator at all. Nevertheless it is found that states having different quantum numbers are mixed, and there is a shift in the energy when interaction of the two fields is considered.

Anomalous Magnetic Moment

Using this approach one can take as starting point the Dirac and electromagnetic fields having, in the state of interest, one electron and a uniform magnetic field but no radiation photons [48,77,186]. The interaction of the fields will couple in virtual states in which the state of the electron is changed and one or more photons are present.

Expressions can be obtained for corrections of various orders to the energy of the system. Any energy shift independent of m_s will cancel out of transitions. We are interested in those corrections which are proportional to m_s and also to the magnetic field strength. Such contributions can be treated as a correction to the g factor. It is found [105] that in terms of the find structure constant $\alpha = e^2/\hbar c$,

$$g = 2[1 + A_1(\alpha/\pi) + A_2(\alpha/\pi)^2 + A_3(\alpha/\pi)^3 + \cdots] \tag{3-9}$$

with

$$
\begin{aligned}
A_1 &= \tfrac{1}{2}, \\
A_2 &= \tfrac{197}{144} + \tfrac{1}{12}\pi^2 + \tfrac{3}{4}\zeta(3) - \tfrac{1}{2}\pi^2 \ln 2 \simeq -0.32847897\ldots, \qquad (3\text{-}10) \\
A_3 &= 1.49\ldots.
\end{aligned}
$$

In the expression for A_2, ζ is the Riemann zeta function. The value for A_3 is reported to include all contributions of the specified order but is obtained numerically.

Comparison of these theoretical values with experiment requires an accurate value for the fine structure constant. The recommended value of Taylor, Parker, and Langenberg [200], $\alpha^{-1} = 137.03602(21)$, leads to a theoretical value

$$g/2 = 1.001159656.$$

A more recent value of Baird *et al.* [9], $\alpha^{-1} = 137.0354(6)$, gives

$$g/2 = 1.001159661.$$

These are to be compared with the currently available experimental value [209]

$$g/2 = 1.001159644(7).$$

The agreement is seen to be excellent, although some small refinement may still be desirable.

If the electron is in a bound state, e.g., in a H atom, additional changes in g will result. The most important of these are inherent in the Dirac theory, and can be dealt with also in the context of Schrödinger plus perturbations. They will be discussed more extensively in the next chapter. There are bound state corrections to the radiative corrections, but these are quite small and will not be considered here.

Modification of the Dirac Equation

We next consider the question of how these quantum electrodynamic effects can be incorporated approximately but systematically into the theory developed in the previous sections. This is a two-stage process involving the modification of the Dirac equation and the reduction of the modified equation to approximate, nonrelativistic form. Again, not all details will be given here.

The effect of quantum electrodynamic or "radiative" corrections can be approximately treated by adding an additional term, sometimes called the Pauli moment, to the Dirac equation. This is most readily done with the equation in an explicitly covarient form corresponding the Eq. (1-9) and gives [17]

$$\left(\sum_{\mu} \pi_\mu \gamma_\mu - imc\right)\psi = \left[g_1\left(\frac{e\hbar}{4mc^2}\right)\sum_{\mu,\nu} \gamma_\mu \gamma_\nu F_{\mu\nu} + \cdots\right]\psi. \tag{3-11}$$

Here the π_μ and γ_μ are the gauge-invariant momentum and Dirac operators of Section 1, $g_1 = g/2 - 1$ is a constant determined by quantum electrodynamics, and $F_{\mu\nu}$ is the antisymmetric electromagnetic field tensor (Appendix A)

$$F_{jk} = B_l, \qquad iF_{j4} = E_j. \tag{3-12}$$

(j, k, l is any cyclic permutation of 1, 2, 3 $= x, y, z$.) The ordinary Dirac equation is recovered if g_1 is set equal to zero. The radiative corrections resulting in the anomalous magnetic moment can be well approximated by treating the term on the right-hand side by first-order perturbation theory. A second term involving second derivatives of the potentials can also be added, giving an approximate treatment of the Lamb shift, but this is not of particular interest here and it will be omitted.

Reduction to Nonrelativistic Form

To be useful in any but the simplest cases this addition to the Dirac equation must be transformed, along with the rest of the equation, to approximate nonrelativistic form. This can be done by a Foldy–Wouthuysen transformation [10] with satisfactory results at least through order α^2, but that treatment will not be reproduced here. We will consider a partitioning approach instead.

The amplified Dirac equation (3-3) can be rewritten

$$(c\boldsymbol{\alpha}\cdot\boldsymbol{\pi} + \beta mc^2 - e\phi - E)\psi = G\psi \tag{3-13}$$

where G gives the effect of the radiative corrections and is

$$G = \begin{pmatrix} G_a & G_b \\ G_d & G_c \end{pmatrix} = -g_1 \frac{e\hbar}{2mc}\begin{pmatrix} \boldsymbol{\sigma}\cdot\mathbf{B} & -i\boldsymbol{\sigma}\cdot\mathbf{E} \\ i\boldsymbol{\sigma}\cdot\mathbf{E} & -\boldsymbol{\sigma}\cdot\mathbf{B} \end{pmatrix}. \tag{3-14}$$

Since G is to be treated by first-order perturbation theory only, we do not consider its effect on the wave function but will be interested in

$$\begin{aligned}\langle -G\rangle &= -\int \psi^* G\psi \, d\tau \\ &= -\left[\int \psi_{\mathrm{u}}^* G_a \psi_{\mathrm{u}} \, d\tau + \int \psi_{\mathrm{u}}^* G_b \psi_l \, d\tau + \int \psi_l^* G_c \psi_{\mathrm{u}} \, d\tau + \int \psi_l^* G_d \psi_l \, d\tau\right],\end{aligned} \tag{3-15}$$

where ψ is determined from the Dirac equation (or an approximation to it) with G absent. The change in sign occurs because G must be transferred to the other side of the equation to be treated by standard perturbation theory formulas. We know that, from Eq. (2-35),

$$\psi_l = \frac{1}{2mc}\,\hat{k}\boldsymbol{\sigma}\cdot\boldsymbol{\pi}\psi_{\mathrm{u}},$$

and ψ_l can thus be eliminated from Eq. (3-6). The result is

$$\langle -G\rangle = \int \psi_{\mathrm{u}}^{*}\left\{g_1 \frac{e\hbar}{2mc}\,\boldsymbol{\sigma}\cdot\mathbf{B} + g_1 \frac{ie\hbar}{4m^2c^2}(\boldsymbol{\sigma}\cdot\boldsymbol{\pi}\hat{k}\boldsymbol{\sigma}\cdot\mathbf{E} - \boldsymbol{\sigma}\cdot\mathbf{E}\hat{k}\boldsymbol{\sigma}\cdot\boldsymbol{\pi}) - g_1\frac{e\hbar}{8m^3c^3}\,\boldsymbol{\sigma}\cdot\boldsymbol{\pi}\hat{k}\boldsymbol{\sigma}\cdot\mathbf{B}\hat{k}\boldsymbol{\sigma}\cdot\boldsymbol{\pi}\right\}\psi_{\mathrm{u}}. \tag{3-16}$$

The first term provides a small correction to the interaction of the electron with a magnetic field. It will affect both the Zeeman term [$\mathbf{B}_0$, Eq. (2-74)] and the dipolar hyperfine term [$\mathbf{B}_\nu$, Eq. (2-75)] in the Hamiltonian obtained previously. When these terms are treated by first-order perturbation theory the change can be effected by inserting an effective g value for the electron. This is most readily done when $\boldsymbol{\sigma}$ is converted to $\mathfrak{s}$. Rather than $\boldsymbol{\sigma} = 2\mathfrak{s}$, we let $\boldsymbol{\sigma} = g_{\mathrm{e}}\mathfrak{s}$ with

$$g_{\mathrm{e}} = 2(1 + g_1) = 2.0023193\ldots.$$

The second term in Eq. (3-7) provides a correction to the spin–orbit interaction. It is of the same form, apart from the distinction between $\hat{k}$ and k_0 and commutators involving them, as $\mathscr{H}_1^{(1)}$ of Table 2-4. Neglecting these differences as leading to higher-order corrections, we see that the effect of this term will be to add a correction to terms arising from $\mathscr{H}_1^{(1)}$, and in particular to the spin–orbit interaction term [Eq. (2-92)]. Note that the coefficient in the second term of Eq. (3-7) differs from that in $\mathscr{H}_1^{(1)}$ by a factor of 2, so the correction will be $2g_1$. Thus in the spin–orbit term we would write $\boldsymbol{\sigma} = 2(1 + 2g_1)\mathfrak{s}$, but only if the term is to be used to first order. Including the effect of g_1 in a second- or higher-order perturbation calculation is not consistent.

In the FW treatment, the Fermi contact term comes from an analysis of the dipolar hyperfine interaction, and the two thus involve the same g factor. In the partitioning approach, the Fermi contact term comes from a term analogous to the spin–orbit term but with the vector potential in place of the momentum. It would thus seem to involve the same g value as the spin–orbit term. This conflict cannot be resolved at the level of the treatment presented here. There are, of course, other small corrections which must also be considered. The hyperfine interaction in the ground state of atomic hydrogen has been extensively studied [68,143,144], but these results will not be further discussed. The finer details of the hyperfine interaction thus remain somewhat ambiguous.

The third term in Eq. (3-7) provides a small correction to a small correction term. We will neglect it.

While we have not dealt extensively in this section with the radiative corrections, we have seen something of their origin and nature and have also seen that they can be incorporated into the effective Hamiltonian via modifications in the values of constants. These results are also included in the Hamiltonian of Appendix F.

Summary of Section 3

In this section we have considered the corrections which arise from a quantum mechanical treatment of the electromagnetic field and of the interaction between an electron and the field. Certain fundamental difficulties have been ignored, and a full treatment was not presented, but an expression for the anomalous magnetic moment through third order was quoted and compared with the experimental value. Its incorporation into the Dirac equation and reduction to approximate nonrelativistic form were considered.

4. Relativistic Many-Electron Theories

The results developed thus far have applied to systems containing only one electron, and most systems of practical interest contain many electrons. How can the theory be appropriately extended?

One approach, and in some respects the most satisfactory one, would be to use quantum electrodynamics. As we have seen, this is a many-electron theory which can deal with relativistic effects. It is not, however, in a form which is useful for our purposes. Each problem must be dealt with individually, and calculations for systems where even the nonrelativistic problem cannot be solved analytically are very difficult.

We must seek instead an approximate theory which will fit into the framework of nonrelativistic quantum mechanics plus perturbative corrections. We will consider two relativistic, two-electron wave equations: the Bethe–Salpeter equation and the Breit equation. The former can in principle be developed to any desired degree of accuracy. The latter is of limited accuracy but is more convenient. Reduction to nonrelativistic form will be considered, and we will find it to be possible only to order α^2. The extension from two electrons to many is possible, at least in low order.

In pursuing this more-or-less standard treatment, we should not forget that there are fundamental problems associated with relativistic quantum mechanics. The concept of localization, which seems essential in a particle theory, may not be compatible with Lorentz invariance. Quantum electrodynamics, although it gives excellent results, is a rather unsatisfying theory. (For some interesting comments on this point, see Dirac [48].)

The Bethe–Salpeter Equation

The Bethe–Salpeter equation is an integro-differential equation (at least in one of its forms) which is essentially a generalization of the Dirac equation to two particles. It is fully covariant (behaves satisfactorily under Lorentz transformations) and can in principle be made accurate to as high an order as desired. Certain difficulties associated with this equation make it unsuitable for our purposes, but we will consider it briefly.

We will not consider a derivation of the Bethe–Salpeter equation because an appropriate background is lacking, as it was for the topics discussed in

Section 3. The most compact form of the equation is obtained by using the four-vector notation employed in the Dirac equation as written in Eq. (1-9) [167]. In this form the Bethe–Salpeter equation is

$$\left(\sum_{\mu=1}^{4} \gamma_\mu^{(1)} \frac{\partial}{\partial x_\mu^{(1)}} + \frac{m^{(1)}c}{\hbar}\right)\left(\sum_{\nu=1}^{4} \gamma_\nu^{(2)} \frac{\partial}{\partial x_\nu^{(2)}} + \frac{m^{(2)}c}{\hbar}\right)\Psi(x^{(1)}, x^{(2)})$$

$$= \int K(x^{(1)}, x^{(2)}, x^{(3)}, x^{(4)})\Psi(x^{(3)}, x^{(4)})\, dx^{(3)}\, dx^{(4)}. \tag{4-1}$$

Here x is the four-vector ($\mathbf{r}$, ict), the γ's are Dirac matrices, and superscripts label particles. The wave function ψ has 16 components, corresponding to a four-valued degree of freedom associated with each particle, and $\gamma^{(k)}$ acts on this degree of freedom for particle k. The operator K includes Dirac matrix operators as well as x-dependent operators. It will be discussed shortly.

To relate this equation to the form of the Dirac equation with which we are more familiar we separate space and time variables for each particle in a particular Lorentz frame. The result is

$$\left(D^{(1)} - i\hbar \frac{\partial}{\partial t^{(1)}}\right)\left(D^{(2)} - i\hbar \frac{\partial}{\partial t^{(2)}}\right)\Psi = \mathscr{K}\Psi. \tag{4-2}$$

where $D^{(k)}$ is the Dirac Hamiltonian [Eq. (2-2)] for the free-particle behavior of the kth particle and $\mathscr{K}$ is $(c/\hbar)^2\beta^{(1)}\beta^{(2)}$ times the integral operator on the right-hand side of Eq. (4-1). It is clear that if we know K we know $\mathscr{K}$ and vice versa.

The operator $\mathscr{K}$ is obtained from quantum electrodynamics. It cannot be expressed exactly, in closed form, but can be obtained as a series valid to any desired order. It does not explicitly include a Coulomb interaction between the particles and cannot because the Coulomb interaction is not Lorentz invariant. It will contain terms that are equivalent through a given order, however, and can for some purposes be approximated as a Coulomb interaction plus corrections. The evaluation of $\mathscr{K}$ and the solution of the resultant equation are problems which arise when the Bethe–Salpeter equation is used directly.

There are other features of the equation which render it unsuitable for our purposes. We note in passing that it involves a product of one-particle operators, rather than the sum which our experience with nonrelativistic quantum mechanics would lead us to expect. More important, however, we note that it involves different time variables for the two particles. This is essential in a fully covariant two-particle theory, but is difficult to interpret physically. It is difficult to eliminate the "relative time" $t_2 - t_1$ from the theory so as to obtain stationary states.

Before leaving the Bethe–Salpeter equation, we note that it can be applied to many situations. The particles being described have not been identified as necessarily electrons, and could in fact be an electron and a proton (the H atom) or a proton and a neutron (the deuteron). Any particles of spin $\frac{1}{2}$, for which the Dirac description is appropriate, may be treated in this way. If nucleons are involved the mesonic field must be considered along with Dirac and electromagnetic fields, and additional difficulties exist.

The Breit Equation

The most obvious starting point for a two-electron relativistic theory is to describe the one-electron behavior of each electron by a Dirac operator and then add the interaction between them. If this were simply the Coulomb interaction, the result for a stationary state of energy E would be

$$\left(D^{(1)} + D^{(2)} + \frac{e^2}{r_{12}} - E\right)\Psi = 0. \tag{4-3}$$

This is not a satisfactory relativistic equation because of the instantaneous character of the Coulomb interaction. In a relativistic classical (i.e., non-quantum) theory, retarded potentials would be introduced to account for the finite velocity of propagation of the interaction. In quantum mechanics we introduce the quantized electromagnetic field and treat its interaction with the electrons by perturbation theory.

We will again omit the details of the quantum electrodynamic calculation. In the treatment presented by Bethe and Salpeter [17], one assumes that eigenfunctions and eigenvalues of Eq. (4-3) are known as the zero-order problem. The two-electron system is assumed to be in some particular zero-order state, and no photons are present. The field interaction term will link this state with zero-order states in which the two electrons are in a different state, and a photon is present. In second order there will be a shift in the energy of the state under consideration. The expression for the shift involves a sum over excited two-electron states and an integral over (virtual or intermediate-state) photon momenta. It will be dominated by contributions for which the photon energy is much larger than the electronic state energy difference, so it is a reasonable approximation to neglect the latter with respect to the former. It is then possible to use the closure relationship to eliminate the sum over states, as in the usual average energy or Unsöld approximation of second-order perturbation theory. The integration over photon momenta can then be done analytically, with the result that the energy shift can be approximated by the expectation value, with respect to the zero-order electronic state, of an operator

$$B = \frac{e^2}{2r_{12}}\left[\boldsymbol{\alpha}_1 \cdot \boldsymbol{\alpha}_2 + \frac{(\boldsymbol{\alpha}_1 \cdot \mathbf{r}_{12})(\boldsymbol{\alpha}_2 \cdot \mathbf{r}_{12})}{r_{12}^2}\right]. \tag{4-4}$$

This operator is known as the Breit operator, and the Breit equation is

$$\left(D^{(1)} + D^{(2)} + \frac{e^2}{r_{12}} - E\right)\Psi = B\Psi. \tag{4-5}$$

It must be noted that the proper use of Eq. (4-5) is not to attempt to solve it exactly, but rather to seek a solution to Eq. (4-3) and then treat B as a perturbation, to first order only.

The discussion above does not constitute a derivation of the Breit equation, but only a sketchy description of a derivation. It may lend greater understanding to make a comparison with classical (i.e., relativistic but nonquantum) theory [100]. The starting point will be the Lagrangian for a particle of charge q in fields described by potentials ϕ and $\mathbf{A}$ (Appendix A).

$$L = -mc^2[1 - (v^2/c^2)]^{1/2} + (q/c)\mathbf{A}\cdot\mathbf{v} - q\phi. \tag{4-6}$$

The potentials are considered to arise from a charge distribution $\rho(\mathbf{r}, t)$ and a current distribution $\mathbf{j}(\mathbf{r}, t)$. When the finiteness of the velocity of light is taken into account they are given by

$$\begin{aligned} \phi(\mathbf{r}, t) &= \int \frac{\rho(\mathbf{r}', t - |\mathbf{r} - \mathbf{r}'|/c)}{|r - r'|}\, d\mathbf{r}', \\ \mathbf{A}(\mathbf{r}, t) &= \frac{1}{c}\int \frac{\mathbf{j}(\mathbf{r}', t - |\mathbf{r} - \mathbf{r}'|/c)}{|\mathbf{r} - \mathbf{r}'|}\, d\mathbf{r}'. \end{aligned} \tag{4-7}$$

We will be interested in the case where ρ and $\mathbf{j}$ are due to other charged particles, and if the velocities of these particles are small compared with c, it will be reasonable to make an expansion of ρ and $\mathbf{j}$ in powers of a time $|\mathbf{r} - \mathbf{r}'|/c$, keeping only the lower-order terms. We let $t' = t - |\mathbf{r} - \mathbf{r}'|/c$ and write

$$\begin{aligned} \rho(\mathbf{r}', t') &= \rho(\mathbf{r}', t) - \frac{\partial}{\partial t}\rho(\mathbf{r}', t)\frac{|\mathbf{r} - \mathbf{r}'|}{c} + \frac{1}{2}\frac{\partial^2}{\partial t^2}\rho(\mathbf{r}', t)\frac{|\mathbf{r} - \mathbf{r}'|^2}{c^2} + \cdots \\ \mathbf{j}(\mathbf{r}', t') &= \mathbf{j}(\mathbf{r}', t) - \frac{\partial}{\partial t}\mathbf{j}(\mathbf{r}', t)\frac{|\mathbf{r} - \mathbf{r}'|}{c} + \cdots. \end{aligned} \tag{4-8}$$

The derivative $\partial/\partial t$ is to be interpreted here as the derivative of ρ or $\mathbf{j}$ with respect to the second argument. The expansion is thus

$$\rho(\mathbf{r}', y) = \rho(\mathbf{r}', y_0) + \left(\frac{\partial\rho}{\partial y}\right)_{y = y_0}(y - y_0) + \frac{1}{2}\left(\frac{\partial^2\rho}{\partial y^2}\right)_{y = y_0}(y - y_0)^2 + \cdots,$$

where $y = t' = t - |\mathbf{r} - \mathbf{r}'|/c$, $y_0 = t$, $y - y_0 = -|\mathbf{r} - \mathbf{r}'|/c$. The order of the operations of integration over spatial variables and differentiation with respect to time can be reversed, so

$$\phi(\mathbf{r}, t) = \int \frac{\rho(\mathbf{r}', t)}{|\mathbf{r} - \mathbf{r}'|} d\mathbf{r}' - \frac{1}{c}\frac{\partial}{\partial t}\int \rho(\mathbf{r}', t)\, d\mathbf{r}' + \frac{1}{2c^2}\frac{\partial^2}{\partial t^2}\int |\mathbf{r} - \mathbf{r}'|\rho(\mathbf{r}', t)\, d\mathbf{r}' + \cdots, \tag{4-9}$$

$$\mathbf{j}(\mathbf{r}, t) = \frac{1}{c}\int \frac{\mathbf{j}(\mathbf{r}', t)}{|\mathbf{r} - \mathbf{r}'|} d\mathbf{r}' - \frac{1}{c^2}\frac{\partial}{\partial t}\int \mathbf{j}(\mathbf{r}', t)\, d\mathbf{r}' + \cdots.$$

A point charge q_l at point $\mathbf{r}_l$, moving with velocity $\mathbf{v}_l$, contributes to ρ and $\mathbf{j}$ terms

$$\rho_l(\mathbf{r}', t) = q_l\delta(\mathbf{r}' - \mathbf{r}_l), \qquad \mathbf{j}_l(\mathbf{r}', t) = q_l\delta(\mathbf{r}' - \mathbf{r}_l)\mathbf{v}_l \tag{4-10}$$

and thus contributes to ϕ and $\mathbf{A}$ terms‡

$$\phi_l(\mathbf{r}, t) = \frac{q_l}{|\mathbf{r} - \mathbf{r}_l|} - \frac{1}{c}\frac{\partial}{\partial t} q_l + \frac{q_l}{2c^2}\frac{\partial^2}{\partial t^2}|\mathbf{r} - \mathbf{r}_l| + \cdots, \qquad \mathbf{A}_l(\mathbf{r}, t) = \frac{q_l}{c}\frac{v_l}{|\mathbf{r} - \mathbf{r}_l|} - \frac{q_l}{c^2}\frac{\partial}{\partial t}\mathbf{v}_l + \cdots. \tag{4-11}$$

The second term in ϕ_l is clearly zero and the contribution of the second term in $\mathbf{A}_l$ will be of higher order in L, where A is multiplied by $1/c$. Before substituting these potentials into the Lagrangian it is convenient to make a gauge transformation

$$\phi_l' = \phi_l - \frac{1}{c}\frac{\partial f}{\partial t}, \qquad \mathbf{A}_l' = \mathbf{A}_l + \nabla f,$$

where f is taken to be

$$f_l = \frac{q_l}{2c}\frac{\partial}{\partial t}|\mathbf{r} - \mathbf{r}_l|. \tag{4-12}$$

Then

$$\phi_l(\mathbf{r}, t) = \frac{q_l}{|\mathbf{r} - \mathbf{r}_l|} + \cdots, \tag{4-13}$$

‡ Now $\partial/\partial t$ acts on the time dependence of $\mathbf{r}_l = \mathbf{r}_l(t)$. By assumption, $\partial\mathbf{r}/\partial t = 0$.

and

$$\mathbf{A}_l(\mathbf{r}, t) = \frac{q_l}{c} \frac{\mathbf{v}_l}{|\mathbf{r} - \mathbf{r}_l|} + \frac{q_l}{2c} \nabla \frac{\partial}{\partial t} |\mathbf{r} - \mathbf{r}_l| + \cdots$$

$$= \frac{q_l}{2c} \left[\frac{\mathbf{v}_l}{|\mathbf{r} - \mathbf{r}_l|} + \frac{\{(\mathbf{r} - \mathbf{r}_l) \cdot \mathbf{v}_l\}(\mathbf{r} - \mathbf{r}_l)}{|\mathbf{r} - \mathbf{r}_l|^3} \right] + \cdots. \tag{4-14}$$

The Lagrangian will include a kinetic energy for the kth particle which can also be expanded:

$$m_k c^2[1 - (v_k^2/c^2)]^{1/2} = -m_k c^2 + \tfrac{1}{2} m_k v_k^2 + (1/8c^2) m_k v_k^4 + \cdots. \tag{4-15}$$

To get the total Lagrangian we must sum over all particles, being careful to count interactions only once. The result through order $1/c^2$ is

$$L = -\sum_k m_k c^2 + \sum_k \tfrac{1}{2} m_k v_k^2 - \sum_{k<l} (q_k q_l / r_{kl})$$

$$+ \frac{1}{c^2} \left\{ \sum_k \tfrac{1}{8} m_k v_k^4 + \sum_{k<l} (q_k q_l / r_{kl}) [\mathbf{v}_k \cdot \mathbf{v}_l + (\mathbf{v}_k \cdot \hat{\mathbf{r}}_{kl})(\mathbf{v}_l \cdot \hat{\mathbf{r}}_{kl})] \right\} + \cdots, \tag{4-16}$$

where

$$r_{kl} = |\mathbf{r}_k - \mathbf{r}_l|, \qquad \hat{\mathbf{r}}_{kl} = (\mathbf{r}_k - \mathbf{r}_l)/r_{kl}. \tag{4-17}$$

Conjugate momenta are introduced as

$$\mathbf{p}_k = \frac{\partial L}{\partial \mathbf{v}_k} = m\mathbf{v}_k + \frac{1}{2c^2} m_k v_k^2 \mathbf{v}_k$$

$$+ \sum_l{}' \frac{q_k q_l}{2c^2 r_{kl}} [\mathbf{v}_l + (\mathbf{v}_l \cdot \hat{\mathbf{r}}_{kl}) \hat{\mathbf{r}}_{kl}] + \cdots, \tag{4-18}$$

where the prime on the summation sign indicates that the term $l = k$ is to be omitted. The Hamiltonian is

$$H = \sum_k \mathbf{v}_k \cdot \mathbf{p}_k - L$$

$$= \sum_k m_k c^2 + \sum_k \tfrac{1}{2} m_k v_k^2 + \sum_{k<l} (q_k q_l / r_{kl})$$

$$+ \frac{1}{c^2} \left\{ \sum_k \tfrac{3}{8} m_k v_k^4 + \sum_{k<l} (q_k q_l / 2r_{kl}) [\mathbf{v}_k \cdot \mathbf{v}_l + (\mathbf{v}_k \cdot \hat{\mathbf{r}}_{kl})(\mathbf{v}_l \cdot \hat{\mathbf{r}}_{kl})] \right\} + \cdots. \tag{4-19}$$

To express H in terms of $\mathbf{p}$ rather than $\mathbf{v}$ we note that

$$\mathbf{v}_k = \frac{1}{m_k}\mathbf{p}_k - \frac{1}{2c^2}v_k^2\mathbf{v}_k - \sum_l{}' \frac{q_k q_l}{2m_k c^2 r_{kl}}[\mathbf{v}_l - (\mathbf{v}_l \cdot \hat{\mathbf{r}}_{kl})\hat{\mathbf{r}}_{kl}] + \cdots$$

$$\simeq \frac{1}{m_k}\mathbf{p}_k - \frac{1}{2m_k^3 c^2}p_k^2\mathbf{p}_k - \sum_l{}' \frac{q_k q_l}{2m_k m_l c^2 r_{kl}}[\mathbf{p}_l - (\mathbf{p}_l \cdot \hat{\mathbf{r}}_{kl})\hat{\mathbf{r}}_{kl}] + \cdots, \quad (4\text{-}20)$$

and that except in the $m_k v_k^2/2$ term of H, only the first term in the expression for $\mathbf{v}_k$ need be retained to give H accurate through order $1/c^2$. The result is

$$H = \sum_k m_k c^2 + \sum_k \frac{p_k^2}{2m_k} + \sum_{k<l} \frac{q_k q_l}{r_{kl}} - \sum_k \frac{p_k^4}{8m_k^3 c^2}$$
$$- \sum_{k<l} \frac{q_k q_l}{2m_k m_l c^2 r_{kl}}[\mathbf{p}_k \cdot \mathbf{p}_l + (\mathbf{p}_k \cdot \hat{\mathbf{r}}_{kl})(\mathbf{p}_l \cdot \hat{\mathbf{r}}_{kl})] + \cdots. \quad (4\text{-}21)$$

The first term in H represents the rest mass contribution to the total energy. The next two terms are the ordinary, nonrelativistic kinetic and potential energy. The fourth term is recognizable from our previous results as the first correction to the kinetic energy for the variation of mass with velocity. The remaining term represents a correction to the interaction energy of the particles.

To lowest order we can still identify $\mathbf{p}$ with $m\mathbf{v}$, and we have seen in Section 1 that in Dirac theory the operator corresponding to $\mathbf{v}$ is $\boldsymbol{\alpha}c$. If we let $q_k = -e$ for each particle and substitute $m_k c\boldsymbol{\alpha}_k$ for $\mathbf{p}_k$ in the last term of Eq. (4-21) it becomes

$$B = -\sum_{k<l} \frac{e^2}{2r_{kl}}[\boldsymbol{\alpha}_k \cdot \boldsymbol{\alpha}_l + (\boldsymbol{\alpha}_k \cdot \hat{\mathbf{r}}_{kl})(\boldsymbol{\alpha}_l \cdot \hat{\mathbf{r}}_{kl})], \quad (4\text{-}22)$$

which, as the notation suggests, is equivalent to the Breit term (4-4).

This comparison is certainly suggestive, but its significance must not be overestimated. The procedures followed are not entirely consistent. The use of retarded potentials would seem to suggest that the Breit interaction is a retardation effect, but other analyses indicate that such is not the case [24]. Whatever its origin, the Breit interaction provides a useful, approximate correction to the interaction of two electrons.

Reduction to Nonrelativistic Form

The wave function in the Breit equation, like that in the Bethe–Salpeter equation, involves four components for each particle. To put it into the Schrödinger-plus-perturbations form we want, we need an equation involving two components per particle. In our reduction of the Dirac equation we found the partitioning method to be preferable, on the whole, to the Foldy–Wouthuysen transformation. We would thus like to apply the partitioning method to the Breit equation. Unfortunately, this cannot be successfully done.

The Breit operator itself presents no difficulties since it is to be treated only by first-order perturbation theory. The partitioning would thus be carried out on Eq. (4-3) and B treated in the way that the Pauli moment term was treated in the amplified Dirac equation. The problem arises in partitioning Eq. (4-3) and is associated with the repulsive Coulomb potential e^2/r_{12}.

Equation (4-3) is equivalent to a set of four equations involving four functions of four components each. These equations can be successively solved formally to generate a single equation for one (the major) four-component function [51]. The inverse operators which arise are much more inconvenient than the $\hat{k}$ of the Dirac reduction, but they might be dealt with at least approximately were it not for one complication. One of the simplest inverse operators is $[e^2/r_{12} - e\phi(\mathbf{r}_1) - e\phi(\mathbf{r}_2) - E]^{-1}$. The potential ϕ will typically involve nuclear Coulomb attractions, but for any ϕ on interest there will be values of $\mathbf{r}_1$ and $\mathbf{r}_2$ for which

$$\frac{e^2}{r_{12}} - e\phi(\mathbf{r}_1) - e\phi(\mathbf{r}_2) = E \simeq 2mc^2, \tag{4-23}$$

and thus the inverse will not exist. A similar problem did not arise in the one-electron case because it was implicitly assumed that $-e\phi(\mathbf{r})$ was everywhere negative [129].

It might be possible to use operator expansion techniques to eliminate the offending terms from the operator inverse. If this were done, however, it would certainly lead to terms with every increasing powers of $1/r_{12}$ and no compensating convergence factors, so the advantage of the partitioning method is lost. An approximate partitioning or "method of the large component" reduction can be made through order $1/c^2$, but in this low order the Foldy–Wouthuysen transformation method is equally valid and perhaps more satisfying. The limitation to order $1/c^2$ is less disturbing in the present case than it would have been in the Dirac case because the Breit equation itself is only an approximation, valid to that same order.

The FW transformation has been carried out for the Breit equation [11,35,36]. The approach is basically that described in Section 2, but new complications arise and of course the algebra is much more tedious. Operators are classified as even–even (EE), even–odd (EO), odd–even (OE), or odd–odd (OO), depending on whether the part of the operator acting on particles one and two, respectively, is even or odd in the sense of Eq. (1-19).

The Breit equation is written

$$[\beta_1 m_1 c^2 + \beta_2 m_2 c^2 + (\mathrm{EE}) + (\mathrm{EO}) + (\mathrm{OE}) + (\mathrm{OO})]\psi = E\Psi \qquad (4\text{-}24)$$

with

$$\begin{aligned} &(\mathrm{EE}) = e_1\phi(\mathbf{r}_1) + e_2\phi(\mathbf{r}_2) + e_1 e_2/r_{12}, \\ &(\mathrm{EO}) = c\boldsymbol{\alpha}_2 \cdot \boldsymbol{\pi}_2, \qquad (\mathrm{OE}) = c\boldsymbol{\sigma}_1 \cdot \boldsymbol{\pi}_1, \qquad (\mathrm{OO}) = -B. \end{aligned} \qquad (4\text{-}25)$$

In these expressions $\phi(\mathbf{r})$ is the potential at point $\mathbf{r}$ from any sources other than the two particles. The corresponding vector potential occurs in

$$\boldsymbol{\pi}_i = \mathbf{p}_i - \frac{e_i}{c}\mathbf{A}(\mathbf{r}_i). \qquad (4\text{-}26)$$

The masses of the two particles are m_1 and m_2 and their charges are e_1 and e_2. For an electron $e_i = -e$. Unit Dirac operators are assumed where appropriate.

A complete factoring of the 16×16 operator into 4×4 blocks is not possible, but it is possible to obtain upper–upper (or lower–lower) separation to any desired order [36]. As in the one-electron case divergent operators appear in higher order, but results are satisfactory through order $1/c^2$. The separated upper–upper part of the Hamiltonian through this order is found to be

$$\begin{aligned} \mathscr{H} = {} & m_1 c^2 + m_2 c^2 + (\mathrm{EE}) + \frac{1}{2m_1 c^2}(\mathrm{OE})^2 + \frac{1}{2m_2 c^2}(\mathrm{EO})^2 \\ & + \frac{1}{8m_1^2 c^4}[[(\mathrm{OE}), (\mathrm{EE})], (\mathrm{OE})] + \frac{1}{8m_2^2 c^4}[[(\mathrm{EO}), (\mathrm{EE})], (\mathrm{EO})] \\ & - \frac{1}{8m_1^3 c^6}(\mathrm{OE})^4 - \frac{1}{8m_2^3 c^6}(\mathrm{EO})^4 \\ & + \frac{1}{8m_1 m_2 c^4}\{[[(\mathrm{OE}), (\mathrm{OO})]_+, (\mathrm{EO})]_+ + [[(\mathrm{EO}), (\mathrm{OO})]_+, (\mathrm{EO})]_+\} \\ & + \frac{m_1 - m_2}{2(m_1^2 - m_2^2)}(\mathrm{OO})^2. \end{aligned} \qquad (4\text{-}27)$$

Since (OO) is the Breit interaction term, which is to be treated in first-order perturbation theory only, the last term in Eq. (4-27) must be neglected. Many of the earlier terms are those which arise in the one-particle case, so that

$$\mathscr{H} = \mathscr{H}_1 + \mathscr{H}_2 + \mathscr{H}_{12}, \qquad (4\text{-}28)$$

where

$$\mathscr{H}_i = m_i c^2 + e_i \phi(\mathbf{r}_i) + \frac{1}{2m_i}(\boldsymbol{\alpha}_i \cdot \boldsymbol{\pi}_i)^2 - \frac{1}{8m_i^3c^2}(\boldsymbol{\alpha}_i \cdot \boldsymbol{\pi}_i)^4 + \frac{1}{8m_i^2c^2}[[(\boldsymbol{\alpha}_i \cdot \boldsymbol{\pi}_i), e_i\phi(\mathbf{r}_i)], (\boldsymbol{\alpha}_i \cdot \boldsymbol{\pi}_i)] \quad (4\text{-}29)$$

is identical with the one-electron FW result. The new terms are found in

$$\mathscr{H}_{12} = \frac{e_1 e_2}{r_{12}} + \frac{1}{8m_1^2c^2}[[(\boldsymbol{\alpha}_1 \cdot \boldsymbol{\pi}_1), e_1e_2/r_{12}], (\boldsymbol{\alpha}_1 \cdot \boldsymbol{\pi}_1)] + \frac{1}{8m_2^2c^2}[[(\boldsymbol{\alpha}_2 \cdot \boldsymbol{\pi}_2), e_1e_2/r_{12}], (\boldsymbol{\alpha}_2 \cdot \boldsymbol{\pi}_2)] - \frac{1}{8m_1m_2c^2}\{[[(\boldsymbol{\alpha}_1 \cdot \boldsymbol{\pi}_1), B]_+, (\boldsymbol{\alpha}_2 \cdot \boldsymbol{\pi}_2)]_+ + [[(\boldsymbol{\alpha}_2 \cdot \boldsymbol{\pi}_2), B]_+, (\boldsymbol{\alpha}_1 \cdot \boldsymbol{\pi}_1)]_+\}. \quad (4\text{-}30)$$

The second and third terms in $\mathscr{H}_{12}$ are identical except for the interchange of 1 and 2. We will consider only the first of them explicitly. It involves

$$[[(\boldsymbol{\alpha}_1 \cdot \boldsymbol{\pi}_1), e_1e_2/r_{12}] = e_1e_2[\boldsymbol{\alpha}_1 \cdot \mathbf{p}_1, 1/r_{12}] = i\hbar e_1e_2(1/r_{12}^3)\boldsymbol{\alpha}_1 \cdot \mathbf{r}_{12} \quad (4\text{-}31)$$

and is thus

$$\begin{aligned}
&\frac{i\hbar e_1e_2}{8m_1^2c^2}\left[\frac{1}{r_{12}^3}(\boldsymbol{\alpha}_1 \cdot \mathbf{r}_{12}), (\boldsymbol{\alpha}_1 \cdot \boldsymbol{\pi}_1)\right] \\
&= \frac{i\hbar e_1e_2}{8m_1^2c^2}\left\{\frac{1}{r_{12}^3}(\mathbf{r}_{12} \cdot \boldsymbol{\pi}_1 + i\boldsymbol{\sigma}_1 \cdot \mathbf{r}_{12} \times \boldsymbol{\pi}_1) - (\boldsymbol{\pi}_1 \cdot \mathbf{r}_{12} + i\boldsymbol{\sigma}_1 \cdot \boldsymbol{\pi}_1 \times \mathbf{r}_{12})\frac{1}{r_{12}^3}\right\} \\
&= \frac{\hbar^2 e_1e_2}{8m_1^2c^2}(-4\pi)\delta(\mathbf{r}_{12}) - \frac{\hbar e_1e_2}{8m_1^2c^2}\left\{\frac{1}{r_{12}^3}\boldsymbol{\sigma}_1 \cdot \mathbf{r}_{12} \times \mathbf{p}_1 - \boldsymbol{\sigma}_1 \cdot \mathbf{p}_1 \times \mathbf{r}_{12}\frac{1}{r_{12}^3}\right\} \\
&\quad - \frac{\hbar e_1^2e_2}{8m_1^2c^3}\left\{\frac{1}{r_{12}^3}\boldsymbol{\sigma}_1 \cdot \mathbf{r}_{12} \times \mathbf{A}(\mathbf{r}_1) - \boldsymbol{\sigma}_1 \cdot \mathbf{A}(\mathbf{r}_1) \times \mathbf{r}_{12}\frac{1}{r_{12}^3}\right\} \quad (4\text{-}32)
\end{aligned}$$

The last term in $\mathscr{H}_{12}$ involves a series of anticommutators which give a very large number of terms. The result given by Chraplyvy [35,36] must be modified to bring the notation into conformity with that used here. The contributions are

$$\begin{aligned}
\mathscr{H}_{12}&(\text{last term}) \\
&= -\frac{e_1 e_2 \hbar}{2m_1 m_2 c^2}\frac{1}{r_{12}^3}[\boldsymbol{\sigma}_1 \cdot (\mathbf{r}_2 - \mathbf{r}_1) \times \boldsymbol{\pi}_2 + \boldsymbol{\sigma}_2 \cdot (\mathbf{r}_1 - \mathbf{r}_2) \times \boldsymbol{\pi}_1] \\
&+ \frac{e_1 e_2 \hbar^2}{4m_1 m_2 c^2}\frac{1}{r_{12}^3}\left[\boldsymbol{\sigma}_1 \cdot \boldsymbol{\sigma}_2 - 3\frac{(\boldsymbol{\sigma}_1 \cdot \mathbf{r}_{12})(\boldsymbol{\sigma}_2 \cdot \mathbf{r}_{12})}{r_{12}^2}\right] \\
&- \frac{8\pi}{3}\frac{e_1 e_2 \hbar^2}{4m_1 m_2 c^2}\boldsymbol{\sigma}_1 \cdot \boldsymbol{\sigma}_2 \delta(\mathbf{r}_{12}) \\
&- \frac{e_1 e_2}{2m_1 m_2 c^2}\left[\frac{p_1 \cdot p_2}{r_{12}} + \frac{(\mathbf{r}_{12} \cdot \mathbf{p}_1)(\mathbf{r}_{12} \cdot \mathbf{p}_2)}{r_{12}^3}\right] \\
&+ \frac{ie_1 e_2 \hbar}{4m_1 m_2 c^2}\left[\frac{(\mathbf{r}_1 - \mathbf{r}_2) \cdot \mathbf{p}_1 + (\mathbf{r}_2 - \mathbf{r}_1) \cdot \mathbf{p}_2}{r_{12}^3}\right. \\
&\left. - 4\pi\delta(\mathbf{r}_{12})\{(\mathbf{r}_1 - \mathbf{r}_2) \cdot \mathbf{p}_1 + (\mathbf{r}_2 - \mathbf{r}_1) \cdot \mathbf{p}_2\}\right].
\end{aligned} \tag{4-33}$$

Other Methods

We have seen that while in principle quantum electrodynamics provides a description of many-electron systems that can be carried to any desired level of accuracy, there are problems associated with attempts to get many-electron relativistic wave equations and to reduce such equations to non-relativistic form. Some of these difficulties can be avoided if the relativistic wave equation is bypassed and an approximate Hamiltonian of nonrelativistic form is obtained directly from quantum electrodynamics.

Such an approach has been reported by Itoh [89]. Unfortunately, he also stopped with terms of order $1/c^2$ although he does not indicate that such a limitation is inherent in the method. The results he obtains are essentially equivalent to those obtained in other ways.

The electron–electron interactions have been derived by essentially classical considerations by a number of authors, including Slater [190].

Discussion of Results

We have seen that at present a two-electron (or many-electron) relativistic treatment is possible in a satisfactory way only to order $1/c^2$, and that to this order the various approaches give equivalent results. They are summarized in Appendix F. The one-electron terms are the same as those considered previously, so only the two-electron terms will be discussed here.

The first term in $\mathscr{H}_{12}$ is just the Coulomb interaction between the two particles. When both particles are electrons it is

$$\mathscr{H}_{12a} = e^2/r_{12}. \tag{4-34}$$

The second and third terms of $\mathscr{H}_{12}$ give rise to two types of contributions, as given in Eq. (4-32). For two electrons these are

$$\mathscr{H}_{12b} = -\frac{\pi e^2 \hbar^2}{m^2 c^2} \delta(\mathbf{r}_{12}) \tag{4-35}$$

and

$$\begin{aligned} \mathscr{H}_{12c} &= \frac{-e^2\hbar}{8m^2c^2}\left\{\frac{1}{r_{12}^3}[\boldsymbol{\sigma}_1 \cdot \mathbf{r}_{12} \times \mathbf{p}_1 - \boldsymbol{\sigma}_2 \cdot \mathbf{r}_{12} \times \mathbf{p}_2] \right. \\ &\quad \left. - [\boldsymbol{\sigma}_1 \cdot \mathbf{p}_1 \times \mathbf{r}_{12} - \boldsymbol{\sigma}_2 \cdot \mathbf{p}_2 \times \mathbf{r}_{12}]\frac{1}{r_{12}^3}\right\}. \\ \mathscr{H}_{12c0} &= \frac{e^3\hbar}{9m^2c^3}\frac{1}{r_{12}^3}[(\boldsymbol{\sigma}_1 \cdot \mathbf{r}_1)(\mathbf{r}_{12} \cdot \mathbf{B}_0) - (\mathbf{r}_{12} \cdot \mathbf{r}_1)(\boldsymbol{\sigma}_1 \cdot \mathbf{B}_0) \\ &\quad - (\boldsymbol{\sigma}_2 \cdot \mathbf{r}_2)(\mathbf{r}_{12} \cdot \mathbf{B}_0) + (\mathbf{r}_{12} \cdot \mathbf{r}_2)(\boldsymbol{\sigma}_2 \cdot \mathbf{B}_0)]. \end{aligned} \tag{4-36}$$

Each of these corresponds directly to a one-electron term. If each electron is considered the source of a Coulomb potential, $\mathscr{H}_{12b}$ is equivalent to the Darwin term $\mathscr{H}_{1av}^{(1)}$ of Eq. (2-88) with $Z = -1$ and a factor of 2 since each electron experiences the field due to the other. The spin–orbit term $\mathscr{H}_{12c}$ is lengthened by the retention of explicit Hermiticity and electron–electron permutational symmetry, but it clearly corresponds to the spin–orbit term $\mathscr{H}_{1cv}^{(2)}$ of Eq. (2-92) with the other electron rather than a nucleus providing the Coulomb field.

The term $\mathscr{H}_{12c0}$ is analogous to $\mathscr{H}_{1ev0}^{(1)}$ of Eq. (2-93). It is a gauge correction term. (See Section 9.) An additional contribution will arise if nuclear dipolar fields are present. It is analogous to the one-electron term $\mathscr{H}_{1evv'}^{(1)}$ of Eq. (2-96) and will not be considered explicitly. These terms are implicit in Eq. (4-3).

The remaining terms in $\mathscr{H}_{12}$ are those which arise from the Breit interaction. They are given in Eq. (4-33). The first of them is a *spin–other orbit* term

$$\mathscr{H}_{12d} = \frac{e^2\hbar}{2m^2c^2}\frac{1}{r_{12}^3}[\boldsymbol{\sigma}_1 \cdot \mathbf{r}_{12} \times \mathbf{p}_2 - \boldsymbol{\sigma}_2 \cdot \mathbf{r}_{12} \times \mathbf{p}_1], \tag{4-37}$$

when both particles are electrons. (Note that $\mathbf{r}_{12} = \mathbf{r}_1 - \mathbf{r}_2$, so $\mathbf{r}_2 - \mathbf{r}_1 = -\mathbf{r}_{12}$.) It can be considered to arise from the interaction of the spin–magnetic moment of one electron with the magnetic field produced by the oribtal motion of the other electron. The most closely analogous one-electron term is the oribtal hyperfine interaction. Another gauge correction term

$$\mathscr{H}_{12\mathrm{d}0} = \frac{e^2\hbar}{4m^2c^3}\frac{1}{r_{12}^3}[(\mathbf{r}_{12}\cdot\mathbf{r}_2)(\boldsymbol{\sigma}_1\cdot\mathbf{B}_0) - (\boldsymbol{\sigma}_1\cdot\mathbf{r}_2)(\mathbf{r}_{12}\cdot\mathbf{B}_0)$$
$$- (\mathbf{r}_{12}\cdot\mathbf{r}_1)(\boldsymbol{\sigma}_2\cdot\mathbf{B}_0) + (\boldsymbol{\sigma}_2\cdot\mathbf{r}_1)(\mathbf{r}_{12}\cdot\mathbf{B}_0)] \qquad (4\text{-}38)$$

also comes from the first term on the right side of Eq. (4-33). An additional term which arises in the presence of nuclear dipole fields will not be considered explicitly.

The next two terms are, in the case of two electrons,

$$\mathscr{H}_{12\mathrm{e}} = \frac{e^2\hbar^2}{4m^2c^2}\frac{1}{r_{12}^3}\left[\boldsymbol{\sigma}_1\cdot\boldsymbol{\sigma}_2 - \frac{3(\boldsymbol{\sigma}_1\cdot\mathbf{r}_{12})(\boldsymbol{\sigma}_2\cdot\mathbf{r}_{12})}{r_{12}^2}\right] \qquad (4\text{-}39)$$

and

$$\mathscr{H}_{12\mathrm{f}} = -\frac{8\pi}{3}\frac{e^2\hbar^2}{4m^2c^2}\boldsymbol{\sigma}_1\cdot\boldsymbol{\sigma}_2\,\delta(\mathbf{r}_{12}). \qquad (4\text{-}40)$$

They correspond to the dipolar and contact hyperfine interaction terms, and $\mathscr{H}_{12\mathrm{e}}$ can be obtained from $\mathscr{H}^{(0)}_{1\mathrm{d}\nu}$ of Eq. (2-74) if $\boldsymbol{\mu}_\nu$ is replaced by $-(e\hbar/2mc)\boldsymbol{\sigma}$. The contact term $\mathscr{H}_{12\mathrm{f}}$ is obtained from an analysis of the dipolar term, as in the FW treatment of the hyperfine interaction.

The remaining terms in Eq. (4-33) are in fact given differently by different methods, but these apparently different forms will result in essentially the same contribution. (Compare the Darwin-type terms in the one-electron case.) Since they are independent of both spins and fields, they are of little interest to us and will not be considered explicitly further.

We have seen that the two-electron terms can be obtained from the one-electron results by treating other electrons to be phenomenological sources of Coulomb and dipolar magnetic fields. Alternatively, one can use the two-particle results with one particle an electron and the other a nucleus to avoid the introduction of *ad hoc* potentials in the one-electron case. This is valid only for spin-$\frac{1}{2}$ nuclei and the "anomalous moment" corrections are very large. This approach does not afford a resolution of the difficulty associated with terms quadratic or higher in the vector potential from a point dipole, because the corresponding terms in this treatment would be of higher than first order in the Breit interaction and must, for consistency, be (arbitrarily) excluded from consideration.

Extension to Many Electrons

In this section we have explicitly considered only two electrons. We could label the electrons by j and k instead of 1 and 2, however, and obtain a many-electron result by summing over all $j < k$. If we were able to consider higher-order terms, we would expect to have factors such as $1/(r_{12}r_{13})$ entering, and we would not be able to limit ourselves to one- and two-electron operators. Through order $1/c^2$, however, these many-electron operators do not arise.

Summary of Section 4

Extension of the previously obtained results to many-electron systems has been pursued in this section. There are a variety of problems associated with such an attempt, and they have not been solved here. Nevertheless, by ignoring the fundamental problems and settling for results through order α^2 only, we have been able to obtain useful results. Spin–spin and spin–other-orbit terms analogous to various of the one-electron hyperfine and spin–orbit terms were obtained. Some can be obtained from the one-electron terms simply by considering each electron as a magnetic dipole source. Others come from the Breit interaction. The latter must be used to first order only.

The reduction to nonrelativistic form was made by an FW transformation. The partitioning method, which had been found preferable in the one-electron case, cannot be used because the repulsive $1/r_{12}$ term in the potential leads to divergent inverse operators.

The terms which contribute to spin or magnetic-field dependent splittings are summarized in Appendix F. Other terms were not considered in detail.

5. Effects of Nuclear Structure

We have thus far treated nuclei as point sources with an electric charge and, possibly, a magnetic dipole or as Dirac particles with anomalous moments. We know however that all nuclei (with the possible exception of the proton) have a finite extent and some degree of structure. In this section we will consider how our results must be modified to take into account a more realistic description of nuclei. We will not examine actual nuclear structures in any detail.

Nuclear Size

If the nuclear charge is spread through a finite volume instead of concentrated at a point, the potential in which electrons move will be modified. It will no longer be a purely Coulomb potential. It can be shown [17] that for a one-electron atom there will be an energy shift given approximately by

$$\Delta E = (2\pi Z e^2/3)|\psi(0)|^2 \langle R^2 \rangle \tag{5-1}$$

where $\psi(0)$ is the value of the electronic wave function at the origin and $\langle R^2 \rangle$ is the mean squared radius of the nuclear charge distribution about its center of mass. This energy shift may be comparable in magnitude to some of the others we have considered, but for given values of the principal and total angular momentum quantum numbers in the atomic case, and presumably correspondingly in molecules, all levels will be shifted by the same amount. There will be no contribution to the transition energies of interest to ESR.

A nuclear charge distribution of finite extent could, in principle, be accommodated in the reduction of the Dirac or Breit equations to nonrelativistic form. In fact, some of the divergence problems we encountered are characteristic of a point source and would disappear for a finite distribution. (Some models are discussed in Moore and Moss [142,143].) To deal with this appropriately we would have to know the nuclear structure. Since we can expect the effect on terms of interest to be small, we will not pursue this matter in detail. It should be noted, however, that the "contact" terms provide probes of structure which are of interest for the investigation of nuclei.

Nuclear Moments [1,164]

While we need not concern ourselves with details of nuclear structure, we must extend our previous treatment slightly. Not only is nuclear charge distributed through a finite volume, but this charge distribution may not be spherically symmetric. Classically the electrostatic interaction energy of an electronic charge distribution ρ_e and a nuclear charge distribution ρ_v is

$$E_{\text{electrostatic}} = \iint \frac{\rho_e(\mathbf{r}_e)\rho_v(\mathbf{R}_v)}{|\mathbf{r}_e - \mathbf{R}_v|} \, d\mathbf{r}_e \, d\mathbf{R}_v. \tag{5-2}$$

We make a multipole expansion by substituting

$$\frac{1}{|\mathbf{r}_e - \mathbf{R}_v|} = 4\pi \sum_{l=0}^{\infty} \sum_{m=-l}^{l} \frac{1}{2l+1} \frac{r_<^l}{r_>^{l+1}} Y_l^{m*}(\theta_e, \phi_e) Y_l^m(\Theta_v, \Phi_v), \tag{5-3}$$

where $r_<$ is the lesser of r_e and R_v and $r_>$ is the greater of these two. We avoid complications by neglecting contributions from $r_e < R_v$, and in this approximation $r_> = r_e$, $r_< = R_v$. The electrostatic energy can then be written‡

$$E_{\text{electrostatic}} \cong \int \rho_e(\mathbf{r}_e) \left[\sum_{l,m} \left\{ \left(\frac{4}{2l+1} \right)^{1/2} r_e^{-l-1} Y_l^{m*}(\theta_e, \phi_e) \right\} \right.$$
$$\left. \times \left\{ \left(\frac{4\pi}{2l+1} \right)^{1/2} \int \rho(\mathbf{R}_v) R_v^l \, Y_l^m(\Theta_v, \Phi_v) \, d\mathbf{R}_v \right\} \right] d\mathbf{r}_e. \tag{5-4}$$

This is just the form that the expectation value of a multiplicative, one-electron operator assumes in quantum mechanics (Appendix D)

$$\int \Psi^* \sum_j f(\mathbf{r}_j) \Psi \, d\tau = \int \rho_e(\mathbf{r}_e) f(\mathbf{r}_e) \, d\mathbf{r}_e. \tag{5-5}$$

The operator describing the interaction of the electrons with the nuclear charge can be written

$$-e\hat{\phi}_v = -e \sum_{l=0}^{\infty} \sum_{m=-l}^{l} \sum_j \left(\frac{4\pi}{2l+1} \right)^{1/2} r_{jv}^{-l-1} Y_l^m(\theta_{jv}, \phi_{jv}) M_m^l(v), \tag{5-6}$$

where the factor $-e$ is inserted to convert the electronic position distribution to a charge distribution and

$$M_m^l(v) = \left(\frac{4\pi}{2l+1} \right)^{1/2} \int \rho_v(\mathbf{R}_v) R_v^l \, Y_l^m(\Theta_v, \Phi_v) \, d\mathbf{R}_v \tag{5-7}$$

is a tensor characterizing the lth moment of the nuclear charge distribution.

The first term, with $l = 0$, has $Y_0^0 = (4\pi)^{-1/2}$ and

$$M_0^0(v) = \int \rho_v(\mathbf{R}_v) \, d\mathbf{R}_v = Z_v e, \tag{5-8}$$

so the contribution to ϕ is

$$-e\hat{\phi}_{v0} = \sum_j -Z_v e^2 / r_{vj}, \tag{5-9}$$

‡ The first integral should extend only over the region "outside" the nucleus and the second only "inside." We ignore these restrictions.

which is of course the Coulomb term. There are theoretical reasons, verified by experimental observations, for believing that the electric dipole moment ($l = 1$) for any nucleus is zero. The quadrupole ($l = 2$) terms will be considered below. Terms with $l > 2$ are possible and probably present for some nuclei, but their effect is too small to be observed so they will not be considered.

Nuclear Quadruple Interaction

A nonnegligible contribution to the potential energy which we have not previously treated arises from the interaction of the electrons with the electric quadrupole moment of the nucleus:

$$\hat{\phi}_{v2} = \sum_j (4\pi/5)^{1/2} r_{jv}^{-3} \sum_m Y_2^{m*}(\theta_{jv}, \phi_{jv}) M_m^2(v). \qquad (5\text{-}10)$$

We can express the electronic portion of this operator also in Cartesian form, but before doing so we should consider the nuclear moment tensor $M_m^2(v)$.

The nuclear quadrupole moment tensor is also an expectation value, this time with respect to the nuclear (internal) wave function. We characterize the nuclear state by spin quantum numbers I and m_I. An additional label can be attached, but we will deal only with nuclear ground states so any other quantum numbers included in this label will not change. (The quantum number I will also be constant, but is included for convenience.) Then

$$M_m^2(v) = \langle I, m_I | (4\pi/5)^{1/2} \sum_k e_k R_k^2 Y_2^m(\Theta_k, \Phi_k) | I, m_I \rangle \qquad (5\text{-}11)$$

where k labels the nucleons of nucleus v, e_k is the nucleon charge (e for a proton and 0 for a neutron), and R_k, $\Theta_k \Phi_k$ are the nucleon coordinates.

We can largely conceal our ignorance of the nuclear wave function by invoking a ploy based on the Wigner–Eckart theorem. This theorem, which is discussed in Appendix C, relates matrix elements of an irreducible tensor operator for different angular momentum states. It says that

$$\langle a'J'M' | T_m^l | aJM \rangle = (-1)^{J'-M'} \begin{pmatrix} J' & l & J \\ -M' & m & M \end{pmatrix} \langle a'J' \| \mathbf{T}^l \| aJ \rangle, \qquad (5\text{-}12)$$

where $|aJM\rangle$ is a state vector characterized by angular momentum quantum numbers J and M and possibly by other quantum numbers contained in a, T_m^l is an irreducible tensor operator, $\left(\begin{smallmatrix} J' & l & J \\ -M' & m & M \end{smallmatrix}\right)$ is a coefficient depending on angular momentum quantum numbers and tensor indices but not on other aspects of either the state vector or the operator, and $\langle a'J' \| \mathbf{T}^l \| aJ \rangle$ is a single, constant factor which does depend on the state, the nature of the operator, J and l, but not on M, M', or m. The operator occurring in Eq. (5-11) is an irreducible tensor operator so the theorem is applicable in this case.

We are interested in matrix elements for which $a' = a$, $J' = J$ and on the dependence of these values on M and the tensor index m. Suppose T^l_m and U^l_m are two different operators. Then from Eq. (5-12) the ratio of corresponding matrix elements will be independent of m and M

$$\frac{\langle aJM'|T^l_m|aJM\rangle}{\langle aJM'|U^l_m|aJM\rangle} = \frac{\langle aJ\|\mathbf{T}^l\|aJ\rangle}{\langle aJ\|\mathbf{U}^l\|aJ\rangle}$$

or

$$\langle aJM'|T^l_m|aJM\rangle = \frac{\langle aJ\|\mathbf{T}^l\|aJ\rangle}{\langle aJ\|\mathbf{U}^l\|aJ\rangle}\langle aJM'|U^l_m|aJM\rangle, \tag{5-13}$$

so that apart from a single constant factor we can replace one tensor operator by the other. We know very little about the nuclear wave function but will assume we know its angular momentum behavior. In the present case we want matrix elements of

$$T^2_m = (4\pi/5)^{1/2}\sum_k e_k R_k^2 Y_2^m(\Theta_k, \Phi_k),$$

which can be rewritten as

$$\begin{aligned} T^2_0 &= \frac{1}{2}\sum_k e_k(3Z_k^2 - R_k^2) \\ T^2_{\pm 1} &= \frac{\sqrt{6}}{2}\sum_k e_k(X_k \pm iY_k)Z_k \\ T^2_{\pm 2} &= \frac{\sqrt{6}}{4}\sum_k e_k(X_k \pm iY_k)^2. \end{aligned} \tag{5-14}$$

We construct a second tensor $U^2_m = Q_m$ from nuclear spin operators

$$\begin{aligned} Q_0 &= \frac{eQ}{I(2I-1)}\frac{1}{2}[3\hat{I}_Z^2 - \hat{I}^2], \\ Q_{\pm 1} &= \frac{eQ}{I(2I-1)}\frac{\sqrt{6}}{2}[(\hat{I}_Z\hat{I}_\pm + \hat{I}_\pm\hat{I}_Z)/2], \\ Q_{\pm 2} &= \frac{eQ}{I(2I-1)}\frac{\sqrt{6}}{4}[(\hat{I}_\pm)^2]. \end{aligned} \tag{5-15}$$

The dependence on the spin operators is such that this is also an irreducible tensor operator with $l = 2$. The constant factor is chosen so that the proportionality constant between T^2_m and Q_m is unity if, for $m_I = I$, we have

$$M^2_0(v) = \langle I, I|T^2_0|I, I\rangle = \langle I, I|Q_0|I, I\rangle = \tfrac{1}{2}eQ. \tag{5-16}$$

The nuclear quadrupole moment is completely characterized by a single constant Q (and the nuclear spin quantum number I.)

If $I = 0$ clearly any matrix elements involving nuclear spin operators will be zero. The combinations of nuclear spin operators occurring in Eq. (5-15) will also produce zero when $I = \frac{1}{2}$. To have an electric quadrupole moment a nucleus must have a spin greater that $\frac{1}{2}$. We are thus justified in using a proportionality constant which is undefined for $I = 0$ or $\frac{1}{2}$.

To express the interaction in a form suitable for incorporation into the Hamiltonian we have been developing, we also delay integration over nuclear spin variables. The nuclear quadrupole interaction will be given by the matrix elements with respect to electronic and nuclear wave functions of an operator involving electronic coordinates and nuclear spin operators. This operator can be written

$$\mathscr{H}_{q,\nu} = -e \sum_j \frac{1}{r_{j\nu}^3} \sum_{m=-2}^{2} Q_m(\nu)\left(\frac{4\pi}{5}\right)^{1/2} Y_2^{-m}(\theta_{j\nu}, \phi_{j\nu}), \tag{5-17}$$

where we have added the index ν to identify the nucleus involved. The quadrupole operator can be expressed in terms of electronic Cartesian coordinates with

$$\begin{aligned} \frac{1}{r_{j\nu}^3}\left(\frac{4\pi}{5}\right)^{1/2} Y_2^0(\theta_{j\nu}, \phi_{j\nu}) &= \frac{1}{r_{j\nu}^5}\frac{1}{2}(3z_{j\nu}^2 - r_{j\nu}^2), \\ \frac{1}{r_{j\nu}^3}\left(\frac{4\pi}{5}\right)^{1/2} Y_2^{\pm 1}(\theta_{j\nu}, \phi_{j\nu}) &= \frac{1}{r_{j\nu}^5}\frac{\sqrt{6}}{2} z_{j\nu}(x_{j\nu} \pm iy_{j\nu}), \\ \frac{1}{r_{j\nu}^3}\left(\frac{4\pi}{5}\right)^{1/2} Y_2^{\pm 2}(\theta_{j\nu}, \phi_{j\nu}) &= \frac{1}{r_{j\nu}^5}\frac{\sqrt{6}}{4}(x_{j\nu} \pm iy_{j\nu})^2. \end{aligned} \tag{5-18}$$

These expressions can also be written in terms of the second derivatives of the potential produced by the electrons at the nucleus, i.e., the gradient of the electric field at the nucleus due to the electrons.

These results can be combined to express the quadrupole interaction operator as

$$\mathscr{H}_{q\nu} = \sum_j \sum_{a,b(=x,y,z)} \hat{I}_{\nu a} q_{ab}^{j\nu} \hat{I}_{\nu b}, \tag{5-19}$$

where

$$q_{ab}^{j\nu} = \frac{-e^2 Q_\nu}{2I_\nu(I_\nu - 1)} \frac{1}{r_{j\nu}^5}(3r_{a,j\nu} r_{b,j\nu} - r_{j\nu}^2 \delta_{ab}). \tag{5-20}$$

Magnetic Interactions

The magnetic interactions of electrons and nuclei could also be expanded in multipole form, but magnetic monopoles do not occur and magnetic quadrupole or higher multipole moments have an effect too small to be observed if they do occur. We have already considered the effect of a nuclear magnetic dipole, but should treat briefly a small nuclear structure effect.

In the hyperfine interaction term we have obtained, the nuclear magnetic dipole moment occurs. This dipole moment can be expressed as

$$\boldsymbol{\mu}_\nu = \hbar\gamma_\nu \mathbf{I}_\nu, \tag{5-21}$$

where γ_ν is the nuclear gyromagnetic ratio and is for our purposes a constant to be obtained from experiment. For nuclei of sufficiently low Z that totally ionized atoms are available, the gyromagnetic ratio is obtainable directly and with great precision from measurements of the nuclear Zeeman splitting. For nuclei of higher Z, an approximate value of γ_ν can be obtained from the nuclear Zeeman splitting in an atom or molecule and a theoretical or experimental estimate of the shielding constant (the absolute NMR chemical shift).

When the hyperfine interaction energies of two atoms which differ only isotopically are compared, the ratio appropriately corrected for differing nuclear spin should be equal to the ratio of the nuclear gyromagnetic ratios. This is found to be not precisely true, however, and the difference is known as the *hyperfine anomaly*. (In molecular radicals the different vibrational behavior of isotopically different species dominates all other effects.)

Consider the simplest possible case, that of the hydrogen and deuterium atoms in their $^2S_{1/2}$ ground states and in the absence of any external fields. The hyperfine interaction with nucleus κ will be‡

$$E_{\mathrm{hf},\kappa} = (8\pi/3) g_e \beta_e \hbar\gamma_\kappa |\psi(0)|^2 \langle \mathscr{S}\cdot\mathscr{I}\rangle_\kappa. \tag{5-22}$$

In the absence of Zeeman interactions, with an S state for which the total electronic angular momentum is $\mathscr{S}$, the electronic and nuclear spins will combine to give a total angular momentum $\mathscr{F} = \mathscr{S} + \mathscr{I}$, and

$$\langle \mathscr{S}\cdot\mathscr{I}\rangle = \langle \tfrac{1}{2}[\hat{F}^2 - \hat{S}^2 - \hat{I}^2]\rangle = \tfrac{1}{2}[f(f+1) - S(S+1) - I(I+1)]. \tag{5-23}$$

Hyperfine transitions are observable between states with different f values at a frequency

$$\nu_\kappa = \Delta E/h = \tfrac{4}{3} g_e \beta_e \gamma_\kappa |\psi(0)|^2 \tfrac{1}{2}\Delta[f(f+1)]. \tag{5-24}$$

‡ There are of course radiative corrections, relativistic corrections, etc. The effect of nuclear mass or structure on these small corrections is very small indeed, so we will not consider them.

For hydrogén $I = \frac{1}{2}$, so $f = 0$ or 1 and $\Delta[f(f + 1)] = 2$. For deuterium $I = 1, f = \frac{1}{2}$ or $\frac{3}{2}$, and $\Delta[f(f + 1)] = 3$. The ratio of hyperfine frequencies is thus

$$\frac{\nu_H}{\nu_D} = \frac{2\gamma_H|\psi_H(0)|^2}{3\gamma_D|\psi_D(0)|^2}. \tag{5-25}$$

The electronic wave functions at the origin have been retained, with subscripts identifying the nuclei, because we must consider the possibility that the two values may differ slightly.

Nuclear magnetic moments are customarily given in units of the nuclear magneton, β_N. The value of that quantity will cancel out of ratios and the values given by Ramsey [164], for example, are relative to the proton value which is taken to be $\mu_H = 2.792743$. The deuteron value is then $\mu_D = 0.8574073(2)$. The ratio of the gyromagnetic ratios is

$$\frac{\gamma_H}{\gamma_D} = \frac{(\mu_H/I_H)}{(\mu_D/I_D)} = 2 \cdot \frac{2.792743}{0.8574073}. \tag{5-26}$$

The experimental values of the hyperfine frequencies are [212]

$$\nu_H = 1{,}420{,}405{,}751.768 \text{ Hz}, \qquad \nu_D = 327{,}384{,}352.5222(17) \text{ Hz},$$

where ν_H is taken to be exact and ν_D is determined relative to it, so that uncertainties in the definition of the second will not affect the ratio. If we compare the two ratios, we find

$$\frac{\nu_H/\nu_D}{2\gamma_H/3\gamma_D} = 0.999\,014\,9. \tag{5-27}$$

The deviation of this quantity from 1 can be attributed to two causes: a slight dependence of the electronic wave function on nuclear mass and a breakdown of the point–dipole approximation.

The effects of finite nuclear mass will be discussed in the next section. We will consider only the simplest result here. For a nonrelativistic, one-electron atom the effect of finite nuclear mass is to replace the bare-electron mass m by a reducted mass $m' = mM/(m + M)$ where M is the nuclear mass. The atomic unit of length, $a_0 = \hbar^2/me^2$ is modified by the substitution of m' for m and the normalization constant of the wave function is proportional to $a_0^{-3/2}$. The effect of this correction on the ratio of values of $|\psi(0)|^2$ will thus be

$$\frac{|\psi_H(0)|^2}{|\psi_D(0)|^2} = \frac{[a(D)]^3}{[a(H)]^3} = \frac{(m'_H)^3}{(m'_D)^3} = 1 + 3\left(\frac{m}{M_D} - \frac{m}{M_H}\right) + \cdots = 0.999\,184. \tag{5-28}$$

Although this accounts for part of the discrepancy, a factor of 0.999831 remains to be explained. While it may be in part due to the need for a more precise treatment of the electronic wave function or nuclear mass dependence in higher-order relativistic corrections to the hyperfine interaction, it also includes a contribution due to nuclear structure and the fact that the electronic wave function actually penetrates the nucleus.

The magnitude of this effect can be expected to increase with nuclear size [6]. On the other hand, other uncertainties increase rapidly with the number of electrons involved so the hyperfine anomaly is unlikely to be of practical significance in what will follow and it will henceforth be neglected.

Summary of Section 5

In this section the effects of nuclear structure have been briefly considered. The most important effect is the nuclear quadrupole interaction, a consequence of the lack of spherical symmetry in the charge distribution of some nuclei. It is an electrostatic interaction, but in the approximation where electron penetration of the nucleus is neglected we can invoke the Wigner–Eckart theorem and express the nuclear quadrupole interaction operator in terms of electronic coordinates and nuclear spin operators.

Other effects of nuclear structure and finite nuclear size are present, as evidenced by the hyperfine anomaly, but they have not been treated in detail.

6. The Separation of Nuclear and Electronic Motions

In this section we will consider the consequences of the fact that nuclei are not fixed, point sources but are particles of finite mass, which move.

Center of Mass in Relativistic Quantum Mechanics

There are difficulties associated with an attempt to separate center-of-mass motion in relativistic quantum mechanics [163]. To begin with, one must define the center of mass and this is nontrivial in the relativistic case; results are not what is expected. Among the difficulties which may arise, depending on the definition used, are operators for the different components of position which do not commute, a center-of-mass position which is not constant in the Lorentz frame where the total momentum is zero, and expressions which do not reduce to their nonrelativistic counterparts in the limit when $c \to \infty$.

If one simply makes the substitution appropriate to the nonrelativistic case in the Breit equation or Eq. (4-3), center-of-mass variables do not separate. A separation of the Bethe–Salpeter equation is possible only if there are no external fields and even then the "internal" wave function depends on a noninterpretable relative time.

Given these difficulties, we will proceed as follows: the relativistic equation is first reduced to approximate, nonrelativistic form. Substitutions are then made which separate the center-of-mass part of the zero-order or Schrödinger part of the equation. The relativistic correction terms are also modified in a consistent way, but the equation no longer separates. The coupling terms are found to be "of higher order," however, and can hopefully be treated by perturbation theory if at all. Similar difficulties exist for many-particle systems even in the nonrelativistic case. We will consider the one-electron atom first and then briefly discuss more complicated systems.

Nonrelativistic, One-Electron Atoms

In nonrelativistic quantum mechanics the Hamiltonian for a one-electron atom can be written

$$\mathscr{H}_0 = T + V, \tag{6-1}$$

where

$$T = -\frac{\hbar^2}{2M_\nu}\nabla_\nu^2 - \frac{\hbar^2}{2m}\nabla_e^2 \tag{6-2}$$

includes the kinetic energy of both the nucleus (mass M_ν, coordinates $\mathbf{r}_\nu$) and the electron (mass m, coordinates $\mathbf{r}_e$), and

$$V = Z_\nu e^2/r \tag{6-3}$$

is the potential energy of interaction. For present purposes the form of V is not critical so long as it depends only on the interparticle coordinate

$$\mathbf{r} = \mathbf{r}_e - \mathbf{r}_\nu. \tag{6-4}$$

We make a change of variables from $\mathbf{r}_\nu$, $\mathbf{r}_e$ to the relative coordinate $\mathbf{r}$ and the center-of-mass coordinate

$$\mathbf{R}_c = (M_\nu/M)\mathbf{r}_\nu + (m/M)\mathbf{r}_e. \tag{6-5}$$

Here $M = M_\nu + m$ is the total mass of the atom. This transformation leaves V unchanged but

$$\boldsymbol{\nabla}_\nu = (M_\nu/M)\boldsymbol{\nabla}_c - \boldsymbol{\nabla}_r, \qquad \boldsymbol{\nabla}_e = (m/M)\boldsymbol{\nabla}_c + \boldsymbol{\nabla}_r \tag{6-6}$$

and the kinetic energy becomes

$$T = -(\hbar^2/2M)\nabla_c^2 - (\hbar^2/2m')\nabla_r^2, \tag{6-7}$$

where $m' = mM_\nu/M$ is the reduced mass. Since V is independent of $\mathbf{R}$, the center-of-mass motion can be separated as that of a free particle of mass M. The remaining motion of the system is the relative motion characterized by the internal Hamiltonian

$$\mathscr{H}_0^{\text{int}} = -\frac{\hbar^2}{2m'}\nabla_r^2 + V(\mathbf{r}). \tag{6-8}$$

This is just the Hamiltonian for a particle of mass m' in a fixed potential $V(\mathbf{r})$.

It is customary to introduce units such that $\hbar = m' = e = 1$. In this system the unit of length $a_0' = \hbar/m'e^2$ and the unit of energy $\varepsilon' = e^2/a_0$ both depend on the nuclear mass via the reduced mass m'.

Effect on Relativistic Corrections for One-Electron Atoms

The relativistic correction terms have been considered in previous sections. We now wish to examine the effect on these corrections terms of the change of variables considered above. For an atom whose nucleus can be approximately described as a Dirac particle with an anomalous moment we can use the results of Section 4 for particles of different mass. In the absence of external fields the correction terms of order c^{-2} can be written

$$\mathcal{H}_1 = -\frac{1}{8c^2}\left(\frac{P_v^4}{M_v^3} + \frac{p_e^4}{m^4}\right),$$

$$\mathcal{H}_2 = \frac{Ze^2\hbar}{4c^2}\left[\frac{g_e'}{m}\frac{1}{r^3}\mathbf{S}\cdot\left(\frac{\mathbf{r}\times\mathbf{p}_e}{m} - 2\frac{\mathbf{r}\times\mathbf{P}_v}{M_v}\right) + \frac{g_v}{M_v}\frac{1}{r^3}\mathbf{I}\cdot\left(2\frac{\mathbf{r}\times\mathbf{p}_e}{m} - \frac{\mathbf{r}\times\mathbf{P}_v}{M_v}\right)\right],$$

$$\mathcal{H}_3 = \frac{Ze^2}{2c^2}\frac{1}{mM_v}\left[\frac{\mathbf{p}_e\cdot\mathbf{P}_v}{r} + \frac{(\mathbf{r}\cdot\mathbf{p}_e)(\mathbf{r}\cdot\mathbf{P}_v)}{r^3}\right] - i\frac{Ze^2\hbar}{4c^2}\frac{1}{mM_v}\left[\frac{\mathbf{r}\cdot(\mathbf{p}_e - \mathbf{P}_v)}{r^3} - 4\pi\delta(\mathbf{r})\mathbf{r}\cdot(\mathbf{p}_e - \mathbf{P}_v)\right], \tag{6-9}$$

$$\mathcal{H}_4 = \frac{Ze^2\hbar^2}{4c^2}\frac{g_e g_v}{mM_v}\left[\frac{3(\mathbf{S}\cdot\mathbf{r})(\mathbf{I}\cdot\mathbf{r})}{r^5} - \frac{\mathbf{S}\cdot\mathbf{I}}{r^3} + \frac{8\pi}{3}\mathbf{S}\cdot\mathbf{I}\delta(\mathbf{r})\right],$$

$$\mathcal{H}_5 = \frac{2\pi Ze^2\hbar^2}{4c^2}\left(\frac{1}{m^2} + \frac{1}{M_v^2}\right)\delta(\mathbf{r}).$$

Here g_e is the electronic g factor and g_v is defined in the present context‡ by

$$\boldsymbol{\mu}_v = g_v\frac{e\hbar}{2M_v c}\mathbf{I}, \tag{6-10}$$

$\mathbf{p}_e$ is the electron momentum and $\mathbf{P}_v$ the nuclear momentum. The grouping and indexing of terms is purely for convenience in referencing. Higher-order terms arising from commutators and factors of k_0 have been omitted.

Since $M_v \gg m$, it will be reasonable to make an expansion in powers of m/M_v and retain only the lowest-order contributions. The results can be expanded in terms of the electron mass m or the reduced mass m', since

$$m' = m\left(1 - \frac{m}{M_v} + \cdots\right), \qquad m = m'\left(1 + \frac{m}{M_v} + \cdots\right). \tag{6-11}$$

The terms which involve momentum operators will be altered by the transformation of Eq. (6-6). All terms will have their expectation values altered because of the change in the distance scale of the zero-order functions. In terms of the reduced mass atomic units

$$\mathcal{H}_0^{\text{int}} = \varepsilon'\left\{-\tfrac{1}{2}a_0'^2\nabla_r^2 - Z\left(\frac{a_0'}{r}\right)\right\}. \tag{6-12}$$

‡ This differs from the usual definition in that the actual nuclear mass replaces the proton mass in the nuclear magneton.

The relativistic correction terms all involve the square of the fine structure constant $\alpha = e^2/\hbar c$ and can be written

$$
\begin{aligned}
\mathscr{H}_1 &= \alpha^2\varepsilon'\left\{-\frac{1}{8}\left[1 - 3\left(\frac{m}{M_v}\right)\right]a_0'^4\nabla_r^4 - \frac{1}{2}\left(\frac{m}{M_v}\right)a_0'^4(\nabla_e\cdot\nabla_r)\nabla_r^2 + \cdots\right\}, \\
\mathscr{H}_2 &= \alpha^2\varepsilon' Z\left\{\frac{g_e'}{4}\left(\frac{a_0'}{r}\right)^3 \mathbf{S}\cdot\left(\frac{\mathbf{r}}{a_0'}\right) \times (-ia_0'\nabla_r)\right. \\
&\quad + \left(\frac{m}{M_v}\right)\frac{g_v}{2}\left(\frac{a_0'}{r}\right)^3 \mathbf{I}\cdot\left(\frac{\mathbf{r}}{a_0'}\right) \times (-ia_0'\nabla_r) \\
&\quad \left. - \left(\frac{m}{M_v}\right)\frac{g_e'}{4}\left(\frac{a_0'}{r}\right)^3 \mathbf{S}\cdot\left(\frac{\mathbf{r}}{a_0'}\right) \times (-ia_0'\nabla_e) + \cdots\right\}, \\
\mathscr{H}_3 &= \alpha^2\varepsilon' Z\left(\frac{m}{M_v}\right)\frac{1}{2}\left\{\left(\frac{a_0'}{r}\right)^3\left[\left(\frac{\mathbf{r}}{a_0'}\right) \times (-ia_0'\nabla_r)\right]^2\right. \\
&\quad + 2\left(\frac{a_0'}{r}\right)^3\left[\left(\frac{r}{a_0'}\right)^2 a_0'\nabla_r)^2 - \left(\frac{\mathbf{r}}{a_0'}\right)\cdot a_0'\nabla_r\right] \\
&\quad \left. + 4\pi a_0'^3\delta\left(\frac{\mathbf{r}}{a_0'}\right)\left(\frac{\mathbf{r}}{a_0'}\right)\cdot(a_0'\nabla_r) + \cdots\right\}, \\
\mathscr{H}_4 &= \alpha^2\varepsilon' Z\left(\frac{m}{M_v}\right)\frac{g_e g_v}{4}\left\{3\left(\frac{a_0'}{r}\right)^5\left[\mathbf{S}\cdot\left(\frac{\mathbf{r}}{a_0'}\right)\right]\left[\mathbf{I}\cdot\left(\frac{\mathbf{r}}{a_0'}\right)\right] - \left(\frac{a_0'}{r}\right)^3\mathbf{S}\cdot\mathbf{I}\right. \\
&\quad \left. + \frac{8\pi}{3}a_0'^3\mathbf{S}\cdot\mathbf{I}\delta\left(\frac{\mathbf{r}}{a_0'}\right) + \cdots\right\}, \\
\mathscr{H}_5 &= \alpha^2\varepsilon' Z\left(\frac{m}{M_v}\right)\left\{a_0'^3\delta\left(\frac{\mathbf{r}}{a_0'}\right) + \cdots\right\}.
\end{aligned}
\tag{6-13}
$$

These expressions are all obtained from those of Eq. (6-9) in a straightforward way, except possibly for $\mathscr{H}_3$. There, vector identities with appropriate commutation corrections have been used to make explicit the orbit–orbit interaction character. In the relative coordinate form, this is seen to involve the square of the orbital angular momentum.

We will not consider explicitly the additional terms which arise when external fields are present.

Other Systems

It is possible in principle to deal with many-electron atoms, with diatomic molecules, and even with polyatomic molecules by similar means, but such treatments become progressively more difficult and the results progressively less satisfactory. The separation of center-of-mass motion is still possible in the nonrelativistic case, and overall rotations can also be treated, but rather than completely separated equations a set of coupled equations results. The separation of electronic and nuclear motions must be dealt with approximately, normally in the Born–Oppenheimer way. Corrections to relativistic corrections will be similar in character to those discussed above and will usually be smaller in their effects.

If one wishes to treat radicals in low-pressure gases, overall molecular rotation and its interaction with electronic orbital angular momentum, if any, and with electronic and nuclear spin angular momenta must be considered. These topics are discussed in connection with microwave spectroscopy [31,88] and high resolution molecular electronic spectroscopy [79]. A complete treatment is beyond the scope of this book and may be considered somewhat less important than topics which are treated, because the great majority of free radical ESR work is done in condensed phases where free molecular rotation does not occur. We will nevertheless consider a brief treatment of H_2^+ as an example. Other diatomic species could be treated in a similar way [41,81,83,84,141,150,151].

The Hydrogen Molecular Ion

We now consider the simplest molecular system, the hydrogen molecular ion H_2^+ (or HD^+, D_2^+), and initially treat only the nonrelativistic, spin-free problem. Atomic units will be used, with the electronic mass m (not a reduced mass) as well as $\hbar$ and e equal to 1. The Hamiltonian is then

$$\mathscr{H} = T + V,$$

$$T = -\frac{1}{2M_a}\nabla_a^2 - \frac{1}{2M_b}\nabla_b^2 - \tfrac{1}{2}\nabla_e^2, \qquad V = \frac{1}{R} - \frac{1}{r_a} - \frac{1}{r_b}. \tag{6-14}$$

Here M_a and M_b are the masses of the nuclei, labeled by a and b, respectively, and e labels the electron. The coordinates of the three particles relative to a space-fixed axis system are $\mathbf{R}_a$, $\mathbf{R}_b$, and $\mathbf{r}_e$. They are shown in Fig. 6-1. Derivatives with respect to these coordinates occur in the Laplacian operators in the kinetic energy T. The interparticle distances appearing in the potential energy V are

$$R = |\mathbf{R}_b - \mathbf{R}_a|, \qquad r_a = |\mathbf{r}_e - \mathbf{R}_a|, \qquad r_b = |\mathbf{r}_e - \mathbf{R}_b|. \tag{6-15}$$

These clearly depend only on interparticle distances, so $\mathscr{H}$ is invariant to translation or overall rotation.

As a consequence of the translational invariance, the total linear momentum will be conserved. It is possible to separate the motion of the center

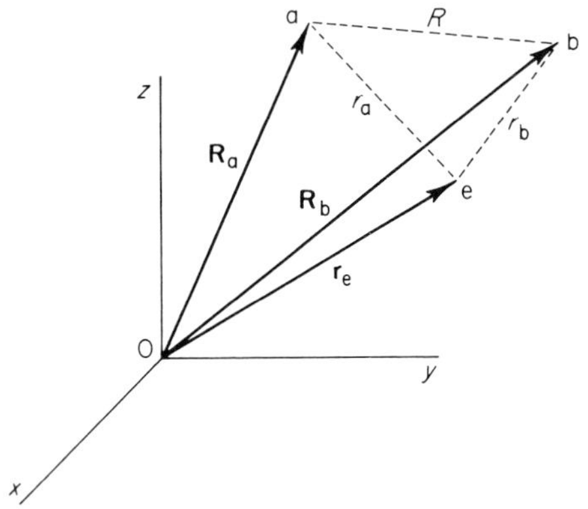

FIG. 6-1. Space-fixed coordinate system and interparticle distances.

of mass from other degrees of freedom. To do this we introduce new variables, three of which are the coordinates of the center of mass. As the remaining variables we take the internuclear vector and the vector from the midpoint of the internuclear axis to the electron

$$\mathbf{R}_{\mathrm{CM}} = \frac{M_{\mathrm{a}}}{M}\mathbf{R}_{\mathrm{a}} + \frac{M_{\mathrm{b}}}{M}\mathbf{R}_{\mathrm{b}} + \frac{1}{M}\mathbf{r}_{\mathrm{e}},$$
$$\mathbf{R} = -\mathbf{R}_{\mathrm{a}} + \mathbf{R}_{\mathrm{b}}, \qquad \mathbf{r}' = -\tfrac{1}{2}\mathbf{R}_{\mathrm{a}} - \tfrac{1}{2}\mathbf{R}_{\mathrm{b}} + \mathbf{r}_{\mathrm{e}}. \tag{6-16}$$

Here $M = M_{\mathrm{a}} + M_{\mathrm{b}} + 1$ is the total mass of the system (in units of the electron mass). There is a corresponding relationship among derivatives

$$\boldsymbol{\nabla}_{R_{\mathrm{a}}} = \frac{M_{\mathrm{a}}}{M}\boldsymbol{\nabla}_{R_{\mathrm{CM}}} - \boldsymbol{\nabla}_{R} - \tfrac{1}{2}\boldsymbol{\nabla}_{r'}, \qquad \boldsymbol{\nabla}_{R_{\mathrm{b}}} = \frac{M_{\mathrm{b}}}{M}\boldsymbol{\nabla}_{R_{\mathrm{CM}}} + \boldsymbol{\nabla}_{R} - \tfrac{1}{2}\boldsymbol{\nabla}_{r'},$$
$$\boldsymbol{\nabla}_{r_e} = \frac{1}{M}\boldsymbol{\nabla}_{R_{\mathrm{CM}}} + \boldsymbol{\nabla}_{r'}. \tag{6-17}$$

These lead to a new expression for the Hamiltonian

$$\mathscr{H} = \mathscr{H}_{\mathrm{CM}} + \mathscr{H}_{\mathrm{int}}, \tag{6-18}$$

where

$$\mathscr{H}_{\mathrm{CM}} = \frac{1}{M}\nabla^2_{R_{\mathrm{CM}}} \tag{6-19}$$

and

$$\mathscr{H}_{\mathrm{int}} = -\frac{1}{2\mu}\nabla^2_{R} - \frac{1}{2}\left(1 + \frac{1}{4\mu}\right)\nabla^2_{r'} - \frac{1}{2\mu'}\nabla_{R}\cdot\boldsymbol{\nabla}_{r'} + V. \tag{6-20}$$

The first term gives the relative nuclear kinetic energy and μ is the reduced mass of the nuclei

$$\frac{1}{\mu} = \frac{1}{M_a} + \frac{1}{M_b}. \tag{6-21}$$

The second term gives the electron kinetic energy relative to the nuclei, with a reduced mass correction. The third term is an interaction term. It is proportional to

$$\frac{1}{\mu'} = \frac{1}{M_a} - \frac{1}{M_b} \tag{6-22}$$

and will thus be absent in the homonuclear case when $M_a = M_b$. Different choices of the internal coordinates are possible, and both the electronic reduced mass and the form of the interaction term depend on choice of coordinates [150,151]. In multi-electron systems there will also be terms involving $\nabla_j \cdot \nabla_k$, where j and k refer to different electrons.

The interparticle distances appearing in V can be expressed as

$$R = |\mathbf{R}|, \qquad r_a = |\mathbf{r}' + \tfrac{1}{2}\mathbf{R}|, \qquad r_b = |\mathbf{r}' - \tfrac{1}{2}\mathbf{R}|. \tag{6-23}$$

As a consequence of the overall orientation independence of $\mathscr{H}$ and $\mathscr{H}_{\text{int}}$, we expect the total angular momentum to be conserved. Angular momentum associated with overall translational motion can be separated and is not of particular interest. The (orbital) angular momentum about the center of mass, which we will denote by **K**, is

$$\begin{aligned} \mathbf{K} &= -i\{(\mathbf{R}_a - \mathbf{R}_{CM}) \times \nabla_{R_a} + (\mathbf{R}_b - \mathbf{R}_{CM}) \times \nabla_{R_b} + (\mathbf{r}_e - \mathbf{R}_{CM}) \times \nabla_{r_e}\} \\ &= -i\{\mathbf{R} \times \nabla_R + \mathbf{r}' \times \nabla_{r'}\}. \end{aligned} \tag{6-24}$$

These two terms are recognizable as the relative angular momentum of the nuclei and the angular momentum of the electron about an origin fixed at the midpoint of the internuclear axis.

We next change from six Cartesian coordinates to three distances and three angles. Unfortunately, it will not be possible to effect a complete separation of the wave function into a single product of a distance-dependent factor and an angle-dependent factor, and a complete result will not be given here in any form, but two possibilities will be briefly explored.

We take the three distance coordinates to be R, the internuclear distance, the perpendicular distance ρ of the electron from the internuclear axis, and z, the component of $\mathbf{r}'$ along the internuclear axis. The three angles are specified by establishing a reference configuration [41]. Consider a coordinate system with its origin at the center of mass and its axes parallel to those of the original, space-fixed axis system. The reference configuration for the molecule is defined by requiring that

1. all nuclei lie in the xz plane,
2. the vector $\mathbf{R}$ is parallel to the z axis, and
3. the (equal) x-components of the nuclear positions are negative.

The three angular coordinates are then taken as the Euler angles of the transformation which returns the molecule to the reference configuration (Appendix C). The distance coordinates and reference configuration are shown in Fig. 6-2.

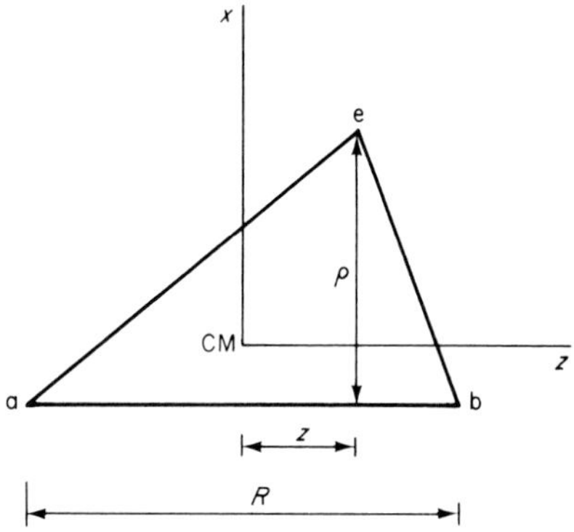

FIG. 6-2. Internal distance coordinates and reference configuration. The y axis is directed out of the plane of the figure.

Intermediate steps will be omitted, but it can be shown that these definitions lead to

$$X = R\sin\beta\cos\alpha, \qquad Y = R\sin\beta\sin\alpha, \qquad Z = R\cos\beta \tag{6-25a}$$

for the components of $\mathbf{R}$, and

$$\begin{aligned} x' &= (\cos\alpha\cos\beta\cos\gamma - \sin\alpha\sin\gamma)\rho + \cos\alpha\sin\beta\, z, \\ y' &= (\sin\alpha\cos\beta\cos\gamma - \cos\alpha\sin\gamma)\rho + \sin\alpha\sin\beta\, z, \\ z' &= -\sin\beta\cos\gamma\,\rho + \cos\beta\, z \end{aligned} \tag{6-25b}$$

for the components of $\mathbf{r}'$. We see that $\mathbf{R}$ has been expressed in spherical-polar coordinates R, β, α. From the figure we see that $\mathbf{r}'$ is expressed in cylindrical coordinates ρ, γ, z defined with respect to the nuclei. The point at which $\gamma = 0$ is somewhat arbitrary but is determined by our specification of the reference configuration.

It is not possible at this point to express an eigenfunction of $\mathscr{H}_{\text{int}}$ as the product of a function of R, ρ, z and a function of α, β, γ. It is possible, however, to express it as a sum of such products. A reasonable choice for the functions of angles are the rotation matrices $D^l_{mm'}(\alpha\beta\gamma)$. (These are discussed in Appendix C.) These are symmetric top eigenfunctions and in the present context we expect the space-fixed component of the angular momentum to be well defined, while the body-fixed z component will be related to the component of the electronic orbital angular momentum along the internuclear axis. Specification of the derivative operators in terms of the new coordinates is possible but quite messy and will not be pursued here. Were these obtained, the properties of the $D^l_{mm'}$ could be used to convert the internal Schrödinger equation to a set of coupled equations involving the functions of R, ρ, and z.

The Born–Oppenheimer Approximation

As an alternative way of treating our example, we consider the Born–Oppenheimer approximation. A formal justification will not be given here, but the qualitative aspects of the simplest form of this method will be reviewed.

The method is based on the observation that electrons move much more rapidly than nuclei. One therefore begins by neglecting all terms involving nuclear momenta. A solution is sought for the electronic Schrödinger equation

$$\mathscr{H}_{\text{el}}(R)\psi_R(\rho, z, \gamma) = E_{\text{el}}(R)\psi_R(\rho, z, \gamma) \tag{6-26}$$

where, in this case,

$$\mathscr{H}_{\text{el}}(R) = -\frac{1}{2}\left[\frac{1}{\rho}\frac{\partial}{\partial\rho}\left(\rho\frac{\partial}{\partial\rho}\right) + \frac{\partial^2}{\partial z^2} + \frac{1}{\rho^2}\frac{\partial^2}{\partial\gamma}\right] - \frac{1}{r_{\text{a}}} - \frac{1}{r_{\text{b}}}. \tag{6-27}$$

It is clear from Eq. (6-23) that r_{a} and r_{b} depend on R. The electronic Hamiltonian, $\mathscr{H}_{\text{el}}$, the wave function, ψ, and the energy, E_{el}, will thus depend parameterically on this variable. In this simple treatment the total wave function is then simply approximated as

$$\Psi(R, \alpha, \beta; \rho, z, \gamma) \simeq \psi_R(\rho z\gamma)\chi(R\alpha\beta), \tag{6-28}$$

where ψ_R is obtained for each R as the solution of Eq. (6-26) and χ is found by solving the Schrödinger equation for the nuclear motion

$$\left\{-\frac{1}{2\mu}\left[\frac{1}{R^2}\frac{\partial}{\partial R}\left(R^2\frac{\partial}{\partial R}\right) + \frac{\mathscr{N}^2(\alpha, \beta)}{2\mu R^2}\right] + U(R)\right\}\chi = E\chi. \tag{6-29}$$

In this equation $\mathscr{N}$ is the relative angular momentum of the nuclei, and

$$U(R) = 1/R + E_{\text{el}}(R). \tag{6-30}$$

An examination of the series of equations (6-26)–(6-30) will show that a number of approximations have been made. The interaction term in Eq. (6-20) has been omitted, even if $M_a \neq M_b$, and the reduced mass correction for the electron has been neglected. The forms of the Laplacian operators in Eqs. (6-27) and (6-29) also involve approximations, neglecting interaction terms associated with the transformation from space-fixed to molecule-fixed coordinates. Although these terms would be significant in a low-pressure, gas-phase study, we will ignore them here.

The electronic Schrödinger equation, Eq. (6-27), can be solved exactly. A transformation is made from ρ, z to ellipsoidal coordinates (which depend parameterically on R)

$$\xi = \frac{r_a + r_b}{R}, \qquad \eta = \frac{r_a - r_b}{R},$$
$$r_a = \left[\left(\frac{R}{2} - z\right)^2 + \rho^2\right]^{1/2}, \qquad r_b = \left[\left(\frac{R}{2} + z\right)^2 + \rho^2\right]^{1/2} \tag{6-31}$$

and the electronic wave function written as $\psi = \Xi(\xi)H(\eta)\Gamma(\gamma)$. The equation separates, and the solution for Γ is found trivially as

$$\Gamma(\gamma) = (1/\sqrt{2\pi})e^{im'\gamma}.$$

The functions Ξ and H and the energy E_{el} are more difficult to obtain and results will not be given here [13].

The Schrödinger equation for nuclear motion, Eq. (6-29), is also separable with

$$\chi = \phi(R)Y_l^m(\beta, \alpha), \tag{6-32}$$

where Y_l^m is the spherical harmonic. We note that the dependence of the total wave function on the angular variables in this approximation is

$$Y_l^m(\beta, \alpha)\frac{1}{\sqrt{2\pi}}e^{im'\gamma} \propto e^{im\alpha}P_l^m(\cos\beta)e^{im'\gamma} \tag{6-33}$$

which is to be compared with the rotation matrix in the other approach

$$D_{mm'}^l(\alpha\beta\gamma) = e^{-im\alpha}d_{mm'}^l(\beta)e^{-im'\gamma}. \tag{6-34}$$

In addition to the change in sign of the m's, which is primarily a matter of convention, $d_{mm'}^l$ differs from P_l^m. Of course Eq. (6-33) arises in a one-term approximation while the rotation matrix in Eq. (6-34) arises as one of several terms in a potentially exact result.

When the spins of the electron and the nuclei are introduced, a new total angular momentum must be defined. The relativistic correction terms should also be introduced. Interparticle distances are independent of the coordinate system used, but momentum operators must be appropriately reexpressed. We will not go into these effects but will consider another factor.

The dominant contributions associated with nuclear motions for condensed-phase ESR studies are the result of changes in the electronic wave function associated with changes in relative nuclear positions. We thus conclude this example with Fig. 6-3, in which the Fermi contact term for either proton in H_2^+ is shown as a function of R. The probability distributions $|\phi(R)|^2$ for the ground and first vibrational states (in the absence of rotation) are shown as well. It is clear that different vibrationally averaged hyperfine interactions will result for the two vibrational states [202].

This treatment has been far from complete, even for the simple case of H_2^+, but hopefully some of the more important features of the separation of electronic and nuclear motions have been illustrated.

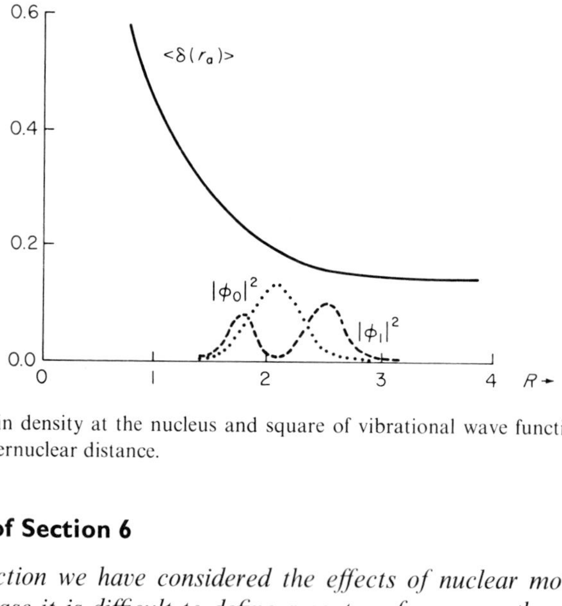

FIG. 6-3. Spin density at the nucleus and square of vibrational wave functions for H_2^+, as functions of internuclear distance.

Summary of Section 6

In this section we have considered the effects of nuclear motions. In the relativistic case it is difficult to define a center of mass, so the approach has been to deal with center of mass and nuclear motions at the Schrödinger level. Appropriate adjustments are then made in relativistic correction terms.

One-electron atoms were considered in detail. The most important effects on relativistic corrections are associated with the difference between bare and reduced electronic masses. An expansion of the corrections in powers of m/M_v *has been given.*

The molecular case was treated much less completely, with H_2^+ *considered as an example. Center of mass motion is readily separated, but a separation of rotational motion which is both complete and exact is not possible. A method for a potentially exact treatment was indicated but not pursued in detail, and the simple Born–Oppenheimer approximation was outlined. The most important effect on relativistic corrections is via the change in zero-order wave functions associated with changed relative nuclear positions.*

CHAPTER II

THE DESCRIPTION OF MAGNETIC ENERGY LEVELS

7. The Spin Hamiltonian as a Summary of Experimental Data

The results of an ESR experiment contain data of various types. We will not be concerned here with dynamic effects other than the ESR transition itself. The data thus consist of a series of transition energies or line positions and the corresponding relative intensities or integrated line amplitudes. (Linewidths are also of interest, but give information about dynamic effects.) It is convenient and customary to analyze the experimental data in terms of the parameters of a spin Hamiltonian. We will be concerned in this section with the correlation between a spin Hamiltonian and a spectrum.

In the most general sense a spin Hamiltonian can be defined as a Hermitian operator containing only (electron and nuclear) spin operators and parameters. The dimension of the electron spin space within which the spin Hamiltonian operates is chosen to correspond to the number of electronic energy levels being considered in the experimental situation, rather than being necessarily related to the S quantum number, if there is one, characterizing the molecules of the sample. An effective spin quantum number is sometimes defined by requiring that $2S_{\text{eff}} + 1 =$ number of (electronic) states. The spin Hamiltonian parameters contain no operators but may be functions of the molecular orientation and of the strengths of external fields.

Using this broad definition, it is clearly possible to reproduce with a spin Hamiltonian any observed set of energy levels. Suppose that the experimental results give a set of relative energy levels as a function of molecular orientation Ω and magnetic field strength B: $\{E_i(\Omega, B)\}$. For *any* orthonormal basis set in the appropriate spin space, $\{|i\rangle\}$, the spin Hamiltonian can be written

$$\mathscr{H} = \sum_i E_i(\Omega, B)|i\rangle\langle i|. \tag{7-1}$$

The coefficients E_i fit the definition of parameters and the projection operators $|i\rangle\langle i|$ can be written as linear combinations of spin operator products. The freedom of choice of the basis functions $\{|i\rangle\}$ can be used to reproduce some of the other desired features, such as relative intensities. It is not immediately clear whether an arbitrary set of observed intensities, taken to give values of $|\langle i|S_x|j\rangle|^2$, can be reproduced in this way. The number of observable intensities (normally many potential transitions do not occur, i.e., they have intensity zero) does correspond to the number of degrees of freedom in choosing a basis set.

In practice additional restrictions are placed on a spin Hamiltonian: it is normally assumed to be of the form

$$\mathscr{H} = \sum_{i,j} \mathbf{v}^i \cdot \mathbf{T}^{ij} \cdot \mathbf{v}^j \tag{7-2}$$

where $\mathbf{v}^i$, $\mathbf{v}^j$, etc., are vectors—either the spin vector operators **S** or **I**, or the magnetic field vector **B**. The parameter sets‡ $\mathbf{T}^{ij}$ depend on molecular orientation but not on field strengths or spin operators. Terms in which $\mathbf{v}^i$ and $\mathbf{v}^j$ are both of the same type, i.e., both electron spin, both nuclear spin, or both field, are often omitted. On the other hand, terms involving higher powers of electron spin operators are sometimes included.

Without additional restrictions a spin Hamiltonian may not be uniquely defined by the observed spectrum. The restrictions are based on convenience and on the presumed derivability of the spin Hamiltonian from an accurate quantum mechanical full Hamiltonian of the sort discussed in Chapter I. This relationship will be considered in the next section.

Since it is not possible to go uniquely from an experimental spectrum to a spin Hamiltonian, and since we cannot hope to make an exhaustive survey of all possible experimental spectra, we will proceed in the other direction: we will consider spin Hamiltonians of several standard types and determine what sort of spectra they can describe.

Isotropic Spin Hamiltonian for $S = \frac{1}{2}$

We begin with the simplest case of the form given in Eq. (7-2), in which the tensors coupling the spins to each other and to the field are orientation independent: $\mathbf{T} = T\mathbf{1}$. To a very good approximation this is true in solution ESR, where the radical tumbles rapidly so that orientation-dependent terms are averaged. We will consider now the energy level structure and the transitions among levels for the isotropic case of a doublet state.

‡ These are commonly called tensors. They sometimes do and sometimes do not transform as tensors under rotations. The term will be used here nevertheless.

If terms quadratic in the spin operators are not present, the general, isotropic spin Hamiltonian for a system with N magnetic nuclei can be written

$$\mathscr{H} = g\beta B S_z - \sum_{\nu=1}^{N} \gamma_\nu B I_z^\nu + \sum_{\nu=1}^{N} A_\nu \mathbf{S}\cdot\mathbf{I}^\nu \tag{7-3}$$

with the direction of the external field, of magnitude B, taken to define the z axis and $g\beta$, γ_ν, and A_ν real constants.‡ We will normally be concerned with the high-field case in which the first term is dominant but will not restrict the discussion to that case.

This Hamiltonian is readily treated. It is convenient to introduce a basis set of spin functions of the simple product form $|m_s; m_1, \ldots, m_N\rangle = |Sm_s\rangle \times |I_1 m_{I,1}\rangle \cdots |I_N m_{I,N}\rangle$ where the unchanging quantum numbers $S, I_1, \ldots, I_N$ have been suppressed and m_i is m_I for the ith nucleus. Then clearly

$$g\beta S_z |m_s; m_1, \ldots, m_N\rangle = g\beta m_s |m_s; m_1, \ldots, m_N\rangle \tag{7-4}$$

and

$$\left(\sum_{\nu=1}^{N} \gamma_\nu B I_z^\nu\right)|m_s; m_1, \ldots, m_N\rangle = \left(\sum_{\nu=1}^{N} \gamma_\nu B m_\nu\right)|m_s; m_1, \ldots, m_N\rangle. \tag{7-5}$$

The effect of the remaining term in $\mathscr{H}$ is more involved but still straightforward since

$$\mathbf{S}\cdot\mathbf{I}^\nu = S_z I_z^\nu + \tfrac{1}{2}(S_+ I_-^\nu + S_- I_+^\nu) \tag{7-6}$$

and for $\mathbf{J} = \mathbf{S}$ or $\mathbf{I}$ (a phase factor depending on m_j is sometimes introduced)

$$J_\pm |m_j\rangle = [j(j+1) - m_j(m_j \pm 1)]^{1/2} |m_j \pm 1\rangle. \tag{7-7}$$

Single Nucleus of Spin $\frac{1}{2}$

As an initial, illustrative example the case of a single nucleus of spin $\frac{1}{2}$ will be considered. The system involves only four states and the matrix of $\mathscr{H}$ is

$$\langle m_s; m_I | \mathscr{H} | m_s'; m_I' \rangle$$

$m_s, m_I/m_s', m_I'$	$\frac{1}{2}, \frac{1}{2}$	$\frac{1}{2}, -\frac{1}{2}$	$-\frac{1}{2}, \frac{1}{2}$	$-\frac{1}{2}, -\frac{1}{2}$
$\frac{1}{2}, \frac{1}{2}$	$\frac{1}{2}g\beta B - \frac{1}{2}\gamma B + \frac{1}{4}A$	0	0	0
$\frac{1}{2}, -\frac{1}{2}$	0	$\frac{1}{2}g\beta B + \frac{1}{2}\gamma B - \frac{1}{4}A$	$\frac{1}{2}A$	0
$-\frac{1}{2}, \frac{1}{2}$	0	$\frac{1}{2}A$	$-\frac{1}{2}g\beta B - \frac{1}{2}\gamma B - \frac{1}{4}A$	0
$-\frac{1}{2}, -\frac{1}{2}$	0	0	0	$-\frac{1}{2}g\beta B + \frac{1}{2}\gamma B + \frac{1}{4}A$

‡ This γ_ν is $g_\nu \beta_N$, where β_N is the nuclear magneton. A nuclear gyromagnetic ratio parameter commonly denoted by γ differs from γ_ν here by a factor of h.

The two states $|1\rangle = |\frac{1}{2}; \frac{1}{2}\rangle$ and $|4\rangle = |-\frac{1}{2}; -\frac{1}{2}\rangle$ are eigenstates of $\mathscr{H}$ with energies

$$\begin{aligned} E_1 &= E_{1/2;\,1/2} = \tfrac{1}{2}g\beta B - \tfrac{1}{2}\gamma B + \tfrac{1}{4}A, \\ E_4 &= E_{-1/2;\,-1/2} = -\tfrac{1}{2}g\beta B + \tfrac{1}{2}\gamma B + \tfrac{1}{4}A. \end{aligned} \tag{7-8}$$

To obtain the other two eigenstates we must diagonalize a 2×2 matrix. This is readily done and the energy levels are

$$E_{2,3} = -\tfrac{1}{4}A \pm \tfrac{1}{2}[(g\beta + \gamma)^2 B^2 + A^2]^{1/2}. \tag{7-9}$$

The corresponding eigenfunctions can be expressed in the form (see Appendix E)

$$\begin{aligned} |2\rangle &= \cos\theta|\tfrac{1}{2}; -\tfrac{1}{2}\rangle + \sin\theta|-\tfrac{1}{2}; \tfrac{1}{2}\rangle, \\ |3\rangle &= -\sin\theta|\tfrac{1}{2}; -\tfrac{1}{2}\rangle + \cos\theta|-\tfrac{1}{2}; \tfrac{1}{2}\rangle, \end{aligned}$$

where

$$\tan 2\theta = |A|/[(g\beta + \gamma)B]. \tag{7-10}$$

Transitions are normally observed when they are induced by an oscillating magnetic field in a direction perpendicular to **B**. The direction of this oscillating field can be taken to be the x direction. The probability of a transition between states j and k is then proportional to $|\langle j|S_x|k\rangle|^2$, and

$$\langle m_s|S_x|m_s'\rangle = \delta_{m_s,\,m_s'+1} + \delta_{m_s,\,m_s'-1}. \tag{7-11}$$

For the states obtained above the nonvanishing matrix elements of S_x are

$$\begin{gathered} \langle 1|S_x|2\rangle = \sin\theta, \qquad \langle 1|S_x|3\rangle = \cos\theta, \qquad \langle 2|S_x|4\rangle = \cos\theta, \\ \langle 3|S_x|4\rangle = -\sin\theta. \end{gathered} \tag{7-12}$$

For the strong field case θ is small. The transitions $1 \to 3$ and $2 \to 4$ with intensity proportional to $\cos^2\theta$ will be strong while $1 \to 2$ and $3 \to 4$ with intensity proportional to $\sin^2\theta$ will be very weak. For the strong transitions

$$\begin{aligned} \Delta E_{1,3} &= E_1 - E_3 = \tfrac{1}{2}g\beta B - \tfrac{1}{2}\gamma B + \tfrac{1}{2}A + \tfrac{1}{2}[(gB + \gamma)^2 B^2 + A^2]^{1/2}, \\ \Delta E_{2,4} &= E_2 - E_4 = \tfrac{1}{2}g\beta B - \tfrac{1}{2}\gamma B - \tfrac{1}{2}A + \tfrac{1}{2}[(gB + \gamma)^2 B^2 + A^2]^{1/2}. \end{aligned} \tag{7-13}$$

It is interesting to note that the splitting between the strong lines

$$\Delta E_{1,3} - \Delta E_{2,4} = A \tag{7-14}$$

is simply equal to the hyperfine coupling constant and is independent of the field strength. (This is a special result for the $I = \frac{1}{2}$ case.) The weak transitions occur at energies

$$\begin{aligned} \Delta E_{1,2} &= E_1 - E_2 = \tfrac{1}{2}g\beta B - \tfrac{1}{2}\gamma B + \tfrac{1}{2}A - \tfrac{1}{2}[(g\beta + \gamma)^2 B^2 + A^2]^{1/2}, \\ \Delta E_{3,4} &= E_3 - E_4 = \tfrac{1}{2}g\beta B - \tfrac{1}{2}\gamma B - \tfrac{1}{2}A - \tfrac{1}{2}[(g\beta + \gamma)^2 B^2 + A^2]^{1/2}. \end{aligned} \tag{7-15}$$

The splitting between these lines, which would be significant in the low-field limit, is again simply A. At high fields these transitions have $\Delta E \sim \gamma B \pm \frac{1}{2}A$, and they would not normally be considered ESR transitions. The interaction of the nuclear spins with the oscillating magnetic field should also be considered. The energy expressions in this case are well known, usually being referred to in one form or another as the Breit–Rabi formula [23].

The high-field limit $g\beta B \gg A, \gamma B$ will be considered below. It is possibly of some interest to consider also the low-field limit. When $B = 0$ the hyperfine interaction couples the electronic and nuclear spins to give a total angular momentum $\mathbf{F} = \mathbf{S} + \mathbf{I}$ with eigenvalues of F^2 being $f(f+1)$. In this case the possible values of f are 0 and 1. The energies and eigenfunctions are

$$f = 0, \qquad E = -\tfrac{3}{4}A, \qquad |f = 0, m_f = 0\rangle = (1/\sqrt{2})(|\tfrac{1}{2}, -\tfrac{1}{2}\rangle - |-\tfrac{1}{2}, \tfrac{1}{2}\rangle),$$

$$\begin{aligned} & & &|f = 1, m_f = 1\rangle = |\tfrac{1}{2}, \tfrac{1}{2}\rangle, \\ f = 1, & &E = \tfrac{1}{4}A, \qquad &|f = 1, m_f = 0\rangle = (1/\sqrt{2})(|\tfrac{1}{2}, -\tfrac{1}{2}\rangle + |-\tfrac{1}{2}, \tfrac{1}{2}\rangle), \\ & & &|f = 1, m_f = -1\rangle = |-\tfrac{1}{2}, -\tfrac{1}{2}\rangle. \end{aligned} \tag{7-16}$$

When B is small but nonzero the energies of the $f = 1$ states are split by an amount proportional to $m_f B$. This approximation rapidly breaks down because $g\beta \gg \gamma$. In the low-field limit transitions having $\Delta f = \pm 1, \Delta m_f = \pm 1$ are allowed and have energies $|\Delta E| = A$. The energy expressions which have been derived above are, of course, valid for any value of B, as eigenvalues of the spin Hamiltonian. Disparity with experimental results would indicate breakdown of the simple spin Hamiltonian description.

Before considering the high-field limit and approximate treatments, we should recognize a consequence of the usual ESR experimental situation. In the treatment above we have obtained expressions for E as a function of B. In principle one could fix B and search spectroscopically for a frequency ν such that $h\nu = \Delta E$ for some allowed transition. In practice this is rarely done, however. Electron spin resonance spectrometers are designed so that the frequency is fixed and the field strength varied to find the resonance values. It is thus desirable to invert the expressions obtained above to find the field strengths leading to transitions for a fixed frequency. For the strong transitions the resonance condition $\Delta E = h\nu$ can be written

$$\tfrac{1}{2}(g\beta - \gamma)B \pm \tfrac{1}{2}A - h\nu = -\tfrac{1}{2}[(g\beta + \gamma)^2 B^2 + A^2]^{1/2}. \tag{7-17}$$

If both sides of this equation are squared, the result is an equation in B which can be solved. It is convenient to divide through by $g\beta$ and define $b = h\nu/g\beta$, $a = A/g\beta$, and $\delta = -\gamma/g\beta$. Of these, b is the resonance field strength in the absence of hyperfine interaction, a is the hyperfine coupling constant in units of magnetic field strength, and δ is a dimensionless parameter of order 10^{-3} or less relating nuclear and electronic gyromagnetic ratios.

The equation corresponding to the resonance condition is then

$$\delta B^2 - (1 + \delta)(b \mp \tfrac{1}{2}a)B + b(b \mp a) = 0. \tag{7-18}$$

It should be noted that if $\delta = 0$,

$$B = b\,\frac{b \mp a}{b \mp \frac{1}{2}a} = b[1 \mp \tfrac{1}{2}a/(b \mp \tfrac{1}{2}a)] = b \mp \tfrac{1}{2}a - a^2/4b + \cdots. \tag{7-19}$$

The expansion is appropriate in the high-field case when $b > a$. If δ is small but nonzero, the general expression obtained by solution of the quadratic equation for B is easily obtained but not particularly illuminating. We note however that the solution of a quadratic equation $px^2 + qx + r = 0$ can be written in the nonstandard form

$$x = -\frac{r}{q}\left[\frac{q^2}{2pr}(1 - [1 - (4qr/q^2)]^{1/2})\right],$$

and if the square root is expanded with p assumed to be small,

$$x = -\frac{r}{q}\left[1 + \frac{pr}{q^2} + 2\left(\frac{pr}{q^2}\right)^2 + \cdots\right].$$

This leads to a result for B in the present situation in which the dependence on δ does not in fact appear through second order in δ and a/b. To this order the expression for B is just that given above. The effect of the nuclear Zeeman interaction on the ESR resonance field strengths is thus essentially negligible.

Relative intensities can be obtained for the strong and weak transitions, respectively, as

$$\cos^2\theta = \frac{1}{2} + \frac{1}{2}\left[1 + \left(\frac{a}{2(1-\delta)B}\right)^2\right]^{-1/2} \simeq 1 - \frac{1}{8}\left[\frac{a}{(1-\delta)B}\right]^2 + \cdots,$$

$$\sin^2\theta = \frac{1}{2} - \frac{1}{2}\left[1 + \left(\frac{a}{2(1-\delta)B}\right)^2\right]^{-1/2} \simeq \frac{1}{8}\left[\frac{a}{(1-\delta)B}\right]^2 + \cdots. \tag{7-20}$$

Here B is in each case the field strength for that transition.

Before we leave this example we should note that the series expansions are equivalent to a perturbation treatment of the original problem. The Hamiltonian can be divided into a zero-order part and a perturbation: $\mathcal{H} = \mathcal{H}_0 + V$, with

$$\mathcal{H}_0 = g\beta BS_z, \qquad V = -\sum_{\nu=1}^{N} \gamma_\nu BI_z^\nu + \sum_{\nu=1}^{N} A_\nu \mathbf{S}\cdot\mathbf{I}^\nu. \tag{7-21}$$

In the high-field limit we expect contributions from V to be small compared with those from $\mathscr{H}_0$. The matrix elements already given are readily separable into contributions from $\mathscr{H}_0$ and V. The zero-order energies are just

$$E^{(0)} = m_s g\beta B = \pm\tfrac{1}{2}g\beta B, \tag{7-22}$$

and each level is doubly degenerate. The perturbation treatment of a system degenerate in zero order requires that the zero-order functions be chosen so as to diagonalize the perturbation within each zero-order degenerate manifold. The eigenvalues of each block of V are the first-order energies.

In the present case the block of V associated with the degenerate $m_s = \frac{1}{2}$ states and that associated with the degenerate $m_s = -\frac{1}{2}$ states are already diagonal in the simple product basis. The first-order energies are

$$\begin{aligned} E^{(1)} &= (-\tfrac{1}{2}\gamma B + \tfrac{1}{4}A), \qquad \text{for} \quad m_s = +\tfrac{1}{2}, \\ E^{(1)} &= (-\tfrac{1}{2}\gamma B - \tfrac{1}{4}A), \qquad \text{for} \quad m_s = -\tfrac{1}{2}. \end{aligned} \tag{7-23}$$

The degeneracy is thus lifted in first order.

For the second-order energies

$$E_j^{(2)} = \sum_{k(\neq j)} \frac{|V_{jk}|^2}{E_j^{(0)} - E_k^{(0)}} \tag{7-24}$$

so that for $E^{(2)}_{m_s, m_I}$

$$E^{(2)}_{1/2, 1/2} = E^{(2)}_{-1/2, -1/2} = 0, \qquad E^{(2)}_{1/2, -1/2} = -E^{(2)}_{-1/2, 1/2} = \frac{A^2}{4g\beta B}. \tag{7-25}$$

The energies of the strong transitions through second order are thus

$$\Delta E_{m_I = +1/2} = g\beta B + \tfrac{1}{2}A - \frac{A^2}{4g\beta B}, \qquad \Delta E_{m_I = -1/2} = g\beta B - \tfrac{1}{2}A - \frac{A^2}{4g\beta B}. \tag{7-26}$$

These are similar to the expressions which are obtained if the square roots in Eq. (7-13) are expanded in powers of $A/(g\beta + \gamma)B$ and powers higher than the second are neglected, except that the denominator of the second term is then $(g\beta + \gamma)B$ rather than $g\beta B$. Identical expressions are obtained from expansion of the square root and from perturbation theory if the nuclear Zeeman term in the Hamiltonian is included in $\mathscr{H}_0$ rather than in V. The perturbation treatment will be further discussed in connection with the many-nuclei case.

Single Nucleus of Arbitrary Spin

The next case to be considered is that of a single nucleus of arbitrary spin, I. The spin Hamiltonian matrix is then of dimension $2(2I + 1)$. The matrix elements are readily determined and it is found that the states $|\frac{1}{2}; I\rangle$ and $|-\frac{1}{2}; -I\rangle$ are eigenfunctions of $\mathscr{H}$ with eigenvalues

$$\begin{aligned} E_{1/2, I} &= \langle \tfrac{1}{2}; I|\mathscr{H}|\tfrac{1}{2}; I\rangle = \tfrac{1}{2}g\beta B - I\gamma B + \tfrac{1}{2}IA, \\ E_{-1/2, -I} &= \langle -\tfrac{1}{2}; -I|\mathscr{H}|-\tfrac{1}{2}; -I\rangle = -\tfrac{1}{2}g\beta B + I\gamma B + \tfrac{1}{2}IA. \end{aligned} \tag{7-27}$$

The remainder of the matrix consists of zeros and 2×2 blocks with matrix elements of the form

$$\begin{aligned} \langle \tfrac{1}{2}; m_I|\mathscr{H}|\tfrac{1}{2}; m_I\rangle &= \tfrac{1}{2}g\beta B - m_I\gamma B + \tfrac{1}{2}m_I A, \\ \langle \tfrac{1}{2}; m_I|\mathscr{H}|-\tfrac{1}{2}; m_I + 1\rangle &= \tfrac{1}{2}A[(I + m_I + 1)(I - m_I)]^{1/2}, \\ \langle -\tfrac{1}{2}; m_I + 1|\mathscr{H}|-\tfrac{1}{2}; m_I + 1\rangle &= -\tfrac{1}{2}g\beta B - (m_I + 1)\gamma B - \tfrac{1}{2}(m_I + 1)A. \end{aligned} \tag{7-28}$$

The spin Hamiltonian can thus be diagonalized analytically, as in the case of $I = \frac{1}{2}$. The result is

$$\begin{aligned} E_{\pm 1/2, m} &= -(m_I + \tfrac{1}{2})\gamma B - \tfrac{1}{4}A \pm \tfrac{1}{2}[(g\beta + \gamma)^2 B^2 \\ &\quad + 2(m_I + \tfrac{1}{2})(g\beta + \gamma)AB + (I + \tfrac{1}{2})^2 A^2]^{1/2} \\ &= \pm\tfrac{1}{2}g\beta B - m\gamma B \pm \tfrac{1}{2}mA \pm \frac{[I(I + 1) - m(m \pm 1)]}{4(g\beta + \gamma)}\frac{A^2}{B}. \end{aligned} \tag{7-29}$$

The subscripts on E refer to the m_s and m_I of the simple product function which is dominant (for $g\beta B \gg A$) in the corresponding eigenfunction. Thus, for $m_s = \frac{1}{2}$ the upper signs are used and $m = m_I$, while for $m_s = -\frac{1}{2}$ the lower signs are used and $m = m_I + 1$ in the notation of Eqs. (7-28). The second expression is obtained by expanding the square root in powers of $A/(g\beta + \gamma)B$. A perturbation treatment through second order gives a result identical to that obtained by expansion if the nuclear Zeeman term is included in $\mathscr{H}_0$. If it is included in V, the denominator contains simply $g\beta$ in place of $g\beta + \gamma$. Although this expression was obtained for $|m_I| \neq I$, it can be readily verified that it is also valid when $|m_I| = I$. The energy differences for the strongly allowed transitions, which can be labeled by the m_I values for the dominant contribution to the corresponding states, are

$$\begin{aligned} \Delta E_{m_I} &= -\gamma B + \tfrac{1}{2}\{[(g\beta + \gamma)^2 B^2 + (2m_I + 1)(g\beta + \gamma)BA \\ &\quad + [I(I + 1) + \tfrac{1}{4}]A^2]^{1/2} + [(g\beta + \gamma)^2 B^2 \\ &\quad + (2m_I - 1)(g\beta + \gamma)BA + [I(I + 1) + \tfrac{1}{4}]A^2]^{1/2}\} \\ &= g\beta B + m_I A + \frac{[I(I + 1) - m_I^2]}{2(g\beta + \gamma)}\frac{A^2}{B} + \cdots. \end{aligned} \tag{7-30}$$

If $h\nu$ is equated to ΔE for fixed ν, an equation again results which determines the field strengths for which transitions occur. Because the sum of two square roots is involved, however, this expression is equivalent to a quartic rather than a quadratic equation for B, and its general solution, though attainable, is not useful. The equation for B reduces to a quadratic if the nuclear Zeeman energy is neglected ($\gamma = 0$) in which case

$$\begin{aligned} B_m &= (1 - a^2/4b^2)^{-1}\{-ma + b[1 - [4(I + \tfrac{1}{2})^2 - 4m^2 + 1](a^2/4b^2) \\ &\quad + (I + \tfrac{1}{2})^2(a^4/4b^4)]^{1/2}\} \\ &= b - ma - [I(I + 1) - m^2]a^2/2b + \cdots \end{aligned} \qquad (7\text{-}31)$$

with b and a as defined previously and m written for m_I.

If the nuclear spin is greater than $\frac{1}{2}$, then terms which are quadratic in the nuclear spin operators may occur in the spin Hamiltonian. The only term of this type which is commonly included is that describing the quadrupole coupling interaction. It is orientation dependent and has a vanishing isotropic component, so discussion of it will be delayed until nonisotropic spin Hamiltonians are considered.

Many Nuclei: Perturbation Treatment‡

If the effects of more than one nucleus are included in the spin Hamiltonian, the hyperfine interaction term will link states in such a way that the spin Hamiltonian matrix in the simple product basis is not separable into 2 × 2 blocks. In consequence the eigenvalues cannot be conveniently obtained in exact, analytic form. A perturbation treatment is straightforward, however, and gives satisfactory results.

The general matrix elements of the parts of $\mathscr{H}$ are easily obtained. It is convenient to represent the nuclear spin state by a single index K, with the understanding that m_ν^K is the value of m_I for the νth nucleus in nuclear spin state K.

$$\langle m_s; K | g\beta B S_z | m_s'; K'\rangle = g\beta B m_s \delta_{m_s, m_s'} \delta_{K,K'}$$

$$\langle m_s; K | \sum_\nu \gamma_\nu B I_z^\nu | m_s'; K'\rangle = \left(\sum_\nu \gamma_\nu m_\nu^K\right) B \delta_{m_s, m_s'} \delta_{K,K'}$$

$$\begin{aligned} &\langle m_s; K | \sum_\nu A_\nu \mathbf{S}\cdot\mathbf{I}^\nu | m_s'; K'\rangle \\ &= m_s\left(\sum_\nu A_\nu m_\nu^K\right)\delta_{m_s, m_s'}\delta_{K,K'} + \tfrac{1}{2}\sum_\mu A_\mu\{[I_\mu(I_\mu + 1) - m_\mu^{K'}(m_\mu^{K'} + 1)]^{1/2} \\ &\quad \times \delta_{m_s, m_s' - 1}\delta_{m_\mu^K, m_\mu^{K'} + 1} + [I_\mu(I_\mu + 1) - m_\mu^{K'}(m_\mu^{K'} - 1)]^{1/2} \\ &\quad \times \delta_{m_s, m_s' + 1}\delta_{m_\mu^K, m_\mu^{K'} - 1}\} \prod_{\nu(\neq\mu)} \delta_{m_\nu^K, m_\nu^{K'}}. \end{aligned} \qquad (7\text{-}32)$$

‡ The nuclear-spin-$\frac{1}{2}$ case has been discussed by Fessenden [54].

As was noted in the perturbation discussion for the case of a single nucleus of spin $\frac{1}{2}$, there is some ambiguity as to whether the nuclear Zeeman term should be included with $\mathscr{H}_0$ or with V. In either case the simple product basis provides an appropriate set of zero-order functions. It is perhaps best to anticipate later problems by dealing with this as a double-perturbation situation. In fact, it is convenient to look not at $\mathscr{H}$ but at $H = \mathscr{H}/B$. Then

$$H = H_0 + \mu H' + \lambda V \tag{7-33}$$

with

$$H_0 = g\beta S_z, \qquad H' = -\sum_\nu \gamma_\nu I_z^\nu, \qquad V = \sum_\nu A_\nu \mathbf{S}\cdot\mathbf{I}^\nu \tag{7-34}$$

and with $\lambda = 1/B$ a natural perturbation parameter but μ a purely formal perturbation parameter to be set equal to 1 in the end. With these definitions and with

$$E = E^{(0,0)} + \mu E^{(1,0)} + \lambda E^{(0,1)} + \mu^2 E^{(2,0)} + \mu\lambda E^{(1,1)} + \lambda^2 E^{(0,2)} + \cdots, \tag{7-35}$$

it is readily shown that

$$E_{m_S,K}^{(0,0)} = g\beta m_s \tag{7-36}$$

and

$$E_{m_S,K}^{(1,0)} = -\sum_\nu \gamma_\nu m_\nu^K, \qquad E_{m_S,K}^{(0,1)} = m_s \sum_\nu A_\nu m_\nu^K. \tag{7-37}$$

Since H' has no off-diagonal matrix elements different from zero, $E^{(2,0)}$ and $E^{(1,1)}$ are zero. The second-order energies with respect to V are given by the usual formula which, in this case, leads to

$$E_{m_S,K}^{(0,2)} = m_s(2g\beta)^{-1} \sum_\mu [I_\mu(I_\mu + 1) - m_\mu^K(m_\mu^K - 2m_s)]A_\mu^2. \tag{7-38}$$

The selection rules still require that the strongly allowed transitions are those for which none of the m_ν^K change, and thus for which (for $m_s = -\frac{1}{2} \rightarrow m_s = +\frac{1}{2}$)

$$\begin{aligned}\Delta E_K &= B(\Delta E^{(0,0)} + \lambda\Delta E^{(0,1)} + \lambda^2 \Delta E^{(0,2)} + \cdots) \\ &= g\beta B + \sum_\nu A_\nu m_\nu^K + (2g\beta B)^{-1} \sum_\mu [I_\mu(I_\mu + 1) - (m_\mu^K)^2]A_\mu^2 + \cdots.\end{aligned} \tag{7-39}$$

The contribution of the nuclear Zeeman energy cancels out through second order in the strongly allowed transitions. This is a straightforward generalization of Eq. (7-30).

Some transitions which are not allowed if zero-order wave functions are used to compute transition probabilities will be weakly allowed when the first-order wave functions are considered. The intensity of an ESR transition will, in the usual experimental situation, be proportional to $|\langle i|S_x|f\rangle|^2$, where $|i\rangle$ and $|f\rangle$ are the initial and final states.

In the present case

$$\psi_{m_S,K} = \psi^{(0)}_{m_S,K} + \lambda\psi^{(1)}_{m_S,K} + \cdots, \tag{7-40}$$

and

$$\psi^{(1)}_{\pm 1/2,K} = \pm \sum_{\mu} \frac{A\mu}{2g\beta}(I_\mu(I_\mu + 1) - m^K_\mu(m^K_\mu \pm 1))^{1/2}\psi^{(0)}_{\mp 1/2,K''}, \tag{7-41}$$

where K'' labels the nuclear spin state for which

$$m^{K''}_\mu = m^K_\mu \pm 1, \qquad m^{K''}_\nu = m^K_\nu, \qquad \nu \neq \mu.$$

If the wave functions through first order are used, there will be nonzero S_x matrix elements of order λ between states $|m_s; K\rangle$ and $|m_s; K''\rangle$ where the labels refer to the dominant, zero-order component. A transition between these states would not be a normal ESR transition, however, because of the small energy difference involved. To obtain additional transitions with $\Delta E^{(0,0)} = g\beta$, we must consider those between $|\frac{1}{2}; K\rangle$ and $|-\frac{1}{2}; K'\rangle$ where K and K' differ in two nuclear spins such that they can have a common K'' in the notation used above. For such transitions the matrix elements of S_x will be of order λ^2 and thus the relative intensity of order λ^4. They will not be observable under most circumstances.

Fixed-Frequency Results

As pointed out above, the usual experimental situation has a fixed frequency with the magnetic field strength varied and the spectrum obtained in terms of field strengths for which transitions occur. It is thus necessary to solve the resonance equation (subject also to selection rules)

$$h\nu = \Delta E(B) \tag{7-42}$$

for the field strength B. This cannot be done analytically in the general case, but a result valid to second order is readily obtained. The resonance equation is obtained from Eq. (7-35) as

$$h\nu = B\Delta E^{(0)} + \Delta E^{(1)} + (1/B)\Delta E^{(2)}$$

or

$$B^2\Delta E^{(0)} + [\Delta E^{(1)} - h\nu]B + \Delta E^{(2)} = 0 \tag{7-43}$$

with $\Delta E^{(0)} = \Delta E^{(0,0)} + \mu\Delta E^{(1,0)} + \cdots$, $\Delta E^{(1)} = \Delta E^{(1,0)} + \mu\Delta E^{(1,1)} + \cdots$, and $\Delta E^{(2)} = \Delta E^{(0,2)} + \cdots$. We have noted that $E^{(2,0)}$ and $E^{(1,1)}$ are zero, and for zero-order-allowed transitions $\Delta E^{(1,0)} = 0$, so all nuclear Zeeman effects drop out. Solving Eq. (7-43) for B, we get

$$B \sim \frac{1}{2\Delta E^{(0)}}[(h\nu - \Delta E^{(1)}) \pm ((h\nu - \Delta E^{(0)})^2 - 4\Delta E^{(0)}\Delta E^{(2)})^{1/2}]. \quad (7\text{-}44)$$

We can separate B into contributions of different orders. If $\Delta E^{(1)}$ and $\Delta E^{(2)}$ are neglected,

$$B \simeq \frac{h\nu \pm \sqrt{(h\nu)^2}}{2\Delta E^{(0)}} = \frac{h\nu}{\Delta E^{(0)}},$$

it being obvious that the + sign must be used. If $\Delta E^{(1)}$ is retained but $\Delta E^{(2)}$ is neglected,

$$B \simeq \frac{h\nu - \Delta E^{(1)}}{2\Delta E^{(0)}} \pm \frac{|h\nu - \Delta E^{(1)}|}{2\Delta E^{(0)}} = \frac{h\nu}{\Delta E^{(0)}} - \frac{\Delta E^{(1)}}{\Delta E^{(0)}}.$$

Finally, then, retaining all of ΔE through $\Delta E^{(2)}$

$$B = \frac{h\nu}{\Delta E^{(0)}} - \frac{\Delta E^{(1)}}{\Delta E^{(0)}} + \frac{h\nu - \Delta E^{(1)}}{2\Delta E^{(0)}}\left[\left(1 - \frac{4\Delta E^{(0)}\Delta E^{(2)}}{(h\nu - \Delta E^{(1)})^2}\right)^{1/2} - 1\right] + \cdots$$

$$= \frac{h\nu}{\Delta E^{(0)}} - \frac{\Delta E^{(1)}}{\Delta E^{(0)}} + \frac{\Delta E^{(2)}}{h\nu - \Delta E^{(1)}} + \cdots.$$

It is thus possible to write

$$B = B_0 + B_1 + B_2 + \cdots, \quad (7\text{-}45)$$

where, in terms of $a_\nu = A_\nu/g\beta$,

$$\begin{aligned} B_0 &= \frac{h\nu}{\Delta E^{(0)}} = \frac{h\nu}{g\beta} = b, \\ B_1 &= -\frac{\Delta E^{(1)}}{\Delta E^{(0)}} = -\sum_\mu a_\mu m_\mu^K, \\ B_2 &= \left\{\frac{1}{2}\sum_\mu [I_\mu(I_\mu + 1) - m_\mu^2]a_\mu^2\right\} \Big/ \left\{\frac{h\nu}{g\beta} - \sum_\nu a_\nu m_\nu\right\} \\ &\simeq \frac{1}{2b}\sum_\mu [I_\mu(I_\mu + 1) - m_\mu^2]a_\mu^2. \end{aligned} \quad (7\text{-}46)$$

The hyperfine coupling constants in units of field strength have been introduced for reasons of obvious simplification.

Equivalent Nuclei

Nuclei μ and ν are equivalent for present purposes if they have $I_\mu = I_\nu$, $\gamma_\mu = \gamma_\nu$, and $A_\mu = A_\nu$. The equality of coupling constants is usually a consequence of molecular symmetry, but may arise accidentally.

Suppose that contributions of second or higher order are negligible. The field strengths at which strongly allowed transitions occur will then be given by

$$B = b - \sum_\mu a_\mu m_\mu = b - \sum_k a_k \left(\sum_{\mu=1}^{N_k} m_{\nu k} \right), \qquad (7\text{-}47)$$

where a_k is the value of a_μ common to the N_k equivalent nuclei in the kth set, and $m_{\nu 1}, \ldots, m_{\nu N_k}$ are their spin projection quantum numbers. More than one state may in general have the same value of $\sum_{\mu=1}^{N_k} m_{\mu k}$, so there will be degeneracy.

The degeneracies which occur, and thus the relative intensities of the lines in the spectrum, depend on the number of equivalent nuclei and their spins. It is convenient to consider only one set of n equivalent nuclei with spin I. There will be $2nI + 1$ distinct values of the field strength at which transitions occur. Let $D_j(n, I)$ be the degeneracy of the jth nuclear spin state and thus the relative intensity of the jth transition in the group. It is convenient to let j assume values $0 \leq j \leq 2nI$.

It is clear that for a single nucleus

$$D_j(1, I) = 1, \qquad 0 \leq j \leq 2I. \qquad (7\text{-}48)$$

The values of D for larger n can then be obtained by recursion. As n is increased by 1, each of the existing states is split into $2I + 1$ levels. Most of these coincide with previously existing levels, however (cf. Fig. 0-2). A little consideration will show that

$$D_k(n + 1, I) = \sum_{j=0}^{2I} D_{k-j}(n, I) \qquad (7\text{-}49)$$

provided it is agreed that by convention

$$D_k(n, I) = 0, \qquad \text{if} \quad k < 0 \quad \text{or} \quad k > 2nI.$$

To find the values of the nonzero D's we introduce a generating function [55].

Consider the coefficient $C_l(n, M)$ defined by

$$f_n^M(x) \equiv (1 + x + x^2 + \cdots + x^M)^n \equiv \sum_{l=0}^{Mn} C_l(n, M)x^l. \qquad (7\text{-}50)$$

It is obvious that

$$f_{n+1}^{M}(x) = (1 + x + \cdots + x^M) f_n^M(x) = \sum_{l=0}^{M(n+1)} C_l(n+1, M) x^l$$

$$= \left(\sum_{k=0}^{nM} C_k(n, M) x^k\right)(1 + x + \cdots + x^M) = \sum_{k=0}^{nM} \sum_{j=0}^{M} C_k(n, M) x^{k+j}, \tag{7-51}$$

and thus that

$$C_l(n+1, M) = \begin{cases} \sum_{j=0}^{l} C_{l-j}(n, M), & \text{for } 1 \leq l \leq M, \\ \sum_{j=0}^{M} C_{l-j}(n, M), & \text{for } M \leq l \leq nM, \\ \sum_{j=l-Mn}^{M} C_{l-j}(n, M), & \text{for } nM \leq l \leq (n+1)M. \end{cases}$$

If a convention is agreed upon setting otherwise undefined C's equal to zero, as for the D's above, then the C's satisfy the same recursion formula as the D's. The values for $n = 1$ are clearly the same so we can identify $D_j(n, I) = C_j(n, 2I)$.

The generating function then provides a way of evaluating the coefficients. It is a power of the sum of a geometric series:

$$f_n^M(x) = \left(\sum_{j=0}^{M} x^j\right)^n = \left[\frac{1 - x^{M+1}}{1 - x}\right]^n \tag{7-52}$$

and thus

$$f_n^M(x) = \sum_{k=0}^{n} \sum_{p=0}^{\infty} (-1)^k \binom{n}{k} \binom{n - 1 + p}{n - 1} x^{(M+1)k+p}$$

$$= \sum_{l=0}^{(M+1)n} \left[\sum_{k=0}^{[l/(M+1)]} (-1)^k \binom{n}{k} \binom{n - 1 + l - (M+1)k}{n - 1}\right] x^l$$

$$+ \sum_{l=(M+1)n+1}^{\infty} \left[\sum_{k=0}^{n} (-1)^k \binom{n}{k} \binom{n - 1 + l - (M+1)k}{n - 1}\right] x^l \tag{7-53}$$

where $[l/(M + 1)]$ is the largest integer not exceeding $l/(M + 1)$. We know that in fact the highest power of x to occur in the expansion of $f_n^M(x)$ is x^{Mn}, and thus each of the terms in square brackets in the second sum on the right side must vanish. This can be verified. The expression in square brackets in the first sum provides an expression for $D_l(n, I)$:

$$D_l(n, I) = \sum_{k=0}^{[l/(2I+1)]} (-1)^k \binom{n}{k} \binom{n - 1 + l - (2I + 1)k}{n - 1}. \tag{7-54}$$

This should again give zero when $l > 2In$, and does. For practical computations it is usually more efficient to generate the D_k's from the recursion formula rather than use the general expression above. In the special case $I = \frac{1}{2}$ it is well known that the general expression reduces to

$$D_l(n, \tfrac{1}{2}) = \binom{n}{l}.$$

Second-Order Hyperfine Terms for Equivalent Nuclei

The degeneracies which exist in first order when there are equivalent nuclei will be at least partially lifted in second order. Some care must be taken in the second-order calculation, however, to assure the correct choice of zero- and first-order functions within the degenerate states.

The spin Hamiltonian can be written, in the presence of equivalent nuclei, as

$$\mathscr{H} = g\beta BS_z - \sum_k \gamma_k B\left(\sum_{\nu=1}^{N_k} I_{\nu k, z}\right) + \sum_k A_k \mathbf{S}\cdot\left(\sum_{\nu=1}^{N_k} \mathbf{I}_{\nu k}\right). \tag{7-55}$$

It is apparent when $\mathscr{H}$ is written in this form that it commutes with $I_k^2 = (\sum_{\nu=1}^{N_k} \mathbf{I}_{\nu k})^2$ for each k. The exact eigenfunctions of $\mathscr{H}$ will thus also be (or at least may be taken to be) eigenfunctions of the various I_k^2. This suggests that the I_k^2 eigenfunctions should provide a good basis set for the perturbation calculation.

Before attempting to determine how the correct treatment of equivalent nuclei is to be carried to second order, it may be well to consider a simple example to see that a problem does in fact exist. We consider the case of two equivalent nuclei of spin $\frac{1}{2}$, using expressions obtained above. The states can be characterized by m_a, m_b for the two nuclei or I, M_I for their combination. The results given in Table 7-1 are equivalent through first

TABLE 7-1

First- and Second-Order Transition Field Strengths for a System with Two Equivalent Spin $\frac{1}{2}$ Nuclei

Simple product function basis			I^2, I_z Eigenfunction basis		
State (m_a, m_b)	B_1	B_2	State (I, M_I)	B_1	B_2
$+\frac{1}{2}, +\frac{1}{2}$	$-a$	$a/2b$	0, 0	0	0
$+\frac{1}{2}, -\frac{1}{2}$	0	$a/2b$	1, 1	$-a$	$a/2b$
$-\frac{1}{2}, +\frac{1}{2}$	0	$a/2b$	1, 0	0	a/b
$-\frac{1}{2}, -\frac{1}{2}$	a	$a/2b$	1, -1	a	$a/2b$

order, each case predicting the well-known 1 : 2 : 1 triplet with a doubly degenerate center line. If second-order effects are not negligible, however, the two predictions differ. If the simple product functions are used, a shift of the whole pattern by $a/2b$ is predicted, but the pattern remains exactly symmetric and the two center lines are still exactly superimposed. If the I^2 eigenfunctions are used, on the other hand, the end lines are still shifted by $a/2b$ but the two components in the center are split, one being entirely unshifted and the other shifting by a/b. We must determine which (if either) of these predictions is correct.

In a perturbation problem it is well known that if a state is degenerate in zero order, the appropriate choice of zero-order function are those which diagonalize each block of the perturbation matrix **V** corresponding to a manifold of degenerate states. (Either the simple product basis or the I_k^2, I_{kz} eigenfunction basis will diagonalize the nuclear Zeeman term, so it presents no complications and will again not contribute to transition energies.) Suppose that the ith degenerate manifold contains g_i states. It is convenient to introduce a second state label so that

$$\mathscr{H}_0 \psi_{ij}^{(0)} = E_i^{(0)} \psi_{i,j}^{(0)}, \qquad j = 1, \ldots, g_i. \tag{7-56}$$

The $\psi_{i,j}^{(0)}$ are to be chosen so that

$$\langle \psi_{i,j}^{(0)} | V | \psi_{i,k}^{(0)} \rangle = E_{i,j}^{(1)} \delta_{jk} \tag{7-57}$$

as indicated, and the first-order energies are the eigenvalues of the blocks of **V**. Some degeneracy may persist, however. If

$$E_{i,j}^{(1)} = E_{i,k}^{(1)}, \qquad j, k = 1, \ldots, g_{ij} \leq g_i, \tag{7-58}$$

a third index can be introduced to label states $\psi_{i,j,k}^{(0)}$ so that

$$\langle \psi_{ijk}^{(0)} | V | \psi_{ijl}^{(0)} \rangle = E_{ij}^{(0)} \delta_{kl}, \qquad k = 1, \ldots, g_{ij}. \tag{7-59}$$

It can be shown [42,80] that for second- and higher-order calculations to proceed correctly, the degenerate states should be chosen so as to satisfy an additional condition

$$\sum_m{}' \frac{\langle \psi_{ijk}^{(0)} | V | \psi_m^{(0)} \rangle \langle \psi_m^{(0)} | \psi_{ijl}^{(0)} \rangle}{E_m^{(0)} - E_i^{(0)}} = 0, \qquad k \neq l. \tag{7-60}$$

The summation extends over states $\psi_m^{(0)}$ which are not degenerate in zero-order with the states under consideration. They may be degenerate within groups among themselves, in which case m might be replaced by a composite index.

The functions chosen to be I^2 eigenfunctions satisfy this condition. This can be seen as follows. The basis functions can be labeled by m_s and by $\{I_n, M_n, q_n\}$, where n labels a group of equivalent nuclei (possibly just one nucleus), I_n is the total nuclear spin for the group in this state, M_n is the M_I for the state of the group, and q_n, $1 \leq q_n \leq f_{i_n}(N_n, I_n)$, labels the particular choice of an I, M eigenfunction from among the f_{i_n} possible I, M eigenfunctions for a set of N_n nuclei of spin i_n.‡ It will be assumed that the states are chosen so that those with different values of q_n are orthogonal. It will then follow that any of the operators I_{nz}, $I_{n\pm}$ which occur in the spin Hamiltonian will have nonvanishing matrix elements only between states of the same I_n and q_n. The structure of the spin Hamiltonian matrix remains such that off-diagonal matrix elements occur only between states with different m_s values.

With these observations in mind we consider the second-order subsidiary condition of Eq. (7-60). For one term in the sum we must consider three states:

$$\psi_{ijk}^{(0)} = |m_s; \{I_n, M_n, q_n\}\rangle, \qquad \psi_{ijl}^{(0)} = |m_s'; \{I_n', M_n', q_n'\}\rangle,$$

$$\psi_{m}^{(0)} = |m_s''; \{I_n'', M_n'', q_n''\}\rangle.$$

If the first matrix element of the numerator product is to be nonzero, it is necessary that $|m_s - m_s''| = 1$, $I_n = I_n''$ and $q_n = q_n''$ for all n, $|M_r - M_r''| = 1$ for some r, and $M_n = M_n''$ for all $n \neq r$. In particular, if $m_s'' = m_s \pm 1$ then $M_r'' = M_r \mp 1$. Similarly for the second matrix element of the product to be nonzero, $I_n' = I_n''$ and $q_n' = q_n''$ for all n, $m_s'' = m_s' \pm 1$, $M_t'' = M_t' \mp 1$ for some t and $M_n'' = M_n'$ for all $n \neq t$. We are interested in the case when $k \neq l$, i.e., the two states are not identical, so it is not possible that $r = t$ or the conditions relating m_s to M would make $M_r = M_r'$ and all the M's would be the same. The condition for a nonzero contribution of the term becomes $M_r' - M_r = M_t - M_t'$, $r \neq t$. The two states contribute to the sum of interest only if they are degenerate in first order. This then requires that $(M_r - M_r')(A_r - A_t) = 0$ and $(M_t - M_t')(A_t - A_r) = 0$, or $A_r = A_t$. This is a combination of conditions, that two nonequivalent nuclei have the same coupling constant, which can be met only accidentally. Such a special case is unlikely and will in fact cause no difficulty. The conclusion is that the I^2 eigenfunction basis satisfies the condition of Eq. (7-60) and is thus the appropriate basis for the second-order calculation.

We conclude that if second-order effects are nonnegligible, the zero-order functions should be chosen to be eigenfunctions of the square of the total nuclear spin for each group of equivalent nuclei. Previously derived expressions with appropriate I values will then give the correct line positions. We must still consider the question of relative intensities. The relative intensities of lines which coincide through second-order will again be determined by

‡ This number will be discussed for the spin $\frac{1}{2}$ case in connection with electron spin coupling in Chapter III. A recursion formula for the general result is presented below.

their degeneracies. We are thus led to consider the question of how many independent states exist for a given I_{total}, M_{total} in a set of N equivalent nuclei of spin I. The formula is well known when $I = \frac{1}{2}$:

$$f_{1/2}(N, I_{\text{total}}) = \begin{pmatrix} N \\ \frac{N}{2} - I_{\text{total}} \end{pmatrix} - \begin{pmatrix} N \\ \frac{N}{2} - I - 1 \end{pmatrix}. \tag{7-61}$$

This result will be discussed in Chapter III in connection with many-electron spin states. Systems with large numbers of equivalent nuclei with $I > \frac{1}{2}$ do not commonly occur and it is probably not worthwhile to obtain general expressions. Required values can be obtained recursively from

$$f_i(1, I = 1) = 1, \qquad f_i(N, I) = \sum_{\substack{I' \ni \\ I' + i \geq I \geq |I' - i|}} f_i(N - 1, I'). \tag{7-62}$$

These results can be summarized as follows: at a fixed frequency, ν, the field strengths B at which resonance will occur are given by

$$B = B_0 + B_1 + B_2 + \cdots$$

with

$$B_0 = \frac{h\nu}{g\beta} = b, \qquad B_1 = -\sum_k a_k M_k, \qquad B_2 = \frac{1}{2b}\sum_k a_k^2[I_k(I_k + 1) - M_k^2]. \tag{7-63}$$

The index k labels a group of equivalent nuclei with coupling constant (in field-strength units) a_k, and I_k, M_k are the total spin and spin-projection quantum numbers for that group in the given nuclear spin state. The relative intensity of the line is given by $f_{i_k}(N_k, I_k)$, the number of distinct states contributing at the same position. If B_2 is negligible the resonance field is independent of I_k and the relative intensity is given by $D_l(N_k, i_k)$ for the kth group. These results reduce to those given previously when each group consists of a single nucleus. Situations which arise from accidental overlap of lines have not been considered and cannot be dealt with in any general way.

The second-order contribution to B is clearly independent of the sign of M_I. Thus a consideration of the field difference

$$\Delta B(|M_k|) = B(|M_k|, M_j\,(j \neq k)) - B(-|M_k|, M_j\,(j \neq k)) = -2|M_k|a_k \tag{7-64}$$

for a given I_k, M_k shows that the coupling constants can be directly related to line position differences even when second-order effects are not negligible.

A still greater simplification occurs when $i = \frac{1}{2}$ [54]. In this case the "center of gravity" of the lines associated with a given M is in fact independent of M. If the second-order splittings are not resolved, the second-order effect is simply a uniform (small) shift of the entire spectrum. A proof of this fact is straightforward, but some additional notation will simplify the presentation. We will consider only one group of nuclei, for simplicity.

Define a quantity proportional to the second-order shift,

$$\delta(I, M) = 2[I(I + 1) - M^2], \tag{7-65}$$

and use $f_{1/2}$ as given by Eq. (7-61). The total number of states with a given M value will be

$$d(N, M) = \sum_{I=M}^{N/2} f_{1/2}(N, I) = \binom{N}{\frac{N}{2} - M}. \tag{7-66}$$

The summation limits follow from the fact that $I \geq M$ and $I_{max} = N/2$ for $i = \frac{1}{2}$. The second equality comes from the fact that $d(N, M)$ must be equal to the number of choices of $N/2 - M$ nuclei to have $m = -\frac{1}{2}$ and $N/2 + M$ nuclei to have $m = +\frac{1}{2}$ from among the N equivalent spin $\frac{1}{2}$ nuclei. If we further define

$$C(N, M) = \sum_{I=M}^{N/2} \delta(I, M) f_{1/2}(N, I), \tag{7-67}$$

then the required center of gravity will be proportional to $C(N, M)/d(N, M)$.

It is convenient to introduce new variables j and k with $M = N/2 - k$ and $I = N/2 - j$. Then

$$f(N, j) = f_{1/2}(N, N/2 - j) = \binom{N}{j} - \binom{N}{j-1},$$

$$\delta(N, j, k) = \delta\left(\frac{N}{2} - j, \frac{N}{2} - k\right) = 2(j + k - N)(j - k) + N - 2j, \tag{7-68}$$

$$C(N, k) = \sum_{j=0}^{k} \delta(N, j, k) f(N, j), \qquad d(N, k) = \sum_{j=0}^{k} f(N, j) = \binom{N}{k}.$$

It should be noted that for $j = 0$, $I = N/2$, and $f(N, 0) = 1$. We now consider $C(N, k + 1)$, which we can write as

$$C(N, k + 1) = \sum_{j=0}^{k} \delta(N, j, k) f(N, j) + \sum_{j=0}^{k} [\delta(N, j, k + 1) - \delta(N, j, k)] f(N, j)$$
$$+ \delta(N, k + 1, k + 1) f(N, k + 1) \tag{7-69}$$

and note that

$$[\delta(N, j, k + 1) - \delta(N, j, k)] = 2(N - 2k - 1)$$

is independent of j so it can be factored out of the sum to give a term proportional to $d(N, k)$. The first term on the right in Eq. (7-69) is just $C(N, k)$, and substitutions can be made in the third term to give

$$C(N, k + 1) = C(N, k) + 2(N - 2k + 1)d(N, k) + (N - 2k - 2)\frac{N - 2k - 1}{k + 1}\binom{N}{k}. \qquad (7\text{-}70)$$

If we now assume that $C(N, k) = Nd(N, k) = N\binom{N}{k}$, we have

$$C(N, k + 1) = \left[N - (N - 2k - 1)\left(2 + \frac{N - 2k - 2}{k + 1}\right)\right]\binom{N}{k}$$

$$= \frac{N(N - k)}{k + 1}\binom{N}{k} = N\binom{N}{k + 1} = Nd(N, k + 1). \qquad (7\text{-}71)$$

When $k = 0$, $C(N, 0) = \delta(N, 0, 0)f(N, 0) = N$, and $d(N, 0) = 1$. The result we have now proved by induction,

$$C(N, k)/d(N, k) = N, \qquad (7\text{-}72)$$

is of the form claimed above.

It would be straightforward to carry the perturbation treatments beyond second-order [80]. The results will be rather messy, however, and a higher-order treatment is not necessary to accurately describe the results in the normal experimental situation. It is of course always possible to proceed by direct numerical diagonalization of the spin Hamiltonian matrix.

Nearly Degenerate Electronic States

In our discussion thus far it has been implicitly assumed, in using a spin Hamiltonian of the form given in Eq. (7-3), that the state we are dealing with is an $\mathcal{S}^2$ eigenfunction. This is not necessarily always the case. As an example we will consider a "biradical"—i.e., a system composed of two weakly interacting doublet subsystems or equivalently a system with nearly degenerate singlet and triplet states [165]. The isotropic description of a pure triplet state can be obtained as a limiting case.

The spin Hamiltonian commonly used in this case is

$$\mathcal{H} = g\beta B(s_{1z} + s_{2z}) + J\mathbf{s}_1 \cdot \mathbf{s}_2 + \sum_\nu \gamma_\nu B I_{\nu z} + \sum_\nu A_{\nu 1}\mathbf{s}_1 \cdot \mathbf{I}_\nu + \sum_\nu A_{\nu 2}\mathbf{s}_2 \cdot \mathbf{I}_\nu. \qquad (7\text{-}73)$$

It includes the terms to be expected for two electrons and an additional term $J\mathbf{s}_1 \cdot \mathbf{s}_2$ in which J is the singlet–triplet separation energy ${}^3E - {}^1E$. Each summation over nuclei ν runs over all the nuclei in the system. Note that if $A_{\nu 1} \neq A_{\nu 2}$ this spin Hamiltonian is not symmetric in the electron indices. It is often the case that the nuclei fall into two groups such that $A_{\nu 1} \simeq 0$ for ν in one group and $A_{\nu 2} \simeq 0$ for ν in the other group. This lack of symmetry seems rather strange. It must be remembered, however, that the only basic requirement for a spin Hamiltonian is that it reproduce the correct matrix. It will be shown in a later section how such a nonsymmetric spin Hamiltonian can arise from a full Hamiltonian which is symmetric with respect to electron interchanges. For the present discussion, as with the previous treatments in this section, we will simply take the spin Hamiltonian as given and investigate the resultant spectral predictions.

To discuss this case it is convenient to write the spin Hamiltonian as

$$\mathscr{H} = \mathscr{H}_0 + \mathscr{H}' + \mathscr{U} + \mathscr{V}_1 + \mathscr{V}_2 \tag{7-74}$$

with

$$\mathscr{H}_0 = g\beta B(s_{1z} + s_{2z}), \qquad \mathscr{H}' = \sum_\nu \gamma_\nu B I_{\nu z},$$

$$\mathscr{U} = J\mathbf{s}_1 \cdot \mathbf{s}_2, \qquad \mathscr{V}_i = \sum_\nu A_{\nu i}\mathbf{s}_i \cdot \mathbf{I}_\nu, \qquad i = 1, 2.$$

The terms $\mathscr{H}'$ and $\mathscr{V}_i$ are expected to be small compared with $\mathscr{H}_0$. The Heisenberg exchange term $\mathscr{U}$ may range from being smaller than $\mathscr{V}_i$ to being larger than $\mathscr{H}_0$. It is convenient to introduce basis functions $|S, M_S, K\rangle$ which are eigenfunctions of $\mathscr{S}^2 = (\mathbf{s}_1 + \mathbf{s}_2)^2$ and $S_z = s_{1z} + s_{2z}$, and of $I_{\nu z}$ for each nucleus. The eigenvalues are $S(S+1)$, M_S, and m_ν^K, respectively.

Since

$$\mathscr{H}_0 = g\beta B S_z \tag{7-75}$$

and

$$\mathscr{U} = \frac{J}{2}(\mathscr{S}^2 - \tfrac{3}{2}), \tag{7-76}$$

these functions will be eigenfunctions of $\mathscr{H}_0$ and $\mathscr{U}$. They are also eigenfunctions of $\mathscr{H}'$, and thus only the $\mathscr{V}_i$ will have off-diagonal matrix elements.

The matrix elements of $\mathscr{H}_0$, $\mathscr{H}'$, and $\mathscr{U}$ are‡

$$\begin{aligned}
\langle S, M_S, K|\mathscr{H}_0|S', M_S', K'\rangle &= g\beta B M_S \delta_{SS'}\delta_{M_S M_S'}\delta_{KK'} \\
\langle S, M_S, K|\mathscr{H}'|S', M_S', K'\rangle &= \left(\sum_\nu m_\nu^K \gamma_\nu\right) B\delta_{SS'}\delta_{M_S M_S'}\delta_{KK'} \\
\langle S, M_S, K|\mathscr{U}|S', M_S', K'\rangle &= (S - \tfrac{3}{4})J\delta_{SS'}\delta_{M_S M_S'}\delta_{KK'}.
\end{aligned} \tag{7-77}$$

‡ The simplified result given for $\mathscr{U}$ is valid only for $S = 0$ or 1, the possible values in this case.

The matrix elements of $\mathscr{V}_1$ and $\mathscr{V}_2$ are also readily determined. The matrix elements of hyperfine operators for spin $\frac{1}{2}$ states have been considered above, and

$$|1, 1, K\rangle = |m_1 = \tfrac{1}{2}, m_2 = \tfrac{1}{2}; K\rangle,$$

$$|1, 0, K\rangle = (1/\sqrt{2})(|m_1 = \tfrac{1}{2}, m_2 = -\tfrac{1}{2}; K\rangle + |m_1 = -\tfrac{1}{2}, m_2 = \tfrac{1}{2}; K\rangle),$$

$$|1, -1, K\rangle = |m_1 = -\tfrac{1}{2}, m_2 = -\tfrac{1}{2}, K\rangle,$$

$$|0, 0, K\rangle = (1/\sqrt{2})(|m_1 = \tfrac{1}{2}, m_2 = -\tfrac{1}{2}, K\rangle - |m_1 = -\tfrac{1}{2}, m_2 = \tfrac{1}{2}; K\rangle). \tag{7-78}$$

It follows that the nonzero matrix elements of $\mathscr{V}_i$ in the S, M_S basis are, on the diagonal

$$\langle 1, M_S, K|\mathscr{V}_i|1, M_S, K\rangle = \frac{1}{2} M_S \sum_\nu A_{\nu i} m_\nu^K$$

and off-diagonal

$$\langle 0, 0, K|\mathscr{V}_i|1, 0, K\rangle = \frac{\varepsilon_i}{2} \sum_\nu A_{\nu i},$$

$$\langle 1, 1, K_\nu^-|\mathscr{V}_i|0, 0, K\rangle = -\frac{\varepsilon_i}{2} \sum_\nu A_{\nu i} f_\nu^-(K),$$

$$\langle 1, 1, K_\nu^-|\mathscr{V}_i|1, 0, K\rangle = \frac{1}{2\sqrt{2}} \sum_\nu A_{\nu i} f_\nu^-(K), \tag{7-79}$$

$$\langle 1, 0, K_\nu^-|\mathscr{V}_i|1, -1, K\rangle = \frac{1}{2\sqrt{2}} \sum_\nu A_{\nu i} f_\nu^-(K),$$

$$\langle 0, 0, K_\nu^-|\mathscr{V}_i|1, -1, K\rangle = \frac{\varepsilon_i}{2\sqrt{2}} \sum_\nu A_{\nu i} f_\nu^-(K),$$

where we have defined $\varepsilon_i = +1$ if $i = 1$, $\varepsilon_i = -1$ if $i = 2$,

$$f_\nu^\pm(K) = [I_\nu(I_\nu + 1) - m_\nu^K(m_\nu^K \pm 1)]^{1/2} \tag{7-80}$$

and $K_\nu^\pm$ differs from K in that m_ν is replaced by $m_\nu \pm 1$. The matrix is symmetric, so only half the elements are given explicitly. The others can be more conveniently expressed in terms of K^+ and $f^+(K)$.

Energies through first order can readily be obtained without the necessity of specifying too precisely what is the zero-order Hamiltonian and what is the perturbation. The Hamiltonian matrix (including all perturbations) is conveniently considered in blocks corresponding to the M_S values. The blocks corresponding to $S = 1$, $M_S = \pm 1$ are diagonal, and the off-diagonal elements of magnitude $A_{\nu i}$ linking them to other blocks are small compared to the differences between corresponding diagonal elements, which are of magnitude $g\beta B$. Consequently, to first order

$$\begin{aligned} E_{1,1,K} &= g\beta B + \tfrac{1}{4}J + \Gamma(K)B + \tfrac{1}{2}\Sigma(K), \\ E_{1,-1,K} &= -g\beta B + \tfrac{1}{4}J + \Gamma(K)B - \tfrac{1}{2}\Sigma(K), \end{aligned} \tag{7-81}$$

where

$$\Gamma(K) = \sum_{\nu} m_{\nu}^{K}\gamma_{\nu} \tag{7-82}$$

is the nuclear Zeeman energy per unit field strength and

$$\Sigma(K) = \sum_{\nu} (A_{\nu 1} + A_{\nu 2})m_{\nu}^{K} \tag{7-83}$$

is related to the hyperfine energy. These terms are the only ones which depend on the nuclear spin state and which split the degeneracies within each of the blocks.

The two blocks with $M_S = 0$ and $S = 0$ or 1 have diagonal elements of order $A_{\nu i}$. Since in some cases $J \lesssim A_{\nu i}$, the methods of degenerate perturbation theory must be used here. There are no nonvanishing matrix elements linking states both having $M_S = 0$ but with differing nuclear spin states. The secular equation within the $M_S = 0$ block thus factors into a set of 2×2 subblocks, one corresponding to each nuclear spin state. These subblocks are

$$\begin{pmatrix} \tfrac{1}{4}J + \Gamma(K)B - E & \tfrac{1}{2}\Delta(K) \\ \tfrac{1}{2}\Delta(K) & -\tfrac{3}{4}J + \Gamma(K)B - E \end{pmatrix} \begin{pmatrix} C_{1,0,K} \\ C_{0,0,K} \end{pmatrix} = 0, \tag{7-84}$$

where

$$\Delta(K) = \sum_{\nu} (A_{\nu 1} - A_{\nu 2})m_{\nu}^{K}$$

would vanish if the two electrons were treated equivalently. The eigenfunctions and eigenvalues, which we label by a and b, are

$$\begin{aligned} |a, K\rangle &= \cos\theta_K |1, 0, K\rangle + \sin\theta_K |0, 0, K\rangle \\ |b, K\rangle &= -\sin\theta_K |1, 0, K\rangle + \cos\theta_K |0, 0, K\rangle \end{aligned} \tag{7-85}$$

with θ_K defined by

$$\tan 2\theta_K = \frac{\Delta(K)}{J} \tag{7-86}$$

and

$$\begin{aligned} E_{a,K} &= \Gamma(K)B - \tfrac{1}{4}J + \tfrac{1}{2}([\Delta(K)]^2 + J^2)^{1/2}, \\ E_{b,K} &= \Gamma(K)B - \tfrac{1}{4}J - \tfrac{1}{2}([\Delta(K)]^2 + J_2)^{1/2}. \end{aligned} \tag{7-87}$$

TABLE 7-2

Transitions in a Biradical

Transition	Relative intensity	ΔE (through first-order)[a]
$\|1, 1, K\rangle \leftarrow \|a, k\rangle$	$\cos^2 \theta_K$	$g\beta B + \frac{1}{2}J + \frac{1}{2}\Sigma(K) - \frac{1}{2}(\Delta^2 + J^2)^{1/2}$
$\|1, 1, K\rangle \leftarrow \|b, K\rangle$	$\sin^2 \theta_K$	$g\beta B + \frac{1}{2}J + \frac{1}{2}\Sigma(K) + \frac{1}{2}(\Delta^2 + J^2)^{1/2}$
$\|a, K\rangle \leftarrow \|1, -1, K\rangle$	$\cos^2 \theta_K$	$g\beta B - \frac{1}{2}J + \frac{1}{2}\Sigma(K) + \frac{1}{2}(\Delta^2 + J^2)^{1/2}$
$\|b, K\rangle \leftarrow \|1, -1, K\rangle$	$\sin^2 \theta_K$	$g\beta B - \frac{1}{2}J + \frac{1}{2}\Sigma(K) - \frac{1}{2}(\Delta^2 + J^2)^{1/2}$

[a] $\Delta = \Delta(K)$.

Transition probabilities are assumed to be proportional to the square of the matrix element of $S_x = s_{1x} + s_{2x}$ between the two states involved. These are readily obtained. The results are given in Table 7-2. Since in this level of approximation transitions occur only between states of the same K, the nuclear Zeeman contribution $\Gamma(K)$ again cancels out completely from the transitions energies.

The behavior in limiting cases is readily understood. If $|J| \gg |\Delta(K)|$ for all K, then $\theta_K \sim 0$ and $|a, K\rangle \sim |1, 0, K\rangle$, $|b, K\rangle \sim |0, 0, K\rangle$. Transitions involving the b or singlet state vanish and those which remain describe the triplet state transitions with $\Delta E = g\beta B + \frac{1}{2}\Sigma(K)$ for both the $-1 \to 0$ and $0 \to 1$ transitions. In the other limit $|J| \ll |\Delta(K)|$ for all K, $|\theta_K| \sim \pi/4$ so

$$|a, K\rangle \sim (1/\sqrt{2})(|1, 0, K\rangle + |0, 0, K\rangle) = |\tfrac{1}{2}, \tfrac{1}{2}, K\rangle;$$
$$|b, K\rangle \sim (1/\sqrt{2})(-|1, 0, K\rangle + |0, 0, K\rangle) = -|-\tfrac{1}{2}, \tfrac{1}{2}, K\rangle.$$

The electrons are essentially decoupled in this case. The four transitions are of equal intensity and occur in pairs. Those involving $1, -1 \to a$ and $b \to 1, 1$ are electron 1 transitions and have

$$\Delta E_1 = g\beta B + \tfrac{1}{2}\Sigma(K) + \tfrac{1}{2}\Delta(K) = g\beta B + \sum_{\nu} A_{\nu 1} m_\nu^K, \tag{7-88}$$

while those involving $a \to 1, 1$ and $1, -1 \to b$ are electron 2 transitions with

$$\Delta E_2 = g\beta B + \tfrac{1}{2}\Sigma(K) - \tfrac{1}{2}\Delta(K) = g\beta B + \sum_{\nu} A_{\nu 2} m_\nu^K. \tag{7-89}$$

Extension to second order is straightforward in the limiting cases by the methods discussed above. For intermediate values of J a second-order contribution to the transition energy can be easily evaluated in any particular case but a general treatment is not sufficiently informative to be worth the trouble involved. When results are retained only through first order, B occurs linearly in the energy-difference expression, so transformation to a fixed-frequency situation is trivial.

Since there are four electronic states involved in this system, one might inquire whether a spin Hamiltonian can be constructed with an effective spin of $\frac{3}{2}$. We will examine the question in the simplest possible case: no hyperfine interactions.

In this case there are just four energy levels

$$E_1 = g\beta B + \tfrac{1}{4}J, \qquad E_2 = \tfrac{1}{4}J, \qquad E_3 = -\tfrac{3}{4}J, \qquad E_4 = -g\beta B + \tfrac{1}{4}J. \quad (7\text{-}90)$$

The appropriate basis functions are $|S = \frac{3}{2}, M_S\rangle$ and they can be taken as eigenfunctions of a spin Hamiltonian

$$\mathscr{H} = (\tfrac{1}{6}g\beta B - \tfrac{1}{2}J)S_z^3 + \tfrac{1}{4}JS_z^2 + (-\tfrac{1}{24}g\beta B + \tfrac{9}{8}J)S_z - \tfrac{5}{16}J, \quad (7\text{-}91)$$

which will reproduce the correct energy levels. The selection rules are not correctly given by matrix elements of S_x, however, because in the two-electron, singlet–triplet basis $S_x = s_{1x} + s_{2x}$ has a matrix

$$\begin{pmatrix} 0 & 1 & 0 & 0 \\ 1 & 0 & 1 & 0 \\ 0 & 1 & 0 & 0 \\ 0 & 0 & 0 & 0 \end{pmatrix},$$

while for the $S = \frac{3}{2}$ basis the matrix of S_x is

$$\begin{pmatrix} 0 & 1 & 0 & 0 \\ 1 & 0 & 1 & 0 \\ 0 & 1 & 0 & 1 \\ 0 & 0 & 1 & 0 \end{pmatrix}.$$

Further, it is not possible to take a linear combination of the $S = \frac{3}{2}$ states as spin Hamiltonian eigenfunctions so as to regain the desired S_x. The $S = \frac{3}{2}$ matrix has eigenvalues $(\frac{3}{2} \pm \sqrt{5}/2)^{1/2}$, $-(\frac{3}{2} \pm \sqrt{5}/2)^{1/2}$ while the singlet–triplet S_x matrix has eigenvalues 0, 0, $\pm\sqrt{2}$. No unitary transformation can change the eigenvalues of a matrix, so the two cannot be made equivalent.

Nonisotropic Spin Hamiltonians

We consider now situations in which the tensors linking the spins to each other and to the field are not necessarily isotropic. For the sake of simplicity, however, we will continue to treat the nuclear Zeeman interaction as isotropic. In addition, we will initially follow the usual procedure and assume all the tensors to be symmetric. At the end of this section the effect of possible antisymmetric components will be briefly considered. The question of the symmetry of these tensors will be considered in Section 9.

For $S = \frac{1}{2}$ and initially neglecting nuclear quadrupole effects, we take the spin Hamiltonian to be

$$\mathscr{H} = \beta \mathbf{S} \cdot \mathbf{g} \cdot \mathbf{B} - \sum_{\nu} \gamma_{\nu} I_z^{\nu} B + \sum_{\nu} \mathbf{S} \cdot \mathbf{A}^{\nu} \cdot \mathbf{I}^{\nu}, \tag{7-92}$$

where again the direction of the magnetic field B is taken to define the z axis. We also consider

$$\mathbf{g} = g_e \mathbf{1} + \Delta \mathbf{g}, \tag{7-93}$$

where g_e is the free electron value 2.002319..., and $\Delta \mathbf{g}$ is presumed to be small for free radicals.

As a first step in obtaining the eigenvalues of this spin Hamiltonian we obtain matrices in a convenient basis and write, as in Eq. (7-33),

$$\mathbf{H} = \mathbf{H}_0 + \mu \mathbf{H}' + \lambda \mathbf{V},$$

$$\mathscr{H}_0 = \beta \mathbf{S} \cdot \mathbf{g} \cdot \hat{\mathbf{B}} = \beta \mathbf{S} \cdot \mathbf{g} \cdot \hat{\mathbf{z}}, \qquad \mathscr{H}' = -\sum_{\nu} \gamma_{\nu} I_z^{\nu}, \qquad \mathscr{V} = \sum_{\nu} \mathbf{S} \cdot \mathbf{A}^{\nu} \cdot \mathbf{I}^{\nu}. \tag{7-94}$$

We note that the eigenvalues of $\mathbf{H}$ must be multiplied by B to obtain eigenvalues of $\mathscr{H}$, $\lambda = 1/B$, μ is a formal parameter to be set equal to 1, and $\hat{\mathbf{z}}$ is a unit vector in the field (z) direction.

We start again with the simple product basis $|m_s, K\rangle$, and determine matrix elements of the various terms. For $\mathscr{H}_0$ we have

$$\langle \tfrac{1}{2}, J | \mathscr{H}_0 | \tfrac{1}{2}, K \rangle = \frac{\beta}{2} (g_e + \Delta g_{zz}) \delta_{JK},$$

$$\langle -\tfrac{1}{2}, J | \mathscr{H}_0 | -\tfrac{1}{2}, K \rangle = -\frac{\beta}{2} (g_e + \Delta g_{zz}) \delta_{JK}, \tag{7-95}$$

$$\langle \tfrac{1}{2}, J | \mathscr{H}_0 | -\tfrac{1}{2}, K \rangle = \langle -\tfrac{1}{2}, J | \mathscr{H}_0 | \tfrac{1}{2}, K \rangle^* = \frac{\beta}{2} (\Delta g_{xz} - i \Delta g_{yz}) \delta_{JK}.$$

The matrix $\mathbf{H}_0$ is thus block diagonal with each nuclear spin state K corresponding to one block, and all the blocks are identical. The matrix elements of $\mathscr{H}'$ are

$$\langle \tfrac{1}{2}, J | \mathscr{H}' | \tfrac{1}{2}, K \rangle = \langle -\tfrac{1}{2}, J | \mathscr{H}' | -\tfrac{1}{2}, K \rangle = -\left(\sum_{\nu} \gamma_{\nu} m_{\nu}^{K} \right) \delta_{JK},$$

$$\langle \tfrac{1}{2}, J | \mathscr{H}' | -\tfrac{1}{2}, K \rangle = \langle -\tfrac{1}{2}, J | \mathscr{H}' | \tfrac{1}{2}, K \rangle = 0. \tag{7-96}$$

The simple product basis thus diagonalizes $\mathbf{H}'$.

In considering the matrix elements of $\mathscr{V}$ it is convenient to partition the basis according to m_s and accordingly partition $\mathbf{V}$ as

$$\mathbf{V} = \begin{pmatrix} \mathbf{V}^{aa} & \mathbf{V}^{ab} \\ \mathbf{V}^{ba} & \mathbf{V}^{bb} \end{pmatrix}. \tag{7-97}$$

The superscripts a and b refer to $m_s = \frac{1}{2}$ and $m_s = -\frac{1}{2}$ respectively. It is readily shown that, if the same ordering of nuclear spin states is used for the a states and the b states, then $\mathbf{V}^{bb} = -\mathbf{V}^{aa}$. It also follows from the Hermiticity of $\mathbf{V}$ that $\mathbf{V}^{ba} = \mathbf{V}^{ab\dagger}$. We again introduce the symbol $K_\nu^\pm$ to denote the nuclear spin state which differs from the state K only in that m_ν^K is replaced by $m_\nu^K \pm 1$, and use $f_\nu^\pm(K)$ as defined by Eq. (7-80). (If $I_\nu = \frac{1}{2}$, the only nonzero value of $f_\nu^\pm$ is 1; while if $I_\nu = 1$, $f_\nu^\pm$ is 0 or $\sqrt{2}$.) The nonzero elements of $\mathbf{V}^{aa}$ can then be written

$$\begin{aligned}
\langle \tfrac{1}{2}, K | \mathscr{V} | \tfrac{1}{2}, K \rangle &= \tfrac{1}{2} \sum_\nu A_{zz}^\nu m_\nu^K, \\
\langle \tfrac{1}{2}, K_\mu^+ | \mathscr{V} | \tfrac{1}{2}, K \rangle &= \tfrac{1}{2} f_\mu^+(K)(A_{xz}^\mu - iA_{yz}^\mu), \\
\langle \tfrac{1}{2}, K_\mu^- | \mathscr{V} | \tfrac{1}{2}, K \rangle &= \tfrac{1}{4} f_\mu^-(K)(A_{xz}^\mu + iA_{yz}^\mu),
\end{aligned} \tag{7-98}$$

while those of $\mathbf{V}^{ab}$ are

$$\begin{aligned}
\langle \tfrac{1}{2}, K | \mathscr{V} | -\tfrac{1}{2}, K \rangle &= \tfrac{1}{2} \sum_\nu (A_{xz}^\nu - iA_{yz}^\nu) m_\nu^K, \\
\langle \tfrac{1}{2}, K_\mu^+ | \mathscr{V} | -\tfrac{1}{2}, K \rangle &= \tfrac{1}{4} f_\mu^+(K)(A_{xx}^\mu - A_{yy}^\mu - 2iA_{xy}^\mu), \\
\langle \tfrac{1}{2}, K_\mu^- | \mathscr{V} | -\tfrac{1}{2}, K \rangle &= \tfrac{1}{4} f_\mu^-(K)(A_{xx}^\mu + A_{yy}^\mu).
\end{aligned} \tag{7-99}$$

If a numerical solution is sufficient, this spin Hamiltonian problem, like all spin Hamiltonian problems, can be readily solved once the matrix elements are given. We want to find a (possibly approximate) analytic solution, however. In addition to providing a basis for understanding, an analytic form is necessary if we are to invert the solution to obtain resonance fields at a fixed frequency. The treatment presented here will differ somewhat from those commonly used in obtaining spin Hamiltonian parameters from experimental data.‡

Since a complete, analytic solution in closed form is not in general possible, a perturbation treatment suggests itself, as in the multinuclear, isotropic case above. There is a difficulty, however. There are only two distinct eigenvalues for $\mathscr{H}_0$, so the methods of degenerate perturbation theory must be used. There are two perturbations: $\mu\mathscr{H}'$ and $\lambda\mathscr{V}$. These two perturbations do not commute and a degenerate, double perturbation problem in which

‡ The simple perturbation methods discussed later provide a basis for some of the commonly used methods. See, e.g., Farach and Poole [53] and Weil and Anderson [205–207].

the permutations do not commute cannot be solved. (That is, a solution as a double power series in the perturbation parameters does not exist.) In the isotropic case, **V** has no off-diagonal matrix elements within the degenerate block in the simple product basis which also diagonalizes **H**′, so blocks of **H**′ and **V** did commute. When **A** is nonisotropic, **V** and **H**′ cannot be simultaneously diagonalized.

Before proceeding with alternate treatments, we will find it instructive to consider the perturbation treatment when $\mathscr{H}'$ is neglected. The results of such a treatment will be usefully valid when hyperfine interactions are much larger than nuclear Zeeman energies.

Zero-Order Problem

In the simple spin product basis, $\mathbf{H}_0$ can be reduced by appropriate permutations of state ordering to a series of identical 2×2 blocks, one for each K. They are

$$\langle i|\mathscr{H}_0|j\rangle$$

$$\begin{array}{ll} i = & j = \quad \tfrac{1}{2}K \qquad\qquad -\tfrac{1}{2}K \\ \tfrac{1}{2}, K & \\ -\tfrac{1}{2}, K & \end{array} \frac{\beta}{2}\begin{pmatrix} g_e + \Delta g_{zz} & \Delta g_{xz} - i\Delta g_{yz} \\ \Delta g_{xz} + i\Delta g_{yz} & -g_e - \Delta g_{zz} \end{pmatrix}$$

and there are thus two distinct zero-order energies

$$E^{(0)} = \pm \frac{\beta}{2}\bar{g}, \tag{7-100}$$

where

$$\bar{g} = [(\Delta g_{xz})^2 + (\Delta g_{yz})^2 + (g_e + \Delta g_{zz})^2]^{1/2}. \tag{7-101}$$

The zero-order eigenfunctions are, correspondingly,

$$\begin{aligned} |1, K\rangle &= \cos\theta|\tfrac{1}{2}, K\rangle + \sin\theta\, e^{-i\chi}|-\tfrac{1}{2}, K\rangle, \\ |2, K\rangle &= -\sin\theta\, e^{i\chi}|\tfrac{1}{2}, K\rangle + \cos\theta|-\tfrac{1}{2}, K\rangle, \end{aligned} \tag{7-102}$$

where θ and χ are defined by

$$\tan 2\theta = \frac{[(\Delta g_{xz})^2 + (\Delta g_{yz})^2]^{1/2}}{g_e + \Delta g_{zz}}, \qquad \tan\chi = \frac{\Delta g_{yz}}{\Delta g_{xz}}. \tag{7-103}$$

Matrix elements of $\mathscr{V}$ (and of $\mathscr{H}'$) in the $\{|1, K\rangle, |2, K\rangle\}$ basis are then readily obtained. If the hyperfine matrix in the new basis is denoted by $\overline{\mathbf{V}}$, and it is again partitioned as in Eq. (7-97), it remains true that $\overline{\mathbf{V}}^{bb} = -\overline{\mathbf{V}}^{aa}$ and $\overline{\mathbf{V}}^{ba} = (\overline{\mathbf{V}}^{ab})^\dagger$.

The nonzero matrix elements of $\bar{\mathbf{V}}^{aa}$ are

$$\begin{aligned}
\bar{V}^{aa}_{KK} &= \langle 1, K|\mathscr{V}|1, K\rangle \\
&= \tfrac{1}{2}\sum_{\nu} [\cos 2\theta\, A^{\nu}_{zz} + \sin 2\theta(\cos\chi\, A^{\nu}_{xz} - \sin\chi\, A^{\nu}_{yz})]m^{K}_{\nu}, \\
\bar{V}^{aa}_{K^{\pm}_{\mu}K} &= \langle 1, K^{\pm}_{\mu}|\mathscr{V}|1, K\rangle \qquad (7\text{-}104)\\
&= \tfrac{1}{2}f^{\pm}_{\mu}[\{\cos 2\theta\, A^{\mu}_{xz} + \sin 2\theta(\cos\chi\, A^{\mu}_{xx} - \sin\chi\, A^{\mu}_{xy})\} \\
&\qquad \mp i\{\cos 2\theta\, A^{\mu}_{yz} - \sin 2\theta(\sin\chi\, A^{\mu}_{yy} - \cos\chi\, A^{\mu}_{xy})\}].
\end{aligned}$$

These matrix elements can be obtained from the expressions for elements of $\mathbf{V}^{aa}$ by replacing $\mathbf{A}^{\nu}$ by an "effective" tensor $\bar{\mathbf{A}}^{\nu}$, with

$$\begin{aligned}
\bar{A}^{\nu}_{zz} &= \cos 2\theta\, A^{\nu}_{zz} + \sin 2\theta(\cos\chi\, A^{\nu}_{xz} - \sin\chi\, A^{\nu}_{yz}), \\
\bar{A}^{\nu}_{xz} &= \cos 2\theta\, A^{\nu}_{xz} + \sin 2\theta(\cos\chi\, A^{\nu}_{xx} - \sin\chi\, A^{\nu}_{xy}), \qquad (7\text{-}105)\\
\bar{A}^{\nu}_{yz} &= \cos 2\theta\, A^{\nu}_{yz} + \sin 2\theta(\cos\chi\, A^{\nu}_{xy} - \sin\chi\, A^{\nu}_{yy}).
\end{aligned}$$

Unfortunately, this same substitution does not lead to correct matrix elements for $\mathbf{V}^{ab}$. The correct matrix elements will be given below.

First-Order Calculation

Since the entire block of states $\{|1, K\rangle\}$ associated with $\bar{\mathbf{V}}^{aa}$ have the same zero-order energy, $E^{(0)} = (\beta/2)\bar{g}$, degenerate perturbation theory is to be used and the first-order energies are the eigenvalues of $\bar{\mathbf{V}}^{aa}$. The $\{|2, K\rangle\}$ states are also degenerate in zero-order with $E^{(0)} = -\beta/2\,\bar{g}$. Since $\bar{\mathbf{V}}^{bb} = -\bar{\mathbf{V}}^{aa}$, the first-order energies will be just the negatives of those for corresponding states in the 1 or a block. The lowest-order selection rule again specifies that the nuclear spin state does not change in allowed transitions, so the first-order contribution to the transition energy is just twice the $\bar{\mathbf{V}}^{aa}$ eigenvalue. Particular results for a single nucleus of spin $\frac{1}{2}$ or 1 will be presented later in connection with a slightly different treatment. The general case is readily treated numerically.

Second-Order Calculation

Let $\mathbf{c}^j$ be the jth eigenvector of $\bar{\mathbf{V}}^{aa}$, with corresponding eigenvalue $E^{(1)}_j$. The matrix $\mathbf{C}$ whose columns are the $\mathbf{c}^j$ can be used to transform to the appropriate zero-order basis for further calculation. Of course $\bar{\mathbf{V}}^{aa}$ is diagonalized. In addition it is convenient to define

$$\mathbf{V}' = \mathbf{C}^{\dagger}\bar{\mathbf{V}}^{ab}\mathbf{C}. \qquad (7\text{-}106)$$

The second-order energies are

$$
\begin{aligned}
E_{1,j}^{(2)} &= \sum_l \frac{V'_{jl} V'^{*}_{jl}}{E_1^{(0)} - E_2^{(0)}} = \frac{1}{\bar{g}\beta} \sum_{i,k,m} C_{ij}^{*} C_{mj} \bar{V}_{ik}^{ab} \bar{V}_{mk}^{ab*} \\
E_{2,j}^{(2)} &= \sum_l \frac{V'^{*}_{lj} V'_{lj}}{E_2^{(0)} - E_1^{(0)}} = -\frac{1}{\bar{g}\beta} \sum_{i,k,m} C_{ij}^{*} C_{mj} \bar{V}_{km}^{ab} \bar{V}_{ki}^{ab*}.
\end{aligned}
\tag{7-107}
$$

Since $\bar{\mathbf{V}}^{ab}$ is not Hermitian, the symmetry between the 1 states and 2 states observed in zero and first order is not in general preserved in second order.

The elements of $\bar{\mathbf{V}}^{ab}$ which are required are

$$
\begin{aligned}
\bar{V}_{KK}^{ab} &= \langle 1, K | V | 2, K \rangle \\
&= \tfrac{1}{2} \sum_{\nu} [\{\sin 2\theta \cos \chi \, A_{zz}^{\nu} + (\cos^2 \theta - \sin^2 \theta \cos 2\chi) A_{xz}^{\nu} \\
&\quad + \sin^2 \theta \sin 2\chi \, A_{yz}^{\nu}\} + i\{\sin 2\theta \sin \chi \, A_{zz} - \sin^2 \theta \sin 2\chi \, A_{xz}^{\nu} \\
&\quad - (\cos^2 \theta - \sin^2 \theta \cos 2\chi) A_{yz}^{\nu}\}] m_{\nu}^{K}, \\
\bar{V}_{K_{\mu}^{\pm}, K}^{ab} &= \langle 1, K_{\mu}^{\pm} | V | 2, K \rangle = \tfrac{1}{4} f_{\mu}^{\pm} [\{(\cos^2 \theta - \sin^2 \theta \cos 2\chi) A_{xx}^{\mu} \\
&\quad \mp (\cos^2 \theta + \sin^2 \theta \cos 2\chi) A_{yy}^{\mu} \pm \sin 2\theta \cos \chi \, A_{xz}^{\mu} \\
&\quad - \sin 2\theta \sin \chi \, A_{yz}^{\mu} + 2\varepsilon_{\pm} \sin^2 \theta \sin 2\chi \, A_{xy}^{\mu}\} \\
&\quad + i\{-\sin^2 \theta \sin 2\chi \, A_{xx}^{\mu} \mp \sin^2 \theta \sin 2\chi \, A_{yy}^{\mu} \pm \sin 2\theta \sin \chi \, A_{xz}^{\mu} \\
&\quad - \sin 2\theta \cos \chi \, A_{yz}^{\mu} - 2(\varepsilon_{\pm} \cos^2 \theta + \varepsilon_{\pm} \sin^2 \theta \cos 2\chi) A_{xy}^{\mu}\}],
\end{aligned}
\tag{7-108}
$$

where $\varepsilon_{\pm} = 0$ for $+$, 1 for $-$, and $\varepsilon_{\mp} = 0$ for $-$, 1 for $+$. The significance of these expressions is less obscure when $\mathbf{g}$ is isotropic so that $\theta = \chi = 0$.

First-order wave functions can also be calculated and the intensities of zero-order forbidden transitions estimated. These results will not be presented here because of the limited validity of the neglect of nuclear Zeeman terms.

Partitioning Treatment

We have already noted the impossibility of a degenerate, double perturbation treatment when the perturbations, $\mathscr{H}'$ and $\mathscr{V}$, do not commute. Unfortunately, for experimentally useful field strengths the proton Zeeman interaction is sometimes comparable in magnitude to proton hyperfine interactions in free radicals. This problem can be dealt with by a partitioning treatment.

In the basis where $\mathbf{H}_0$ is diagonal, $\mathbf{H}'$ remains diagonal; it is in fact the same as in the simple product basis since these two bases differ by a transformation mixing only states with the same nuclear spin contributions. In the $\{|1, K\rangle, |2, K\rangle\}$ basis, the complete spin Hamiltonian matrix eigenvalue equation‡

$$
(\mathbf{H}_0 + \mathbf{H}' + \lambda \bar{\mathbf{V}} - E\mathbf{1})\mathbf{c} = 0 \tag{7-109}
$$

‡ The formal perturbation parameter μ has been set equal to 1.

can be written in partitioned form as

$$\begin{pmatrix} \frac{1}{2}\bar{g}\beta\mathbf{1}^{aa} + \mathbf{H}'^{aa} + \lambda\bar{\mathbf{V}}^{aa} - E\mathbf{1}^{aa} & \lambda\bar{\mathbf{V}}^{ab} \\ \lambda\bar{\mathbf{V}}^{ba} & -\frac{1}{2}\bar{g}\beta\mathbf{1}^{bb} + \mathbf{H}'^{bb} + \lambda\bar{\mathbf{V}}^{bb} - E\mathbf{1}^{bb} \end{pmatrix}\begin{pmatrix} \mathbf{c}^a \\ \mathbf{c}^b \end{pmatrix} = 0. \tag{7-110}$$

In fact

$$\mathbf{H}'^{bb} = -\mathbf{H}'^{aa}, \qquad \bar{\mathbf{V}}^{bb} = -\bar{\mathbf{V}}^{aa}, \qquad \mathbf{1}^{bb} = \mathbf{1}^{aa}, \tag{7-111}$$

and it is notationally convenient to drop the aa superscript. Context will distinguish between the aa blocks of $\mathbf{H}'$, $\bar{\mathbf{V}}$ or the unit matrix and the corresponding full matrices. The partitioned equation can then be written

$$\begin{aligned} [\mathbf{H}' + \lambda\bar{\mathbf{V}} - (-\tfrac{1}{2}\bar{g}\beta + E)\mathbf{1}]\mathbf{c}^a + \lambda\bar{\mathbf{V}}^{ab}\mathbf{c}^b &= 0, \\ \lambda\bar{\mathbf{V}}^{ba}\mathbf{c}^a + [\mathbf{H}' - \lambda\bar{\mathbf{V}} - (\tfrac{1}{2}\bar{g}\beta + E)\mathbf{1}]\mathbf{c}^b &= 0. \end{aligned} \tag{7-112}$$

For those solutions with $E \sim \frac{1}{2}\bar{g}\beta$, we define

$$E = \tfrac{1}{2}\bar{g}\beta + e^a \tag{7-113}$$

and solve the second equation for $\mathbf{c}^b$

$$\mathbf{c}^b = [\lambda\bar{\mathbf{V}} - \mathbf{H}' + (\bar{g}\beta + e^a)\mathbf{1}]^{-1}\lambda\mathbf{V}^{ba}\mathbf{c}^a. \tag{7-114}$$

Substitution into the first equation then gives

$$\{\lambda\bar{\mathbf{V}} + \mathbf{H}' + \lambda^2\bar{\mathbf{V}}^{ab}[\lambda\bar{\mathbf{V}} - \mathbf{H}' + (\bar{g}\beta + e^a)\mathbf{1}]^{-1}\bar{\mathbf{V}}^{ba} - e^a\mathbf{1}\}\mathbf{c}^a = 0. \tag{7-115}$$

When $E \sim -\frac{1}{2}\bar{g}\beta$, we define

$$E = -\tfrac{1}{2}\bar{g}\beta - e^b \tag{7-116}$$

and a formal solution of the first equation of the set (7-112) followed by substitution into the second gives

$$\{\lambda\bar{\mathbf{V}} - \mathbf{H}' + \lambda^2\bar{\mathbf{V}}^{ba}[\lambda\bar{\mathbf{V}} + \mathbf{H}' + (\bar{g}\beta + e^b)\mathbf{1}]^{-1}\bar{\mathbf{V}}^{ab} - e^b\mathbf{1}\}\mathbf{c}^b = 0. \tag{7-117}$$

Equations (7-115) and (7-117) are exact, but are not standard eigenvalue equations because of the inclusion of the eigenvalue (e^a or e^b) in the inverse operator. Approximate equations of standard (and simpler) form can be obtained by neglecting e^a or e^b, $\bar{\mathbf{V}}$, and $\mathbf{H}'$ with respect to $g\beta\mathbf{1}$ in the inverse operator. Since the inverse operator itself is multiplied by λ^2, neglect of these terms will introduce an error of higher than second order. It is convenient to define

$$\begin{aligned} \mathbf{P}^a &= \bar{\mathbf{V}}^{ab}\bar{\mathbf{V}}^{ba} = \bar{\mathbf{V}}^{ab}(\bar{\mathbf{V}}^{ab})^\dagger, \\ \mathbf{P}^b &= \bar{\mathbf{V}}^{ba}\bar{\mathbf{V}}^{ab} = (\bar{\mathbf{V}}^{ab})^\dagger\bar{\mathbf{V}}^{ab} \end{aligned} \tag{7-118}$$

The approximate equations can then be written

$$\begin{aligned} [\lambda\bar{\mathbf{V}} + \mathbf{H}' + (\bar{g}\beta)^{-1}\lambda^2\mathbf{P}^a - e^a\mathbf{1}]\mathbf{c}^a &= 0, \\ [\lambda\bar{\mathbf{V}} - \mathbf{H}' + (\bar{g}\beta)^{-1}\lambda^2\mathbf{P}^b - e^b\mathbf{1}]\mathbf{c}^b &= 0. \end{aligned} \tag{7-119}$$

The first of these equations, it is to be recalled, is used for states with energies near $\frac{1}{2}\bar{g}\beta$ and the second for states with energies near $-\frac{1}{2}\bar{g}\beta$. In either case the first two terms describe the hyperfine and nuclear Zeeman interactions, respectively, and the diagonalization of their sum leads to a first-order treatment. Inclusion of the third term is equivalent to a second-order treatment insofar as it is possible in this case. A discussion of the energy levels which arise will be deferred until somewhat later.

The diagonalization of these matrices again leads to energy levels as a function of field strength. We wish to be able to determine those field strengths for which $\Delta E = h\nu$ for allowed transitions at a fixed frequency, ν. An approximate solution to this problem is possible. We divide λ into two parts

$$\lambda = B^{-1} = \lambda_0 + \Delta\lambda \tag{7-120}$$

with

$$\lambda_0 = (B_0)^{-1}, \qquad B_0 = h\nu/\bar{g}\beta, \tag{7-121}$$

and normally $\Delta\lambda \ll \lambda_0$. The problem is then to determine a value of $\Delta\lambda$ corresponding to each transition. Substituting and multiplying the equations by B_0, we obtain

$$\begin{aligned} &\left\{\bar{\mathbf{V}} + B_0\mathbf{H}' + (\bar{g}\beta B_0)^{-1}\mathbf{P}^a + \frac{\Delta\lambda}{\lambda_0}[\bar{\mathbf{V}} + 2(\bar{g}\beta B_0)^{-1}\mathbf{P}^a]\right.\\ &\qquad\left. + \left(\frac{\Delta\lambda}{\lambda_0}\right)^2(\bar{g}\beta B_0)^{-1}\mathbf{P}^a - e^a B_0\mathbf{1}\right\}\mathbf{c}^a = 0,\\ &\left\{\bar{\mathbf{V}} - B_0\mathbf{H}' + (\bar{g}\beta B_0)^{-1}\mathbf{P}^b + \frac{\Delta\lambda}{\lambda_0}[\bar{\mathbf{V}} + 2(\bar{g}\beta B_0)^{-1}\mathbf{P}^b]\right.\\ &\qquad\left. + \left(\frac{\Delta\lambda}{\lambda_0}\right)^2(\bar{g}\beta B_0)^{-1}\mathbf{P}^b - e^b B_0\mathbf{1}\right\}\mathbf{c}^b = 0. \end{aligned} \tag{7-122}$$

These can now be treated as a perturbation problem with perturbation parameter $\Delta\lambda/\lambda_0$. A treatment to higher than first order will again be difficult if degeneracies or near degeneracies occur in the "zero-order" treatment of this problem, so we will consider only the first-order treatment.

We suppose that the zero-order problem has been solved (typically numerically). The matrix $\mathbf{C}^a$ with columns $\mathbf{c}^a$ diagonalizes $\bar{\mathbf{V}} + B_0\mathbf{H}' + (\bar{g}\beta B_0)^{-1}\mathbf{P}^a$ giving eigenvalues $B_0 e_i^{a,0}$ and similarly, $\mathbf{C}^b$ diagonalizes $\bar{\mathbf{V}} - B_0\mathbf{H}' + (g\beta B_0)^{-1}\mathbf{P}^b$ giving eigenvalues $B_0 e_j^{b,0}$. These eigenvalues are the zero-order energies of the present problem, but it must be recalled that $\pm\frac{1}{2}\bar{g}\beta B_0$ must be added to them. The first-order energies will be

$$\begin{aligned} e_i^{a,1} &= [\mathbf{C}^{a\dagger}(\bar{\mathbf{V}} + 2(\bar{g}\beta B_0)^{-1}\mathbf{P}^a)\mathbf{C}^a]_{ii},\\ e_j^{b,1} &= [\mathbf{C}^{b\dagger}(\bar{\mathbf{V}} + 2(\bar{g}\beta B_0)^{-1}\mathbf{P}^b)\mathbf{C}^b]_{jj}. \end{aligned} \tag{7-123}$$

The transitions of interest are those between a level of a type and one of b type. In this approximation the relative transition probability will be given by

$$|\langle a, j|S_x|b, k\rangle|^2 = \left|\sum_l C_{lj}^{a*}C_{lk}^{b}\right|^2. \tag{7-124}$$

The transition energy will be

$$\Delta E = e_j^a + e_k^b + \bar{g}\beta \tag{7-125}$$

from the way in which e^a and e^b were defined. This energy arises from a Hamiltonian which has been divided through by B, however. The resonance condition is thus

$$h\nu = B\Delta E \tag{7-126}$$

or

$$\lambda\nu = h^{-1}\Delta E. \tag{7-127}$$

This leads, for the $a, j \to b, k$ transition, to

$$\lambda_0\left(1 + \frac{\Delta\lambda}{\lambda_0}\right)\nu = h^{-1}\left[\bar{g}\beta + e_j^{a,0} + \frac{\Delta\lambda}{\lambda_0}e_j^{a,1} + e_k^{b,0} + \frac{\Delta\lambda}{\lambda_0}e_k^{b,1} + \cdots\right] \tag{7-128}$$

which can be solved for $\Delta\lambda/\lambda_0$:

$$\frac{\Delta\lambda}{\lambda_0} \simeq \frac{e_j^{a,0} + e_k^{b,0}}{\bar{g}\beta - e_j^{a,1} - e_k^{b,1}}. \tag{7-129}$$

The field strengths at which transitions occur are given by

$$B = \lambda^{-1} = \left[\lambda_0\left(1 + \frac{\Delta\lambda}{\lambda_0}\right)\right]^{-1} = B_0\left(1 + \frac{\Delta\lambda}{\lambda_0}\right)^{-1}. \tag{7-130}$$

Another First-Order Treatment

A slightly different first-order or linearized treatment is possible and will give useful results in some cases. We begin with a different decomposition of the spin Hamiltonian of Eq. (7-92),

$$\mathscr{H} = \mathscr{H}^{(0)} + \mathscr{H}^{(1)} + \mathscr{H}^{(2)}, \tag{7-131}$$

where

$$\mathscr{H}^{(0)} = g_0\beta BS_z, \tag{7-132}$$

and g_0 can be either g_e or the isotropic part of $\mathbf{g}$. (If the latter choice is made, $\Delta\mathbf{g} = \mathbf{g} - g_0\mathbf{1}$ has zero trace.) As in the partitioning treatment we define

$$B_0 = h\nu/g_0\beta, \qquad B = B_0 + \Delta B. \tag{7-133}$$

The remaining terms in $\mathscr{H}$ are then

$$\begin{aligned}\mathscr{H}^{(1)} &= \beta \mathbf{S} \cdot \mathbf{\Delta g} \cdot \hat{\mathbf{z}} B_0 - \sum_\nu \gamma_\nu I_z^\nu B_0 + \sum_\nu \mathbf{S} \cdot \mathbf{A} \cdot \mathbf{I}^\nu, \\ \mathscr{H}^{(2)} &= \beta \mathbf{S} \cdot \mathbf{\Delta g} \cdot \hat{\mathbf{z}} \Delta B - \sum_\nu \gamma_\nu I_z^\nu \Delta B.\end{aligned} \tag{7-134}$$

The notation and grouping of terms suggest that we are considering shifts due to anisotropy in **g**, hyperfine interactions, and nuclear Zeeman interactions all to be at least potentially of the same magnitude. On the other hand, it is assumed that $\Delta B \ll B$, so g anisotropy and nuclear Zeeman terms involving ΔB will be small. We will now investigate the approximation obtained by neglecting $\mathscr{H}^{(2)}$ and treating $\mathscr{H}^{(1)}$ to first order only. In this approximation the energies will be linear in B and the transformation from fixed-field to fixed-frequency expressions is trivial.

The zero-order energies are

$$E_{m_s}^{(0)} = g_0 \beta B m_s. \tag{7-135}$$

The first-order energies are obtained by diagonalizing the block of $\mathscr{H}^{(1)}$ within each m_s manifold. These blocks are readily obtained from previous results, and can be summarized as

$$\mathbf{H}_{m_s}^{(1)} = m_s \Delta g_{zz} \beta B_0 \mathbf{1} + 2m_s \mathbf{V}^{aa} + \mathbf{\Gamma}, \tag{7-136}$$

where $\mathbf{V}^{aa}$ is given by Eq. (7-98) and $\mathbf{\Gamma}$ is a diagonal matrix with

$$\Gamma_{K,K'} = -\delta_{K,K'} \sum_\nu \gamma_\nu m_\nu^K B_0. \tag{7-137}$$

A numerical treatment is always possible. We will consider explicitly the cases of a single nucleus of spin $\frac{1}{2}$ or 1 where an analytic treatment is also possible.

For a single, spin $\frac{1}{2}$ nucleus we can readily obtain not only the eigenvalues but also the eigenvectors of the blocks, and can thus evaluate approximate transitions probabilities. The first-order energies are, for $m_s = \frac{1}{2}$

$$\begin{aligned}E_1^{(1)} &= \tfrac{1}{2}\Delta g_{zz}\beta B_0 + \tfrac{1}{4}[A_{xz}^2 + A_{yz}^2 + (A_{zz} - 2\gamma B_0)^2]^{1/2}, \\ E_2^{(1)} &= \tfrac{1}{2}\Delta g_{zz}\beta B_0 - \tfrac{1}{4}[A_{xz}^2 + A_{yz}^2 + (A_{zz} - 2\gamma B_0)^2]^{1/2}\end{aligned} \tag{7-138}$$

and for $m_s = -\frac{1}{2}$

$$\begin{aligned}E_3^{(1)} &= -\tfrac{1}{2}\Delta g_{zz}\beta B_0 + \tfrac{1}{4}[A_{xz}^2 + A_{yz}^2 + (A_{zz} + 2\gamma B_0)^2]^{1/2}, \\ E_4^{(1)} &= -\tfrac{1}{2}\Delta g_{zz}\beta B_0 - \tfrac{1}{4}[A_{xz}^2 + A_{yz}^2 + (A_{zz} + 2\gamma B_0)^2]^{1/2}.\end{aligned} \tag{7-139}$$

Relative intensities of transitions will be given by

$$\begin{aligned}|\langle 1|S_x|4\rangle|^2 &= |\langle 2|S_x|3\rangle|^2 = \tfrac{1}{2}(1 + \xi), \\ |\langle 1|S_x|3\rangle|^2 &= |\langle 2|S_x|4\rangle|^2 = \tfrac{1}{2}(1 - \xi),\end{aligned} \tag{7-140}$$

where

$$\xi = \frac{A_{xz}^2 + A_{yz}^2 + A_{zz}^2 - \gamma^2 B_0^2}{[(A_{xz}^2 + A_{yz}^2)^2 + (A_{zz}^2 - \gamma^2 B_0^2)^2 + 2(A_{xz}^2 + A_{yz}^2)(A_{zz}^2 + \gamma^2 B_0^2)]^{1/2}}. \tag{7-141}$$

The calculation leading to this result is straightforward, following similar calculations presented for the isotropic case, but is lengthy and will not be included here. We note that if **A** is isotropic or if γB_0 is neglected, $\xi = 1$. We thus expect the $1 \to 4$ and $2 \to 3$ transitions to be much stronger than the others.

The energies of the "strong" transitions are

$$\begin{aligned} \Delta E &= \Delta E^{(0)} + E_f^{(1)} - E_i^{(1)} \\ &= g_0 \beta B + \Delta g_{zz} \beta B_0 \pm \tfrac{1}{4}[(A_{xz}^2 + A_{yz}^2 + (A_{zz} - 2\gamma B_0)^2)^{1/2} \\ &\quad + (A_{xz}^2 + A_{yz}^2 + (A_{zz}^2 + 2\gamma B_0)^2)^{1/2}]. \end{aligned} \tag{7-142}$$

The splitting between the observed lines is the difference between the transition energies

$$\begin{aligned} \Delta(\Delta E) = \tfrac{1}{2}[&(A_{xz}^2 + A_{yz}^2 + (A_{zz} - 2\gamma B_0)^2)^{1/2} \\ &+ (A_{xz}^2 + A_{yz}^2 + (A_{zz} + 2\gamma B_0)^2)^{1/2}]. \end{aligned} \tag{7-143}$$

The first-order result of our previous perturbation treatment is obtained by neglecting the nuclear Zeeman term, i.e., setting $\gamma = 0$. That splitting is

$$a = (A_{xz}^2 + A_{yz}^2 + A_{zz}^2)^{1/2}. \tag{7-144}$$

If γB_0 is small but not completely negligible we can make an expansion to obtain

$$\begin{aligned} \Delta(\Delta E) &= a + 2\frac{(\gamma B_0)^2}{a} - 2\frac{(\gamma B_0)^2[A_{zz}^2 + (\gamma B_0)^2]}{a^3} + \cdots \\ &= a + 2\frac{(\gamma B_0)^2(A_{xz}^2 + A_{yz}^2)}{a^3} - \cdots. \end{aligned} \tag{7-145}$$

We note that the lowest-order contribution of the nuclear Zeeman term is dependent on the anisotropy of the hyperfine tensor.‡

First-order energies in this approximation can also be readily obtained in the case of a single nucleus of spin 1. They are

$$\begin{aligned} E_{m_s=1/2}^{(1)} &= \tfrac{1}{2}\Delta g_{zz}\beta B_0,\ \tfrac{1}{2}\Delta g_{zz}\beta B_0 \pm \tfrac{1}{2}[A_{xz}^2 + A_{yz}^2 + (A_{zz} - 2\gamma B_0)^2]^{1/2}, \\ E_{m_s=-1/2}^{(1)} &= -\tfrac{1}{2}\Delta g_{zz}\beta B_0,\ -\tfrac{1}{2}\Delta g_{zz}\beta B_0 \pm \tfrac{1}{2}[A_{xz}^2 + A_{yz}^2 + (A_{zz} + 2\gamma B_0)^2]^{1/2} \end{aligned} \tag{7-146}$$

‡ It is of some interest that the transition energies to this order are independent of the sign of the nuclear Zeeman term. This is comforting to those of us who sometimes get it wrong.

and lead to splittings similar to those obtained previously. Relative intensities could be obtained in this case, but not as conveniently as when $I = \frac{1}{2}$. They will not be given here. In either case, splittings in terms of field strength will be $\Delta(\Delta E)/g_0\beta$ to first order.

Any of the techniques considered above could be extended in a straightforward way to deal with systems having $S > \frac{1}{2}$, but extension may be difficult if the spin Hamiltonian contains terms $\mathbf{S}\cdot\mathbf{D}\cdot\mathbf{S}$. Still another approach, the eigenfield method, will be considered after we have treated some additional terms to low order.

Nuclear Quadrupole and Spin Dipolar Terms

In some cases, two other orientation dependent terms may be appropriately included in useful spin Hamiltonians. They are the nuclear quadrupole term $\mathscr{H}_q = \sum_\nu \mathbf{I}^\nu \cdot \mathbf{Q}^\nu \cdot \mathbf{I}^\nu$ and the electron spin–spin dipolar term $\mathbf{S}\cdot\mathbf{D}\cdot\mathbf{S}$. Neither has a net isotropic contribution, so they have not been considered previously. The two are very different in origin and in the situations where they are likely to be significant, but a formal similarity makes it convenient to treat them together.

We begin by considering a general spin operator term of the form

$$\mathscr{T} = \mathbf{J}\cdot\mathbf{T}\cdot\mathbf{J} = \sum_{a,b} T_{ab} J_a J_b, \tag{7-147}$$

where $\mathbf{J}$ is $\mathbf{S}$ or $\mathbf{I}$ and $\mathbf{T}$ is a tensor coupling them. Since $\mathbf{T}$ couples an angular momentum to itself, we expect it to be symmetric. In addition, any isotropic part of $\mathbf{T}$ would contribute only a term proportional to J^2 and thus constant within the manifold of states characterized by a given value of the quantum number j. We will thus consider only the case where $\mathbf{T}$ is symmetric and of zero trace.

The operator $\mathscr{T}$ can also be expressed in terms of $J_\pm = J_x \pm iJ_y$ as

$$\begin{aligned}\mathscr{T} &= \mathscr{A}J_+^2 + \mathscr{B}(J_+J_z + J_zJ_+) + \mathscr{C}(3J_z^2 - J^2) \\ &\quad + \mathscr{B}^*(J_-J_z + J_zJ_-) + \mathscr{A}^*J_-^2,\end{aligned} \tag{7-148}$$

where (for $T_{ij} = T_{ji}, \sum_i T_{ii} = 0$)

$$\mathscr{A} = \tfrac{1}{4}(T_{xx} - T_{yy}) - \frac{i}{2}T_{xy}, \qquad \mathscr{B} = \tfrac{1}{2}(T_{xz} - iT_{yz}), \qquad \mathscr{C} = \tfrac{1}{2}T_{zz}. \tag{7-149}$$

It follows that

$$\begin{aligned}\mathscr{T}|j,m\rangle = {} & \mathscr{A}[j(j+1)-m(m+1)]^{1/2}[j(j+1)\\ & -(m+1)(m+2)]^{1/2}|j,m+2\rangle\\ & +\mathscr{B}[j(j+1)-m(m+1)]^{1/2}(2m+1)|j,m+1\rangle\\ & +\mathscr{C}[3m^2-j(j+1)]|j,m\rangle\\ & +\mathscr{B}^*[j(j+1)-m(m-1)]^{1/2}(2m-1)|j,m-1\rangle\\ & +\mathscr{A}^*[j(j+1)-m(m-1)]^{1/2}[j(j+1)\\ & -(m-1)(m-2)]^{1/2}|j,m-2\rangle. \qquad (7\text{-}150)\end{aligned}$$

If $j = 0$ or $\frac{1}{2}$, each term in $\mathscr{T}$ gives zero acting on each $|j, m\rangle$. For $j = 1$ and $j = \frac{3}{2}$, the matrices $\langle jm|\mathscr{T}|jm'\rangle$ are given in Table 7-3. Results for larger values of j are also readily obtained. It is possible in principle to obtain the eigenvalues of any Hermitian 3×3 (or 4×4) matrix analytically. Unless some simplifications occur, however, the resultant expressions are not likely to be very informative or otherwise useful except in numerical treatments. We will consider shortly the special case in which the coordinate system coincides with the principal axis system of **T**.

TABLE 7-3

Matrices for the Operator $\mathscr{T}$

$\langle jm|\mathscr{T}|jm'\rangle$

$j = 1$

$m \backslash m'$	1	0	−1
1	$\mathscr{C}$	$\sqrt{2}\mathscr{B}^*$	$2\mathscr{A}^*$
0	$\sqrt{2}\mathscr{B}$	$-2\mathscr{C}$	$-\sqrt{2}\mathscr{B}^*$
−1	$2\mathscr{A}$	$-\sqrt{2}\mathscr{B}$	$\mathscr{C}$

$j = \frac{3}{2}$

$m \backslash m'$	$\frac{3}{2}$	$\frac{1}{2}$	$-\frac{1}{2}$	$-\frac{3}{2}$
$\frac{3}{2}$	$3\mathscr{C}$	$2\sqrt{3}\mathscr{B}$	$2\sqrt{3}\mathscr{A}$	0
$\frac{1}{2}$	$2\sqrt{3}\mathscr{B}^*$	$-3\mathscr{C}$	0	$2\sqrt{3}\mathscr{A}$
$-\frac{1}{2}$	$2\sqrt{3}\mathscr{A}^*$	0	$-3\mathscr{C}$	$-2\sqrt{3}\mathscr{B}$
$-\frac{3}{2}$	0	$2\sqrt{3}\mathscr{A}^*$	$-2\sqrt{3}\mathscr{B}^*$	$3\mathscr{C}$

In the nuclear quadrupole case $\mathbf{J} = \mathbf{I}$ and $\mathscr{T}$ is $\mathscr{H}_q$, with $\mathbf{T} = \mathbf{Q}$. The matrix of $\mathscr{H}_q$ over all electron and nuclear spin states is diagonal in and independent of m_s. This term is independent of the magnetic field strength, so it is readily combined with the hyperfine interaction term in the division corresponding to Eqs. (7-33) and (7-94). The matrix $\mathbf{V}$ is thus augmented by a quadrupole contribution. If $\mathbf{U}$ is the matrix with elements $\langle K | \mathscr{H}_q | K' \rangle$, it is clear that $\mathbf{V}^{ab}$ will be unchanged but that

$$\mathbf{V}^{aa} \to \mathbf{V}^{aa} + \mathbf{U}, \qquad \mathbf{V}^{bb} \to -\mathbf{V}^{bb} + \mathbf{U}.$$

Any of the methods developed previously can then be applied.

The effect of the nuclear quadrupole term is readily dealt with numerically. To gain some feeling for what it does, we will consider an example in a somewhat special case. We will assume that $\mathbf{g}$ is isotropic and that only a single nucleus need be treated. Further, we assume that the principal axes of $\mathbf{A}$ and $\mathbf{Q}$ coincide and that the laboratory axis system coincides with this common principal axis system. It is then possible to give a simple treatment through first order.

The zero-order energy is of course $E^{(0)} = g\beta B m_s$. Three terms contribute in first order: the hyperfine, quadrupolar, and nuclear Zeeman terms. We introduce a field-independent approximation to the nuclear Zeeman term by substituting $B_0 = h\nu/g\beta$ for B and define

$$a = A_{zz}, \qquad b = \gamma B_0, \qquad q = Q_{zz}, \qquad \delta = Q_{xx} - Q_{yy}.$$

The zero-order functions which diagonalize the matrix corresponding to the sum of these three contributions within degenerate blocks are given in Table 7-4 for the case $I = 1$. The expressions simplify somewhat if the nuclear

TABLE 7-4

Zero-Order Functions and First-Order Energies Including Quadrupole Interaction with an $I = 1$ Nucleus

State[a]	$E^{(1)}$
$\lvert \frac{1}{2}, a\rangle = \cos\theta_+ \lvert \frac{1}{2}, 1\rangle + \sin\theta_+ \lvert \frac{1}{2}, -1\rangle$	$\frac{1}{2}q + [\frac{1}{4}\delta^2 + (b + \frac{1}{2}a)^2]^{1/2}$
$\lvert \frac{1}{2}, 0\rangle$	$-q$
$\lvert \frac{1}{2}, b\rangle = -\sin\theta_+ \lvert \frac{1}{2}, 1\rangle + \cos\theta_+ \lvert \frac{1}{2}, -1\rangle$	$\frac{1}{2}q - [\frac{1}{4}\delta^2 + (b + \frac{1}{2}a)^2]^{1/2}$
$\lvert -\frac{1}{2}, a\rangle = \cos\theta_- \lvert -\frac{1}{2}, 1\rangle + \sin\theta_- \lvert -\frac{1}{2}, -1\rangle$	$\frac{1}{2}q - [\frac{1}{4}\delta^2 + (b - \frac{1}{2}a)^2]^{1/2}$
$\lvert -\frac{1}{2}, 0\rangle$	$-q$
$\lvert -\frac{1}{2}, b\rangle = -\sin\theta_- \lvert -\frac{1}{2}, 1\rangle + \cos\theta_- \lvert -\frac{1}{2}, -1\rangle$	$\frac{1}{2}q + [\frac{1}{4}\delta^2 + (b - \frac{1}{2}a)^2]^{1/2}$
$\tan 2\theta_\pm = \dfrac{\delta}{2b \pm a}$	

[a] Expressed in terms of $\lvert m_s, M_I\rangle$ basis.

Zeeman contribution is assumed to be small ($b \ll (a^2 + \delta^2)^{1/2}$). This is likely to be the case for an $I = 1$ nucleus. The resultant transitions are listed in Table 7-5, through first order in $b/(a^2 + \delta^2)^{1/2}$.

We note that q cancels out completely, to this order, and if $\delta = 0$ the results are just those obtained previously. If **Q** has cylindrical symmetry, δ will be zero if the symmetry axis is parallel to the field but nonzero if the symmetry axis is perpendicular to the field.

TABLE 7-5

ESR Transition Energies and Intensities, $I = 1$ Nucleus Including Quadrupole Interaction

Transition	$\Delta E^{(1)a}$	Relative intensity
$a \to a$	$(a^2 + \delta^2)^{1/2}$	$a^2/(a^2 + \delta^2)$
$b \to a$	$\dfrac{2ab}{(a^2 + \delta^2)^{1/2}}$	$\delta^2/(a^2 + \delta^2)$
$0 \to 0$	0	1
$a \to b$	$-\dfrac{2ab}{(a^2 + \delta^2)^{1/2}}$	$\delta^2/(a^2 + \delta^2)$
$b \to b$	$-(a^2 + \delta^2)^{1/2}$	$a^2/(a^2 + \delta^2)$

[a] All transitions have $\Delta E^{(0)} = g\beta B$. In terms of field strength, $B = B_0 - \Delta E^{(1)}/g\beta$.

Similar expressions for states and energies can readily be found when $I = \frac{3}{2}$, but they remain fairly complicated even when $b = 0$ and are probably better dealt with numerically.

In the spin dipolar case, $\mathbf{J} = \mathbf{S}$ and **T** is commonly written **D**. The operator is then independent of and degenerate in all nuclear spin quantum numbers. Since the term is independent also of the magnetic field strength, it would be tempting to combine it again with the hyperfine term, but its magnitude is often sufficiently large that low-order perturbation theory would then fail to give adequate answers.

As an indication of the nature of the effect of this term, we consider a simple situation in which **g** is isotropic and the magnetic field direction coincides with one principal axis of **D** so that the parameter $\mathscr{B}$ of Eq. (7-149) is zero. The electronic Zeeman and spin–spin terms together can be described by

$$\mathscr{H}_0^{\mathrm{T}} = g\beta BS_z + \mathbf{S}\cdot\mathbf{D}\cdot\mathbf{S}. \tag{7-151}$$

For a triplet state $S = 1$ and the matrix of $\mathscr{H}_0^{\mathrm{T}}$ is

$$\begin{pmatrix} \mathscr{C} + g\beta B & 0 & 2\mathscr{A}^* \\ 0 & -2\mathscr{C} & 0 \\ 2\mathscr{A} & 0 & \mathscr{C} - g\beta B \end{pmatrix}.$$

It is clear that the $m_s = 0$ state is an eigenfunction of $\mathscr{H}_0^{\mathrm{T}}$ with eigenvalue $-2\mathscr{C} = -D_{zz}$. The $m_s = \pm 1$ states are mixed, except in the limit of very high field strength. The eigenvalues are

$$\begin{aligned} E_0^{\mathrm{T}}(\pm) &= \mathscr{C} \pm [(g\beta B)^2 + 4|\mathscr{A}|^2]^{1/2} \\ &= \tfrac{1}{2}D_{zz} \pm [(g\beta B)^2 + \tfrac{1}{4}(D_{xx} - D_{yy})^2 + D_{xy}^2]^{1/2}. \end{aligned} \tag{7-152}$$

The eigenfunctions could readily be found as well, and other terms in the full spin Hamiltonian treated by perturbation theory, although a power series in B will not result.

This is true for general orientations as well. It is of course straightforward to obtain general, numerical energy levels for a fixed-field strength. The field strengths at which transitions will occur for a fixed-microwave frequency can be easily obtained by the method used here only if a first-order treatment is sufficient for the hyperfine interaction.

The Eigenfield Method [14,15]

The effect of nuclear quadrupole interactions could be included in a straightforward way in the perturbation or partitioning treatments considered earlier. The nuclear quadrupole term in the spin Hamiltonian is independent of the magnetic field strength, so it should be included along with the hyperfine term in the construction of $\mathbf{V}$. It would not contribute to $\mathbf{V}^{ab}$ or $\mathbf{V}^{ba}$, but would contribute to $\mathbf{V}^{aa}$ and $\mathbf{V}^{bb}$ as

$$\begin{aligned} \mathbf{V}^{aa} &= \mathbf{V}^{aa}(\text{hyperfine}) + \mathbf{V}^{aa}(\text{quadrupole}) \\ \mathbf{V}^{bb} &= -\mathbf{V}^{aa}(\text{hyperfine}) + \mathbf{V}^{aa}(\text{quadrupole}). \end{aligned} \tag{7-153}$$

One more matrix diagonalization would thus be required, but there would be no essential change in the method.

Unfortunately, this is not the case if a zero-field splitting such as the spin–spin dipolar interaction is included in the spin Hamiltonian. Such a term is independent of field and nuclear spin state and its magnitude may be comparable to or larger than the electronic Zeeman interaction. The basic perturbation approach used heretofore then breaks down. There is of course no difficulty in obtaining energy levels for a given field strength. The problem is again that of efficiently determining the field strengths at which transitions will occur with a given energy.

A solution to this problem, as well as an alternative way of treating the cases already considered, is given by the eignenfield method developed by Belford and co-workers [14]. The presentation here is based on their work, but the notation is changed to coincide more closely with that which we have been using.

We begin by noting that all of the spin Hamiltonian terms we have considered are either independent of the magnetic field or linear in it. As usual, we will take the direction of the external magnetic field to define the laboratory z axis, so that only the magnitude of the field, B, will occur. The total spin Hamiltonian is written

$$\mathscr{H} = \mathscr{F} + B\mathscr{G}, \tag{7-154a}$$

where, with the terms we have thus far considered,

$$\begin{aligned} \mathscr{F} &= \mathbf{S}\cdot\mathbf{D}\cdot\mathbf{S} + \sum_{\nu} \mathbf{S}\cdot\mathbf{A}^{\nu}\cdot\mathbf{I}^{\nu} + \sum_{\nu} \mathbf{I}^{\nu}\cdot\mathbf{Q}^{\nu}\cdot\mathbf{I}^{\nu}, \\ \mathscr{G} &= \beta\mathbf{S}\cdot\mathbf{g}\cdot\hat{\mathbf{z}} - \sum_{\nu} \gamma_{\nu} I_z^{\nu}. \end{aligned} \tag{7-154b}$$

Some of these terms could be omitted or other terms added without changing the major features of the treatment. The only essential characteristic is that $\mathscr{H}$ be of the form given in Eq. (7-154a), with $\mathscr{F}$ and $\mathscr{G}$ independent of B.

We introduce a basis set which might at least initially be the simple product basis, to convert the problem to a matrix problem. The matrix eigenvalue equation is

$$\mathbf{H}\mathbf{C}^{j} = E_{j}\mathbf{C}^{j}, \tag{7-155}$$

where $\mathbf{H}$ is the matrix of $\mathscr{H}$ and the index j labels a particular eigenvalue E_j and eigenvector $\mathbf{C}^j$. Suppose that there is another solution labeled by k

$$\mathbf{H}\mathbf{C}^{k} = E_{k}\mathbf{C}^{k}. \tag{7-156}$$

This is an equation relating two column vectors. We can write its transpose, complex conjugate as the row vector equation

$$\mathbf{C}^{k\dagger}\mathbf{H} = E_{k}\mathbf{C}^{k\dagger}. \tag{7-157}$$

Since $\mathscr{H}$ is Hermitian, $\mathbf{H}^{\dagger} = \mathbf{H}$. Equation (7-155) is now multiplied from the right by $\mathbf{C}^{k\dagger}$, Eq. (7-157) is multiplied from the left by $\mathbf{C}^{j}$, and the results subtracted to give

$$\mathbf{H}\mathbf{C}^{j}\mathbf{C}^{k\dagger} - \mathbf{C}^{j}\mathbf{C}^{k\dagger}\mathbf{H} = (E_j - E_k)\mathbf{C}^{j}\mathbf{C}^{k}. \tag{7-158}$$

The product of vectors $\mathbf{C}^{j}\mathbf{C}^{k\dagger}$ is "in the wrong order" so that the result is a matrix rather than a scalar.

$$\mathbf{U}^{jk} = \mathbf{C}^{j}\mathbf{C}^{k\dagger}; \qquad U_{pq}^{jk} = C_p^{j} C_q^{k*}. \tag{7-159}$$

We also separate **H** into **F** + B**G**, where **F** and **G** are the matrices of $\mathscr{F}$ and $\mathscr{G}$, respectively, and introduce $\Delta E_{jk} = E_k - E_j$. Equation (7-158) can then be written

$$\mathbf{F}\mathbf{U}^{jk} - \mathbf{U}^{jk}\mathbf{F} + \Delta E_{jk}\mathbf{U}^{jk} = B(\mathbf{U}^{jk}\mathbf{G} - \mathbf{G}\mathbf{U}^{jk}). \tag{7-160}$$

We are interested in finding those values of B for which (at least for some values of j and k) $\Delta E_{jk} = h\nu$. Equation (7-160) looks now almost like an eigenvalue equation. To take advantage of this we think of **U** as a vector U whose elements are labeled by a composite index pq, i.e., we think of the ordered pair of indices p, q as a single index. The equation can be written in terms of components as

$$\sum_r F_{pr}U_{rq} - \sum_r U_{pr}F_{rq} + h\nu U_{pq} = B\left(\sum_r U_{pr}G_{rq} - G_{pr}U_{rq}\right), \tag{7-161}$$

where $h\nu$ has been substituted for ΔE_{jk} and the label jk has been dropped on U. With the insertion of appropriate Kronecker deltas and relabeling of summation indices we can rewrite this as

$$\sum_{rs} (F_{pr}\delta_{sq} - \delta_{pr}F_{sq} + h\nu\delta_{pr}\delta_{sq})U_{rs} - B\sum_{rs} (\delta_{pr}G_{sq} - G_{pr}\delta_{sq})U_{rs} = 0 \tag{7-162}$$

or as

$$(\mathbf{P} - B\mathbf{Q})\mathrm{U} = 0 \tag{7-163}$$

where U is the column vector with elements U_{rs}, and **P** and **Q** are matrices (supermatrices) with elements

$$\begin{aligned} P_{(pq)(rs)} &= F_{pr}\delta_{sq} - \delta_{pr}F_{sq} + h\nu\delta_{pr}\delta_{sq}, \\ Q_{(pq)(rs)} &= \delta_{pr}G_{sq} - G_{pr}\delta_{sq}. \end{aligned} \tag{7-164}$$

From the Hermiticity of **F** and **G** it can readily be shown that **P** and **Q** are Hermitian, i.e., $P^*_{(pq)(rs)} = P_{(rs)(pq)}$ and similarly for **Q**.

Equation (7-163) is a generalized eigenvalue equation, with the field strength B (at which transitions of energy $h\nu$ can occur) as eigenvalue. Equations similar to this occur most often in quantum chemistry when a nonorthogonal basis set is used. The matrix corresponding to **Q** is then the basis set overlap matrix. There is an important difference, however, in that an overlap matrix is positive definite while **Q** has some eigenvalues which are positive, some which are negative, and some which are zero.

Suppose that the original matrices **H**, **F**, and **G** were $n \times n$. Then C is a vector of n elements, and the $n \times n$ matrix **U** has become a vector with n^2 elements. The matrices **P** and **Q** are $n^2 \times n^2$. Consider now a basis in which

G is diagonal. Since $\mathbf{G} = \mathbf{H}^0 + \mathbf{H}'$ of the previous discussion, the $|1, K\rangle$, $|2, K\rangle$ basis of Eq. (7-102) will be appropriate. Let

$$G_{pq} = \Gamma_p \delta_{pq} \tag{7-165}$$

in this basis. Then

$$\begin{aligned} Q_{(pq)(rs)} &= \delta_{pr}\Gamma_s\delta_{sq} - \Gamma_p\delta_{pr}\delta_{sq} \\ &= (\Gamma_p - \Gamma_q)\delta_{pr}\delta_{qs} = (\Gamma_p - \Gamma_q)\delta_{(pq)(rs)}, \end{aligned} \tag{7-166}$$

i.e., **Q** is a diagonal matrix with diagonal elements (eigenvalues) which are differences between eigenvalues of **G**. The n eigenvalues of **Q** are the n differences $\Gamma_p - \Gamma_q$ for $1 \leq p, q \leq n$. If there is one eigenvalue $\Gamma_t - \Gamma_u$ when $p = t$ and $q = u$, then there will be another eigenvalue $\Gamma_u - \Gamma_t$ when $p = u$ and $q = t$. There will be a minimum of n zero eigenvalues, when $p = q$. If g has degenerate eigenvalues there will be additional zero eigenvalues of **Q** corresponding to $\Gamma_p - \Gamma_q = 0$ with $p \neq q$.

The generalized eigenvalue equation (7-163) will have only as many eigenvalues B as **Q** has nonzero eigenvalues. To see this we consider the equation

$$\det(\mathbf{P} - B\mathbf{Q}) = 0, \tag{7-167}$$

which must be satisfied if Eq. (7-163) is to be solved. We can think of expanding the determinant in the basis where **Q** is diagonal. Clearly the highest power of B to occur is equal to the number, $r(Q)$, of nonzero elements of **Q**. Equation (7-167) is thus an equation of degree $r(Q)$ in B, and it will have $r(Q)$ roots.

In addition, despite the fact that **P** and **Q** are Hermitian, the eigenvalues B may be complex. This can be illustrated by a simple 2×2 example. (This is not really of the form we are considering, since $2 \neq n^2$, but it serves to illustrate the point.) Let

$$\mathbf{P} = \begin{pmatrix} \alpha & \beta \\ \beta & \alpha \end{pmatrix}, \qquad \mathbf{Q} = \begin{pmatrix} 1 & 0 \\ 0 & -1 \end{pmatrix},$$

where α and β are real. Then Eq. (7-167) becomes

$$0 = \begin{vmatrix} \alpha - B & \beta \\ \beta & \alpha + B \end{vmatrix} = \alpha^2 - B^2 - \beta^2$$

from which

$$B = \pm(\alpha^2 - \beta^2)^{1/2}$$

so that B will be imaginary if $\beta^2 > \alpha^2$.

We have seen that some of the eigenvalues of **Q** are zero and others occur in pairs of equal magnitude and opposite sign. Normally, the eigenvalues of

H itself are, apart from labeling, independent of the sign of B. It is then necessary to consider only the positive solutions of Eq. (7-167) or its equivalent. Any complex solutions can also be ignored as corresponding to situations not physically attainable. Each real, positive solution B_{jk} corresponds to a potentially interesting resonance field strength. To complete the investigation it is necessary to consider relative intensities.

If for a given field strength B_{jk} a transition occurs for which $\Delta E_{jk} = h\nu$ it will (in the normal experimental situation) be observed with a relative intensity proportional to $|\langle j|\mathscr{S}_x|k\rangle|^2$. The state functions ψ_j and ψ_k are given in terms of basis functions by the expansion coefficients vectors $\mathbf{C}^j$ and $\mathbf{C}^k$. Thus

$$\langle j|\mathscr{S}_x|k\rangle = \sum_{p,q} C_p^{j*} C_q^k S_{pq}^x, \tag{7-168}$$

where S_{pq}^x is the p, q matrix element of $\mathscr{S}_x$ in the basis with respect to which **H**, **F**, and **G** are defined. If we have a solution $\mathbf{U}^{jk}$ of Eq. (7-163) corresponding to B_{jk}, the intensity of the transition will thus be

$$I_{jk} = K\left|\sum_{pq} U_{qp}^{jk} S_{pq}^x\right|^2 = K|\mathrm{tr}\{\mathbf{U}^{jk}\mathbf{S}^x\}|^2. \tag{7-169}$$

The proportionality constant K is independent of B for fixed ν, and thus relative intensitives are determined.

The eigenfield method allows us to treat zero field splittings on the same basis as other terms in the spin Hamiltonian. It also provides a nonperturbative and in principle exact solution, limited by the numerical accuracy with which the generalized eigenvalue equation can be solved. Computational techniques are discussed by Belford *et al.* [14] and other general treatments of the algorithms required are also available (e.g., Wilkinson [211]). These advantages are not gained without cost, however. The problem has been changed from the diagonalization of several matrices of dimension n to the solution of a generalized eigenvalue problem of order n^2. Even for ordinary matrix diagonalizations, computing time required increases approximately as (dimension)^3, so the eigenfield method rapidly becomes unworkable in a practical sense as n increases. As one way of avoiding this problem, a perturbation approximation to the eigenfield method has been developed [15].

Effects of Orientation

We have thus far treated the components of the various coupling tensors in the spin Hamiltonian as being fixed, given quantities. We will now consider briefly the variation of these components, and the resultant spectral variations, produced by changes in the orientation of the radical. These results can be expressed elegantly in terms of irreducible tensors and rotation matrices, but we will employ here only simpler, direct methods.

If $\mathbf{T}^{\mathrm{m}}$ is any of the coupling tensors we have considered, expressed in the molecule-(radical-)fixed coordinate system and $\mathbf{T}^{l}$ is the same tensor in the laboratory-fixed system with respect to which **B** and the microwave magnetic field direction are defined,

$$\mathbf{T}^{l} = \mathbf{R}^{\mathrm{T}}\mathbf{T}^{\mathrm{m}}\mathbf{R}, \tag{7-170}$$

where $\mathbf{R}$ is the matrix for the rotation relating the two systems and $\mathbf{R}^{\mathrm{T}}$ is its transpose. (See Appendix C.) We will confine our attention to two cases: for one we will assume that the molecule-fixed coordinate system is the principal axis system of $\mathbf{T}^{\mathrm{m}}$; for the other we will continue to treat $\mathbf{T}^{\mathrm{m}}$ as general, but consider only rotations about a single axis.

Let us begin by considering the effect of a rotation by an angle η about the x axis. (With the laboratory directions as defined previously this is the most common experimental situation.) In this case

$$\mathbf{R} = \begin{pmatrix} 1 & 0 & 0 \\ 0 & \cos\eta & \sin\eta \\ 0 & -\sin\eta & \cos\eta \end{pmatrix}. \tag{7-171}$$

We assume $\mathbf{T}^{\mathrm{m}}$ is symmetric, and find

$$\begin{aligned}
T^{l}_{xx} &= T^{\mathrm{m}}_{xx} \\
T^{l}_{xy} &= T^{\mathrm{m}}_{xy}\cos\eta - T^{\mathrm{m}}_{xz}\sin\eta \\
T^{l}_{xz} &= T^{\mathrm{m}}_{xy}\sin\eta + T^{\mathrm{m}}_{xz}\cos\eta \\
T^{l}_{yy} &= T^{\mathrm{m}}_{yy}\cos^2\eta - 2T^{\mathrm{m}}_{yz}\sin\eta\cos\eta + T^{\mathrm{m}}_{zz}\sin^2\eta \\
T^{l}_{yz} &= (T^{\mathrm{m}}_{yy} - T^{\mathrm{m}}_{zz})\sin\eta\cos\eta + T^{\mathrm{m}}_{yz}(\cos^2\eta - \sin^2\eta) \\
T^{l}_{zz} &= T^{\mathrm{m}}_{yy}\sin^2\eta + 2T^{\mathrm{m}}_{yz}\sin\eta\cos\eta + T^{\mathrm{m}}_{zz}\cos^2\eta.
\end{aligned} \tag{7-172}$$

The parameter determining the zero-order energy is

$$\bar{g} = [(g^{l}_{xz})^2 + (g^{l}_{yz})^2 + (g^{l}_{zz})^2]^{1/2},$$

and in a first-order treatment we found a useful parameter to be

$$a = [(A^{l}_{xz})^2 + (A^{l}_{yz})^2 + (A^{l}_{zz})^2]^{1/2}.$$

We thus consider

$$\begin{aligned}
t^2 &\equiv (T^{l}_{xz})^2 + (T^{l}_{yz})^2 + (T^{l}_{zz})^2 \\
&= T^{l}_{zx}\cdot T^{l}_{xz} + T^{l}_{zy}\cdot T^{l}_{yz} + T^{l}_{zz}\cdot T^{l}_{zz} = [(\mathbf{T}^{l})^2]_{zz}.
\end{aligned} \tag{7-173}$$

This can be expressed as

$$\begin{aligned} t^2 &= [(\mathbf{T}^m)^2]_{yy} \sin^2 \eta + 2[(\mathbf{T}^m)^2]_{yz} \sin \eta \cos \eta + [(\mathbf{T}^m)^2]_{zz} \cos^2 \eta \\ &= \tfrac{1}{2}\{[(\mathbf{T}^m)^2]_{yy} + [(\mathbf{T}^m)^2]_{zz}\} - \tfrac{1}{2}\{[(\mathbf{T}^m)^2]_{yy} - [(\mathbf{T}^m)^2]_{zz}\} \cos 2\eta \\ &\quad + [(\mathbf{T}^m)^2]_{yz} \sin 2\eta. \end{aligned} \tag{7-174}$$

If we neglect orientation dependence of **g** in treating **A**, treat hyperfine interactions to first order only, and neglect nuclear Zeeman and quadrupole terms, Eq. (7-174) provides the basis for an essentially complete description of the effect on the spectrum of a rotation of the radical about the laboratory x axis. When hyperfine interactions are treated to first order only, the center of the spectrum is predicted to be just where it would be if there were no hyperfine interactions. This position, in terms of field strength for fixed frequency, is

$$\begin{aligned} B_0 = h\nu/\bar{g}\beta = (h\nu/\beta)[\tfrac{1}{2}\{(g^2)_{yy} + (g^2)_{zz}\} \\ - \tfrac{1}{2}\{(g^2)_{yy} - (g^2)_{zz}\} \cos 2\eta + (g^2)_{yz} \sin 2\eta]^{-1/2}, \end{aligned} \tag{7-175}$$

where $g^2 = (\mathbf{g}^m)^2$. This is clearly a periodic function of η with period π. It can be rewritten as

$$B_0 = [C_0 + C_1 \cos(2\eta - \phi)]^{-1/2} \tag{7-176}$$

for appropriate C_0, C_1, and ϕ, so

$$dB_0/d\eta = C_1 \sin(2\eta - \phi)[C_0 + C_1 \cos(2\eta - \phi)]^{-3/2} \tag{7-177}$$

will have just two zeros, corresponding to one maximum and one minimum in $B_0(\eta)$. (It can be shown that $C_0 > |C_1| > 0$, so the denominators in B_0 and $dB_0/d\eta$ are real and nonvanishing.) A similar result will hold for the splittings between hyperfine components in this approximation.

Another useful way of examining the dependence of the spectrum on tensor orientation is to assume an "initial" orientation in which the coordinate system coincides with the principal axes of the tensor and then consider a general rotation. We will still be interested in t^2, as given in Eq. (7-174), and find it to be

$$t^2 = T_X^2 \sin^2 \beta \cos^2 \gamma + T_Y^2 \sin^2 \beta \sin^2 \gamma + T_Z^2 \cos^2 \beta, \tag{7-178}$$

where T_X, T_Y, and T_Z are the principal values of **T**, and β and γ are the second and third Euler angles characterizing the rotation. (This first Euler angle, α, determines a rotation about the field direction, which has no effect.)

A complete and general, analytic treatment without approximation would be impossible. In the few cases where an exact, analytic solution would be possible, it is probably too messy to be useful. If in fact the tensors are known in any coordinate system, a numerical treatment is possible.

Effective Fields

When a first-order treatment of the hyperfine interaction is adequate, useful insights can sometimes be gained from a consideration of what are known as effective fields. Zero-order states are obtained as in Eqs. (7-100)–(7-103) by exact diagonalization of the electronic Zeeman term in the spin Hamiltonian. Electron spin and nuclear spin dependence is separated, however, so that

$$|j, K\rangle = |j\rangle|K\rangle, \qquad j = 1, 2. \qquad (7\text{-}179)$$

Each nucleus is then assumed to interact with an effective field which depends on the electron spin state

$$\mathscr{H}_\nu = -\gamma_\nu \mathbf{I}_\nu \cdot \mathbf{b}_{\text{eff}}(j, \nu), \qquad \mathbf{b}_{\text{eff}}(j, \nu) = \mathbf{B} - \langle j|\mathbf{S}\cdot\mathbf{A}^\nu|j\rangle. \qquad (7\text{-}180)$$

The result is a pseudo-Zeeman problem which is readily solved. Within each electronic state the hyperfine levels are equally spaced, and the splitting can be determined from B and the elements of $\mathbf{g}$ (see Weil and Anderson [206]). This method is not readily extended to higher order, and can become quite complicated if several nuclei are present which do not have the principal axes of their hyperfine tensors parallel [205].

Nonsymmetric Tensor Components

As we will see in Section 9, the tensors in a spin Hamiltonian may in fact not be symmetric. It does appear that any antisymmetric component is likely to be small in magnitude compared with the symmetric component. We will now briefly examine the consequences of the presence of antisymmetric components.

We being by reexamining the case of no hyperfine interactions, but where $\Delta\mathbf{g}$ is possibly not symmetric. No assumption about the symmetry of $\Delta\mathbf{g}$ was made in obtaining Eqs. (7-100) and (7-101), so they remain valid. However, Eq. (7-173) must be modified. If $\mathbf{T}^l = \mathbf{T}^{l,\text{s}} + \mathbf{T}^{l,\text{a}}$ where $\mathbf{T}^{l,\text{s}}$ is symmetric and $\mathbf{T}^{l,\text{a}}$ is antisymmetric, we find

$$t^2 = (T^l_{xz})^2 + (T^l_{yz})^2 + (T^l_{zz})^2 = (\mathbf{T}^{l,\text{s}})^2_{zz} + (\mathbf{T}^{l,\text{a}})^2_{zz} = (T^l)^2_{zz}. \qquad (7\text{-}181)$$

Both $(\mathbf{T}^{l,\text{s}})^2$ and $(\mathbf{T}^{l,\text{a}})^2$ are symmetric. The antisymmetric part of $(\mathbf{T}^l)^2$, $\mathbf{T}^{l,\text{a}}\mathbf{T}^{l,\text{s}} + \mathbf{T}^{l,\text{s}}\mathbf{T}^{l,\text{a}}$, does not contribute to the diagonal zz component. Equation (7-157) remains valid if $(\mathbf{T}^{\text{m}})^2$ is taken to be $(\mathbf{T}^{\text{m},\text{s}})^2 + (\mathbf{T}^{\text{m},\text{a}})^2$, and in Eq. (7-158) $\mathbf{g}^2$ must be taken to be $(\mathbf{g}^\text{s})^2 + (\mathbf{g}^\text{a})^2$. Spectra for an appropriate series of orientations can be analyzed to obtain all elements of $(\mathbf{g}^\text{s})^2 + (\mathbf{g}^\text{a})^2$, but $\mathbf{g}^\text{s}$ and $\mathbf{g}^\text{a}$ cannot be separately obtained. An antisymmetric component of $\mathbf{g}$ is thus not distinguishable from a shift in the symmetric component values via the energy levels produced. The relative intensity for any orientation is proportional to $g_{zz}^2/(g_{xz}^2 + g_{yz}^2 + g_{zz}^2)$ which also provides no way to obtain the antisymmetric component.

If a first-order treatment of the hyperfine interaction is sufficient, then by similar arguments only $(\mathbf{A}^s)^2 + (\mathbf{A}^a)^2$ will be observable. We are thus led to the conclusion that any antisymmetric component in the hyperfine tensor will have an effect only in the (relatively small) second- or higher-order contributions to the energy. Since the antisymmetric part is itself expected to be a small part of the total tensor, it is likely to be unobservable.

Powder Spectra

Thus far we have considered the spectra arising from isotropic spin Hamiltonians, appropriate for most liquids, and anisotropic spin Hamiltonians for well-defined radical orientations. Some experiments are carried out with radicals contained in powder, polycrystalline, or glassy matrices. In such a situation the orientation of each radical is fixed but there is a random distribution of orientations within the sample. We will treat briefly the spectra which result.

Consider a subset of radicals in the sample which are all in (essentially) the same orientation. The contribution of this subset to the spectrum is of the form determined in the preceding subsection. It can be characterized as consisting of a series of lines (one or more per nuclear spin state), each with a certain position and relative intensity. These depend on the spin Hamiltonian parameters in a laboratory-fixed coordinate system and thus on radical orientation. We will use j to label a transition, with relative intensity A_j and position B_j. In fact, a transition is not infinitely sharp, but is characterized by a lineshape function f centered about the line position. The function f, or at least parameters it contains, may depend on j and on orientation.

The total spectrum arising from the sample is obtained as a function of field strength by summing over transitions and integrating over orientations, Ω:

$$I(B) = C \int d\Omega \sum_j A_j(\Omega) f_j(\Omega; B - B_j(\Omega)). \tag{7-182}$$

The constant C is normally chosen so that

$$\int I(B)\, dB = 1. \tag{7-183}$$

In complicated cases the spectrum can in principle be calculated by determining each A_j, B_j, and f_j for a variety of orientations and using numerical integration to approximate $I(B)$.

In order to gain some further understanding of possible spectra, we will make approximations and treat a few simple cases. We neglect the dependence of f on j and Ω. This will normally be a good approximation unless there are significant unresolved hyperfine interactions, and it is perhaps easier in that case to include such interactions explicitly by increasing the number of distinct transitions considered. We will also neglect the dependence of A_k on orientation and assume that B_k is not affected by rotations about the field direction. These approximations are not necessary but simplify matters and are valid for the simple cases we will consider.

Let us look first at the case of a radical with no magnetic or quadrupolar nuclei, so that we consider only the electronic Zeeman interaction. There is a single transition with

$$B_0(\Omega) = (h\nu/\beta)[g_X^2 \sin^2\theta \cos^2\phi + g_Y^2 \sin^2\theta \sin^2\phi + g_Z^2 \cos^2\theta]^{-1/2} \tag{7-184}$$

from Eqs. (7-178) and (7-100), etc. The Euler angles are now written as θ and ϕ rather than β and γ, and it is convenient to define

$$b_0 = h\nu/\beta, \qquad \gamma^2 = g_X^2 \cos^2\phi + g_Y^2 \sin^2\phi. \tag{7-185}$$

We can then write

$$b = B_0(\theta, \phi) = b_0[\gamma^2 + (g_Z^2 - \gamma^2)\cos^2\theta]^{-1/2} \tag{7-186}$$

and

$$\begin{aligned} I(B) &= C \int_0^{2\pi} d\phi \int_0^{\pi} \sin\theta \, d\theta \, f(B - B_0(\theta, \phi)) \\ &= C \int_0^{2\pi} d\phi \int_{-1}^{1} d\mu \, f(B - B_0(\mu, \phi)), \end{aligned} \tag{7-187}$$

where $\mu = \cos\theta$. We then change the variables of integration from μ, ϕ to b, ϕ and get

$$I(B) = C \int_0^{2\pi} d\phi \int_{b_1}^{b_2} db \left(\frac{\partial \mu}{\partial b}\right)_\phi f(B - b), \tag{7-188}$$

where

$$\begin{aligned} \left(\frac{\partial \mu}{\partial b}\right)_\phi &= \frac{\partial}{\partial b}\left[\frac{(b_0/b)^2 - \gamma^2}{g_Z^2 - \gamma^2}\right]^{1/2} \\ &= \frac{1}{b}\left(\frac{b_0}{b}\right)^2 (\gamma^2 - g_Z^2)^{-1/2}(\gamma^2 - (b_0/b)^2)^{-1/2}. \end{aligned} \tag{7-189}$$

The limits of integration are determined by the extreme values b assumes as μ varies from -1 to 1, but we note that the integrand in Eq. (7-187) is an even function of μ, so we rewrite the integral as $2\int_0^1 d\mu$ and absorb the 2 into C. Then

$$b_1 = b(\mu = 0, \phi) = b_0/\gamma, \qquad b_2 = b(\mu = 1, \phi) = b_0/g_Z. \quad (7\text{-}190)$$

At this point it would again be possible to proceed numerically. To obtain analytic results we neglect linewidth and replace $f(B - b)$ by $\delta(B - b)$. Then

$$I(B) = \frac{b_0^2 C}{B^3} \int_0^{2\pi} d\phi h(b_0/B, \phi), \quad (7\text{-}191)$$

where

$$h(x, \phi) = \begin{cases} (\gamma^2 - g_Z^2)^{-1/2}(\gamma^2 - x^2)^{-1/2}, & \text{for } x \text{ between } g_Z \text{ and } \gamma, \\ 0, & \text{otherwise.} \end{cases} \quad (7\text{-}192)$$

and the ϕ dependence of h is through γ.

The normalization constant C can now be evaluated. We integrate over B to obtain

$$\int I(B)\, dB = -C \int dx \int_0^{2\pi} d\phi\, xh(x, \phi)$$

$$= C \int_0^{2\pi} d\phi\, (\gamma^2 - g_Z^2)^{-1/2} \int_{g_z}^{\gamma} dx\, x(\gamma^2 - x^2)^{-1/2} = 2\pi C. \quad (7\text{-}193)$$

We thus take $C = \frac{1}{2}\pi$.

The result is greatly simplified if **g** has axial symmetry so that $g_X = g_Y$. Then $\gamma = g_X = g_Y = g_\perp$ is independent of ϕ. Denoting g_Z by $g_\parallel$ in this case, we have

$$I(B) = \frac{b_0^2}{B^3}(g_\perp^2 - g_\parallel^2)^{-1/2}\left(g_\perp^2 - \left(\frac{b_0}{B}\right)^2\right)^{-1/2}$$

$$= \frac{b_0^2}{(g_\perp^2 - g_\parallel^2)^{1/2}} \frac{1}{B^2(B^2 g_\perp^2 - b_0^2)^{1/2}} \quad (7\text{-}194)$$

for B between $b_0/g_\parallel$ and $b_0/g_\perp$. $I(B)$ is zero for B outside this range. The spectral intensity becomes infinite at $B = b_0/g_\perp$, but the integral over all B is finite. The effect of using a lineshape function of finite width rather than a δ function will be to broaden the features of the spectrum.

If **g** does not have axial symmetry, a more complicated treatment is necessary. We begin by noting that γ^2 is of period π and that $\gamma^2(\pi - \phi) = \gamma^2(\phi)$. We can thus write

$$I(B) = \frac{2x^3}{\pi b_0} \int_0^{\pi/2} h(x, \phi)\, d\phi \quad (7\text{-}195)$$

where again $x = b_0/B$. We can perform the ϕ integration by making use of the indefinite integral [65, p. 177]

$$\int (1 - p^2 \sin^2 \phi)^{-1/2}(1 - q^2 \sin^2 \phi)^{-1/2}\, d\phi$$
$$= (1 - p^2)^{-1/2} F(\alpha, ((q^2 - p^2)/(1 - p^2))^{1/2}) \qquad (7\text{-}196)$$

for $0 < p^2 < q^2 < 1$ and $0 < \phi < \pi/2$, with

$$\alpha = \arcsin\left[\frac{(1 - p^2)^{1/2} \sin \phi}{(1 - p^2 \sin^2 \phi)^{1/2}}\right] \qquad (7\text{-}197)$$

and F the elliptic integral

$$F(\alpha, k) = \int_0^{\alpha} \frac{du}{(1 - k^2 \sin^2 u)^{1/2}}. \qquad (7\text{-}198)$$

In particular, $F(\pi/2, k) = K(k)$ is the complete elliptic integral of the first kind, and α will be $\pi/2$ when $\phi = \pi/2$. We note also that $F(0, k) = 0$.

Let us identify the three principal axes of g as g_i, $i = 1, 2, 3$, such that $g_1 < g_2 < g_3$. Since we are averaging over all orientations, we can choose the molecule-fixed principal axis system labels to suit our convenience, and can use different labelings for different values of the field strength. In particular, if $g_1 < x < g_2$, we take $g_X = g_3$, $g_Y = g_2$, and $g_Z = g_1$, while if $g_2 < x < g_3$ we take $g_X = g_1$, $g_Y = g_2$, and $g_Z = g_3$. Of course for $x < g_1$ or $x > g_3$, $I(B) \equiv 0$. With these choices of axes, we have, when $g_1 < x < g_3$,

$$I(B) = \frac{2x^3}{\pi b_0} \int_0^{\pi/2} [(g_X^2 - g_Z^2) - (g_X^2 - g_Y^2) \sin^2 \phi]^{-1/2}$$
$$\times [(g_X^2 - x^2) - (g_X^2 - g_Y^2) \sin^2 \phi]^{-1/2}\, d\phi$$
$$= \frac{2x^3}{\pi b_0} (g_X^2 - g_Z^2)^{-1/2} (g_X^2 - x^2)^{-1/2}$$
$$\times \int_0^{\pi/2} (1 - p^2 \sin^2 \phi)^{-1/2}(1 - q^2 \sin^2 \phi)^{-1/2}\, d\phi, \qquad (7\text{-}199)$$

where

$$p^2 = \frac{g_X^2 - g_Y^2}{g_X^2 - g_Z^2}, \qquad q^2 = \frac{g_X^2 - g_Y^2}{g_X^2 - x^2}. \qquad (7\text{-}200)$$

Equations (7-176)–(7-178) then give

$$I(B) = \frac{2x^3}{b_0} (g_X^2 - x^2)^{-1/2} (g_Y^2 - g_Z^2)^{-1/2} K(k), \qquad (7\text{-}201)$$

where

$$k = \left[\frac{(g_X^2 - g_Y^2)(x^2 - g_Z^2)}{(g_Y^2 - g_Z^2)(g_X^2 - x^2)}\right]^{1/2} \tag{7-202}$$

When g_1, g_2, and g_3 are substituted for g_X, g_Y, and g_Z, we find that the k obtained in one case is the reciprocal of that obtained in the other case. The results, expressed again in terms of B and constants $b_i = b_0/g_i$, are

$$I(B) = \begin{cases} 0, & \text{if } B < b_3, \\ \dfrac{2}{\pi}\dfrac{b_1 b_2 b_3}{(b_2^2 - b_3^2)}\dfrac{K(k)}{B^2(b_1^2 - B^2)^{1/2}}, & \text{if } b_3 < B < b_2, \\ \dfrac{2}{\pi}\dfrac{b_1 b_2 b_3}{(b_1^2 - b_2^2)}\dfrac{K(1/k)}{B^2(B^2 - b_3^2)^{1/2}}, & \text{if } b_2 < B < b_1, \\ 0, & \text{if } B > b_1, \end{cases} \tag{7-203}$$

with

$$k = \left[\frac{(b_1^2 - b_2^2)(B^2 - b_3^2)}{(b_2^2 - b_3^2)(b_1^2 - B^2)}\right]^{1/2} \tag{7-204}$$

The complete elliptic integral K changes monotonically from $K(0) = \pi/2$ (when $B = b_1$ or b_3) to $K(1) = \infty$ (when $B = b_2$). Thus $I(B)$ becomes infinite at $B = b_2$, but again its integral over all B is finite [97].

When a first-order treatment is sufficient to characterize the effects of hyperfine interactions and nuclear Zeeman and quadrupolar effects are negligible, we have seen that the hyperfine splitting is given by the parameter a of Eq. (7-144). This parameter has the same orientation dependence as $\bar{g}$, so the results we have obtained can be carried over with the principal values of **A** replacing those of **g**. In more complicated situations, numerical treatment is straightforward, based on Eq. (7-182).

Summary of Section 7

In this rather lengthy section the relationships between spin Hamiltonian parameters and observed spectra have been explored. Energy levels and selection rules can be calculated for a given spin Hamiltonian and used to predict positions and relative intensities of absorption lines as a function of magnetic field strength at fixed frequency. In simple cases the relationships are such that spin Hamiltonian parameters can be evaluated directly from measurements on experimental spectra. In more complicated cases it would be necessary to proceed by simulation and successive approximations.

For the isotropic spin Hamiltonians appropriate to radicals in solution, most results can be obtained analytically in useful form. For a doublet state including hyperfine interaction with a single nucleus, exact energy levels can be obtained analytically, but when $I > \frac{1}{2}$ *approximations must be made to obtain transitions as a function of field strength at fixed microwave frequency. When hyperfine interactions with several nuclei are involved, closed form, analytic results are not attainable but a perturbation treatment is adequate if carried to second order or sometimes even only to first order. It was found that nuclear Zeeman effects can be neglected. Expressions have also been obtained for relative line intensities when there are equivalent nuclei of arbitrary spin, and second order effects for such systems have been included.*

A biradical or nearly degenerate singlet–triplet system was considered as an example of the use of pseudo-spin operators to duplicate the effect of spin-independent near degeneracies. Rather complicated spectra may result when the singlet–triplet separation is comparable in magnitude to hyperfine interactions. The difficulties of extending this approach and of using effective spin quantum numbers were also considered.

Significantly greater problems arise when anisotropic terms are included in the spin Hamiltonian. A variety of methods including several perturbation methods, a partitioning approach, effective fields and the eigenfield method of obtaining transition field strengths were considered. In general, nuclear Zeeman terms must be included. Zero-field-splitting and nuclear quadrupole effects may also be important and were discussed. Dependence of predicted spectra on radical orientation was treated. The possibility that $\mathbf{g}$ *and* $\mathbf{A}$ *may not be symmetric tensors was considered, but in free radical ESR it is unlikely that the presence of an antisymmetric component could be distinguished from an altered value in the symmetric component.*

Finally, spectra to be expected for systems of radicals in glassy or polycrystalline media were considered. Numerical treatments are always possible, and analytic results were obtained for the simplest cases where only the electronic Zeeman interaction need be considered and where, further, linewidth is neglected.

8. The Relationship of the Spin Hamiltonian to Calculated Energy Levels

The previous section included a discussion of the relationship between spin Hamiltonian parameters and experimentally observable energy levels. A large number of experimental observables can be summarized in terms of a relatively small number of parameters. To complete the connection between theory and observation, we must link these parameters to energy levels calculated according to the theory developed in Chapter I. We will be concerned in this section with general aspects of this relationship. Expressions for specific spin Hamiltonian parameters in terms of operators and wave functions or the equivalent will be given in later sections.

Partitioning Treatment

Of the various ways in which a spin Hamiltonian can be related to more fundamental theory, that which seems to offer the best combination of generality with rigor employs the method of partitioning [123]. The matrix form of the partitioning technique used in previous sections can be generalized by use of an operator formulation, but we will continue to use the matrix form. The matrices will differ from those considered earlier in that they are in principle of infinite dimension. In practice, of course, only finite matrices are used in any calculation.

We begin by supposing that the system of interest can be characterized by a full Hamiltonian of the type considered in Chapter I. This full Hamiltonian is divided into two parts:

$$\mathscr{H} = \mathscr{H}_0 + \mathscr{H}'. \tag{8-1}$$

The zero-order part, $\mathscr{H}_0$, is usually taken to be just the nonrelativistic Schrödinger Hamiltonian but could include relativistic corrections which do not depend on spins or external magnetic fields; $\mathscr{H}_0$ is assumed to be independent of these. The eigenfunctions of $\mathscr{H}_0$ can then be chosen to be eigenfunctions of $\mathscr{S}^2$ and $\mathscr{S}_Z$ as well, and states differing only in their M_S values will be degenerate. We label these sets of states by an index k, using distinct labels for states which differ in something other than just M_S values.

$$\mathscr{H}_0\psi_{kSM}^{(0)} = E_k^{(0)}\psi_{kSM}^{(0)}, \qquad \mathscr{S}^2\psi_{kSM}^{(0)} = S(S+1)\psi_{kSM}^{(0)}, \quad \mathscr{S}_Z\psi_{kSM}^{(0)} = M\psi_{kSM}^{(0)}. \tag{8-2}$$

We will assume that the total zero-order functions can be expressed as products of the $\mathscr{H}_0$ eigenfunctions and nuclear spin functions. We are thus omitting any description of the nuclear spatial behavior, except to the extent that the electronic wave function (in the Born–Oppenheimer approximation) depends parametrically on the nuclear coordinates, and permutational symmetry involving nuclei of a given type is reduced to that contained in any point group symmetry of the molecule of interest. We must bear this approximation in mind; we may later make a partial correction by including an average over nuclear vibrational motions when spin Hamiltonian parameters are evaluated. We will normally take the nuclear spin functions to be of the simple product type and label them by the K introduced in the previous section.

The minimum degeneracy of the zero-order state is $(2S + 1)\Pi_\nu(2I_\nu + 1)$, associated with different possible values of M_S and the M_ν^K. There may be additional degeneracies or near degeneracies associated with $\mathscr{H}_0$, and it is best at this point to consider all nearly degenerate states together. By nearly degenerate states we mean states split by an amount of magnitude comparable to the splittings produced by $\mathscr{H}'$. We will use a label a to designate the manifold of degenerate or nearly degenerate states of interest, and a label b to designate all remaining states. We will assume that the $\psi_{kSM}^{(0)}$ are known (at least approximately) for the a states, but not necessarily for the b states. The total degeneracy of the a group is

$$d_a = \sum_{k \in a} (2S_k + 1) \prod_\nu (2I_\nu + 1), \tag{8-3}$$

and we define an average a group energy

$$E_a^{(0)} = \sum_{k \in a} (2S_k + 1)E_k^{(0)} / \sum_{k \in a} (2S_k + 1). \tag{8-4}$$

In the most common situation for free radical work, the a group consists only of a single set of S, M_S states and $E_a^{(0)} = E_k^{(0)}$ for that set.

We write the total, time-independent Schrödinger equation whose solutions we seek as

$$(\mathscr{H} - E)\phi = 0. \tag{8-5}$$

The wave function is expressed as a linear combination of (electronic function)–(nuclear spin function) products. The basis set of electronic functions consists of the $\psi_{kSM}^{(0)}$ eigenfunctions for the a group and an orthonormal set of functions $\{\chi_{tSM}\}$ spanning the b space. (Each χ_{tSM} is orthogonal to all ψ_{kSM} of the a group.) As the notation suggests, they are assumed to be $\mathscr{S}^2$, $\mathscr{S}_Z$ eigenfunctions. We denote the nuclear spin functions by θ_K.

$$\phi = \sum_{k \in a} \sum_M \sum_K C_{kMK}^a \psi_{kM}^{(0} \theta_K + \sum_t \sum_M \sum_K C_{tMK}^b \chi_{tM} \theta_K. \tag{8-6}$$

The label S has been suppressed because states with differing S values will have different k (or t) indices.

Equation (8-5) then becomes a matrix equation, which we partition by separating the a and b group contributions.

$$\begin{pmatrix} \mathbf{H}^{aa} - E\mathbf{1}^{aa} & \mathbf{H}^{ab} \\ \mathbf{H}^{ba} & \mathbf{H}^{bb} - E\mathbf{1}^{bb} \end{pmatrix} \begin{pmatrix} \mathbf{c}^{a} \\ \mathbf{c}^{b} \end{pmatrix} = 0. \tag{8-7}$$

We are interested in solutions of dominantly a character, so E will not be equal to an eigenvalue of $\mathbf{H}^{bb}$ and the second of the two equations can be formally solved to give

$$\mathbf{c}^{b} = (E\mathbf{1}^{bb} - \mathbf{H}^{bb})^{-1}\mathbf{H}^{ba}\mathbf{c}^{a}. \tag{8-8}$$

This result is substituted into the first of the two equations, making it

$$[\mathbf{H}^{aa} + \mathbf{H}^{ab}(E\mathbf{1}^{bb} - \mathbf{H}^{bb})^{-1}\mathbf{H}^{ba} - E\mathbf{1}^{aa}]\mathbf{c}^{a} = 0. \tag{8-9}$$

It is convenient to write $\mathbf{H}^{aa}$ as

$$\mathbf{H}^{aa} = E_a^{(0)}\mathbf{1}^{aa} + \mathbf{H}^{(1)} \tag{8-10}$$

with

$$\mathbf{H}^{(1)} = (\mathbf{H}_0^{aa} - E_a^{(0)}\mathbf{1}^{aa}) + \mathbf{H}'^{aa}. \tag{8-11}$$

If the degeneracy of the a levels is exact, the term in parentheses vanishes.

We define

$$\varepsilon = E - E_a^{(0)} \tag{8-12}$$

and write Eq. (8-9) as

$$[\mathbf{H}^{(1)} + \mathbf{H}'^{ab}(E\mathbf{1}^{bb} - \mathbf{H}^{bb})^{-1}\mathbf{H}'^{ba} - \varepsilon\mathbf{1}^{aa}]\mathbf{c}^{a} = 0. \tag{8-13}$$

The replacement of $\mathbf{H}^{ab}$ and $\mathbf{H}^{ba}$ by $\mathbf{H}'^{ab}$ and $\mathbf{H}'^{ba}$ is possible since our choice of basis assures that $\mathbf{H}_0^{ab} = \mathbf{H}_0^{ba} = 0$. The second term in Eq. (8-13) can be approximated by neglecting ε relative to $E_a^{(0)}$ and $\mathbf{H}'^{bb}$ relative to $\mathbf{H}_0^{bb}$, so that

$$(E\mathbf{1}^{bb} - \mathbf{H}^{bb})^{-1} \simeq (E_a^{(0)}\mathbf{1}^{bb} - \mathbf{H}_0^{bb})^{-1} \equiv \mathbf{R}^{0}. \tag{8-14}$$

This approximation will be valid through "second order," and we write

$$\mathbf{H}^{(2)} = \mathbf{H}^{ab}\mathbf{R}^{0}\mathbf{H}^{ba}. \tag{8-15}$$

If we take the b group basis functions to be $\mathscr{H}_0$ eigenfunctions, this term leads to the ordinary, second-order Rayleigh–Schrödinger perturbation energy expression. Higher-order correction terms can be obtained, but they are seldom required. We will usually be concerned only with the lowest order contribution to any particular spin Hamiltonian parameter; errors resulting from the approximate nature of the zero-order functions will be substantially greater than higher-order corrections.

We have now succeeded in replacing the general problem represented by Eq. (8-5) by an approximate problem involving a matrix of dimension d_a:

$$(\mathbf{H}^{(1)} + \mathbf{H}^{(2)} - \varepsilon \mathbf{1}^a)\mathbf{c}^a = 0. \tag{8-16}$$

Spin Hamiltonian

The next step will be to obtain an equivalent matrix problem from a spin Hamiltonian. This is always possible in a purely formal sense, but some restrictions are necessary if the result is to be of the form we seek, with readily interpretable parameters.

The perturbation operator $\mathscr{H}'$ is a sum of terms. A typical term can be written as

$$\mathscr{H}^x = \sum_\mu \hbar^x(\mu) N^x(\mu) \tag{8-17}$$

where

$$\hbar^x(\mu) = \sum_\kappa (-1)^\kappa \hbar^x_\kappa(\mu), \qquad \hbar^x_\kappa(\mu) = \sum_p h^x(\mu\kappa; p) s^{[k]}_{-\kappa}(p). \tag{8-18}$$

In these expressions the superscript x identifies the particular term being considered, μ labels nuclei, and $N^x(\mu)$ is a nuclear spin operator for nucleus μ. If $\mathscr{H}^x$ does not include nuclear spin dependence we take $\hbar^x$ and h^x to be independent of μ and let $\sum_\mu N^x(\mu) = 1$. The operators $\hbar^x(\mu)$ act on electronic variables only, The spatial part of the electronic operator is $h^x(\mu\kappa; p)$. It may include the external magnetic field. The index p labels electrons or electron pairs, as may be appropriate for this particular term. Finally, $s^{(k)}_{-\kappa}(p)$ is the $-\kappa$ component of an irreducible tensorial set of electron spin operators. If $\mathscr{H}^x$ is a one-electron operator, $p \leftrightarrow j$, then $k = 1$ and the $s^{(1)}_{-\kappa}(j)$ are just the (spherical) tensorial components of the spin operator for electron j. If the term involves a two-electron operator, $p \leftrightarrow i < j$ and

$$s^{(k)}_{-\kappa}(p) = [\mathbf{s}(i) \times \mathbf{s}(j)]^{(k)}_{-\kappa}. \tag{8-19}$$

The construction of such irreducible product operators is discussed in Appendix C. The tensorial order k is assumed to be determined by x; terms with different k's will have different x's. (In the spin–other-orbit operators, p must be considered a one-electron label in $s^{(k)}_{-\kappa}$ but a two-electron label in h^x. This does not cause any major difficulties and will be discussed in the next section.) The terms in $\mathscr{H}'$ which are independent of electronic coordinates can be treated in a separate and essentially trivial way.

We now denote the electronic part of the wave function by $|nSM\rangle$ and the nuclear spin part by $|K\rangle$, with

$$|nSM; K\rangle = |nSM\rangle |K\rangle. \tag{8-20}$$

We note again that S is determined by n, but it will usually be written explicitly, nevertheless. As indicated previously, the nuclear spin states will normally be the simple product states considered in the previous section, but their precise form is not of significance here, so long as $\langle K | K' \rangle = \delta_{KK'}$ and a complete set of states is included.

Because of the assumed product form of the functions, matrix elements also factor

$$\langle nSM; K | \mathscr{H}^{x} | n'S'M'; K' \rangle = \langle nSM | \hbar^{x}(\mu) | n'S'M' \rangle \langle K | N^{x}(\mu) | K' \rangle. \quad (8\text{-}21)$$

In dealing with the electronic portion of this matrix element, we will again make use of the Wigner–Eckart theorem. The "rotations" under which the state functions and operators transform among themselves, respectively, must in this context be regarded as hypothetical operators affecting electron spin functions and operators only. The functions we are dealing with are spin eigenfunctions but not, in general, eigenfunctions of a total angular momentum. The method is similar to that used in Chapter I in the discussion of the nuclear quadrupole term. In the ESR literature (mostly with respect to transition metal complexes) it is frequently known as the "method of equivalent operators." The coefficients multiplying the spin part of the operator must also undergo appropriate transformations, and we will have to determine what these are. The treatment presented here is based in large part on that of Griffith [66].

In the electronic matrix element we introduce a "resolution of the identity"

$$1 = \sum_{n''S''M''} |n''S''M''\rangle\langle n''S''M''|, \quad (8\text{-}22)$$

where the sum extends over all members of a complete set of electronic states.[‡] Then

$$\langle nSM | \hbar_{\kappa}^{x}(\mu) | n'S'M' \rangle$$
$$= \sum_{p} \sum_{n''S''M''} \langle nSM | h^{x}(\mu\kappa; p) | n''S''M'' \rangle \langle n''S''M'' | s_{-\kappa}^{(k)}(p) | n'S'M' \rangle. \quad (8\text{-}23)$$

From its definition, h^x is spin independent, so it will commute with all spin operators. Its matrix elements between states with different spin quantum numbers will thus be zero, and within a manifold of states differing only in M values, will be independent of M. That is,

$$\langle nSM | h^{x}(\mu\kappa; p) | n''S''M'' \rangle = \langle nS\overline{M} | h^{x}(\mu\kappa; p) | n''S\overline{M} \rangle \delta_{S''S} \delta_{M''M}. \quad (8\text{-}24)$$

The matrix element is expressed in terms of a reference state with quantum number $\overline{M}$, which can be chosen for convenience.

[‡] For the set to be complete, functions of all permutational symmetries must be included. Only the antisymmetric functions have physical significance, but the others are also required mathematically because individual terms in the sum over p do not commute with permutation operators.

Of the spin matrix elements we need consider only those with $S'' = S$ and $M'' = M$, since others will be multiplied by zero coefficients. They can, by the Wigner–Eckart theorem, be expressed in terms of reduced matrix elements and angular momentum coupling coefficients:

$$\langle n''SM|s_{-\kappa}^{(k)}(p)|n'S'M'\rangle = \langle n''S\|s^{(k)}(p)\|n'S'\rangle\begin{pmatrix} S & k & S' \\ -M & -\kappa & M' \end{pmatrix}(-1)^{S-M}. \tag{8-25}$$

The coefficient in parentheses is a Wigner 3-j symbol (cf. Appendix C). The reduced or double bar matrix element is independent of m-type indices. It is evaluated by use of the equation above for any one, convenient choice of M, κ, and M'

$$\langle n''S\|s^{(k)}(p)\|n'S'\rangle = (-1)^{\bar{M}-S}\begin{pmatrix} S & k & S' \\ -\bar{M} & -\bar{\kappa} & \bar{M}' \end{pmatrix}^{-1}\langle n''S\bar{M}|s_{-\bar{\kappa}}^{(k)}(p)|n'S'\bar{M}'\rangle. \tag{8-26}$$

The full electronic matrix element can then be written

$$\langle nSM|\sum_p h^x(\mu\kappa;p)s_{-\kappa}^{(k)}(p)|n'S'M'\rangle = A_\kappa^x(\mu, nn')(-1)^{S-M}\begin{pmatrix} S & k & S' \\ -M & -\kappa & M' \end{pmatrix}, \tag{8-27}$$

where

$$A_\kappa^x(\mu, nn') = \sum_{n''(S''\neq S),\,p}\langle nS\bar{M}|h^x(\mu\kappa;p)|n''S\bar{M}\rangle\langle n''S\|s^{(k)}(p)\|n'S'\rangle \tag{8-28}$$

is independent of M and M' but depends on κ via h^x. The notation implies that only those states n'' with $S'' = S$ are included in the sum. The expression for $A_\kappa^x(\mu)$ can be simplified by inserting the expression for the reduced matrix element and reintroducing the sum over S'' and M'' in intermediate states. This will have no effect since the added terms will all be zero, but the complete sum over states can then be removed.

$$\begin{aligned}
&A_\kappa^x(\mu, nn') \\
&= \sum_p\sum_{n''}\langle nS\bar{M}|h^x(\mu\kappa;p)|nS\bar{M}\rangle(-1)^{\bar{M}-S}\begin{pmatrix} S & k & S' \\ -\bar{M} & -\bar{\kappa} & \bar{M}' \end{pmatrix}^{-1} \\
&\quad\times\langle n''S\bar{M}|s_{-\bar{\kappa}}^{(k)}(p)|n'S'\bar{M}'\rangle \\
&= (-1)^{\bar{M}-S}\begin{pmatrix} S & k & S' \\ -\bar{M} & -\bar{\kappa} & \bar{M}' \end{pmatrix}^{-1}\sum_p\sum_{n''S''M''}\langle nS\bar{M}|h^x(\mu\kappa;p)|n''S''M''\rangle \\
&\quad\times\langle n''S''M''|s_{-\kappa}^{(k)}(p)|n'S'\bar{M}'\rangle \\
&= (-1)^{\bar{M}-S}\begin{pmatrix} S & k & S' \\ -\bar{M} & -\bar{\kappa} & \bar{M}' \end{pmatrix}^{-1}\langle nS\bar{M}|\sum_p h^x(\mu\kappa;p)s_{-\bar{\kappa}}^{(k)}(p)|n'S'\bar{M}'\rangle.
\end{aligned} \tag{8-29}$$

The reference values $\overline{M}$, $\overline{M}'$, and $\bar{\kappa}$ should clearly be chosen so that the 3-j coefficient is nonzero. Again it should be noted that the κ-dependence of A is via h^x rather than $s^{(k)}_{-\kappa}$. We note also that either all of the quantum numbers are integer or all of them are half-integer, so κ, $\bar{\kappa}$, and k must be integer. This is of course the case for the operators of interest.

First-Order Contribution

For the simple case when only a single n and S are included in the a group, the first-order contribution to the spin Hamiltonian can now be obtained. We have

$$\langle nSM; K|\mathscr{H}^x|nSM'; K'\rangle$$
$$= \sum_{\mu}\left\{\sum_{\kappa}(-1)^{\kappa}A^x_{\kappa}(\mu, nn)(-1)^{S-M}\begin{pmatrix} S & k & S' \\ -M & -\kappa & M' \end{pmatrix}\right\}\langle K|N^x(\mu)|K'\rangle \tag{8-30}$$

and seek a purely spin operator which has the same matrix elements. We introduce spin operators $\mathscr{S}$, which are either the N-electron spin operators acting on the N-electron wave functions, or effective spin operators acting on the spin functions of the basis with respect to which the spin Hamiltonian is defined. The distinction is not important in the present context. In terms of the spin basis

$$\langle SM|\mathscr{S}^{(k)}_{-\kappa}|SM'\rangle = (-1)^{S-M}\begin{pmatrix} S & k & S \\ -M & -\kappa & M' \end{pmatrix}\langle S\|s^{(k)}\|S\rangle. \tag{8-31}$$

We can thus write

$$\langle nSM; K|\mathscr{H}^x|nSM'; K'\rangle$$
$$= \sum_{\kappa\mu}(-1)^{\kappa}A^x_{\kappa}(\mu, nn)\frac{\langle SM|\mathscr{S}^{(k)}_{-\kappa}|SM'\rangle}{\langle S\|\mathscr{S}^{(k)}\|S\rangle}\langle K|N^x(\mu)|K'\rangle$$
$$= \langle SMK|\sum_{\kappa\mu}(-1)^{\kappa}B^x_{\kappa}(\mu)\mathscr{S}^{(k)}_{-\kappa}N^x(\mu)|SM'K'\rangle, \tag{8-32}$$

where

$$B^x_{\kappa}(\mu) = \frac{A^x_{\kappa}(\mu, nn)}{\langle S\|\mathscr{S}^{(k)}\|S\rangle}. \tag{8-33}$$

In the expression for $A^x_{\kappa}(\mu; nn)$ it is reasonable to take $\overline{M}' = \overline{M}$ since $S' = S$, and in that case $\bar{\kappa}$ must be zero or the 3-j coefficient will vanish. We evaluate $\langle S\|\mathscr{S}^{(k)}\|S\rangle$ from Eq. (8-31) and get

$$B^x_{\kappa}(\mu) = \langle S\overline{M}|\mathscr{S}^{(k)}_0|S\overline{M}\rangle^{-1}\langle nS\overline{M}|\sum_p h^x(\mu\kappa: p)s^{(k)}_0(p)|nS\overline{M}\rangle, \tag{8-34}$$

where $\overline{M}$ is chosen for convenience.

The functions $|SMK\rangle$ on the right side of Eq. (8-32) are purely (electronic and nuclear) spin functions and the operator

$$H^x = \sum_{\kappa,\mu} (-1)^\kappa B_\kappa^x(\mu) \mathscr{S}_{-\kappa}^{(k)} N^x(\mu) \tag{8-35}$$

involves only parameters and spin operators. It is the first-order contribution to the spin Hamiltonian corresponding to the term $\mathscr{H}^x$ in the full Hamiltonian. Although the index μ has thus far been used to label nuclei, it is convenient now to let it include also a label for the components of the nuclear spin operator for that nucleus. We assume that these components are chosen so as to be individually Hermitian—e.g., if $N^x(\mu)$ is a component of $\mathbf{I}_\mu$, we take the Cartesian rather than the spherical components. The electron spin operators are, of course, expressed in terms of irreducible (spherical) components. It would be possible at this point to transform back to Cartesian components. A more familiar expression would in many cases result.

We know that $\mathscr{H}^x$ is Hermitian, and we will now verify that H^x is also. We have

$$(\mathscr{S}_{-\kappa}^{(k)})^\dagger = (-1)^{-\kappa} \mathscr{S}_\kappa^{(k)}, \tag{8-36}$$

and by assumption $N^x(\mu)$ is Hermitian. These operators commute with each other and with the numbers $B_\kappa^x(\mu)$. In addition, κ is an integer so $(-1)^{\kappa^*} = (-1)^{-\kappa} = (-1)^\kappa$. Thus

$$\begin{aligned} H^{x\dagger} &= \sum_{\kappa,\mu} (-1)^\kappa (B_\kappa^x(\mu))^* (-1)^\kappa \mathscr{S}_\kappa^{(k)} N^x(\mu) \\ &= \sum_{\kappa,\mu} (-1)^\kappa [(-1)^\kappa B_{-\kappa}^x(\mu)]^* \mathscr{S}_{-\kappa}^{(k)} N^x(\mu). \end{aligned} \tag{8-37}$$

From Eq. (8-34),

$$\begin{aligned} (-1)^\kappa B_{-\kappa}^x(\mu)^* &= (-1)^\kappa \langle S\overline{M} | (\mathscr{S}_0^{(k)})^\dagger | S\overline{M}\rangle^{-1} \\ &\quad \times \langle nS\overline{M} | \left(\sum_p h^x(\mu\kappa; p) s_0^{(k)}(p) \right)^\dagger | nS\overline{M}\rangle. \end{aligned} \tag{8-38}$$

It follows from the Hermiticity of $\mathscr{H}^x$ and $N^x(\mu)$ that

$$\hbar^x(\mu) = \sum_{\kappa,p} (-1)^\kappa h^x(\mu\kappa; p) s_{-\kappa}^{(k)}(p) \tag{8-39}$$

is Hermitian. Since the $s_{-\kappa}^{(k)}(p)$ are independent and satisfy Eq. (8-36), it follows that

$$h^x(\mu\kappa; p)^\dagger = (-1)^\kappa h^x(\mu\ -\kappa; p). \tag{8-40}$$

Thus

$$(-1)^\kappa B_{-\kappa}^x(\mu)^* = B_\kappa^x(\mu), \tag{8-41}$$

and since $(\mathscr{S}_0^{(k)})^\dagger = \mathscr{S}_0^{(k)}$, H^x is Hermitian.

Any term in the full Hamiltonian which does not depend on electronic variables can be taken over directly into the spin Hamiltonian, although nuclear coordinates should be averaged over nuclear vibrational motions. To the extent that parameters such as $B_\kappa^x(\mu)$ depend on nuclear coordinates, these should be averaged in the same way. In the case being considered here, where the only degeneracy of the zero-order problem is that associated with M_S and the M_I's, terms involving electronic spatial operators but not spins can also be easily dealt with. The spin Hamiltonian parameters arising from them are just the expectation values of the corresponding operators. (See, e.g., the nuclear quadrupole term in the next section.)

Second-Order Contributions

The matrix elements of the second-order-part of the spin Hamiltonian will, from Eq. (8-15), need to reproduce expressions like

$$\langle SMK | H^{xy} | S'M'K' \rangle = \sum_{\substack{n'', n''' \\ (\ni S''' = S'')}} \sum_{M'', K''} \langle nSMK | \mathscr{H}^x | n''S''M''K'' \rangle R^0_{n''n'''} \times \langle n'''S''M''K'' | \mathscr{H}^y | n'S'M'K' \rangle. \qquad (8\text{-}42)$$

Since $\mathscr{H}_0$ is spin independent, $\mathbf{R}^0$ is diagonal in spin quantum numbers and only one set of intermediate M'', K'' indices are required. The quantum number S'' is included as a label but not as a summation index because it is determined by n''. The sum over n''' is restricted to those values for which $S''' = S''$ (otherwise the matrix element of $\mathbf{R}^0$ would be zero).

We will consider here only the case where the a group consists of a single n, S manifold, so $n' = n$ and $S' = S$. The expressions above can then be written

$$\langle SMK | H^{xy} | SM'K' \rangle = \sum_{\substack{n'', n''' \\ (\ni S''' = S'')}} \sum_{M'', K''} \sum_{\mu, \nu} \langle nSM | h^x(\mu) | n''S''M'' \rangle R^0_{n''n'''} \times \langle n'''S''M'' | h^y(\nu) | nSM' \rangle \langle K | N^x(\mu) | K'' \rangle \langle K'' | N^y(\nu) | K' \rangle. \quad (8\text{-}43)$$

The total second-order contribution will involve sums over x and y. For some terms $x = y$ and for others $x \neq y$. In the latter case only the sum $H^{xy} + H^{yx}$ will occur.

Let us consider first the case in which one of the pair $\mathscr{H}^x$, $\mathscr{H}^y$ is in fact independent of electronic spin. (The case where both are independent of electronic spin can be dealt with trivially.) It is probably best to introduce new notation and call such an operator $\mathscr{H}^z$:

$$\mathscr{H}^z = \sum_{\nu} \hbar^z(\nu) N^z(\nu),$$
$$\hbar^z(\nu) = \sum_{q} h^z(\nu; q). \tag{8-44}$$

The electronic matrix elements of such an operator will be of the form

$$\langle nSM | \hbar^z(\nu) | n'S'M' \rangle = \langle nS\overline{M} | \hbar^z(\nu) | n'S\overline{M} \rangle \delta_{SS'} \delta_{MM'}, \tag{8-45}$$

where $\overline{M}$ is any convenient value of M. The matrix element is independent of it.

From the above and Eqs. (8-18) and (8-27), we have

$$\begin{aligned}
&\langle SMK | H^{xz} | SM'K' \rangle \\
&= \sum_{\mu\nu} \Bigg\{ \sum_{\substack{n'', n''' \\ (\ni S''' = S'')}} R^0_{n''n'''} \sum_{M''} \left[\sum_{\kappa} (-1)^\kappa A^x_\kappa(\mu, nn'')(-1)^{S-M} \begin{pmatrix} S & k & S'' \\ -M & -\kappa & M'' \end{pmatrix} \right] \\
&\quad \times [\langle n'''S\overline{M} | \hbar^z(\nu) | nS\overline{M} \rangle \delta_{SS''} \delta_{M''M}] \langle K | N^x(\mu) N^y(\nu) | K' \rangle \Bigg\} \\
&= \sum_{\mu\nu} \sum_{\kappa} (-1)^\kappa \Bigg\{ \sum_{\substack{n'', n''' \\ (\ni S''' = S'' = S)}} R^0_{n''n'''} A^x_\kappa(\mu, nn'') \langle n'''S\overline{M} | \hbar^z(\nu) | nS\overline{M} \rangle \Bigg\} \\
&\quad \times (-1)^{S-M} \begin{pmatrix} S & k & S \\ -M & -\kappa & M' \end{pmatrix} \langle K | N^x(\mu) N^z(\nu) | K' \rangle,
\end{aligned} \tag{8-46}$$

and we can take

$$H^{xz} = \sum_{\mu\nu} \sum_{\kappa} (-1)^\kappa C^{xz}_\kappa(\mu\nu) \mathscr{S}^{(k)}_{-\kappa} N^x(\mu) N^z(\nu), \tag{8-47}$$

where

$$\begin{aligned}
C^{xz}_\kappa(\mu\nu) &= \langle S\overline{M} | \mathscr{S}^{(k)}_0 | S\overline{M} \rangle^{-1} \sum_{\substack{n''n''' \\ (\ni S''' = S'' = S)}} \langle nS\overline{M} | \sum_p h^x(\mu\kappa; p) s^{(k)}_0(p) | n''S\overline{M} \rangle \\
&\quad \times R^0_{n''n'''} \langle n'''S\overline{M} | \hbar^z(\nu) | nS\overline{M} \rangle.
\end{aligned} \tag{8-48}$$

This is obviously very similar to the first-order result, except that the expectation value of Eq. (8-34) is replaced by an appropriate second-order expression.

To complete the treatment of this case we examine H^{zx}. We have

$$\langle SMK|H^{zx}|SM'K'\rangle$$

$$= \sum_{\mu\nu}\left\{\sum_{\substack{n'',n''' \\ (\ni S'''=S'')}} R^0_{n''n'''}\sum_{M''}[\langle nS\overline{M}|\mathscr{h}^z(\nu)|n''S\overline{M}\rangle\delta_{SS''}\delta_{MM''}]\right.$$

$$\times\left[\sum_{\kappa}(-1)^{\kappa}A^x_{\kappa}(\mu,n''n)(-1)^{S''-M''}\begin{pmatrix} S'' & k & S \\ -M'' & -\kappa & M'\end{pmatrix}\right]$$

$$\left.\times\langle K|N^z(\nu)N^x(\mu)|K'\rangle\right\},$$

$$= \sum_{\mu\nu}\sum_{\kappa}(-1)^{\kappa}\left\{\sum_{\substack{n'',n''' \\ (\ni S'''=S''=S)}} R^0_{n''n'''}\langle nS\overline{M}|\mathscr{h}^z(\nu)|n''S\overline{M}\rangle A^x_{-\kappa}(\mu,n'''n)\right\}$$

$$\times(-1)^{S-M}\begin{pmatrix} S & k & S \\ -M & \kappa & M'\end{pmatrix}\langle K|N^z(\nu)N^x(\mu)|K'\rangle. \tag{8-49}$$

As one step in the transformation to the second of these expressions, the index of summation κ has been changed to $-\kappa$. This is possible because it has the symmetric range $-k$ to k, and is an integer so $(-1)^{-\kappa} = (-1)^{\kappa}$. We can then take

$$H^{zx} = \sum_{\mu\nu}\sum_{\kappa}(-1)^{\kappa}\tilde{C}^{zx}_{-\kappa}(\nu\mu)\mathscr{S}^{(k)}_{\kappa}N^z(\nu)N^x(\mu) \tag{8-50}$$

for appropriate parameters $\tilde{C}^{zx}_{-\kappa}(\nu\mu)$. The change in sign of κ has been made so that we can identify H^{zx} with $H^{zx\dagger}$. Using the arguments presented in the treatment of H^x we find

$$(H^{xz})^{\dagger} = \sum_{\mu\nu}(-1)^{\kappa}[(-1)^{\kappa}\tilde{C}^{zx}_{-\kappa}(\nu\mu)]^*\mathscr{S}^{(k)}_{-\kappa}N^x(\mu)N^z(\nu), \tag{8-51}$$

which will be equal to H^{xz} provided that

$$(-1)^{\kappa}\tilde{C}^{zx}_{-\kappa}(\nu\mu)^* = C^{xz}_{\kappa}(\mu\nu). \tag{8-52}$$

Equations (8-49) and (8-50) constitute an implicit definition of $\tilde{C}^{zx}_{-\kappa}(\nu\mu)$ as

$$\tilde{C}^{zx}_{-\kappa}(\nu\mu) = \sum_{\substack{n'',n''' \\ (\ni S'''=S''=S)}} R^0_{n''n'''}\langle nS\overline{M}|\mathscr{h}^z(\nu)|n''S\overline{M}\rangle A^x_{-\kappa}(\mu,n'''n). \tag{8-53}$$

Since $\mathbf{R}^0$ is a Hermitian matrix and $\mathscr{h}^z(\nu)$ is a Hermitian operator,

$$(-1)^{\kappa}\tilde{C}^{zx}_{-\kappa}(\nu\mu)^* = \sum_{\substack{n'',n''' \\ (\ni S'''=S''=S)}} R^0_{n'''n''}\langle n''S\overline{M}|\mathscr{h}^z(\nu)|nS\overline{M}\rangle(-1)^{\kappa}A^x_{-\kappa}(\mu,n'''n)^*. \tag{8-54}$$

Let us now consider A_κ^x as defined in Eq. (8-29). We take $\bar{\kappa} = 0$ for convenience and note that this requires that $\overline{M}' = \overline{M}$. The 3-$j$ coefficients are real and $\overline{M} - S$ will always be an integer, so

$$A_\kappa^x(\mu, nn')^* = (-1)^{\overline{M}-S}\begin{pmatrix} S & k & S' \\ -\overline{M} & 0 & \overline{M} \end{pmatrix}^{-1} \langle nS\overline{M}|\sum_p h^x(\mu\kappa; p)s_0^{(k)}(p)|n'S'\overline{M}\rangle^*$$

$$= (-1)^{S'-S+\overline{M}-S'}\begin{pmatrix} S' & k & S \\ -\overline{M} & 0 & \overline{M} \end{pmatrix}^{-1}$$

$$\times \langle n'S'\overline{M}|\left(\sum_p h^x(\mu\kappa; p)s_0^{[k]}(p)\right)^\dagger |nSM\rangle. \tag{8-55}$$

(See Appendix C). We use Eq. (8-40) and obtain

$$A_\kappa^x(\mu, nn')^* = (-1)^{S'-S+\kappa}(-1)^{\overline{M}-S'}\begin{pmatrix} S' & k & S \\ -\overline{M} & 0 & \overline{M} \end{pmatrix}^{-1}$$

$$\times \langle n'S'\overline{M}|\sum_p h^x(\mu-\kappa; p)s_0^{(k)}(p)|nSM\rangle$$

$$= (-1)^{S'-S+\kappa}A_{-\kappa}^x(\mu, n'n). \tag{8-56}$$

In the present situation $S' = S$ so, interchanging summation indices n'' and n''',

$$(-1)^\kappa \tilde{C}_{-\kappa}^{zx}(\nu\mu)^* = \sum_{\substack{n''n''' \\ (\ni S''' = S'' = S)}} R_{n''n'''}^0 \langle n'''S\overline{M}|\hbar^z(\nu)|nS\overline{M}\rangle A_\kappa^x(\mu, nn'')$$

$$= C_\kappa^{xz}(\mu\nu), \tag{8-57}$$

and thus $H^{zx} = H^{xz\dagger}$ so $H^{xz} + H^{zx}$ is Hermitian.

A more complicated situation arises in those second-order terms for which both $\mathscr{H}^x$ and $\mathscr{H}^y$ include electron spin operators. It is convenient to write Eq. (8-43) as

$$\langle SMK|H^{xy}|SM'K'\rangle = \sum_{\mu\nu}\sum_{\substack{n'',n''' \\ (\ni S''' = S'')}} P_{\mu\nu}^{xy}(n'', n''')R_{n''n'''}^0\langle K|N^x(\mu)N^y(\nu)|K'\rangle, \tag{8-58}$$

where

$$P_{\mu\nu}^{xy}(n'', n''') = \sum_{M''}\langle nSM|\hbar^x(\mu)|n''S''M''\rangle\langle n'''S''M''|\hbar^y(\nu)|nSM'\rangle$$

$$= \sum_{M''}\left[\sum_\kappa (-1)^\kappa A_\kappa^x(\mu, nn'')(-1)^{S-M}\begin{pmatrix} S & k & S'' \\ -M & -\kappa & M'' \end{pmatrix}\right]$$

$$\times\left[\sum_\lambda (-1)^\lambda A_\lambda^y(\nu, n'''n)(-1)^{S''-M''}\begin{pmatrix} S'' & l & S \\ -M'' & -\lambda & M' \end{pmatrix}\right] \tag{8-59}$$

from Eqs. (8-18) and (8-27). As the notation suggests, we have taken

$$\hbar^y(v) = \sum_\lambda (-1)^\lambda \sum_q h^y(v\lambda; q) s^{(l)}_{-\lambda}(q). \tag{8-60}$$

The properties of the 3-j coefficients allow us to rewrite Eq. (C-30) of Appendix C as

$$\sum_\phi (-1)^{f-\phi} \begin{pmatrix} d & b & f \\ \delta & \beta & \phi \end{pmatrix} \begin{pmatrix} f & a & e \\ -\phi & \alpha & \varepsilon \end{pmatrix}$$
$$= \sum_{c,\gamma} (-1)^{d+e-2f-\alpha-\beta-2\delta}(2c+1) \begin{Bmatrix} a & b & c \\ d & e & f \end{Bmatrix} \begin{pmatrix} a & b & c \\ \alpha & \beta & \gamma \end{pmatrix} \begin{pmatrix} d & c & e \\ \delta & -\gamma & \varepsilon \end{pmatrix}, \tag{8-61}$$

and thus

$$P^{xy}_{\mu\nu}(n'', n''') = \sum_{\kappa,\lambda} (-1)^{\kappa+\lambda} A^x_\kappa(\mu, nn'') A^y_\lambda(\nu, n'''n)$$
$$\times \sum_{M''} (-1)^{S-M+S''-M''} \begin{pmatrix} S & k & S'' \\ -M & -\kappa & M'' \end{pmatrix} \begin{pmatrix} S'' & l & S \\ -M'' & -\lambda & M' \end{pmatrix}$$
$$= \sum_{\kappa,\lambda} (-1)^{\kappa+\lambda} A^x_\kappa(\mu, nn'') A^y_\lambda(\nu, n'''n) \sum_{c,\gamma} (-1)^{3S+M-2S''+\kappa+\lambda}(2c+1)$$
$$\times \begin{Bmatrix} l & k & c \\ S & S & S'' \end{Bmatrix} \begin{pmatrix} l & k & c \\ -\lambda & -\kappa & \gamma \end{pmatrix} \begin{pmatrix} S & c & S \\ -M & -\gamma & M' \end{pmatrix}. \tag{8-62}$$

By further manipulation we are lead to

$$\langle SMK | H^{xy} | SM'K' \rangle = \sum_{\mu,\nu} \sum_{c,\gamma} (-1)^\gamma \Bigg[\sum_{\substack{n'', n''' \\ (\ni S''' = S'')}} R^0_{n''n'''}$$
$$\times \sum_{\kappa,\lambda} (-1)^{\kappa+\lambda} A^x_\kappa(\mu, nn'') A^y_\lambda(\nu, n'''n)(-1)^{2S''}(2c+1)$$
$$\times \begin{Bmatrix} k & l & c \\ S & S & S'' \end{Bmatrix} \begin{pmatrix} k & l & c \\ \kappa & \lambda & -\gamma \end{pmatrix} \Bigg]$$
$$\times (-1)^{S-M} \begin{pmatrix} S & c & S \\ -M & -\gamma & M' \end{pmatrix} \langle K | N^x(\mu) N^y(\nu) | K' \rangle, \tag{8-63}$$

and we can take

$$H^{xy} = \sum_{\mu\nu} \sum_{c\gamma} (-1)^\gamma D^{xy}_{c\gamma}(\mu\nu) \mathscr{S}^{(c)}_{-\gamma} N^x(\mu) N^y(\nu), \tag{8-64}$$

where

$$D_{c\gamma}^{xy}(\mu\nu) = \langle S\overline{M}|\mathscr{S}_0^{(c)}|S\overline{M}\rangle^{-1}\Bigg[\sum_{\substack{n'', n''' \\ (\ni S''' = S'')}} R^0_{n''n'''} \sum_{\kappa, \lambda} (-1)^{\kappa+\lambda} A^x_\kappa(\mu, nn'')$$

$$\times A^y_\lambda(\nu, n'''n)(-1)^{2S''}(2c+1)\begin{Bmatrix} k & l & c \\ S & S & S'' \end{Bmatrix}\begin{pmatrix} k & l & c \\ \kappa & \lambda & -\gamma \end{pmatrix}\Bigg]. \qquad (8\text{-}65)$$

The sum over c extends over those values for which the 3-j and 6-j coefficients are nonzero, depending on k and l. It is possible that one pair of terms $\mathscr{H}^x$, $\mathscr{H}^y$ can lead to more than one term in the second-order spin Hamiltonian in the sense that more than one c value may occur. The sum over γ extends from $-c$ to c.

If we take the adjoint of Eq. (8-64) and change the sign of the summation index γ, we find

$$H^{xy\dagger} = \sum_{\mu\nu}\sum_{c\gamma}(-1)^\gamma[(-1)^\gamma D^{xy}_{c,-\gamma}(\mu\nu)]^* \mathscr{S}^{(c)}_{-\gamma} N^y(\nu)N^x(\mu). \qquad (8\text{-}66)$$

(Note that when μ and ν refer to the same nucleus, N^x and N^y may not commute.) From Eq. (8-65), however,

$$(-1)^\gamma D^{xy}_{c,-\gamma}(\mu\nu)^* = (-1)^\gamma\langle S\overline{M}|\mathscr{S}_0^{(c)}|S\overline{M}\rangle^{-1}\Bigg[\sum_{\substack{n'', n''' \\ (\ni S''' = S'')}} R^0_{n'''n''} \sum_{\kappa\lambda}(-1)^{\kappa+\lambda}$$

$$\times (-1)^{S''-S'+\kappa} A^x_{-\kappa}(\mu, n''n)(-1)^{S-S''+\lambda} A^y_{-\lambda}(\nu, nn''')$$

$$\times (-1)^{2S''}(2c+1)\begin{Bmatrix} k & l & c \\ S & S & S'' \end{Bmatrix}\begin{pmatrix} k & l & c \\ \kappa & \lambda & \gamma \end{pmatrix}\Bigg]$$

$$= (-1)^\gamma\langle S\overline{M}|\mathscr{S}_0^{(c)}|S\overline{M}\rangle^{-1}\Bigg[\sum_{\substack{n'', n''' \\ (\ni S''' = S'')}} R^0_{n''n'''} \sum_{\kappa, \lambda}(-1)^{\kappa+\lambda}$$

$$\times A^y_\lambda(\nu, nn'')A^x_\kappa(\mu, n'''n)(-1)^{2S''}(2c+1)$$

$$\times \begin{Bmatrix} l & k & c \\ S & S & S'' \end{Bmatrix}\begin{pmatrix} l & k & c \\ \lambda & \kappa & -\gamma \end{pmatrix}\Bigg]$$

$$= D^{yx}_{c\gamma}(\nu\mu). \qquad (8\text{-}67)$$

In obtaining the second expression we have interchanged the summation indices n'' and n''', changed the signs of the summation indices κ and λ, made use of the fact that for nonzero terms $\kappa + \lambda = \gamma$, and used the symmetry properties of the 3-j and 6-j coefficients. We conclude, finally, that

$$H^{xy\dagger} = \sum_{\mu\nu}\sum_{c\gamma}(-1)^\gamma D^{yx}_{cn}(\nu\mu)\mathscr{S}^{(c)}_{-\gamma} N^y(\nu)N^x(\mu) = H^{yx}, \qquad (8\text{-}68)$$

so that H^{xx} and $(H^{xy} + H^{yx})$ are Hermitian.

In order to establish certain properties of some of the spin Hamiltonian parameters, we need a relationship between $A_\kappa^x(\mu, nn')$ and $A_\kappa^x(\mu, n'n)$ in addition to that given in Eq. (8-56). To obtain this relationship we will use the Kramers conjugation operator, which is discussed in Appendix C. In what follows we drop the nuclear spin labels μ, ν. In many cases of interest, they do not in fact occur; where they are needed they can be reinserted unambiguously. An overbar will be used to denote the Kramers conjugate. For our spin angular momentum eigenfunctions

$$\overline{|nSM\rangle} \equiv K|nSM\rangle = (-1)^M |nS\ -M\rangle \tag{8-69}$$

and for operators

$$\overline{\mathcal{H}^x} \equiv K\mathcal{H}^x K^{-1} = (-1)^{\eta_x}\mathcal{H}^x \tag{8-70}$$

where η_x (= 0 or 1) is characteristic of the operator involved. For a matrix element we use a scalar product notation to avoid ambiguity and find

$$\overline{(\phi, F\psi)} = (\bar{\phi}, \overline{F\psi}) = (K\phi, KF\psi) = (K\phi, KFK^{-1}K\psi) = (\bar{\phi}, \bar{F}\bar{\psi}). \tag{8-71}$$

For any number, including a matrix element, the Kramers conjugate is equal to the complex conjugate

$$\overline{(\phi, F\psi)} = (\phi, F\psi)^*. \tag{8-72}$$

From the above we find

$$\overline{\langle nSM|\mathscr{h}^x|n'S'M'\rangle} = (-1)^{M'-M+\eta_x}\langle nS\ -M|\mathscr{h}^x|n'S'\ -M'\rangle \tag{8-73}$$

or, from Eq. (8-27)

$$\begin{aligned}
&\overline{\langle nSM|\mathscr{h}_x|n'S'M'\rangle}\\
&\quad = (-1)^{M'-M+\eta_x}\sum_\kappa (-1)^\kappa A_\kappa^x(nn')(-1)^{S+M}\begin{pmatrix} S & k & S' \\ M & -\kappa & -M' \end{pmatrix}\\
&\quad = (-1)^{S+M'+\eta_x}\sum_\kappa (-1)^\kappa A_\kappa^x(nn')(-1)^{S+S'+k}\begin{pmatrix} S & k & S' \\ -M & \kappa & M' \end{pmatrix}\\
&\quad = (-1)^{2S+S'+M'+\eta_x+k}\sum_\kappa (-1)^\kappa A_{-\kappa}^x(nn')\begin{pmatrix} S & k & S' \\ -M & -\kappa & M' \end{pmatrix}.
\end{aligned} \tag{8-74}$$

But this must be the same as the complex conjugate

$$\langle nSM|\mathscr{h}^x|n'S'M'\rangle^* = \sum_\kappa (-1)^\kappa [A_\kappa^x(nn')]^*(-1)^{M-S}\begin{pmatrix} S & k & S' \\ -M & -\kappa & M' \end{pmatrix}. \tag{8-75}$$

Since the 3-j coefficients form an orthogonal set and $(-1)^{3S} = (-1)^{-S}$, we can conclude that

$$[A_\kappa^x(nn')]^* = (-1)^{S'-S+K+\eta_x+\kappa}A_{-\kappa}^x(nn'). \tag{8-76}$$

By comparison with Eq. (8-56), then,

$$A_\kappa^x(n'n) = (-1)^{k+\eta_x} A_\kappa^x(nn'), \tag{8-77}$$

which is the relationship we need.

We now examine $D_{c\gamma}^{xy}$ as given in Eq. (8-65). Let us assume that $R_{n''n'''}^0 = (E_n^{(0)} - E_{n''}^{(0)})^{-1}\delta_{n''n'''}$, i.e., that the b-group states are $\mathscr{H}_0$ eigenfunctions. This is certainly possible in principle, although it may not be the most convenient choice computationally. We then have

$$\begin{aligned} D_{c\gamma}^{xy} &= \langle S\bar{M}|\mathscr{S}_0^{[c]}|S\bar{M}\rangle^{-1}(2c+1)(-1)^{l+\eta_y} \\ &\quad \times \sum_{n''} (E_n^{(0)} - E_{n''}^{(0)})^{-1}(-1)^{2S''} \begin{Bmatrix} k & l & c \\ S & S & S'' \end{Bmatrix} \\ &\quad \times \sum_{\kappa,\lambda} (-1)^{\kappa+\lambda} A_\kappa^x(nn'') A_\lambda^y(nn'') \begin{pmatrix} k & l & c \\ \kappa & \lambda & -\gamma \end{pmatrix} \\ &= \langle S\bar{M}|\mathscr{S}_0^{[c]}|S\bar{M}\rangle^{-1}(2c+1)^{1/2}(-1)^{k+\eta_y} \\ &\quad \times \sum_{n''} (E_n^{(0)} - E_{n''}^{(0)})^{-1}(-1)^{2S''} \begin{Bmatrix} k & l & c \\ S & S & S'' \end{Bmatrix} \\ &\quad \times [\mathbf{A}^x(nn'') \times \mathbf{A}^y(nn'')]_\gamma^{[c]}, \end{aligned} \tag{8-78}$$

where

$$\begin{aligned} &[\mathbf{A}^x(nn'') \times \mathbf{A}^y(nn'')]_\gamma^{[c]} \\ &\quad = (-1)^{l-k+\gamma}(2c+1)^{1/2} \sum_{\kappa,\lambda} A_\kappa^x(nn'') A_\lambda^y(nn'') \begin{pmatrix} k & l & c \\ \kappa & \lambda & -\gamma \end{pmatrix}. \end{aligned} \tag{8-79}$$

The form of the last expression is chosen to conform to the usual definition of a tensor product (cf. Appendix C), and we have used the fact that $\kappa + \lambda = \gamma$ for nonzero terms.

In cases where $x = y$, $k = l$ and we find

$$\begin{aligned} &[\mathbf{A}^x(nn'') \times \mathbf{A}^x(nn'')]_\gamma^{[c]} \\ &\quad = (-1)^\gamma(2c+1)^{1/2} \sum_{\kappa\lambda} A_\kappa^x(nn'') A_\lambda^x(nn'') \begin{pmatrix} k & k & c \\ \kappa & \lambda & -\gamma \end{pmatrix} \\ &\quad = (-1)^\gamma(2c+1)^{1/2}(-1)^{2k+c} \sum_{\kappa\lambda} A_\kappa^x(nn'') A_\lambda^x(nn'') \begin{pmatrix} k & k & c \\ \lambda & \kappa & -\gamma \end{pmatrix}. \end{aligned} \tag{8-80}$$

This is possible only if $(-1)^{2k+c} = 1$, i.e., $(-1)^c = 1$ or c is even, or if the quantity is in fact zero. We conclude that

$$D_{c\gamma}^{xx} \equiv 0, \qquad c \text{ odd}. \tag{8-81}$$

When two different operators are involved, we can use the invariance of the 6-j coefficient under permutations of its columns to write

$$\begin{aligned} D_{c\gamma}^{xy} + D_{c\gamma}^{yx} = {} & \langle S\overline{M}|\mathscr{S}_0^{(c)}|S\overline{M}\rangle^{-1}(2c+1) \\ & \times \sum_{n''} (E_n^{(0)} - E_{n''}^{(0)})^{-1}(-1)^{2S''+\gamma}\begin{Bmatrix} k & l & c \\ S & S & S'' \end{Bmatrix} \\ & \times \sum_{\kappa,\lambda}\Bigg[(-1)^{l+\eta_y}A_\kappa^x(nn'')A_\lambda^y(nn'')\begin{pmatrix} k & l & c \\ \kappa & \lambda & -\gamma \end{pmatrix} \\ & + (-1)^{k+\eta_x}A_\lambda^y(nn'')A_\kappa^x(nn'')\begin{pmatrix} l & k & c \\ \lambda & \kappa & -\gamma \end{pmatrix}\Bigg] \\ = {} & \langle S\overline{M}|\mathscr{S}_0^{(c)}|S\overline{M}\rangle^{-1}(2c+1)\sum_{n''}(E_n^{(0)} - E_{n''}^{(0)})^{-1} \\ & \times (-1)^{2S''+\gamma+l+\eta_y}\begin{Bmatrix} k & l & c \\ S & S & S'' \end{Bmatrix} \\ & \times \sum_{\kappa\lambda} A_\kappa(nn'')A_\lambda(nn'')\begin{pmatrix} k & l & c \\ \kappa & \lambda & \gamma \end{pmatrix}[1 + (-1)^{\eta_x-\eta_y+c}] \\ = {} & 0, \qquad \text{if} \quad \eta_c - \eta_y + c \text{ is odd.} \end{aligned} \tag{8-82}$$

In this case only odd or only even values of c occur, depending on the relative parities of η_x and η_y.

The parameter sets $B_\kappa^x(\mu)$, $C_{c\gamma}^{xz}(\mu\nu)$, and $D_{c\gamma}^{xy}(\mu\nu)$ occur as coefficients of irreducible tensorial spin operators. The transformation behavior considered has been that of the electron spin operators only, however, and it has not been shown that these parameters transform among themselves under actual rotations like the elements of tensorial sets. To examine their behavior we will need to consider two types of rotations, a rotation of the coordinate system, which relabels or alters individual terms but will leave overall energy levels unchanged, and a rotation of the radical relative to the magnetic field direction, which will in general change energy levels. These properties will be considered for specific spin Hamiltonian parameters in the next section.

States with Additional Degeneracies

We have thus far considered only cases in which the manifold of states of interest consists of a single n, S set with all degeneracy being associated with different M_S or M_I values. The formalism is not restricted to this case. It is always possible to find a spin Hamiltonian, acting on a space of spin functions with effective electron spin quantum number $S_{\text{eff}} = \frac{1}{2}(d_a - 1)/\prod_\nu(2I_\nu + 1)$, which reproduces the matrix $\mathbf{H}^{(1)} + \mathbf{H}^{(2)}$ of Eq. (8-16). One approach was discussed at the beginning of Section 7. An alternative method has been presented by Griffith, using irreducible tensor operators to span the space.

Suppose that terms quadratic in **B** and quadratic or bilinear in nuclear spins need not be considered. The matrix $\mathbf{H}^{(1)} + \mathbf{H}^{(2)}$ can then be replaced by a sum of matrices

$$\mathbf{H}^{(1)} + \mathbf{H}^{(2)} = \mathbf{H}^0 + \sum_a \mathbf{H}^{B_a} B_a + \sum_{\nu, a} \mathbf{H}^{I_{\nu a}} I_{\nu a}, \tag{8-83}$$

where B_a is the ath component ($a = x, y$, or z) of the field **B** and $I_{\nu a}$ is the ath component of the nuclear spin operator for nucleus ν. For each of the matrices $\mathbf{H}^0$, $\mathbf{H}^{B_a}$, $\mathbf{H}^{I_{\nu a}}$, one then finds a spin operator acting on the effective spin space which reproduces that matrix. The determination of such operators in terms of irreducible tensorial sets is discussed by Griffith. A less elegant but straightforward method is to introduce what might be called "single element operators" or basis operators having only a single nonzero element each.

Let the $2S_{\text{eff}} + 1$ states of the effective spin space be denoted by $|\mathcal{M}\rangle$. An operator $\mathcal{F}^{m'm}$ whose only nonzero matrix element is $\langle \mathcal{M}' | \mathcal{F}^{m'm} | \mathcal{M} \rangle = 1$ can be constructed as a product of projection operators

$$\mathcal{O}_M = \prod_{M'' \neq M} \left(\frac{\mathcal{S}_z - M''}{M - M''} \right) \tag{8-84}$$

and spin raising or lowering operators with appropriate renormalization. The fact that $|M| \leq S_{\text{eff}}$ can be used to eliminate some of the projection operators. This will not be developed in detail here, but some examples are given in Table 8-1. The choice of such operators is of course not unique. The spin Hamiltonian terms can then be expressed as

$$H^x = \sum_{m, m'} H^x_{mm'} \mathcal{F}^{mm'}(x). \tag{8-85}$$

Such a spin Hamiltonian will correctly reproduce energy levels as a function of **B** and nuclear spin states. It is not clear, however, how selection rules or relative intensities of transitions are to be obtained from the "eigenfunctions" in the effective spin space. It seems likely that one possible procedure would be to construct the matrix of $\mathcal{S}_x$ (assuming that the microwave magnetic field is in the x direction) in the actual $|nSM\rangle$ basis, and to subject this matrix to the same transformation which is used to diagonalize the spin Hamiltonian. The squares of matrix elements between resultant states would then be taken to give relative intensities of the corresponding transitions.

Treatments involving effective spin are of importance in transition metal EPR. They seldom arise, except in a trivial way with $S_{\text{eff}} = S$, for free radical

TABLE 8-1

Some Single-Element Operators[a]

$S = \frac{1}{2}$

m' \ m	$\frac{1}{2}$	$-\frac{1}{2}$
$\frac{1}{2}$	$\frac{1}{2} + \mathcal{S}_z$	$\mathcal{S}_+$
$-\frac{1}{2}$	$\mathcal{S}_-$	$\frac{1}{2} - \mathcal{S}_z$

$S = 1$

m' \ m	1	0	-1
1	$\frac{1}{2}(\mathcal{S}_z^2 + \mathcal{S}_z)$	$\frac{1}{\sqrt{2}}\mathcal{S}_z\mathcal{S}_+$	$\frac{1}{2}\mathcal{S}_+^2$
0	$\frac{1}{\sqrt{2}}\mathcal{S}_-\mathcal{S}_z$	$1 - \mathcal{S}_z^2$	$-\frac{1}{\sqrt{2}}\mathcal{S}_+\mathcal{S}_z$
-1	$\frac{1}{2}\mathcal{S}_-^2$	$-\frac{1}{\sqrt{2}}\mathcal{S}_z\mathcal{S}_-$	$\frac{1}{2}(\mathcal{S}_z^2 - \mathcal{S}_z)$

$S = \frac{3}{2}$

m' \ m	$\frac{3}{2}$	$\frac{1}{2}$	$-\frac{1}{2}$	$-\frac{3}{2}$
$\frac{3}{2}$	$\frac{1}{48}(-3 - 2\mathcal{S}_z + 12\mathcal{S}_z^2 + 8\mathcal{S}_z^3)$	$\frac{1}{2\sqrt{3}}(\mathcal{S}_z^2 - \frac{1}{4})\mathcal{S}_+$	$\frac{1}{2\sqrt{3}}(\mathcal{S}_z - \frac{1}{2})\mathcal{S}_+^2$	$\frac{1}{6}\mathcal{S}_+^3$
$\frac{1}{2}$	$\frac{1}{2\sqrt{3}}\mathcal{S}_-(\mathcal{S}_z^2 - \frac{1}{4})$	$\frac{1}{48}(27 + 54\mathcal{S}_z - 12\mathcal{S}_z^2 - 24\mathcal{S}_z^3)$	$-\frac{1}{2}(\mathcal{S}_z + \frac{1}{2})\mathcal{S}_+(\mathcal{S}_z - \frac{1}{2})$	$\frac{1}{2\sqrt{3}}\mathcal{S}_+^2(\mathcal{S}_z + \frac{1}{2})$
$-\frac{1}{2}$	$\frac{1}{2\sqrt{3}}\mathcal{S}_-^2(\mathcal{S}_z - \frac{1}{2})$	$-\frac{1}{2}(\mathcal{S}_z - \frac{1}{2})\mathcal{S}_-(\mathcal{S}_z + \frac{1}{2})$	$\frac{1}{48}(27 - 54\mathcal{S}_z^2 - 12\mathcal{S}_z + 24\mathcal{S}_z^3)$	$\frac{1}{2\sqrt{3}}\mathcal{S}_+(\mathcal{S}_z^2 - \frac{1}{4})$
$-\frac{3}{2}$	$\frac{1}{6}\mathcal{S}_-$	$\frac{1}{2\sqrt{3}}(\mathcal{S}_z + \frac{1}{2})\mathcal{S}_-^2$	$\frac{1}{2\sqrt{3}}(\mathcal{S}_z^2 - \frac{1}{4})\mathcal{S}_-$	$\frac{1}{48}(-3 + 2\mathcal{S}_z + 12\mathcal{S}_z^2 - 8\mathcal{S}_z^3)$

[a] For each S, the operator $\mathcal{F}^{m'm}$ in row m' and column m has the property $\langle SM'|\mathcal{F}^{m'm}|SM\rangle = \delta_{M'm'}\delta_{Mm}$.

ESR, where most commonly one deals with a single M_s manifold with $S = \frac{1}{2}$ or 1. One other situation which is sometimes encountered is that of a "biradical," with nearly degenerate singlet and triplet states.

BIRADICALS

To treat the biradical case, let us consider a system in which there are just two electrons interacting with two spin one-half nuclei. We will include only the electronic Zeeman and isotropic hyperfine terms, and consider only two electronic zero-order energies associated with the a set, one for a singlet and the other for a triplet, with energy separation

$$J = {}^3E^{(0)} - {}^1E^{(0)}. \tag{8-86}$$

The "full" Hamiltonian for this model problem can be written

$$\begin{aligned} \mathscr{H} &= \mathscr{H}_0 + g\beta B(s_{1z} + s_{2z}) + \mathscr{V}, \\ \mathscr{V} &= C\left\{\sum_{i=1}^{2}[\delta(\mathbf{r}_{ia})\mathbf{s}_i \cdot \mathbf{I}_a + \delta(\mathbf{r}_{ib})\mathbf{s}_i \cdot \mathbf{I}_b]\right\}. \end{aligned} \tag{8-87}$$

This Hamiltonian is of course symmetric with respect to interchange of electron labels. The total wave function for each state is written as the product of an electronic part and a nuclear spin part. We take the nuclear spin functions to be eigenfunctions of $\mathscr{I}^2$ and $\mathscr{I}_z$ where $\mathscr{I} = I_a + I_b$. Since only two electrons are involved, the electronic function can be factored into a spatial part and spin part as well, with

$$\begin{aligned} \mathscr{H}_0\,{}^3\psi(\mathbf{r}_1, \mathbf{r}_2) &= {}^3E^{(0)}\,{}^3\psi(\mathbf{r}_1, \mathbf{r}_2), \\ \mathscr{H}_0\,{}^1\psi(\mathbf{r}_1, \mathbf{r}_2) &= {}^1E^{(0)}\,{}^1\psi(\mathbf{r}_1, \mathbf{r}_2). \end{aligned} \tag{8-88}$$

The spatial electronic wave function will depend parametrically on nuclear position coordinates, but we will not consider the nuclear spatial function. The wave function we are considering may thus be either symmetric or antisymmetric with respect to interchange of nuclei, and each electronic spatial function will be assumed to have a definite symmetry in this respect. (The nuclei are equivalent under point group symmetry operations.)

In this case $\mathscr{H}_0$ can be replaced by a Heisenberg exchange term in the spin Hamiltonian. Apart from an additive constant which we ignore

$$\mathscr{H}_0 = J\mathbf{S}_1 \cdot \mathbf{S}_2 \tag{8-89}$$

We can take the electronic Zeeman term directly into the spin Hamiltonian if $g = g_e$, or use previously discussed methods (cf. also next section) to get an effective g.

When the spin operators in $\mathscr{V}$ act on the spin functions of the basis, the result is to produce linear combinations of these spin basis functions. The coefficients of the nonzero results involve combinations of δ functions:

$$\Delta_{++} = \frac{c}{4}(\delta_{1a} + \delta_{1b} + \delta_{2a} + \delta_{2b}), \qquad \Delta_{+-} = \frac{c}{4}(\delta_{1a} - \delta_{1b} + \delta_{2a} - \delta_{2b}),$$

$$\Delta_{-+} = \frac{c}{4}(\delta_{1a} + \delta_{1b} - \delta_{2a} - \delta_{2b}), \qquad \Delta_{--} = \frac{c}{4}(\delta_{1a} - \delta_{1b} - \delta_{2a} + \delta_{2b}), \tag{8-90}$$

where $\delta_{1a} = \delta(\mathbf{r}_{1a})$, etc. The spatial matrix elements of these operators (assuming real functions) then involve

$$e_r = \int {}^3\psi\, \Delta_r\, {}^3\psi\, d\tau, \qquad f_r = \int {}^3\psi\, \Delta_r\, {}^1\psi\, d\tau. \tag{8-91}$$

None of the terms in $\mathscr{H}$ link states with different values of $M = M_S + M_I$. It is thus possible to consider $\mathscr{V}$ in terms of blocks with definite M. The results are given in Table 8-2. Note that only four distinct elements actually occur: e_{++}, e_{+-}, f_{-+}, and f_{--}. Clearly $\mathscr{V}$ can be replaced by an operator (cf. the "single element operator" discussed above).

$$\mathscr{V} = \sum_{i,j} V_{ij} |i\rangle\langle j|. \tag{8-92}$$

In this case $|i\rangle\langle j|$ can be expressed as a product of spin operators for electrons and nuclei. For any spin one-half system, with states labeled by $m = \frac{1}{2}$, and $j = S$ or I

$$\begin{aligned} |\tfrac{1}{2}\rangle\langle\tfrac{1}{2}| &= \tfrac{1}{2} + j_z, \\ |\tfrac{1}{2}\rangle\langle -\tfrac{1}{2}| &= j_+ = (j_x + ij_y), \\ |-\tfrac{1}{2}\rangle\langle\tfrac{1}{2}| &= j_- = (j_x - ij_y), \\ |-\tfrac{1}{2}\rangle\langle\tfrac{1}{2}| &= \tfrac{1}{2} - j_z. \end{aligned} \tag{8-93}$$

(Compare Table 8-1, $S = \frac{1}{2}$.) When terms are combined and cancelled where possible, the net result is that $\mathscr{V}$ can be replaced by a spin operator

$$V_{\text{spin}} = e_{++}\mathscr{E}_{++} + e_{+-}\mathscr{E}_{+-} + f_{-+}\mathscr{F}_{-+} + f_{--}\mathscr{F}_{--}, \tag{8-94}$$

where

$$\begin{aligned} \mathscr{E}_{++} &= (\mathbf{S}_1 + \mathbf{S}_2)\cdot(\mathbf{I}_a + \mathbf{I}_b), & \mathscr{E}_{+-} &= (\mathbf{S}_1 + \mathbf{S}_2)\cdot(\mathbf{I}_a - \mathbf{I}_b), \\ \mathscr{F}_{-+} &= (\mathbf{S}_1 - \mathbf{S}_2)\cdot(\mathbf{I}_a + \mathbf{I}_b), & \mathscr{F}_{--} &= (\mathbf{S}_1 - \mathbf{S}_2)\cdot(\mathbf{I}_a - \mathbf{I}_b), \end{aligned} \tag{8-95}$$

or

$$V_{\text{spin}} = A_{1a}\mathbf{S}_1\cdot\mathbf{I}_a + A_{1b}\mathbf{S}_1\cdot\mathbf{I}_b + A_{2a}\mathbf{S}_2\cdot\mathbf{I}_a + A_{2b}\mathbf{S}_2\cdot\mathbf{I}_b, \tag{8-96}$$

TABLE 8-2

Matrix Elements of V[a]

$M = 2, -2$	$\langle 1, 1; 1, 1 \vert V \vert 1, 1; 1, 1\rangle = e_{++}$ $\langle 1, -1; 1, -1 \vert V \vert 1, -1; 1, -1\rangle = e_{++}$

$M = 1$[b]	$\vert 1, 0; 1, -1\rangle$ $\vert 1, 1; 1, 0\rangle$	$\vert 1, -1; 1, 0\rangle$ $\vert 1, 0; 1, 1\rangle$	$\vert 0, 0; 1, -1\rangle$ $\vert 0, 0; 1, 1\rangle$	$\vert 1, -1; 0, 0\rangle$ $\vert 1, 1; 0, 0\rangle$
$\vert 1, 0; 1, -1\rangle$ $\vert 1, 1; 1, 0\rangle$	0	e_{++}	$-f_{-+}$	e_{+-}
$\vert 1, -1; 1, 0\rangle$ $\vert 1, 0; 1, 1\rangle$	e_{++}	0	f_{-+}	$-e_{+-}$
$\vert 0, 0; 1, -1\rangle$ $\vert 0, 0; 1, 1\rangle$	$-f_{-+}$	f_{-+}	0	f_{--}
$\vert 1, -1; 0, 0\rangle$ $\vert 1, 1; 0, 0\rangle$	e_{+-}	$-e_{+-}$	f_{--}	0

$M = 0$	$\vert 1, 1; 1, -1\rangle$	$\vert 1, 0; 1, 0\rangle$	$\vert 1, -1; 1, 1\rangle$	$\vert 0, 0; 1, 0\rangle$	$\vert 1, 0; 0, 0\rangle$	$\vert 0, 0; 0, 0\rangle$
$\vert 1, 1; 1, -1\rangle$	$-e_{++}$	e_{++}	0	$-f_{-+}$	e_{+-}	$-f_{--}$
$\vert 1, 0; 1, 0\rangle$	e_{++}	0	e_{++}	0	0	f_{--}
$\vert 1, -1; 1, 1\rangle$	0	e_{++}	$-e_{++}$	f_{-+}	$-e_{+-}$	$-f_{--}$
$\vert 0, 0; 1, 0\rangle$	$-f_{-+}$	0	f_{-+}	0	f_{--}	0
$\vert 1, 0; 0, 0\rangle$	e_{+-}	0	$-e_{-+}$	f_{--}	0	0
$\vert 0, 0; 0, 0\rangle$	$-f_{--}$	f_{--}	$-f_{--}$	0	0	0

[a] Basis functions are labeled by $|S, M_S; I, M_I\rangle$ and $M = M_S + M_I$. Blocks not shown are zero. The parameters e_{++}, e_{+-}, f_{-+}, and f_{--} are defined in the text.

[b] Use all upper states or all lower states for both row and column indices.

where

$$A_{1a} = e_{++} + e_{+-} + f_{-+} + f_{--}, \qquad A_{1b} = e_{++} - e_{+-} + f_{-+} - f_{--},$$
$$A_{2a} = e_{++} + e_{--} - f_{-+} - f_{--}, \qquad A_{2b} = e_{++} - e_{--} - f_{-+} + f_{--}. \tag{8-97}$$

Having gone to a spin Hamiltonian

$$H = J\mathbf{S}_1 \cdot \mathbf{S}_2 + g\beta B(\mathbf{S}_{1z} + \mathbf{S}_{2z}) + V_{\text{spin}}, \tag{8-98}$$

we note that there is no longer permutational symmetry with respect to electron labels.

If we further simplify the model by using a minimal basis, valence-bond approximation for ψ,

$$^1\psi \sim a(\mathbf{r}_1)b(\mathbf{r}_2) + b(\mathbf{r}_1)a(\mathbf{r}_2), \qquad ^3\psi \sim a(\mathbf{r}_1)b(\mathbf{r}_2) - b(\mathbf{r}_1)a(\mathbf{r}_2), \tag{8-99}$$

where a is an atomic orbital on nucleus a, and b is an equivalent orbital on nucleus b, so that

$$a(r_a = 0) = b(r_b = 0) \neq 0, \qquad a(r_b = 0) = a(r_a = 0) \sim 0, \quad \text{(8-100)}$$

we find that

$$A_{1a} = A_{2b} \neq 0, \qquad A_{1b} = A_{2a} \sim 0, \quad \text{(8-101)}$$

and the spin Hamiltonian is of particularly simple form.

This treatment of a simple model does not constitute a derivation of a general biradical spin Hamiltonian but does suggest how it arises. One approach to the many-electron case would be to combine what has been done here with the density matrix method to be developed in Section 10.

A spin Hamiltonian acting on a spin space with $S_{\text{eff}} = \frac{3}{2}$ could be derived in terms of the single-element operators discussed above. It would be much more complicated than that given in Eqs. (8-98), (8-96), etc., and has little to recommend it.

Possible Extensions

If we think of the biradical as two weakly interacting doublet systems, an extension which immediately suggests itself is that to three or more doublet systems which interact weakly. As a simple model one can think of three hydrogen atoms separated by moderate distances. There will be a total of eight degenerate or nearly degenerate states in such a system, which can be divided into a quartet and two doublets.

If the three interacting systems are symmetrically equivalent (e.g., three H atoms in an equilateral triangle) there will be a spatially induced degeneracy in addition to that associated with different M_s values. The two independent doublet functions will be associated with these spatially degenerate states and a simple spin Hamiltonian term which will reproduce the zero-order energies can be written

$$H^0 = J(\mathbf{S}_1 \cdot \mathbf{S}_2 + \mathbf{S}_1 \cdot \mathbf{S}_3 + \mathbf{S}_2 \cdot \mathbf{S}_3) = \tfrac{1}{2}J\mathcal{S}^2 - \tfrac{9}{8}J, \quad \text{(8-102)}$$

where $\mathcal{S} = \mathbf{S}_1 + \mathbf{S}_2 + \mathbf{S}_3$ and

$$J = \tfrac{2}{3}({}^4E^{(0)} - {}^2E^{(0)}), \quad \text{(8-103)}$$

and the zero point of the energy scale is the average energy for all eight states involved.

If the system has lower symmetry (e.g., three H atoms in a linear configuration or in a isosceles or scalene triangle) there will be three distinct energies, ${}^4E^{(0)}$, ${}^2E_1^{(0)}$, and ${}^2E_2^{(0)}$. It will not be possible to reproduce these energies with a spin Hamiltonian that treats all electrons equivalently. The way in which the spin Hamiltonian is chosen becomes arbitrary in some respects. If we express the energies relative to their degeneracy weighted average as

$$^4E^{(0)} = a/2, \qquad ^2E_1^{(0)} = -a/2 + b/2, \qquad ^2E_2^{(0)} = -a/2 - b/2 \quad (8\text{-}104)$$

and seek H^0 of the form

$$H^0 = J_{12}\mathbf{S}_1 \cdot \mathbf{S}_2 + J_{13}\mathbf{S}_1 \cdot \mathbf{S}_3 + J_{23}\mathbf{S}_2 \cdot \mathbf{S}_3, \quad (8\text{-}105)$$

we can take

$$J_{12} = J_{13} = \tfrac{1}{3}(2a + b), \qquad J_{23} = \tfrac{2}{3}(a - b). \quad (8\text{-}106)$$

The hyperfine interactions terms will be messy, even in the simplest cases.

If more than three systems are interacting, a zero-order spin Hamiltonian term of the Heisenberg form [Eq. (8-105)] is not in general possible, and of course the hyperfine terms will be still worse. Extension of the simple, biradical-type spin Hamiltonian thus seems impossible.

Other Near Degeneracies

In transition metal EPR, situations frequently occur in which the states of interest would, for the uncomplexed metal ion, have exact degeneracies corresponding to different M_L values. In a complex, L is no longer a good quantum number because the potential seen by the ion is not spherical, but some or all of the states may remain nearly degenerate. In particular, the spin–orbit interaction must be treated by degenerate, first-order perturbation theory, and S_{eff} will differ from S. These situations have been extensively discussed in the transition metal EPR literature and will not be further treated here.

Summary of Section 8

In this section a connection has been made between the full Hamiltonian obtained in Chapter I *and the eigenfunctions of the zero-order, spin-free Hamiltonian on the one hand, and a spin Hamiltonian acting within an effective spin space on the other. A basis set was introduced so that the original problem was expressed in matrix form. The size of the matrix is very large, in principle infinite, but the partitioning method can be used to obtain an equivalent result for the manifold of states of interest in terms of a matrix with dimension equal to the number of states in that manifold. The exact energy in the inverse operator occurring in the partitioning method was then approximated by a zero-order energy giving a result that is valid through second order.*

By using the theory of tensor operators and the Wigner–Eckart theorem we have been able to replace the space and spin operators originally present by purely spin operators and parameters. The parameters are given in terms of reference-state matrix elements and angular momentum coupling coefficients.

The possibility of states with degeneracy in addition to that associated with M_S *and the various* M_I *was also considered briefly in the general case and more fully for the biradical case. It was shown that for a system with nearly degenerate singlet and triplet states a spin Hamiltonian including a Heisenberg exchange term and treating electrons inequivalently reproduces the energy levels of the symmetric, full Hamiltonian. Extension to more complicated situations would be difficult, however.*

9. Perturbation Expressions for Spin Hamiltonian Parameters

We are now prepared to combine the results of the preceding section with those of Chapter I to obtain explicit expressions for specific spin Hamiltonian parameters. It is convenient to organize the presentation according to the results, i.e., the spin Hamiltonian parameters. We begin by asserting a form for the spin Hamiltonian. After a discussion of why this form is appropriate, and of possible omissions, we will examine the terms one at a time. Practical aspects of the calculations of the parameters will be discussed in Chapter III.

Form of the Spin Hamiltonian

The full Hamiltonian presented in Chapter I and summarized in Appendix F can be written in the symbolic form

$$\mathcal{H} = \mathcal{H}_0 + \mathcal{H}_B + \mathcal{H}_I + \mathcal{H}_S + \mathcal{H}_{B^2} + \mathcal{H}_{I^2} + \mathcal{H}_{S^2} + \mathcal{H}_{BI} + \mathcal{H}_{BS} + \mathcal{H}_{IS}. \tag{9-1}$$

Subscripts B, S, and I indicate operators containing these entities. When we examine the explicit terms, we note that powers of B or any I higher than the second do not occur, electron spin operators of tensorial rank greater than two do not occur, and in any term the sum of powers of B, I, and the tensorial rank of electron spin operators does not exceed two. We will see that for a state which has as its maximum degeneracy that associated with M_S and the M_I, the terms in $\mathcal{H}_B$, $\mathcal{H}_I$, and $\mathcal{H}_S$ do not contribute in first order. These considerations lead us to a spin Hamiltonian of the form

$$H = H^0(B, S) + \mathbf{S} \cdot \mathbf{D} \cdot \mathbf{S} + \mathbf{S} \cdot \mathbf{g} \cdot \mathbf{B} + \sum_\nu \mathbf{I}^\nu \cdot \gamma^\nu \cdot \mathbf{B} + \sum_\nu \mathbf{S} \cdot \mathbf{A}^\nu \cdot \mathbf{I}^\nu + \sum_{\mu,\nu} \mathbf{I}^\mu \cdot \mathbf{q}^{\mu\nu} \cdot \mathbf{I}^\nu. \tag{9-2}$$

The dots indicate a scalar product which can be expressed in either Cartesian or spherical form.

The first term in this spin Hamiltonian can be further subdivided as

$$H^0(B, S) = H_0^0 + \mathbf{B} \cdot \mathbf{d} \cdot \mathbf{B} + \mathbf{S} \cdot \mathbf{J} \cdot \mathbf{S} + \cdots. \tag{9-3}$$

All contributions to the energy which are independent of spin state and field strength are included in H_0^0, which is a multiple of the unit operator in the spin space. The effect of this term is unobservable in an ESR experiment and it is usually omitted, providing a redefinition of the zero point of the energy scale. The *diamagnetic* term $\mathbf{B} \cdot \mathbf{d} \cdot \mathbf{B}$ clearly introduces a field dependence into the energy, but is also a multiple of the unit operator in the effective spin space so it produces no splittings, and its effect is not observable in ESR. The parameter $\mathbf{d}$ is essentially the magnetic susceptibility. It includes first-order contributions from $\mathcal{H}_{B^2}$ and second-order contributions from $\mathcal{H}_B$. Both must be considered together. (Compare the discussion of gauge invariance below.) This term will henceforth be neglected.

The *Heisenberg* term $\mathbf{S} \cdot \mathbf{J} \cdot \mathbf{S}$ may sometimes be included to mimic the effect of near degeneracies, as in the biradical case. By definition it does not arise from true spin interactions in $\mathcal{H}$. If large values of S_{eff} are employed, additional terms involving higher powers of S may be included to mimic the effects of near degeneracies arising from only small deviations from spherical symmetry. Such situations are rare in free radical ESR, and we will not consider such terms further.

We come next to the question of why there are no terms in the spin Hamiltonian linear in (only one of) B, I, or S. To begin with, we note that each of the terms in $\mathcal{H}_B$, $\mathcal{H}_I$, and $\mathcal{H}_S$ is pure imaginary. (They are Hermitian, but of the form i times a real, anti-Hermitian operator.) The expectation value of any Hermitian operator is real, and thus the expectation value of any of these operators with respect to a real wave-function, which will also of necessity be pure imaginary, must be zero.

The electronic states we are considering are described by wave functions ψ_{nSM} which are (at least approximate) eigenfunctions of the *real* operator $\mathcal{H}_0$. It follows that ψ_{nSM}^* is an eigenfunction of $\mathcal{H}_0$ with the same energy. In the representation we are using, ψ_{nSM}^* is also an eigenfunction of $\mathcal{S}^2$ and $\mathcal{S}_z$ with quantum numbers S and M, respectively. Then either $\psi_{nSM}^* \propto \psi_{nSM}$, in which case appropriate choice of a constant phase factor will make ψ_{nSM} real; or there is degeneracy in excess of that associate with M. (This is M_S; nuclear spin degeneracy does not enter this discussion.) We assume the latter not to be the case and conclude that first-order contributions from $\mathcal{H}_B$, $\mathcal{H}_I$, and $\mathcal{H}_S$, which would lead to spin Hamiltonian terms of the type under discussion, vanish identically.

The exclusion of terms involving powers higher than the second of B, I, and S or their combinations from the spin Hamiltonian is not rigorous, but is a convenient and very good approximation. It is clear that such terms could arise if we went to higher than second order in perturbation theory. Such contributions may reasonably be supposed to be small. Some contributions of this type could also arise in second order, but the associated coefficients will be very small for those combinations of terms which can in principle be nonzero. The details will not be considered here.

A study of additional spin Hamiltonian terms, including those of higher order, would be of interest. For consistency, however, the starting point would have to be a Hamiltonian valid to order higher than α^2. In what is being considered here, we will not go beyond order α^2 except where additional factors of $1/c$ arise in connection with vector potentials. In a few cases terms will be included whose formal order is equal to that of other terms which are neglected. Such terms are included only when necessitated by internal consistency requirements in particular spin Hamiltonian parameters.

Spin Hamiltonian Parameters

Zero Field Splitting

The term $\mathbf{S}\cdot\mathbf{D}\cdot\mathbf{S}$ in the spin Hamiltonian is usually referred to as the zero field splitting term, since it leads to energy differences for otherwise degenerate states independent of magnetic field strength (and of nuclear spin state). Two terms in the full Hamiltonian can contribute in first order to such a spin Hamiltonian term: the spin–spin dipolar and contact terms. A second-order contribution can arise involving spin–orbit operators.

The spin–spin contact term involves a spin–tensorial operator of rank zero and would give a contribution of the same form to the spin Hamiltonian. From Eqs. (8-34) and (8-35)

$$H^{\text{SS contact}} = B_0^{\text{SS contact}} \mathscr{S}_0^{(0)}, \tag{9-4}$$

where

$$B_0^{\text{SS contact}} = \langle S\overline{M}|\mathscr{S}_0^{(0)}|S\overline{M}\rangle^{-1} \frac{32\pi}{3} \beta^2 \langle nS\overline{M}| - \sum_{j<k} \delta(r_{jk})\mathscr{S}_0^{(0)}(jk)|nS\overline{M}\rangle. \tag{9-5}$$

This will be just a constant contribution, independent of M_S, and it is normally neglected. In a biradical it would contribute to the singlet–triplet separation but normally only by an amount negligible with respect to the J defined in Eq. (8-86).

The spin–spin dipolar term provides the most important contribution to the zero field splitting. Using the spherical–tensorial form of this term and taking the reference state with $\overline{M} = S$ we find

$$B_\kappa^{\text{SS dipolar}} = \frac{(-12)\sqrt{6}}{S(2S-1)} \beta^2 \langle nS\overline{M}| \sum_{j<k} \frac{1}{r_{jk}^5} [\mathbf{r}_{jk} \times \mathbf{r}_{jk}]_\kappa^{(2)} [\mathbf{s}_j \times \mathbf{s}_k]_0^{(2)} |nS\overline{M}\rangle. \tag{9-6}$$

nominator vanishes if $S < 1$, but the considerations of the previous show that the entire contribution is zero in this case. (Compare Eq. (8-27) and note that the 3-j coefficient will vanish unless $2S \geq 2$ in this case.) The spin factor is common to all κ values. It is possible to take linear combinations of the B_κ, which will be expectation values of operators involving corresponding linear combinations of the $[\mathbf{r}_{jk} \times \mathbf{r}_{jk}]_\kappa^{(2)}$. These combinations can be taken so as to return to a Cartesian form

$$D'_{ab} = \frac{4\beta^2}{S(2S-1)} \langle nSS| \sum_{i<j} \frac{r_{ij}^2 \delta_{ab} - 3(r_{ij})_a (r_{ij})_b}{r_{ij}^5} \times (2s_{jz}s_{kz} - s_{jx}s_{kx} - s_{jy}s_{ky})|nSS\rangle. \tag{9-7}$$

The single prime on D indicates a first-order contribution. The subscripts a and b range over the Cartesian component indices x, y, and z. Clearly $D'_{ab} = D'_{ba}$ and $\sum_a D'_{aa} = 0$.

Second-order contributions to the zero field splitting are likely to be smaller than the first-order contributions, but may not be negligible. To consider them we must look at the spin–orbit operators. These are in fact three "spin–orbit" operators. Each can be written in the form

$$\mathscr{H}_{\mathrm{SO}} = i\beta^2 \sum_j \mathbf{F}_j \cdot \mathbf{s}_j. \tag{9-8}$$

For the ordinary, one-electron spin–orbit operator

$$\mathbf{F}_j^{\mathrm{SO}} = -g'_e \sum_\nu Z_\nu k_0^2(\mathbf{r}_{j\nu}) \frac{\mathbf{r}_{j\nu} \times \nabla_j}{r_{j\nu}^3}, \tag{9-9}$$

where $\mathbf{r}_{j\nu} \times \nabla_j$ is proportional to the operator for the electronic angular momentum about nucleus ν. The spin-other-orbit term has

$$\mathbf{F}_j^{\mathrm{SOO}} = 4 \sum_{k(\neq j)} \frac{(\mathbf{r}_k - \mathbf{r}_j) \times \nabla_k}{r_{jk}^3} \tag{9-10}$$

while the electron–electron spin–orbit term has

$$F_j^{\mathrm{eeSO}} = g'_e \sum_{k(\neq j)} \frac{(\mathbf{r}_j - \mathbf{r}_k) \times \nabla_j}{r_{jk}^3}. \tag{9-11}$$

The last two are sometimes combined in a single "spin–other-orbit" term

$$\mathscr{H}_{\mathrm{SOO}} = i\beta^2 \sum_{j,k}{}' \frac{(\mathbf{r}_{jk} \times \nabla_j)}{r_{jk}^3} \cdot (g'_e \mathbf{s}_j + 4\mathbf{s}_k) \tag{9-12}$$

but at other times it is convenient to treat them separately. Recall that in the convention used here $\mathbf{r}_{jk} = \mathbf{r}_j - \mathbf{r}_k$. Since both operators in the second-order expression involve spin, Eqs. (8-64) and (8-65) or their equivalent must be used. We note, however, that nuclear spins and the magnetic field are not involved. Whatever combination of spin–orbit operators is used, $k = l = 1$. In addition, each of the spin–orbit operators has the same behavior under Kramers conjugation, so the only possible values of c are 0 and 2.

A term with $c = 0$ would have an effect independent of M_S and would therefore be uninteresting, for the reasons discussed above. Such terms will not be considered.

In treating the second-order, second rank contribution, we must consider all possible combinations of the spin–orbit operators. It is also convenient to separate contributions corresponding to different values of S''. The treatment leading to the $A^x(nn'')$ tells us, in Eq. (8-27), that $|S - k| \leq S'' \leq S + k$. We define σ such that $S'' = S + \sigma$, $\sigma = -1, 0$, or 1. (Note that only $S \geq 1$ will be of interest.) Then

$$\mathbf{D}'' = \sum_{\sigma} \sum_{x,y} \mathbf{D}''(\sigma; xy), \tag{9-13}$$

where x and y range independently over labels identifying the three spin–orbit terms.

In the spherical–tensorial basis, from Eq. (8-65) and in analogy with the treatment leading to Eq. (8-92), we find (for $c = 2$)

$$D_{2\gamma}^{xy}(\sigma) = \langle S\overline{M}|\mathscr{S}_0^{(2)}|S\overline{M}\rangle^{-1}(-1)^{2S+2\sigma}\sqrt{5}\begin{Bmatrix} 1 & 1 & 2 \\ S & S & S+\sigma \end{Bmatrix}$$
$$\times \sum_{\substack{n'', n''' \\ (\ni S''' = S'' = S+\sigma)}} R^0_{n'', n'''} \times [\mathbf{A}^x(nn'') \times \mathbf{A}^y(n'''n)]^{(2)}_\gamma, \tag{9-14}$$

where

$$[\mathbf{A}^x(nn'') \times \mathbf{A}^y(n'''n)]^{(2)}_\gamma = (-1)^\gamma\sqrt{5}\sum_{\kappa,\lambda} A^x_\kappa(nn'')A^y_\lambda(n'''n)\begin{pmatrix} 1 & 1 & 2 \\ \kappa & \lambda & -\gamma \end{pmatrix}. \tag{9-15}$$

Equation (8-64) then gives the corresponding spin Hamiltonian term as the scalar product of $D_{2\gamma}^{xy}$ and $\mathscr{S}_{-\gamma}^{(2)}$. If we express the scalar product in Cartesian rather than spherical form, we can define D_{ab}^{xy} such that

$$H^{xy} = \sum_{a,b} S_a D_{ab}^{xy} S_b. \tag{9-16}$$

Since it is equivalent to a second rank spherical tensor, D_{ab}^{xy} must be symmetric in a and b and traceless ($\sum_a D_{aa}^{xy} = 0$).

We now insert the definition of A^x_κ from Eq. (8-29) and transform back to Cartesian form. We find the total second-order contribution to be

$$D''_{ab} = \sum_\sigma C(\sigma) \sum_{x,y} \sum_{\substack{n'',n'' \\ (\ni S'''=S''=S+\sigma)}} R^0_{n'',n'''} \times \left[\tfrac{1}{2}(X^{n''n'''}_{ab} + X^{n''n'''}_{ba}) - \tfrac{1}{3} \sum_c X^{n''n'''}_{cc} \delta_{ab} \right], \tag{9-17}$$

where

$$X^{n''n'''}_{ab} = -\beta^4 \langle nS\overline{M} | \sum_j F^x_{ja} S_{jz} | n''S + \sigma\overline{M} \rangle \langle n'''S + \sigma\overline{M} | \sum_k F^y_{kb} S_{kz} | nS\overline{M} \rangle \tag{9-18}$$

and

$$C(\sigma) = \frac{(-1)^{2\overline{M}+\sigma}\sqrt{30}}{[3\overline{M}^2 - S(S+1)]} \begin{Bmatrix} 1 & 1 & 2 \\ S & S & S+\sigma \end{Bmatrix} \begin{pmatrix} S & 1 & 2+\sigma \\ -\overline{M} & 0 & \overline{M} \end{pmatrix}^{-2}. \tag{9-19}$$

Expressions for $C(\sigma)$ in terms of S, $\overline{M}$, and σ, suggested choices of $\overline{M}$, and numerical values for $S = 1$ are given in Table 9-1. Of course the same choice of $\overline{M}$ must be used in the evaluation of $C(\sigma)$ and the $X^{n''n'''}_{ab}$ for that σ.

Electron Zeeman Term: The g Tensor

We consider now the term describing the interaction of electron magnetic moments with the external field. The relevant parameter is the g tensor [197]. It is convenient to separate the free-electron contribution and write

$$\mathbf{g} = g_e \mathbf{1} + \Delta\mathbf{g}. \tag{9-20}$$

The g_e term arises in a trivial way. Since the ordinary Zeeman operator has no spatial dependence for a uniform field, it can be taken directly into the spin Hamiltonian. Two other terms contribute in first order: the kinetic energy and gauge corrections to the Zeeman interaction. Second-order contributions arise from spin–orbit and orbital Zeeman cross terms.

The kinetic energy correction term is present even for a "free" electron, and is contained in Eq. (1-67), for example. The κ dependence of the spatial part comes only in **B** and can be factored out of all integrals over electronic coordinates. The contribution to $\Delta\mathbf{g}$ is thus isotropic.

$$\Delta g^{\text{KE}}_{ab} = \delta_{ab} g_e \beta \frac{1}{m^2c^2} \langle nS\overline{M} | \sum_j (-\tfrac{1}{2}\nabla_j^2) s_{jz} | nS\overline{M} \rangle. \tag{9-21}$$

The expectation value is proportional to the kinetic energy only in a one-electron system or other cases where S is equal to half the number of electrons.

TABLE 9-1

Coefficients for Zero-Field-Splitting Parameters

	$\sigma = +1$	$\sigma = 0$	$\sigma = -1$
$C(\sigma)$[a]	$\dfrac{x}{[3\overline{M}^2 - S(S+1)][(S+1)^2 - \overline{M}]}$	$\dfrac{-x}{[3\overline{M}^2 - S(S+1)]\overline{M}^2}$	$\dfrac{x}{[3\overline{M}^2 - S(S+1)]}$
Suggested $\overline{M}$	S	S	0
$C(\sigma)$ with that choice	$\left[\dfrac{(2S+2)(2S+3)}{(2S-1)(2S)(2S+1)}\right]^{1/2}$	$-\dfrac{1}{S^2}\left[\dfrac{(2S+1)(2S+2)(2S+3)}{(2S-1)(2S)}\right]^{1/2}$	$-2\left[\dfrac{(2S-1)(2S+1)(2S+3)}{(2S)(2S+2)}\right]^{1/2}$
Value of $C(\sigma)$ for $S = 1$ and $\overline{M}$ as above	$\sqrt{\frac{10}{3}}$	$\sqrt{30}$	$\sqrt{\frac{15}{2}}$

[a] $x = \frac{1}{2}[(2S-1)(2S)(2S+1)(2S+2)(2S+3)]^{1/2}$.

The gauge-correction terms have been called that because they must be retained to give a gauge-invariant result for the g tensor. The same origin must be used in defining the angular momentum in the orbital Zeeman term (which contributes to **g** in second order) and in expressing the vector potential. These terms make anisotropic contributions to $\Delta\mathbf{g}$ in first order. Before considering them in detail we must examine the question of gauge invariance and the choice of origin. In Chapter I we noted that a gauge change in Dirac or Schrödinger operators is offset by a phase change in the wave function, so the Dirac or Schrödinger equation remains unchanged. A similar argument cannot be used here, because we are involved in a perturbation calculation with fixed zero-order functions. We can nevertheless find gauge invariant combinations of terms.

It will be convenient at this point to work directly with matrix elements rather than with spin Hamiltonian parameters. We will also assume that the excited states are eigenstates of $\mathscr{H}_0$ so that $R^0_{n''n'''} = \delta_{n''n'''}(E_a^{(0)} - E_{n''}^{(0)})^{-1}$ As remarked previously, the conclusions we draw will in fact be independent of this choice, but it makes the algebra simpler. The first-order matrix elements of interest are

$$\begin{aligned}
\langle M|H^{(1)}_{\mathrm{SO}}|M'\rangle &= \langle nSM|g'_e\beta^2\frac{e}{\hbar c}\sum_{j,\nu}\frac{Z_\nu}{r_j^3}\mathbf{s}_j\cdot\mathbf{r}_{j\nu}\times\mathbf{A}(\mathbf{r}_j)|nSM'\rangle,\\
\langle M|H^{(1)}_{\mathrm{SOO}}|M'\rangle &= \langle nSM|\beta^2\frac{4e}{\hbar c}\sum_{j,k}{}'\frac{1}{r_{jk}^3}\mathbf{s}_j\cdot\mathbf{r}_{jk}\times\mathbf{A}(\mathbf{r}_k)|nSM'\rangle, \qquad (9\text{-}22)\\
\langle M|H^{(1)}_{\mathrm{eeSO}}|M'\rangle &= \langle nSM|-g'_e\beta^2\frac{e}{\hbar c}\sum_{j,k}{}'\frac{1}{r_{jk}^3}\mathbf{s}_j\cdot\mathbf{r}_{jk}\times\mathbf{A}(\mathbf{r}_j)|nSM'\rangle
\end{aligned}$$

These terms arise from the operators in Eqs. (2-93), (4-36), and (4-38), respectively, but we have expressed them in their earlier forms involving the vector potential. The labeling corresponds to that used on the spin–orbit operators. We will see that a one-to-one correspondence exists.

The second-order terms can be expressed in the general form

$$\begin{aligned}
\langle M|H^{(2)}_{xz}|M'\rangle = &\sum_{n''M''}(E_n^{(0)} - E_{n''}^{(0)})^{-1}\langle nSM|i\beta^2\sum_j\mathbf{F}_j^x\cdot\mathbf{s}_j|n''S''M''\rangle\\
&\times\langle n''S''M''|-i\beta\sum_k(\boldsymbol{\nabla}_k\cdot\mathbf{A}(\mathbf{r}_k)+\mathbf{A}(\mathbf{r}_k)\cdot\boldsymbol{\nabla}_k)|nSM'\rangle,\\
\langle M|H^{(2)}_{zx}|M'\rangle = &\sum_{n''M''}{}'(E_n^{(0)} - E_{n''}^{(0)})^{-1}\langle nSM|-i\beta\sum_k(\boldsymbol{\nabla}_k\cdot\mathbf{A}(\mathbf{r}_k) \qquad (9\text{-}23)\\
&+\mathbf{A}(\mathbf{r}_k)\cdot\boldsymbol{\nabla}_k|n''S''M''\rangle\times\langle n''S''M''|i\beta^2\sum_j\mathbf{F}_j^x\cdot\mathbf{s}_j|nSM'\rangle
\end{aligned}$$

where the prime on the summation sign means $n'' \neq n$. The operator involving $\mathbf{F}_j^x$ is any of the spin–orbit operators with $\mathbf{F}_j^x$ given by Eqn. (9-9)–(9-11). The other operator is the orbital Zeeman term reexpressed in terms of a general **A** so as to make no assumptions about the choice of gauge. The sums extend over the complete set of excited states, but in fact only those terms with $S'' = S$ and $M'' = M$ in the second sum will be nonzero.

In order to treat the effect of a gauge transformation, we now employ an argument based on the treatment of Griffith [67, Appendix A] and Davies [45]. Let

$$\tilde{g}(\mathbf{r}_1, \mathbf{r}_2, \ldots) = \sum_k g(\mathbf{r}_k) \tag{9-24}$$

be a function of the position coordinates of the electrons. Consider

$$\begin{aligned}
\langle t|\mathscr{H}_0\tilde{g} - \tilde{g}\mathscr{H}_0|u\rangle &= (E_t^{(0)} - E_u^{(0)})\langle t|\tilde{g}|u\rangle \\
&= -\frac{\hbar^2}{2m}\langle t|\sum_j \nabla_j^2\tilde{g} - \tilde{g}\sum_j \nabla_j^2|u\rangle \\
&= -\frac{\hbar^2}{2m}\langle t|\sum_j [\nabla_j^2 g(\mathbf{r}_j) - g(\mathbf{r}_j)\nabla_j^2]|u\rangle \\
&= -\frac{\hbar^2}{2m}\langle t|[\operatorname{div}_j \operatorname{grad}_j g(\mathbf{r}_j) + 2\operatorname{grad}_j g(\mathbf{r}_j)\cdot\mathbf{V}_j]|u\rangle.
\end{aligned} \tag{9-25}$$

Here t and u label zero-order eigenstates, so the first equality is obvious. The second follows from the fact that the potential terms in $\mathscr{H}_0$ commute with the functions $\tilde{g}$, and the third from the fact that $[\nabla_j^2, g(\mathbf{r}_k)] = 0$ if $j \neq k$. In the last line, div_j and grad_j represent derivatives with respect to the components of $\mathbf{r}_j$ which act on $g(\mathbf{r}_j)$ but not on $|u\rangle$. Of course $\mathbf{V}_j$ does act on $|u\rangle$. On comparing the first and last expressions and inserting the definition of $\tilde{g}$, we find

$$\frac{\langle t|\sum_j [\operatorname{div}_j \operatorname{grad}_j g(\mathbf{r}_j) + 2\operatorname{grad}_j g(\mathbf{r}_j)\cdot\mathbf{V}_j]|u\rangle}{E_u^{(0)} - E_t^{(0)}} = \frac{2m}{\hbar^2}\langle t|\sum_k g(\mathbf{r}_k)|u\rangle. \tag{9-26}$$

Armed with this relationship we proceed with an examination of gauge transformations.

Suppose that the vector potential is subjected to a gauge transformation

$$\mathbf{A}(\mathbf{r}) \to A(\mathbf{r}) + \operatorname{grad} f(\mathbf{r}). \tag{9-27}$$

(Note that this means $\mathbf{A}(\mathbf{r}_j) \to \mathbf{A}(\mathbf{r}_j) + \text{grad}_j f(\mathbf{r}_j)$.) There will be corresponding changes in the first- and second-order matrix elements. In the first-order terms the changes will be

$$\Delta(\langle M | H_{\text{SO}}^{(1)} | M' \rangle) = g_e' \beta^2 \frac{e}{\hbar c} \sum_\nu Z_\nu \langle nSM | \sum_j \frac{1}{r_{j\nu}^3} \mathbf{s}_j \cdot \mathbf{r}_{j\nu} \times \text{grad}_j f(\mathbf{r}_j) | nSM' \rangle$$

$$\Delta(\langle M | H_{\text{SO}}^{(1)} | M' \rangle) = \beta^2 \frac{4e}{\hbar c} \langle nSM | \sum_{j,k}' \frac{1}{r_{jk}^3} \mathbf{s}_j \cdot \mathbf{r}_{jk} \times \text{grad}_k f(\mathbf{r}_k) | nSM' \rangle,$$

$$\Delta(\langle M | H_{\text{eeSO}}^{(1)} | M' \rangle) = -g_e' \beta^2 \frac{e}{\hbar c} \langle nSM | \sum_{j,k}' \frac{1}{r_{jk}^3} \mathbf{s}_j \cdot \mathbf{r}_{jk} \times \text{grad}_j f(\mathbf{r}_j) | nSM' \rangle. \tag{9-28}$$

For the changes in the second-order terms we use Eq. (9-26) with $g = f$ and with $t \leftrightarrow n''S''M''$, $u \leftrightarrow nSM'$ to obtain

$$\begin{aligned}
&\Delta(\langle M | H_{xz}^{(2)} | M' \rangle) \\
&\quad = \beta^3 \sum_{n''M''}' \langle nSM | \sum_j \mathbf{F}_j^x \cdot \mathbf{s}_j | n''S''M'' \rangle \\
&\qquad \times \frac{\langle n''S''M'' | \sum_k (2 \,\text{grad}_k f(\mathbf{r}_k) \cdot \nabla_k + \text{div}_k \,\text{grad}_k f(\mathbf{r}_k) | nSM' \rangle}{E_n^{(0)} - E_{n''}^{(0)}} \\
&\quad = \beta^3 \frac{2m}{\hbar^2} \sum_{n''M''} \langle nSM | \sum_j \mathbf{F}_j^x \cdot \mathbf{s}_j | n''S''M'' \rangle \langle n''S''M'' | \sum_k f(\mathbf{r}_k) | nSM' \rangle \\
&\quad = \beta^2 \frac{e}{\hbar c} \langle nSM | \Big(\sum_j \mathbf{F}_j^x \cdot \mathbf{s}_j \Big) \Big(\sum_k f(\mathbf{r}_k) \Big) | nSM' \rangle
\end{aligned} \tag{9-29}$$

The last equality requires that the sum over states be extended to include $n'' = n$. If $|nSM\rangle$ is spatially nondegenerate, i.e., its only degeneracy is that associated with M_S, then it can be taken to be real and

$$\langle nSM | \sum_j \mathbf{F}_j^x \cdot \mathbf{s}_j | nSM \rangle = 0,$$

by the argument used at the beginning of this section. The extension is therefore possible. Taking $t \leftrightarrow nSM$, $u \leftrightarrow n''S''M''$ we obtain, similarly,

$$\begin{aligned}
&\Delta(\langle M | H_{zx}^{(2)} | M' \rangle) \\
&\quad = \beta^3 \sum_{n''M''}' \frac{\langle nSM | \sum_k (2 \,\text{grad}_k f(\mathbf{r}_k) \cdot \nabla_k + \text{div}_k \,\text{grad}_k f(\mathbf{r}_k) | n''S''M'' \rangle}{E_n^{(0)} - E_{n''}^{(0)}} \\
&\qquad \times \langle n''S''M'' | \sum_j \mathbf{F}_j^x \cdot \mathbf{s}_j | nSM' \rangle \\
&\quad = \beta^3 \Big(-\frac{2m}{\hbar^2} \Big) \sum_{n''M''} \langle nSM | \sum_k f(\mathbf{r}_k) | n''S''M'' \rangle \langle n''S''M'' | \sum_j \mathbf{F}_j^x \cdot \mathbf{s}_j | nSM' \rangle \\
&\quad = \beta^2 \frac{e}{\hbar c} \langle nSM | - \Big(\sum_k f(\mathbf{r}_k) \Big) \Big(\sum_j \mathbf{F}_j^x \cdot \mathbf{s}_j \Big) | nSM' \rangle.
\end{aligned} \tag{9-30}$$

The total second-order contribution will include the sum $H^{(2)}_{xz} + H^{(2)}_{zx}$, and the change in this sum resulting from the gauge transformation is

$$\Delta(\langle M|H^{(2)}_{xz} + H^{(2)}_{zx}|M'\rangle) = \beta^2 \frac{e}{\hbar c} \langle nSM|\left[\sum_j \mathbf{F}^x_j \cdot \mathbf{s}_j, \sum_k f(\mathbf{r}_k)\right]|nSM'\rangle. \tag{9-31}$$

For the one-electron spin–orbit operator (ignoring k_0 for simplicity)

$$\begin{aligned}\left[\sum_j \mathbf{F}^{\mathrm{SO}}_j \cdot \mathbf{s}_j, \sum_k f(\mathbf{r}_k)\right] &= g'_e\left[\sum_{\nu, j} Z_\nu \frac{\mathbf{r}_{j\nu} \times \boldsymbol{\nabla}_j}{r^3_{j\nu}} \cdot \mathbf{s}_j, \sum_k f(\mathbf{r}_k)\right] \\ &= g'_e \sum_\nu Z_\nu \sum_j \left[\frac{\mathbf{r}_{j\nu} \times \boldsymbol{\nabla}_j}{r^3_{j\nu}} \cdot \mathbf{s}_j, f(\mathbf{r}_j)\right] \\ &= g'_e \sum_\nu Z_\nu \sum_j \frac{1}{r^3_{j\nu}} \mathbf{s}_j \cdot \mathbf{r}_{j\nu} \times \mathrm{grad}_j\, f(\mathbf{r}_j) \end{aligned} \tag{9-32}$$

and the change in the second-order contribution is

$$\begin{aligned}\Delta(\langle M|H^{(2)}_{\mathrm{SO},z} + H^{(2)}_{z,\mathrm{SO}}|M'\rangle) &= -g'_e\beta^2 \frac{e}{\hbar c} \sum_\nu Z_\nu \langle nSM|\sum_j \frac{1}{r^3_{j\nu}} \mathbf{s}_j \cdot \mathbf{r}_{j\nu} \\ &\qquad \times \mathrm{grad}_j\, f(\mathbf{r}_j)|nSM'\rangle \\ &= -\Delta(\langle M|H^{(1)}_{\mathrm{SO}}|M'\rangle), \end{aligned} \tag{9-33}$$

so that the sum of the first- and second-order contributions is invariant under the gauge transformation. We can in fact make a stronger statement. For each term associated with a particular nucleus, labeled by ν, the sum of the first- and second-order contributions is gauge invariant. A change in the choice of origin for the vector potential is a gauge transformation, and the same origin must be used in both the first- and second-order terms, for $\mathbf{A}(\mathbf{r}_j)$ and for $\boldsymbol{l}_j = \hbar^{-1}(\mathbf{r}_j \times \mathbf{P}_j)$. However, we see from the above that different choices can be made for different values of ν, provided they are made consistently. This will be done shortly in the expressions for $\Delta\mathbf{g}$.

For the spin–other-orbit term we have

$$\begin{aligned}\left[\sum_j \mathbf{F}^{\mathrm{SOO}}_j \cdot \mathbf{s}_j, \sum_k f(\mathbf{r}_k)\right] &= 4\left[\sum_{j,l}{}' \frac{\mathbf{r}_{lj} \times \boldsymbol{\nabla}_l}{r^3_{jl}} \cdot \mathbf{s}_j, \sum_k f(\mathbf{r}_k)\right] \\ &= 4\sum_{j,k}{}' \left[\frac{\mathbf{r}_{kj} \times \boldsymbol{\nabla}_k}{r^3_{jk}} \cdot \mathbf{s}_j, f(\mathbf{r}_k)\right] \\ &= 4\sum_{j,k}{}' \frac{1}{r^3_{jk}} \mathbf{s}_j \cdot \mathbf{r}_{kj} \times \mathrm{grad}_k\, f(\mathbf{r}_k) \end{aligned} \tag{9-34}$$

and

$$\Delta(\langle M | H^{(2)}_{\mathrm{SOO},z} + H^{(2)}_{z,\mathrm{SOO}} | M' \rangle = 4\beta^2 \frac{e}{\hbar c} \langle nSM | \sum_{j,k}{}' \frac{1}{r_{jk}^3} \mathbf{s}_j \cdot \mathbf{r}_{kj} \times \operatorname{grad}_k f(\mathbf{r}_k) | nSM' \rangle = -\Delta(\langle M | H^{(1)}_{\mathrm{SOO}} | M' \rangle), \tag{9-35}$$

since $\mathbf{r}_{jk} = -\mathbf{r}_{kj}$. Similarly, for the electron–electron spin–orbit term

$$\left[\sum_j \mathbf{F}_j^{\mathrm{eeSO}} \cdot \mathbf{s}_j, \sum_k f(\mathbf{r}_k)\right] = g'_e \left[\sum_{j,l}{}' \frac{\mathbf{r}_{jl} \times \boldsymbol{\nabla}_j}{r_{jl}^3} \cdot \mathbf{s}_j, \sum_k f(\mathbf{r}_k)\right] = g'_e \sum_{j,k}{}' \left[\frac{\mathbf{r}_{jk} \times \boldsymbol{\nabla}_j}{r_{jk}^3} \cdot \mathbf{s}_j, f(\mathbf{r}_j)\right] = g'_e \sum_{j,k}{}' \frac{1}{r_{jk}^3} \mathbf{s}_j \cdot \mathbf{r}_{jk} \times \operatorname{grad}_j f(\mathbf{r}_j) \tag{9-36}$$

and

$$(\langle M | H^{(2)}_{\mathrm{eeSO},z} + H^{(2)}_{z,\mathrm{eeSO}} | M' \rangle) = g'_e \beta^2 \frac{e}{\hbar c} \langle nSM | \sum_{j,k}{}' \frac{1}{r_{jk}^3} \mathbf{s}_j \cdot \mathbf{r}_{jk} \times \operatorname{grad}_j f(\mathbf{r}_j) | nSM' \rangle = -\Delta(\langle M | H^{(1)}_{\mathrm{eeSO}} | M' \rangle). \tag{9-37}$$

Each of these sums of first- and second-order contributions is thus also gauge invariant.

Let us now consider the contributions to the g tensor making convenient choice of origin in a consistent way.

$$\Delta g'_{ab}(\mathrm{SO}) = g'_e \beta \frac{e^2}{4mc^2} \frac{1}{\overline{M}} \sum_\nu Z_\nu \langle nS\overline{M} | \sum_j \frac{1}{r_{j\nu}^3} [r_{j\nu}^2 \delta_{ab} - (\mathbf{r}_{j\nu})_a (\mathbf{r}_{j\nu})_b] s_{jz} | nS\overline{M} \rangle \tag{9-38}$$

$$g''_{ab}(\mathrm{SO}) = g'_e \beta^3 \frac{1}{\overline{M}} \sum_\nu Z_\nu \sum_{\substack{n'',n''' \\ (\ni S''' = S'' = S)}} \Bigg\{ \langle nSM | \sum_j \frac{k_0^2(r_{j\nu})}{r_{j\nu}^3} \times (\boldsymbol{l}_{j\nu})_a s_{jz} | n''S\overline{M} \rangle R^0_{n''n'''} \langle n'''S\overline{M} | \sum_k (\boldsymbol{l}_{k\nu})_b | nSM \rangle + \langle nS\overline{M} | \sum_k (\boldsymbol{l}_{k\nu})_b | n''S\overline{M} \rangle R^0_{n''n'''} \langle nS\overline{M} | \sum_j \frac{k_0^2(r_{j\nu})}{r_{j\nu}^3} (\boldsymbol{l}_{j\nu})_a s_{jz} | nS\overline{M} \rangle \Bigg\}. \tag{9-39}$$

The first-order contribution is symmetric in the indices a and b, but the second-order contribution is not obviously so.

The two-electron spin–orbit contributions can be combined at this point to give

$$\Delta g'_{ab}(2\text{el} = \beta^2 \frac{e}{2\hbar c}\frac{1}{\overline{M}}\langle nS\overline{M}|\sum_{jk}{}' \frac{1}{r_{jk}^3}[\mathbf{r}_{jk}\cdot(4\mathbf{r}_k - g'_e\mathbf{r}_j)\delta_{ab} - (4\mathbf{r}_k - g'\mathbf{r}_j)_a(\mathbf{r}_{jk})_b]s_{jz}|nS\overline{M}\rangle \tag{9-40}$$

and

$$\Delta g''_{ab}(2\text{el}) = \beta^3\frac{1}{\overline{M}}\sum_{\substack{n''n'''\\(\ni S'''=S''=S)}}\Big\{\langle nS\overline{M}|\sum_{j,k}{}'\frac{1}{r_{jk}^3}[\mathbf{r}_{jk}\times(g'_e\nabla_j - 4\nabla_k)]s_{jz}|n''S\overline{M}\rangle R^0_{n''n'''}\langle n'''S\overline{M}|\sum_l(\mathbf{r}_l\times\nabla_l)_b|nSM\rangle + \text{c.c.}\Big\} \tag{9-41}$$

where " +c.c." indicates addition of the complex conjugate of the preceding term.

The total result for Δg_{ab} is the sum of contributions

$$\Delta g_{ab} = \Delta g_{ab}^{\text{KE}} + \Delta g'_{ab}(\text{SO}) + \Delta g''_{ab}(\text{SO}) + \Delta g'_{ab}(2\text{el}) + \Delta g''_{ab}(2\text{el}). \tag{9-42}$$

Like any other second order, Cartesian tensor, $\Delta\mathbf{g}$ can be separated into an isotropic part and a traceless part. It is not clear that the traceless part will necessarily be symmetric in general, but we have seen in Section 7 that the tensor which is readily observable is $\mathbf{gg}^{\mathrm{T}}$, and this is necessarily symmetric.

Nuclear Zeeman Terms

The nuclear Zeeman term in the full Hamiltonian can be taken over directly into the spin Hamiltonian to give a first-order nuclear Zeeman term independent of the electronic wave function. Since, as we have seen in Section 7, the effect of the nuclear Zeeman term is usually small in ESR it is probably sufficient to stop with this contribution. There are, however, additional first- and second-order contributions as well. They lead to the shielding tensor and chemical shift effects in NMR.

The nuclear Zeeman spin Hamiltonian parameter γ^{ν} of Eq. (9-2) is customarily expressed as‡

$$\gamma^{\nu} = g_{\nu}\beta_{\text{N}}(\mathbf{1} - \boldsymbol{\sigma}^{\nu}) \tag{9-43}$$

‡ As commonly used, γ differs from the value implied here by a factor of h.

where β_N is the nuclear magneton, g_ν is the g factor appropriate to the bare nucleus, and $\boldsymbol{\sigma}^\nu$ is the nuclear shielding tensor. It is the sum of a first-order contribution, coming from the cross term between the nuclear moment contribution and the external field contribution in the square of the vector potential, and a second-order contribution linking the orbital hyperfine and orbital Zeeman terms. As in the case of the g tensor contributions, these terms are not individually gauge invariant, but their sum is, and in calculating $\boldsymbol{\sigma}^\nu$, it is convenient to choose the origin for the angular momentum and for that part of $\mathbf{A}$ coming from the uniform field to be at nucleus ν. Then (neglecting k_0)

$$\sigma_{ab}^{\nu'} = \frac{e^2}{2mc^2} \langle nS\overline{M} | \sum_j \frac{1}{r_{j\nu}^3} [r_{j\nu}^2 \delta_{ab} - (\mathbf{r}_{j\nu})_a (\mathbf{r}_{j\nu})_b] | nS\overline{M} \rangle \tag{9-44}$$

and

$$\sigma_{ab}^{\nu''} = \beta^2 \sum_{\substack{n'', n'' \\ (\ni S''' = S'' = S)}} \left\{ \langle nS\overline{M} | \sum_j \frac{k_0(\mathbf{r}_{j\nu})}{r_{j\nu}^3} (\boldsymbol{l}_{j\nu})_a | n''S\overline{M} \rangle R_{n''n'''}^0 \right.$$
$$\times \langle n'''S\overline{M} | \sum_k (\boldsymbol{l}_{k\nu})_b | nS\overline{M} \rangle$$
$$\left. + \langle nS\overline{M} | \sum_k (\boldsymbol{l}_{k\nu})_b | n''S\overline{M} \rangle R_{n''n'''}^0 \langle n'''S\overline{M} | \sum_j \frac{k_0(\mathbf{r}_{j\nu})}{r_{j\nu}^3} (\boldsymbol{l}_{j\nu})_a | nS\overline{M} \rangle \right\}. \tag{9-45}$$

These results are independent of the choice of $\overline{M}$ since they do not involve electron spin operators at all.

It might appear that another second-order contribution could arise involving electron spin Zeeman and hyperfine interactions with the spin dependence coupled to rank zero. We note, however, that the Zeeman term can be written as $g_e \beta \mathbf{S} \cdot \mathbf{B}$ where $\mathbf{S}$ is the total spin operator, and thus $\langle nSM | g_e \beta \mathbf{S} \cdot \mathbf{B} | n'S'M' \rangle = 0$ if $n' \neq n$.

Hyperfine Interaction Terms

The hyperfine interaction includes a sum of two first-order contributions corresponding to the Fermi contact and dipolar hyperfine terms in the Hamiltonian. There are also second-order contributions arising as cross terms between the orbital hyperfine operator and any of the spin–orbit operators. The second-order contributions are expected to be negligible in free radical work, but we will consider them briefly.

The contribution from the Fermi contact hyperfine operator is clearly isotropic

$$A_{ab}^{\nu'}(\text{contact}) = \frac{8\pi}{3} \delta_{ab} g_e' \beta g_\nu \beta_N \frac{1}{\overline{M}} \langle nS\overline{M} | \sum_j \delta(\mathbf{r}_{j\nu}) s_{jz} | nS\overline{M} \rangle. \tag{9-46}$$

The contribution of the dipolar hyperfine operator is

$$A_{ab}^{\nu'}(\text{dipolar}) = g_e \beta g_\nu \beta_N \frac{1}{\overline{M}} \langle nS\overline{M}| \sum_j \frac{k_0(\mathbf{r}_{j\nu})}{r_{j\nu}^3} \left[\delta_{ab} - 3\frac{(\mathbf{r}_{j\nu})_a(\mathbf{r}_{j\nu})_b}{r_{j\nu}^2}\right] s_{jz} |nS\overline{M}\rangle. \tag{9-47}$$

It is apparent that $A_{ab}^{\nu'}(\text{dipolar}) = A_{ba}^{\nu'}(\text{dipolar})$ and that $\sum_a A_{aa}^{\nu'}(\text{dipolar}) = 0$.

If second-order contributions to **A** are to be considered, then for consistency certain additional but small first-order contributions should be included. These are analogous to the "gauge correction" terms contributing to $\Delta\mathbf{g}$ but with the vector potential due to the nuclear moment replacing that due to the uniform external field. A special case of one of these has already been considered insofar as it corresponds in the partitioning approach to the Fermi contact term. The much smaller, general contribution is

$$A_{ab}^{\nu'}(\text{SO correction}) = g_\nu \beta_N g_e' \beta^2 \frac{e}{\hbar c} \frac{1}{\overline{M}} \langle nS\overline{M}| \sum_j \sum_{\nu'(\neq \nu)} \frac{Z_{\nu'} k_0^2(r_{j\nu'})}{r_{j\nu}^3 r_{j\nu'}^3}$$
$$\times [(\mathbf{r}_{j\nu} \cdot \mathbf{r}_{j\nu'})\delta_{ab} - (\mathbf{r}_{j\nu'})_a(\mathbf{r}_{j\nu})_b] s_{jz} |nS\overline{M}\rangle. \tag{9-48}$$

Similar corrections associable with the two-electron spin–orbit terms can be combined to give

$$A_{ab}^{\nu'}(\text{2el corrections})$$
$$= g_\nu \beta_N \beta^2 \frac{e}{\hbar c} \frac{1}{\overline{M}} \langle nS\overline{M}| \sum_{j,k}{}' \frac{1}{r_{jk}^3 r_{j\nu}^3}$$
$$\times [\mathbf{r}_{jk} \cdot (4\mathbf{r}_{k\nu} - g_e' \mathbf{r}_{j\nu})\delta_{ab} - (4\mathbf{r}_{k\nu} - g_e' r_{j\nu})_a (\mathbf{r}_{j\nu})_a (\mathbf{r}_{jk})_b] s_{jz} |nS\overline{M}\rangle. \tag{9-49}$$

The corresponding second-order contributions are

$$A_{ab}^{\nu''}(\text{SO}) = g_\nu \beta_N g_e' \beta^2 \frac{1}{\overline{M}} \sum_{\substack{n'', n''' \\ (\ni S''' = S'' = S)}} \left\{ \langle nS\overline{M}| \sum_j \sum_{\nu'} Z_{\nu'} \frac{k_0^2}{r_{j\nu'}^3} (\boldsymbol{l}_{j\nu'})_a \right.$$
$$\left. \times s_{jz} |n''S\overline{M}\rangle R_{n''n'''}^0 \langle n'''S\overline{M}| \sum_k \frac{k_0}{r_{k\nu}^3} (\boldsymbol{l}_{k\nu})_b |nS\overline{M}\rangle + \text{c.c.} \right\} \tag{9-50}$$

$$A_{ab}^{\nu''}(\text{2el}) = g_\nu \beta_N \beta^2 \frac{1}{\overline{M}} \sum_{\substack{n'', n''' \\ (\ni S''' = S'' = S)}} \left\{ \langle nS\overline{M}| \sum_{j,k}{}' \frac{1}{r_{jk}^3} [\mathbf{r}_{jk} \times (4\nabla_k - g_e' \nabla_j)]_a \right.$$
$$\left. \times s_{jz} |n''S\overline{M}\rangle R_{n''n'''}^0 \langle n'''S\overline{M}| \sum_l \frac{k_0}{r_{l\nu}^3} (\boldsymbol{l}_{l\nu})_b |nS\overline{M}\rangle + \text{c.c.} \right\}. \tag{9-51}$$

In principle $\mathbf{A}^{\nu}$ is the sum of all these contributions, and there is no guarantee that the second-order contributions will be symmetric in their Cartesian indices. In practice, the only significant contributions in free radicals are likely to be the first-order contact and dipolar contributions, which are symmetric.

Nuclear Spin–Nuclear Spin Coupling Terms

Terms which are quadratic or bilinear in nuclear spin operators can arise in both first and second order. The only really important contribution for our purposes is that from the nuclear quadrupole term, which will contribute in first order. The direct dipole–dipole interaction can be taken directly into the spin Hamiltonian. It and second-order contributions leading to coupling of nuclear spins will be considered briefly. They are of importance in NMR but are not normally so in ESR.

The nuclear quadrupole contribution gives

$$q_{ab}^{\nu\nu}(\text{quadrupole}) = \frac{-e^2 Q_\nu}{2I_\nu(2I_\nu - 1)} \langle nS\overline{M}| \sum_j \left(\frac{3(\mathbf{r}_{j\nu})_a(\mathbf{r}_{j\nu})_b - r_{j\nu}^2 \delta_{ab}}{r_{j\nu}^5} \right) |nS\overline{M}\rangle. \tag{9-52}$$

Here I_ν is the nuclear spin quantum number and the result is independent of $\overline{M}$.

The direct dipolar interaction between nuclei gives

$$q_{ab}^{\nu\nu'}(\text{dipole}) = g_\nu g_{\nu'} \beta_{\mathrm{N}}^2 \left[\frac{\delta_{ab}}{R_{\nu\nu'}^3} - 3\frac{(\mathbf{R}_{\nu\nu'})_a(\mathbf{R}_{\nu\nu'})_b}{R_{\nu\nu'}^5} \right] \qquad (\nu \neq \nu'). \tag{9-53}$$

This quantity is entirely independent of the electronic variables, but should be appropriately averaged over nuclear motions. It is traceless so its spherical average is zero.

A final first-order contribution is that due to the square of the vector potential from the nuclear moments:

$$q_{ab}^{\nu\nu'}(A^2) = g_\nu g_{\nu'} \beta_{\mathrm{N}}^2 \frac{e^2}{2mc^2} \langle nS\overline{M}| \sum_j \frac{k_0}{r_{j\nu}^3 r_{j\nu'}^3} [(\mathbf{r}_{j\nu} \cdot \mathbf{r}_{j\nu'})\delta_{ab} - (\mathbf{r}_{j\nu'})_a(\mathbf{r}_{j\nu})_b] |nS\overline{M}\rangle. \tag{9-54}$$

It is not clear how this term should be treated, since the integrals involved are divergent when $\nu = \nu'$, as pointed out in Section 2. In other cases the term is very small. It should probably be ignored until a more satisfactory treatment of nuclear moments and their interaction with electrons is available.

A second-order contribution arises from the orbital hyperfine term

$$q_{ab}^{\nu\nu'}(\text{orbital}) = g_\nu g_{\nu'} \beta_N^2 \beta^2 \sum_{\substack{n'', n''' \\ (\ni S''' = S'' = S)}} \left\{ \langle nS\bar{M} | \sum_j \frac{k_0}{r_{j\nu}^3} (\mathbf{l}_{j\nu})_a | n''S\bar{M} \rangle \right.$$

$$\left. \times R^0_{n''n'''} \langle n'''S\bar{M} | \sum_k \frac{k_0}{r_{k\nu'}^3} (\mathbf{l}_{k\nu'})_b | nS\bar{M} \rangle \right\}. \qquad (9\text{-}55)$$

Other second-order contributions can arise involving the hyperfine interaction. They are not really of the form of the other terms considered here, since they involve an electron spin operator as well as two nuclear spin operators, but if the electron spin tensorial rank c is zero, the distinction is not very significant. For the term arising from the contact hyperfine interaction, for example,

$$q_{ab\ 0}^{\nu\nu'[0]} = \langle S\bar{M} | \mathscr{S}_0^{[0]} | S\bar{M} \rangle^{-1} \left[\sum_{\substack{n'', n''' \\ (\ni S''' = S'')}} R^0_{n''n'''} \sum_{\kappa, \lambda} (-1)^{\kappa+\lambda} \right.$$

$$\left. \times A_\kappa(\nu; nn'') A_\lambda(\nu'; n'''n) (-1)^{2S''} \begin{Bmatrix} 1 & 1 & 0 \\ S & S & S'' \end{Bmatrix} \begin{pmatrix} 1 & 1 & 0 \\ \kappa & \lambda & 0 \end{pmatrix} \right], \qquad (9\text{-}56)$$

where

$$A_\kappa(\nu; nn'') = (-1)^{\bar{M}-S} \begin{pmatrix} S & 1 & S'' \\ -\bar{M} & 0 & \bar{M} \end{pmatrix}^{-1} \langle nS\bar{M} | \sum_j \delta(\mathbf{r}_{j\nu}) s_{jz} | n''S''\bar{M} \rangle. \qquad (9\text{-}57)$$

The contributions will not be further pursued here. They are discussed in connection with NMR theory.

Orientation Dependence of Spin Hamiltonian Parameters

Before leaving the subject of theoretical expressions for the spin Hamiltonian parameters, we should examine further the questions of how the parameters depend on molecular orientation and of the sense (if any) in which they should be considered "tensors."

Thus far, the only transformations which have been explicitly considered in this or the preceding section are those of electron spin operators and the corresponding spin eigenfunctions. The eigenfunctions we are working with are not eigenfunctions of total angular momentum. On the other hand, it is clear that our choice of a coordinate system orientation cannot affect the actual, observable energy levels. Rather than being concerned with the formal transformation properties of the full spin Hamiltonian eigenvalue equation, however, we will here consider the consequences of rotating the molecular radical relative to the laboratory-fixed coordinate system.

A physical, laboratory-fixed coordinate system orientation is determined by the directions of the static magnetic field and the microwave magnetic field (except in the special case where they are parallel). In the common case where they are perpendicular, we may choose to have these directions define the z and x axes, respectively, but whether we do or not, they provide spatially fixed, physically meaningful reference directions. The expressions developed in this section for spin Hamiltonian parameters involve components of position or momentum operators defined with respect to this coordinate system, and the Cartesian components of the spin operators (as well of course as those of **B**) are defined with respect to it.

Consider now the actual rotation of the molecular radical, leaving field directions unchanged. The spin operators are unchanged but the components of the spin Hamiltonian parameters will change, and the energy levels will in general change. Recall that we are working with an electronic wave function in the Born–Oppenheimer approximation, and that apart from possibly adding vibrational corrections at some point, we are thinking of the nuclei as being fixed relative to one another. We can therefore define a molecule-fixed coordinate system. The zero-order Hamiltonian does not include any field dependence, and thus the molecule-fixed coordinate system is the appropriate frame of reference for the zero-order wave functions. Since they are degenerate in M_S, we are free to take the axis with respect to which spin quantization is defined to be either laboratory fixed or molecule fixed. In any case the spin Hamiltonian parameters are expressed here in such a way that each component of a given parameter involves s_z in the same way.

The conclusions to be drawn from these observations can be stated as follows: the components of each spin Hamiltonian parameter are to be calculated in a molecule-fixed coordinate system. The operators involved for the particular parameter and the point group symmetry of the radical will determine the number of independent components to be evaluated. The axis of spin quantization for this calculation may be taken to be the molecular z axis. If the radical is so oriented that the molecular axis system coincides with the laboratory-fixed axis with fields along z and x, the parameters are "ready for use." For other orientations, each parameter must be transformed like a Cartesian tensor of second degree, i.e., for the parameter set C_{ab}

$$C_{ab}^{\text{lab}} = \sum_{a'b'} R_{aa'}(\omega)R_{bb'}(\omega)C_{a'b'}^{\text{mol}}, \tag{9-58}$$

where $\mathbf{R}(\omega)$ is the rotation matrix describing the rotation from molecule-fixed to laboratory-fixed axes, with Euler angles α, β, $\gamma \equiv \omega$.‡

‡ It should be noted that if the effective spin in the spin Hamiltonian differs from the true electron spin quantum number for the state of interest, then the parameters of the spin Hamiltonian may not transform as tensors when the molecule is rotated.

Any symmetric, Cartesian tensor can be diagonalized and one can give either six independent components in some fixed coordinate system or three principal values and the three angles relating the principal axis system to the fixed coordinate system. Except when they are completely determined by symmetry, there is no reason to suppose that the principal axes of different tensors in the spin Hamiltonian will coincide.

As we saw in the previous section, if a tensor in the spin Hamiltonian is $\mathbf{T} = \mathbf{T}^{s} + \mathbf{T}^{a}$, where $\mathbf{T}^{s}$ is symmetric and $\mathbf{T}^{a}$ is antisymmetric, and if second-order effects are small enough that the contribution of $\mathbf{T}^{a}$ to them can be neglected, then $\mathbf{T}$ can be replaced by a symmetric, effective tensor

$$\mathbf{T}^{\text{eff}} = (\mathbf{T}^{s2} - \mathbf{T}^{a2})^{1/2} \tag{9-59}$$

with no observable effect on the spectrum predicted.

Summary of Section 9

In this section terms in the spin Hamiltonian which are quadratic or bilinear in magnetic field, electron spin, and nuclear spins have been considered. Terms which would be linear in only one of these are shown to be zero in the absence of orbital degeneracy. Terms which might involve combined powers higher than the second have been neglected. They would arise in higher order or possibly, in the case of higher powers of $\mathcal{S}$, if degeneracies not actually associated with spin are important. Expressions have been obtained for spin Hamiltonian parameters in terms of matrix elements involving eigenfunctions of the zero-order, spin-free Hamiltonian.

Usually the nonzero contribution of lowest order is dominant, but in some cases it is necessary to treat first- and second-order contributions together in order to retain gauge invariance. In particular, coordinate origins for orbital angular momentum and for the vector potential must be chosen in a consistent way.

One normally wishes to determine matrix elements in a coordinate system fixed in the molecule (with "frozen" nuclear positions) while external fields define a laboratory-fixed coordinate system. Spin Hamiltonian parameters are written as "tensors" and will transform as tensors when the effective spin of the spin Hamiltonian is the same as the true spin of the system. When these two differ the parameters may not transform as tensors, but these problems do not normally arise in free radical ESR and have not been considered.

10. Summarizing Calculated Data in Terms of Density Matrix Components

An alternative way of considering the relationship between spin Hamiltonian parameters and electronic wave functions has been presented by McWeeny [123]. It is based on the use of reduced density matrices and has the advantage, as we shall see in the next chapter, of providing a convenient conceptual framework applicable to very complicated, good wave functions as well as to simple models. Basic ideas of reduced density matrix theory are reviewed in Appendix D. In this section we will be primarily concerned with the spin dependence of reduced density matrices and how this can be put to good use in connection with spin Hamiltonian parameters. (See also McWeeny [124].)

Spin Components of Reduced Density Matrices

When the wave functions one is dealing with are eigenfunctions of $\mathscr{S}^2$ and $\mathscr{S}_z$, as are our zero-order functions, the reduced density matrices can be divided in a straightforward way into spin components. Within a manifold of states differing just in their M_S values, only a rather small number of components are independent, the others being expressible in terms of them.

The spin components and relationships among them can be obtained in several ways. One is to examine the spin–tensorial properties of operators of which the density matrices can be regarded as matrix elements. A second-quantized formulation leads to very compact expressions. We will deal instead, here, with operators involving δ functions [126]. A more purely group-theoretic approach is presented by Bingel and Kutzelnigg [18].

One-Electron Reduced Density Matrix

The one-electron reduced density matrix between states t and u (they may be the same or different) is (cf. Appendix D)

$$\gamma(tu|x_1;x_1') = N\int \Psi_u(x_1, x_2, \ldots, x_N)\Psi_t^*(x_1', x_2, \ldots, x_N)\, dx_2 \cdots dx_N. \tag{10-1}$$

Here the variable x_j stands for the space and spin coordinates of electron j and N is the number of electrons. This can be expressed as a matrix element

$$\gamma(tu|\bar{x}_1;\bar{x}_1') = \langle t|\hat{\gamma}(\bar{x}_1;\bar{x}_1')|u\rangle \qquad (10\text{-}2)$$

of an operator $\hat{\gamma}$ which is an integral operator for electron 1 with kernel

$$g(\bar{x}_1,\bar{x}_1'|x_1,x_1') = \delta(x_1-\bar{x}_1')\delta(\bar{x}_1-x_1'). \qquad (10\text{-}3)$$

Then

$$\begin{aligned}\hat{\gamma}(\bar{x}_1;\bar{x}_1')\Psi_u(x_1,x_2,\ldots,x_N) &= \int g(\bar{x}_1,\bar{x}_1'|x_1,x_1')\Psi_u(x_1',x_2,\ldots,x_N)\,dx_1'\\ &= \delta(x_1-\bar{x}_1')\Psi_u(\bar{x}_1,x_2,\ldots,x_N). \qquad (10\text{-}4)\end{aligned}$$

(It is possible to make g an N-electron kernel involving all electrons equivalently, $(1/N)\sum_j \delta(x_j-\bar{x}_1')\delta(\bar{x}_1-x_j')\prod_{k(\neq j)}\delta(x_k-x_k')$. This would clearly make no difference in the results.)

We now examine the spin dependence of $\hat{\gamma}$. We begin by writing

$$g = g_r g_s \qquad (10\text{-}5)$$

where we divide x into the spatial variables $\mathbf{r}$ and the spin variable ξ, and

$$g_r = g_r(\bar{\mathbf{r}}_1,\bar{\mathbf{r}}_1'|\mathbf{r}_1,\mathbf{r}_1') = \delta(\mathbf{r}_1-\bar{\mathbf{r}}_1')\delta(\bar{\mathbf{r}}_1-\mathbf{r}_1'), \qquad (10\text{-}6)$$

$$g_s = g_s(\bar{\xi}_1,\bar{\xi}_1'|\xi_1,\xi_1') = \delta(\xi_1-\bar{\xi}_1')\delta(\bar{\xi}_1-\xi_1'). \qquad (10\text{-}7)$$

The meaning of a delta function of spin variables is defined, as is that of any other delta function, in terms of how it behaves in an integral. In the present case we use the representation of a delta function as a sum over a complete, orthonormal set of functions

$$\delta(y-y') = \sum_k \chi_k(y)\chi_k^*(y') \qquad \text{(complete, orthonormal set).} \qquad (10\text{-}8)$$

In the case of one-electron spin functions, the complete orthonormal set consists of only two functions and we can write

$$\begin{aligned}\delta(\xi_1-\bar{\xi}_1') &= \alpha(\xi_1)\alpha^*(\bar{\xi}_1') + \beta(\xi_1)\beta^*(\bar{\xi}_1'),\\ \delta(\bar{\xi}_1-\xi_1') &= \alpha(\bar{\xi}_1)\alpha^*(\xi_1') + \beta(\bar{\xi}_1)\beta^*(\xi_1').\end{aligned} \qquad (10\text{-}9)$$

It is readily verified that these have the desired effect. In any N-electron function the spin dependence of electron 1 can be explicitly separated, e.g.,

$$\Psi_u(x_1,x_2,\ldots,x_N) = \Psi_u^a(\mathbf{r}_1,x_2,x_N)\alpha(\xi_1) + \Psi_u^b(\mathbf{r}_1,x_2,\ldots,x_N)\beta(\xi_1). \qquad (10\text{-}10)$$

Then

$$\int \delta(\bar{\xi}_1 - \xi_1)\Psi_u \, d\xi_1$$

$$= \Psi_u^a(\mathbf{r}_1, x_2, \ldots, x_N) \int [\alpha(\bar{\xi}_1)\alpha^*(\xi_1) + \beta(\bar{\xi}_1)\beta^*(\xi_1)]\alpha(\xi_1)\, d\xi_1$$

$$+ \Psi_u^b(\mathbf{r}_1, x_2, \ldots, x_N) \int [\alpha(\bar{\xi}_1)\alpha^*(\xi_1) + \beta(\bar{\xi}_1)\beta^*(\xi_1)]\beta(\xi_1) d\xi_1$$

$$= \Psi_u^a(\mathbf{r}_1, x_2, \ldots, x_N)\alpha(\bar{\xi}_1) + \Psi_u^b(\mathbf{r}_1, x_2, \ldots, x_N)\beta(\bar{\xi}_1). \quad (10\text{-}11)$$

If we insert the expressions from Eq. (10-9) into Eq. (10-7), expand, and rearrange, we obtain

$$g_s = \alpha(\bar{\xi}_1)\alpha^*(\bar{\xi}_1')\alpha(\xi_1)\alpha^*(\xi_1') + \alpha(\bar{\xi}_1)\beta^*(\bar{\xi}_1')\beta(\xi_1)\alpha^*(\xi_1')$$
$$+ \beta(\bar{\xi}_1)\alpha^*(\bar{\xi}')\alpha(\xi_1)\beta^*(\xi_1') + \beta(\bar{\xi}_1)\beta^*(\bar{\xi}_1')\beta(\xi_1)\beta^*(\xi_1'). \quad (10\text{-}12)$$

This can then be reexpressed in terms of ordinary spin operators for electron 1 [cf. Eq. (8-93)] as

$$g_s = \tfrac{1}{2}[\alpha(\bar{\xi}_1)\alpha^*(\bar{\xi}_1') + \beta(\bar{\xi}_1)\beta^*(\bar{\xi}_1')] + \beta(\bar{\xi}_1)\alpha^*(\bar{\xi}_1')s_{1+}$$
$$+ [\alpha(\bar{\xi}_1)\alpha^*(\bar{\xi}_1') - \beta(\bar{\xi}_1)\beta^*(\bar{\xi}_1')]s_{1z} + \alpha(\bar{\xi}_1)\beta^*(\bar{\xi}_1')s_{1-}. \quad (10\text{-}13)$$

The one-electron reduced density matrix can then be separated into spin components as (now dropping the overbar)

$$\gamma(tu|x_1; x_1') = \gamma^0(tu|\mathbf{r}_1; \mathbf{r}_1') \cdot \tfrac{1}{2}[\alpha(\xi_1)\alpha^*(\xi_1') + \beta(\xi_1)\beta^*(\xi_1')]$$
$$+ \gamma^+(tu|\mathbf{r}_1; \mathbf{r}_1') \cdot \tfrac{1}{2}\beta(\xi_1)\alpha^*(\xi_1')$$
$$+ \gamma^z(tu|\mathbf{r}_1; \mathbf{r}_1') \cdot \tfrac{1}{2}[\alpha(\xi_1)\alpha^*(\xi_1') - \beta(\xi_1)\beta^*(\xi_1')]$$
$$+ \gamma^-(tu|\mathbf{r}_1; \mathbf{r}_1') \cdot \tfrac{1}{2}\alpha(\xi_1)\beta^*(\xi_1'). \quad (10\text{-}14)$$

If $\mathscr{F}$ is any one-electron operator

$$\mathscr{F} = \sum_j [f_j^0 + f_j^+ s_1^{[1]}(j) + f_j^z s_0^{[1]}(j) + f_j^- s_{-1}^{[1]}(j)], \quad (10\text{-}15)$$

where the f's are spatial operators, its matrix elements can then be written[‡]

$$\langle t|\mathscr{F}|u\rangle = \int' f_1^0 \gamma^0(tu|\mathbf{r}_1; \mathbf{r}_1') + \int' f_1^+ \tfrac{1}{2}\gamma^+(tu|\mathbf{r}_1; \mathbf{r}_1')$$
$$+ \int' f_1^z \tfrac{1}{2}\gamma^z(tu|\mathbf{r}_1; \mathbf{r}_1') + \int' f_1^- \tfrac{1}{2}\gamma^-(tu|\mathbf{r}_1; \mathbf{r}_1'). \quad (10\text{-}16)$$

(See Appendix D for discussion of the meaning of the prime on the integral sign.)

‡ The factors $\frac{1}{2}$ associated with γ^κ here and in Eq. (10-14) are a consequence of the normalization convention, Eq. (10-36), chosen for convenience elsewhere. The normalization is not uniform in the literature.

If the states labeled by t and u are $\mathscr{S}^2$, $\mathscr{S}_z$ eigenfunctions, then several of the density matrix components will vanish in any given case, and components between states of different M_S's for the same S's will be related by the Wigner–Eckart theorem. This follows from the fact that they are matrix elements of irreducible, spin–tensorial operators

$$\begin{aligned} \gamma^0(tu|\mathbf{r}_1;\mathbf{r}_1') &= \langle t|\hat{\gamma}_r|u\rangle, \\ \gamma^\kappa(tu|\mathbf{r}_1;\mathbf{r}_1') &= 2\langle t|\hat{\gamma}_r s_\kappa^{[1]}|u\rangle, \qquad \kappa = +, z, -, \end{aligned} \tag{10-17}$$

where $\hat{\gamma}$ is the one-electron integral operator with g_r as kernel. Then

$$\gamma^0(tu|\mathbf{r}_1, \mathbf{r}_1') = \gamma^0(tS_t\overline{M}, uS_u\overline{M}|\mathbf{r}_1;\mathbf{r}_1')\delta_{M_tM_u}\delta_{S_tS_u}, \tag{10-18}$$

where $\overline{M}$ is any convenient reference value of M_t and M_u. For the spin-dependent components, S_t and S_u can be the same or differ by 1 for a nonzero result. For given S values there is only one independent γ^κ; components for various choices of κ and the M's are all proportional (or zero). These results are summarized in Table 10-1.

TABLE 10-1

Relationships between Spin Components of One-Electron Reduced Density Matrices[a]

	Charge density	
	$\gamma^0(nSM, n'S'M'|\mathbf{r}_1;\mathbf{r}_1') = \delta_{SS'}\delta_{MM'}\gamma^0(nSS, n'SS|\mathbf{r}_1;\mathbf{r}_1')$	
	Spin density	
$S' = S$	Proportional to $\gamma^z(nSS, n'SS|\mathbf{r}_1;\mathbf{r}_1')$	
	Component	Proportionality constant
	$\gamma^z(nSM, n'SM|\mathbf{r}_1;\mathbf{r}_1')$	M/S
[b]	$\gamma^z(nSM, n'SM \pm 1|\mathbf{r}_1;\mathbf{r}_1')$	$[(S \mp M)(S \pm M + 1)]^{1/2}/S$
	(If $S = S' = 0$, $\gamma^z \equiv 0$.)	
$S' = S + 1$	Proportional to $\gamma^z(nSS, n'S + 1S|\mathbf{r}_1;\mathbf{r}_1')$	
	Component	Proportionality constant
	$\gamma^z(nSM, n'S + 1M|\mathbf{r}_1;\mathbf{r}_1')$	$\left[\dfrac{(S - M + 1)(S + M + 1)}{2S + 1}\right]^{1/2}$
	$\gamma^z(nSM, n'S + 1M \pm 1|\mathbf{r}_1;\mathbf{r}_1')$	$\mp\left[\dfrac{(S \pm M + 2)(S \pm M + 1)}{2S + 1}\right]^{1/2}$
	(If $|M - M'| > 1$ or $|S - S'| > 1$, $\gamma^z \equiv 0$.)	
Results for $S' < S$ can be obtained from	$\gamma^z(tu|\mathbf{r}_1;\mathbf{r}_1') = [\gamma^z(ut|\mathbf{r}_1;\mathbf{r}_1')]^*$	

[a] From McWeeny and Mizuno, [126].

[b] When $M' \neq M$, γ^z is $\gamma^\pm$.

The spinless component γ^0 is the *charge density matrix*. It can be obtained from γ by integration over spin

$$\gamma^0(tu|\mathbf{r}_1;\mathbf{r}'_1) = \int \gamma(tu|\mathbf{r}_1\xi_1;\mathbf{r}'_1\xi_1)\,d\xi_1. \tag{10-19}$$

Its diagonal elements

$$\rho^0(tu|\mathbf{r}) = \gamma^0(tu|\mathbf{r};\mathbf{r}) \tag{10-20}$$

provided the ordinary transition charge density ($t \neq u$) or charge density in one state ($t = u$). The component γ^z is the *spin density matrix*. It can be obtained from γ as

$$\gamma^z(tu|\mathbf{r}_1;\mathbf{r}'_1) = \int' 2s_{1z}\gamma(tu|x_1;x'_1)\,d\xi_1, \tag{10-21}$$

and its diagonal elements

$$\rho^z(tu|\mathbf{r}) = \gamma^z(tu|\mathbf{r},\mathbf{r}) \tag{10-22}$$

provided the spin density. These components will be further discussed in what follows.

Two-Electron Reduced Density Matrix

The two-electron reduced density matrix can be divided into spin components by techniques similar to those used for the one-particle density matrix. There are a total of 16 components, but by use of spin angular momentum properties and permutational symmetry relating the two electrons, all the nonzero components in any particular case can be expressed in terms of not more than three independent components. The intermediate algebra becomes quite extensive and will not be reproduced here. Some of the results are given in Table 10-2.

One of the independent components is the *two-electron charge density* Γ^0. It can be obtained from the density matrix Γ by integrating over spin variables

$$\Gamma^0(tu|\mathbf{r}_1,\mathbf{r}_2;\mathbf{r}'_1,\mathbf{r}'_2) = \int \Gamma(tu|\mathbf{r}_1\xi_1,\mathbf{r}_2\xi_2;\mathbf{r}'_1\xi_1,\mathbf{r}'_2\xi_2)\,d\xi_1\,d\xi_2 \tag{10-23}$$

and determines the matrix element of any two-electron spin-free operator. The charge density matrix is related to it by

$$\gamma^0(tu|\mathbf{r}_1;\mathbf{r}'_1) = \frac{2}{N-1}\int \Gamma^0(tu|\mathbf{r}_1,\mathbf{r}_2;\mathbf{r}'_1,\mathbf{r}_2)\,d\mathbf{r}_2. \tag{10-24}$$

The second independent component is the *conditional spin density matrix* Γ^z. It arises when the spin of only one electron is involved in a two-electron operator. It can be obtained from Γ as

$$\Gamma^z(tu|\mathbf{r}_1, \mathbf{r}_2; \mathbf{r}'_1, \mathbf{r}'_2) = \int' 2s_{1z}\Gamma(tu|x_1, x_2; x'_1 x'_2)\, d\xi_1\, d\xi_2 \qquad (10\text{-}25)$$

and is related to the spin density by

$$\gamma^z(tu|\mathbf{r}_1; \mathbf{r}'_1) = \frac{2}{N-1}\int \Gamma^z(tu|\mathbf{r}_1, \mathbf{r}_2; \mathbf{r}'_1, \mathbf{r}_2)\, d\mathbf{r}_2. \qquad (10\text{-}26)$$

The third independent component is the *spin–spin coupling density matrix* Γ^{SS}. It is required when the spins of both electrons are involved in an essential way. It can be obtained from Γ as

$$\Gamma^{SS}(tu|\mathbf{r}_1, \mathbf{r}_2; \mathbf{r}'_1, \mathbf{r}'_2) = \int' (3s_{1z}s_{2z} - \mathbf{s}_1 \cdot \mathbf{s}_2)\Gamma(tu|x_1, x_2; x'_1, x'_2)\, d\xi_1\, d\xi_2. \qquad (10\text{-}27)$$

There is no corresponding component of the one-electron density matrix.

Relationship to Spin Hamiltonian Parameters

The density matrix spin components provide a way of obtaining expressions for spin Hamiltonian parameters and for gaining some additional feeling for what these parameters mean. The use of spin components allows us to express the parameters in terms of purely spatial quantities. Relationships between components for different M values provide an alternative to some of the development of Section 8. We will consider especially the interpretive aspects of the first-order contributions, and look briefly at the second-order contributions.

First-Order Contributions

Relatively few quantities of interest to ESR are determined by the charge density matrix. Of course the zero-order energies or matrix elements of $\mathbf{R}^0$ can be determined from the γ^0 and Γ^0 for the various states involved, but they are a result of the zero-order calculation, which will be examined in Chapter III. The nuclear quadrupole parameter is determined by γ^0 (in fact by ρ^0), since it depends only on the electronic charge distribution. The same is true of the first-order contribution to the nuclear shielding tensor.

The reduced density matrix of greatest interest is the spin density. It follows from the expressions presented above that for a given state, γ^z is

TABLE 10-2

Relationships between Spin Components for Two-Electron Reduced Density Matrices[a]

	Two-electron charge density	
	$\Gamma^0(nSM, n'S'M' \mid \mathbf{r}_1, \mathbf{r}_2 : \mathbf{r}'_1, \mathbf{r}'_2) = \delta_{SS'}\delta_{MM'}\Gamma^0(nSS, n'SS \mid \mathbf{r}_1, \mathbf{r}_2 : \mathbf{r}'_1, \mathbf{r}'_2)$	
	Conditional spin density	
$S' = S$	Proportional to $\Gamma^z(nSS, n'SS \mid \mathbf{r}_1, \mathbf{r}_2 : \mathbf{r}'_1, \mathbf{r}'_2)$	
	Component	Proportionality constant
	$\Gamma^z(nSM, n'SM \mid \mathbf{r}_1, \mathbf{r}_2 : \mathbf{r}'_1, \mathbf{r}'_2)$	M/S
	$\Gamma^z(nSM, n'SM \pm 1 \mid \mathbf{r}_1, \mathbf{r}_2 : \mathbf{r}'_1, \mathbf{r}'_2)$	$[(S \mp M)(S \pm M + 1)]^{1/2}/S$
	(If $S' = S = 0$, $\Gamma^z \equiv 0$.)	
$S' = S + 1$	Proportional to $\Gamma^z(nSS, n'S + 1S \mid \mathbf{r}_1, \mathbf{r}_2 : \mathbf{r}'_1, \mathbf{r}'_2)$	
	Component	Proportionality constant
	$\Gamma^z(nSM, n'S + 1M \mid \mathbf{r}_1 \mathbf{r}_2 : \mathbf{r}'_1 \mathbf{r}'_2)$	$\left[\dfrac{(S - M + 1)(S + M + 1)}{2S + 1}\right]^{1/2}$
	$\Gamma^z(nSM, n'S + 1M \pm 1 \mid \mathbf{r}_1 \mathbf{r}_2 : \mathbf{r}'_1 \mathbf{r}'_2)$	$\left[\dfrac{(S \pm M + 2)(S \pm M + 1)}{2S + 1}\right]^{1/2}$
	(If $\lvert M - M' \rvert > 1$ or $\lvert S - S' \rvert > 1$, $\Gamma^z \equiv 0$.)	
	Spin–spin coupling	
$S' = S$	Proportional to $\Gamma^{SS}(nSS, n'SS \mid \mathbf{r}_1, \mathbf{r}_2 : \mathbf{r}'_1, \mathbf{r}'_2)$	
	Component	Proportionality constant
	$\Gamma^{SS}(nSM, n'SM \mid \mathbf{r}_1, \mathbf{r}_2 : \mathbf{r}'_1, \mathbf{r}'_2)$	$\dfrac{3M^2 - S(S + 1)}{S(2S - 1)}$
	$\Gamma^{SS}(nSM, n'SM \pm 1 \mid \mathbf{r}_1, \mathbf{r}_2 : \mathbf{r}'_1, \mathbf{r}'_2)$	$3(1 \pm 2M)[(S \mp M)(S \pm M + 1)]^{1/2}$ [illegible]

	$\Gamma^{SS}(nSM, n'SM \pm 2 \mid \mathbf{r}_1, \mathbf{r}_2 : \mathbf{r}_1', \mathbf{r}_2')$	$\dfrac{3[(S \mp M - 1)(S \mp M)(S \pm M + 1)(S \pm M + 2)]^{1/2}}{S(2S - 1)}$
	(If $S' = S < 1$, $\Gamma^{SS} \equiv 0$)	
$S' = S + 1$	Proportional to $\Gamma^{SS}(nSS, n'S + 1S \mid \mathbf{r}_1, \mathbf{r}_2 : \mathbf{r}_1', \mathbf{r}_2')$	
	Component	Proportionality constant
	$\Gamma^{SS}(nSM, n'S + 1M \mid \mathbf{r}_1, \mathbf{r}_2 : \mathbf{r}_1', \mathbf{r}_2')$	$\dfrac{M}{S}\left[\dfrac{(S - M + 1)(S + M + 1)}{2S + 1}\right]$
	$\Gamma^{SS}(nSM, n'S + 1M \pm 1 \mid \mathbf{r}_1, \mathbf{r}_2 : \mathbf{r}_1', \mathbf{r}_2')$	$\pm \dfrac{(S \mp 2M)}{2S}\left[\dfrac{(S \pm M + 2)(S \pm M + 1)}{2S + 1}\right]^{1/2}$
	$\Gamma^{SS}(nSM, n'S + 1M \pm 1 \mid \mathbf{r}_1, \mathbf{r}_2 : \mathbf{r}_1', \mathbf{r}_2')$	$\mp \dfrac{1}{S}\left[\dfrac{(S \mp M)(S \pm M + 1)(S \pm M + 2)(S \pm M + 3)}{2S + 1}\right]^{1/2}$
	(If $S = 0$, $S' = 1$, $\Gamma^{SS} \equiv 0$)	
$S' = S + 2$	Proportional to $\Gamma^{SS}(nSS, n'S + 2S \mid \mathbf{r}_1, \mathbf{r}_2 : \mathbf{r}_1', \mathbf{r}_2')$	
	Component[b]	Proportionality constant
	$\Gamma^{SS}(nSM, n'S + 2M \mid \mathbf{r}_1, \mathbf{r}_2 : \mathbf{r}_1', \mathbf{r}_2')$	$\dfrac{1}{2}\left[\dfrac{(S - M + 2)(S - M + 1)(S + M + 2)(S + M + 1)}{(S + 1)(2S + 1)}\right]^{1/2}$
	$\Gamma^{SS}(nSM, n'S + 2M \pm 1 \mid \mathbf{r}_1, \mathbf{r}_2 : \mathbf{r}_1', \mathbf{r}_2')$	$\dfrac{1}{2}\left[\dfrac{(S \mp M + 1)(S \pm M + 3)(S \pm M + 2)(S \pm M + 1)}{(S + 1)(2S + 1)}\right]^{1/2}$
	$\Gamma^{SS}(nSM, N'S + 2M \pm 2 \mid \mathbf{r}_1, \mathbf{r}_2 : \mathbf{r}_1', \mathbf{r}_2')$	$\dfrac{1}{2}\left[\dfrac{(S \pm M + 1)(S \pm M + 2)(S \pm M + 3)(S \pm M + 4)}{(S + 1)(2S + 1)}\right]^{1/2}$
	(If $\lvert M - M' \rvert > 2$ or $\lvert S - S' \rvert > 2$, $\Gamma^{SS} \equiv 0$)	

[a] From McWeeny and Mizuno, [126].
[b] When $M' = M \pm 1$, Γ^z is $\Gamma^{\pm}$, defined analogously to $\gamma^{\pm}$. The significance of Γ^{SS} when $M' \neq M$ is discussed by McWeeny and Mizuno [126].

proportional to M_S, and transition values between states differing only in M_S are determined by 3-j coefficients and one reference-state spin density. In a state of definite M_S, γ^+ and γ^- vanish, and γ can be written

$$\gamma(x; x') = \gamma^{++}(\mathbf{r}; \mathbf{r}')\alpha(\xi)\alpha^*(\xi') + \gamma^{--}(\mathbf{r}; \mathbf{r}')\beta(\xi)\beta^*(\xi'), \tag{10-28}$$

where

$$\gamma^{++} = \tfrac{1}{2}(\gamma^0 + \gamma^z), \qquad \gamma^{--} = \tfrac{1}{2}(\gamma^0 - \gamma^z). \tag{10-29}$$

The state labels $t = u$ have been suppressed. It can be shown (cf. Appendix D) that there are functions $\psi_k(x)$ such that

$$\gamma(x; x') = \sum_k \lambda_k \psi_k(x)\psi_k^*(x') \tag{10-30}$$

with $0 \leq \lambda_k \leq 1$. One must then have

$$\psi_k(x) = \phi_k^+(\mathbf{r})\alpha(\xi) \qquad \text{or} \qquad \psi_k(x) = \phi_k^-(\mathbf{r})\beta(\xi), \tag{10-31}$$

and γ^{++} and γ^{--} can be separately expanded in a similar way

$$\begin{aligned} \gamma^{++}(\mathbf{r}; \mathbf{r}') &= \sum_{k(+)} \lambda_k^+ \phi_k^+(\mathbf{r})\phi_k^+(\mathbf{r}')^*, \\ \gamma^{--}(\mathbf{r}; \mathbf{r}') &= \sum_{k(-)} \lambda_k^- \phi_k^-(\mathbf{r})\phi_k^-(\mathbf{r}')^*. \end{aligned} \tag{10-32}$$

It follows that the diagonal elements of these components are everywhere nonnegative

$$\begin{aligned} \rho^{++}(\mathbf{r}) = \gamma^{++}(\mathbf{r}; \mathbf{r}) &= \sum_{k(+)} \lambda_k^+ |\phi_k^+(\mathbf{r})|^2 \geq 0, \\ \rho^{--}(\mathbf{r}) = \gamma^{--}(\mathbf{r}; \mathbf{r}) &= \sum_{k(-)} \lambda_k^- |\phi_k^-(\mathbf{r})|^2 \geq 0. \end{aligned} \tag{10-33}$$

The charge density

$$\rho^0(\mathbf{r}) = \rho^{++}(\mathbf{r}) + \rho^{--}(\mathbf{r}) \tag{10-34}$$

is clearly nowhere negative, as is to be expected. For the spin density, however,

$$\rho^z(\mathbf{r}) = \rho^{++}(\mathbf{r}) - \rho^{--}(\mathbf{r}), \tag{10-35}$$

and the sign at any point depends on the relative values of ρ^{++} and ρ^{--} at that point. The overall normalization condition is

$$\int \rho^z(\mathbf{r})\, d\mathbf{r} = \int \gamma^z(\mathbf{r}; \mathbf{r})\, d\mathbf{r} = 2M_S. \tag{10-36}$$

Customarily the reference state is taken with $M_S = S \geq 0$. A region of *negative spin density* is thus one where $\rho^z(\mathbf{r}) < 0$ or $\rho^{++}(\mathbf{r}) < \rho^{--}(\mathbf{r})$. We will consider ways in which this can occur in the next chapter.

A probabilistic interpretation of the spin density can be given. Just as the charge density (electron density) at a point is proportional to the probability of finding an electron at that point, so the spin density at a point is proportional to the probability of finding an electron there with spin up minus that of finding one there with spin down. (The components ρ^{++} and ρ^{--} give probability densities for spin-up and spin-down electrons, respectively.)

The first-order contributions to the hyperfine parameters are clearly determined by the spin density. The Fermi contact term depends only on the spin densities at the nuclei, while the dipole contribution involves an integration over the spin density distribution. The kinetic energy contribution to $\Delta\mathbf{g}$ is also determined by the spin density matrix. In this case momentum operators are involved, so γ^z is required rather than just ρ^z.

There are no first-order contributions dependent on the conditional spin density, but this component will be needed in second-order contributions involving the two-electron spin–orbit operators. The first-order contribution to the zero-field splitting is determined by the spin–spin coupling function

$$P^{SS}(\mathbf{r}_1, \mathbf{r}_2) = \Gamma^{SS}(\mathbf{r}_1, \mathbf{r}_2; \mathbf{r}_1, \mathbf{r}_2) \tag{10-37}$$

and indeed it is the spin–spin interaction term which gives significance to this component. We note that $\Gamma^{SS} \equiv 0$ unless $S \geq 1$.

Second-Order Contributions

It is of course not possible to express the second-order contributions to the spin Hamiltonian parameters as simply as the first-order contributions were expressed. The matrix elements which enter into the second-order expressions can be simply expressed in terms of density matrices, however, by letting $t \leftrightarrow nSM$ and $u \leftrightarrow n''S''M''$ or $t \leftrightarrow N'''S''M''$ and $u \leftrightarrow nSM'$. The M dependence can be expressed in terms of 3-j coefficients, using the results of Tables 10-1 and 10-2.

Matrix elements of the orbital Zeeman and orbital hyperfine operators can be expressed in terms of γ^0. Those of the electron spin hyperfine and one-electron spin–orbit operators can be expressed in terms of γ^z. The only two-electron operators entering into the second-order contributions we have considered are the spin–other-orbit and electron–electron spin–orbit operators. Matrix elements of these can be expressed in terms of Γ^z, but some additional discussion is required.

A symmetric, two-electron operator is one which treats all electrons equivalently and can be written in the form

$$\mathscr{F} = \sum_{j<k} F_{jk} = \tfrac{1}{2} \sum_{j,k}{}' F_{jk}, \tag{10-38}$$

where $F_{jk} = F_{kj}$. For such an operator

$$\langle t|\mathscr{F}|u\rangle = \int' F_{12}\Gamma(x_1, x_2 ; x_1', x_2')\, dx_1\, dx_2. \tag{10-39}$$

In order to put the spin–orbit operators into this form, they must be rewritten in a symmetrized way: [cf. Eqs. (9-8)–(9-11)]

$$\begin{aligned}\mathscr{H}''_{\mathrm{SO}} = \sum_{j,k}' \mathbf{F}_{jk}\cdot\mathbf{s}_j &= \tfrac{1}{2}\sum_{j,k}' (\mathbf{F}_{jk}\cdot\mathbf{s}_j + \mathbf{F}_{kj}\cdot\mathbf{s}_k) \\ &= \sum_{j<k}(\mathbf{F}_{jk}\cdot\mathbf{s}_j + \mathbf{F}_{kj}\cdot\mathbf{s}_k),\end{aligned} \tag{10-40}$$

where

$$\mathbf{F}_{jk}^{\mathrm{SO}} = 4\frac{(\mathbf{r}_k - \mathbf{r}_j)\times\mathbf{\nabla}_j}{r_{jk}^3}, \qquad \mathbf{F}_{jk}^{\mathrm{eeSO}} = g_e'\frac{(\mathbf{r}_j - \mathbf{r}_k)\times\mathbf{\nabla}_j}{r_{jk}^3} \tag{10-41}$$

are not symmetric in j and k, but the quantity in parentheses in Eq. (10-40) is. Then

$$\langle t|\mathscr{H}''_{\mathrm{SO}}|u\rangle = \int' (\mathbf{F}_{12}\cdot\mathbf{s}_1 + \mathbf{F}_{21}\cdot\mathbf{s}_2)\Gamma(x_1, x_2 ; x_1', x_2')\, dx_1\, dx_2. \tag{10-42}$$

The first term reduces to an integral over $(F_{12})_z\Gamma^z$, but the second term requires a component of Γ involving the spin of electron 2 only. It can be shown that this component, which we denote by $\tilde{\Gamma}^z$, is related to Γ^z by

$$\tilde{\Gamma}^z(\mathbf{r}_1, \mathbf{r}_2 ; \mathbf{r}_1', \mathbf{r}_2') = \Gamma^z(\mathbf{r}_2, \mathbf{r}_1 ; \mathbf{r}_2', \mathbf{r}_1'). \tag{10-43}$$

Then by relabeling the variables of integration we can show that the contribution from the second term is equal to that from the first term, so only Γ^z and $(F_{12})_z$ are required.

Some additional algebra can be performed in general with respect to second-order contributions in density matrix terms. Suppose we have a second-order term of the form

$$H''_{tu} = \sum_{v,v'(\neq t,u)} \langle t|\mathscr{F}|v\rangle R^0_{vv'}\langle v'|\mathscr{G}|u\rangle, \tag{10-44}$$

where

$$\mathscr{F} = \sum_j f_j, \qquad \mathscr{G} = \sum_k g_k \tag{10-45}$$

are symmetric, one-electron operators. We define a *resolvent density*

$$G(x_1, x_1' : \bar{x}_1, \bar{x}_1') = \sum_{v,v'} \gamma(tv|x_1 ; x_1')R^0_{vv'}\gamma(v'u|\bar{x}_1 ; \bar{x}_1'). \tag{10-46}$$

Then

$$H''_{tu} = \int' \int' f_1 \bar{g}_1 G(x_1, x'_1 : \bar{x}_1, \bar{x}'_1)\, dx_1\, d\bar{x}_1, \tag{10-47}$$

where the convention is that f_1 acts on x_1, $\bar{g}_1$ acts on $\bar{x}_1$, and after the action of the operators but before integration the primes of x'_1 and $\bar{x}'_1$ are dropped. (Compare Appendix D.) It is clear that similar resolvent densities could be defined where one or both of the operators involve two electrons.

It is possible to separate resolvent densities into spin components, and to apply angular momentum coupling theory to eliminate M dependence except via 3-j symbols. The method could be developed as an alternative to the second-order treatment of Section 8. The final results will, of course, be equivalent. It is also possible that an investigation of resolvent density matrix components may facilitate development of simple pictures for second-order contributions. This has not yet been explored. This approach could, clearly, be related to one based on the use of Green's functions.

Summary of Section 10

This section has explored the way in which spin Hamiltonian parameters can be expressed in terms of the spin components of one- and two-electron reduced density matrices. Each such component depends on spatial variables only and provides a simple way of treating even very complicated wave functions. The one-electron reduced density matrix has charge density and spin density components. Many of the important spin Hamiltonian parameters are determined by the spin density matrix. The two-electron reduced density matrix has three independent components: charge density, conditional spin density, and spin–spin coupling density.

The density matrix analysis is particularly useful when first-order contributions are considered. An extension to include second-order contributions was shown to be possible but was not pursued.

CHAPTER III

CALCULATIONS

11. Wave Functions for Open-Shell Systems

In this section we will consider some of the general aspects of the problem of obtaining (approximate) eigenfunctions of $\mathscr{H}_0$. We will normally seek functions which are also eigenfunctions of $\mathscr{S}^2$ and $\mathscr{S}_z$. Such functions are certainly possible because the three operators commute. Although $\mathscr{H}_0$ is itself spin-free, we have seen in Chapter II that its eigenfunctions provide the necessary information to determine the parameters of interest to us.

Many of the effects of interest, including in particular the hyperfine interactions, can be determined from the ground state wave function or reduced density matrix components for, e.g., the state with $M_S = S$. We will be particularly interested in the determination of the spin density matrix. For effects which must be treated to second order, either excited state wave functions or at least the matrix of $\mathscr{H}_0$ in some basis set orthogonalized to the ground state wave function will be required. We will deal explicitly with excited states only briefly, but much of what is said about the ground state applies to excited states as well.

The problems associated with the determination of good, approximate, ground state, zero-order eigenfunctions for the systems of interest to ESR include all the problems associated with any determination of molecular electronic properties. We will be able to survey them only briefly here and will concentrate on certain aspects which, although they are general, assume much greater significance in the cases of the systems and properties we are interested in.

Because we are dealing with open-shell systems, questions of spin couplings and their relationship to permutational symmetry will be more important to us than they are in the case of singlet systems. Because terms like the Fermi contact interaction involve the spin density at a point, our results will be even more sensitive than is commonly the case to the choice of basis functions. The spin coupling problem will be treated first, since it can be dealt with extensively in a general, formal way. We will then consider some problems common to most molecular electronic calculations and the problems associated with the point character of some of our operators. The latter are probably the most difficult to deal with.

This section will conclude with a brief survey of some nonvariational methods and a comparison of a number of calculations on the lithium atom, illustrating some of the problems which have been considered.

Spin Couplings and Antisymmetry

It is clear that any spin operator will commute with the spin-free Hamiltonian $\mathcal{H}_0$. In addition, $\mathcal{H}_0$ must be symmetric with respect to any permutation of electron labels, so it commutes with all electron permutation operators. Electrons are Fermions and thus only antisymmetric wave functions are admissible.

$$\hat{P}\Psi = (-1)^p\Psi, \tag{11-1}$$

where $\hat{P}$ is any permutation operator acting on electron labels and p is its parity. (The parity can be taken as the number of pairwise interchanges required to produce $\hat{P}$. This number is not unique, but for a given $\hat{P}$ is always odd or always even.) If Ψ is to be a spin eigenfunction,

$$\mathcal{S}^2\Psi = S(S+1)\Psi. \tag{11-2}$$

Because $\hat{P}$ operates on both spatial and spin coordinate labels, these two conditions are not independent.

Spin and permutational symmetries may be treated at the same time or separately. Even in the latter case their interaction is unavoidable. The requirement of antisymmetry, applied to functions of different spin quantum number, forces different spatial behavior and thus different energies. As we have seen, these differences can sometimes be described by an effective spin Hamiltonian, but they do not correspond to true spin interactions as do the magnetic interactions. It is essential that this distinction not be lost. The spatial functions can be considered alone, without any involvement of spin functions, if appropriate permutational symmetry requirements, depending in part on spin quantum numbers, are imposed. This is the basis of the spin-free quantum mechanics developed by Matsen and co-workers [136]. We are interested in actual spin properties, however, and will follow the more usual practice of including spin explicitly.

We will first consider some properties of many-electron spin eigenfunctions by themselves, and then investigate their combination with spatial functions to produce antisymmetric total wave functions.

Spin Eigenfunctions

We will use the one-electron spin functions α and β as a basis, constructing many-electron functions as products of one-electron functions. We retain the convention that the first factor is the spin function for electron 1, the second for electron 2, etc.

$$\alpha\beta\alpha\cdots \equiv \alpha(1)\beta(2)\alpha(3)\cdots. \tag{11-3}$$

(Recall that at this point we are not concerned with permutational symmetry.) The 2^N possible products form a basis for the spin space of N electrons.

Since $[\mathcal{S}^2, \mathcal{S}_z] = 0$ and $[\mathcal{H}_0, \mathcal{S}_z] = 0$, we can choose our spin functions to be eigenfunctions of $\mathcal{S}_z$ as well as of $\mathcal{S}^2$. The simple product functions are already eigenfunctions of $\mathcal{S}_z$. If there are μ α functions and ν β functions in the product ($\mu + \nu = N$) then the eigenvalue of $\mathcal{S}_z$ is $M_S = \frac{1}{2}(\mu - \nu)$ (in units of $\hbar$). Unfortunately, a little more effort must be expended to obtain eigenfunctions of $\mathcal{S}^2$.

There are many possible ways of obtaining $\mathcal{S}^2$ eigenfunctions.‡ One obvious way would be to construct the matrix of $\mathcal{S}^2$ in the product basis and diagonalize it. This is not practical if more than a few electrons are involved, nor does it provide a unique prescription, since degenerate eigenvalues occur. Three of the other possible methods will be considered here: genealogical construction using simple angular momentum coupling techniques, the use of Löwdin spin projection operators, and Rumer diagram methods. Each of these methods is capable of producing a complete set of independent functions, but only the first normally produces an orthogonal set. These methods and others can be related to the theory of the symmetric group. This relationship and group-theoretic projection operators will not be considered here.

In order to avoid getting lost in a morass of general formalism, it is useful to consider occasionally some examples. We will frequently consider a three-electron system as the simplest nontrivial case.

There are eight spin product functions for three electrons. They are

$$\begin{array}{llll} \alpha\alpha\alpha, & M_S = \frac{3}{2}, & \begin{array}{l}\alpha\beta\beta,\\ \beta\alpha\beta,\\ \beta\beta\alpha,\end{array} & M_S = -\frac{1}{2}, \\[2ex] \begin{array}{l}\alpha\alpha\beta,\\ \alpha\beta\alpha,\\ \beta\alpha\alpha,\end{array} & M_S = \frac{1}{2}, & \beta\beta\beta, & M_S = -\frac{3}{2}. \end{array}$$

‡ Many, many references would be possible. One recent discussion is that of Pauncz [155, Chapter 2].

It can be directly verified that $\alpha\alpha\alpha$ and $\beta\beta\beta$ are already eigenfunctions of $\mathscr{S}^2$ with $S = \frac{3}{2}$. Since the maximum value of S for N electrons is $N/2$ and the minimum value is $\frac{1}{2}$ for odd N (0 if N is even), the only other S possible is $\frac{1}{2}$. Applying $\mathscr{S}_-$ to $\alpha\alpha\alpha$ yields a function

$$\mathscr{S}_-\alpha\alpha\alpha = (\alpha\alpha\beta + \alpha\beta\alpha + \beta\alpha\alpha), \tag{11-4}$$

which has $S = \frac{3}{2}$, $M_S = \frac{1}{2}$. The other two linearly independent combinations of the three $M_S = \frac{1}{2}$ products orthogonal to $\mathscr{S}_-\alpha\alpha\alpha$ must be eigenfunctions of $\mathscr{S}^2$ with $S = \frac{1}{2}$, since there is no other possibility. Because they are degenerate in both S and M_S, there is no criterion at this point for choosing one set of linear combinations over another. We could take, for example, $(\alpha\beta\alpha - \beta\alpha\alpha)/\sqrt{2}$ and $(2\alpha\alpha\beta - \alpha\beta\alpha - \beta\alpha\alpha)/\sqrt{6}$. Alternatively we could consider the matrix of $\mathscr{S}^2$ in the basis of $M_S = \frac{1}{2}$ products. ($\mathscr{S}^2$ will have no nonzero matrix elements between functions with different M_S values.) The matrix is

$$\mathscr{S}^2 = \begin{pmatrix} \frac{7}{4} & 1 & 1 \\ 1 & \frac{7}{4} & 1 \\ 1 & 1 & \frac{7}{4} \end{pmatrix},$$

and it is readily verified that the vector (1, 1, 1) is an (unnormalized) eigenvector with eigenvalue $\frac{15}{4} = \frac{3}{2}(\frac{3}{2} + 1)$ while $(0, 1, -1)$ and $(2, -1, -1)$ are eigenvectors with eigenvalue $\frac{3}{4} = \frac{1}{2}(\frac{1}{2} + 1)$ each.

A similar treatment gives one $S = \frac{3}{2}$ and two $S = \frac{1}{2}$ functions from the $M_S = -\frac{1}{2}$ group. The eight three-electron product functions can thus be combined to give eight spin eigenfunctions as given in Table 11-1. We will return to this example for each of the three general methods of constructing spin eigenfunctions to be considered.

TABLE 11-1

Spin Eigenfunctions for Three Electrons

M_S	$S = \frac{3}{2}$	$S = \frac{1}{2}$
$\frac{3}{2}$	$\alpha\alpha\alpha$	
$\frac{1}{2}$	$(1/\sqrt{3})(\alpha\alpha\beta + \alpha\beta\alpha + \beta\alpha\alpha)$	$(1/\sqrt{2})(\alpha\beta\alpha - \beta\alpha\alpha)$ $(1/\sqrt{6})(2\alpha\alpha\beta - \alpha\beta\alpha - \beta\alpha\alpha)$
$-\frac{1}{2}$	$(1/\sqrt{3})(\alpha\beta\beta + \beta\alpha\beta + \beta\beta\alpha)$	$(1/\sqrt{2})(\alpha\beta\beta - \beta\alpha\beta)$ $(1/\sqrt{6})(-\alpha\beta\beta - \beta\alpha\beta + 2\beta\beta\alpha)$
$-\frac{3}{2}$	$\beta\beta\beta$	

Genealogical Construction: Vector Coupling [99,178]

The method of genealogical construction of spin eigenfunctions by successive couplings of angular momenta starts with one electron and adds additional electrons, one at a time, until the spin eigenfunctions for the desired number of electrons are obtained. Angular momenta are appropriately coupled at each stage. (The coupling of angular momenta is reviewed in Appendix C.) An angular momentum eigenfunction $|j, m\rangle$ can be constructed from products of angular momentum eigenfunctions as

$$|j, m\rangle = \sum_{m_1} C(jm; j_1 m_1 j_2 m - m_1)|j_1, m_1\rangle|j_2, m - m_1\rangle, \qquad (11\text{-}5)$$

where the C's are the Clebsch–Gordan coefficients. For the construction of spin eigenfunctions we take the functions $|j_2, m_2\rangle$ to be the one-electron functions $|\frac{1}{2}, \frac{1}{2}\rangle = \alpha$ and $|\frac{1}{2}, -\frac{1}{2}\rangle = \beta$. We can usually construct spin eigenfunctions for N electrons from those for $N - 1$ electrons in two ways

$$|N; S, M\rangle = \left(\frac{S + M}{2S}\right)^{1/2} |N - 1; S - \tfrac{1}{2}; M - \tfrac{1}{2}\rangle\alpha + \left(\frac{S - M}{2S}\right)^{1/2} |N - 1; S - \tfrac{1}{2}; M + \tfrac{1}{2}\rangle\beta \qquad (11\text{-}6a)$$

or

$$|N; S, M\rangle = -\left(\frac{S - M + 1}{2S + 1}\right)^{1/2} |N - 1; S + \tfrac{1}{2}, M - \tfrac{1}{2}\rangle\alpha + \left(\frac{S + M + 1}{2S + 2}\right)^{1/2} |N - 1; S + \tfrac{1}{2}, M + \tfrac{1}{2}\rangle\beta. \qquad (11\text{-}6b)$$

In cases where $M = 0$ or $M = S$, or where $S = 0$ or $N/2$, only one of the equations may be applicable or an equation may reduce to a single term.

With initial one-electron functions $|1; \frac{1}{2}, \frac{1}{2}\rangle = \alpha$ and $|1; \frac{1}{2}, -\frac{1}{2}\rangle = \beta$,

$$\begin{aligned} |2; 1, 1\rangle &= 1 \cdot \alpha\alpha + 0 = \alpha\alpha, \\ |2; 1, 0\rangle &= \frac{1}{\sqrt{2}}\beta\alpha + \frac{1}{\sqrt{2}}\alpha\beta = \frac{1}{\sqrt{2}}(\alpha\beta + \beta\alpha), \\ |2; 1, -1\rangle &= 0 + 1 \cdot \beta\beta = \beta\beta, \end{aligned} \qquad (11\text{-}7)$$

and

$$|2; 0, 0\rangle = -\frac{1}{\sqrt{2}}\beta\alpha + \frac{1}{\sqrt{2}}\alpha\beta = \frac{1}{\sqrt{2}}(\alpha\beta - \beta\alpha). \qquad (11\text{-}8)$$

We then move on to the three-electron functions, considering only those with $M_S = \pm\frac{1}{2}$. We find

$$|3;\tfrac{3}{2},\tfrac{1}{2}\rangle = \sqrt{\tfrac{2}{3}}|2;1,0\rangle\alpha + \sqrt{\tfrac{1}{3}}|2\cdot 1,1\rangle\beta$$
$$= \sqrt{\tfrac{2}{3}}\frac{1}{\sqrt{2}}(\alpha\beta + \beta\alpha)\alpha + \sqrt{\tfrac{1}{3}}\,\alpha\alpha\cdot\beta = \frac{1}{\sqrt{3}}(\alpha\alpha\beta + \alpha\beta\alpha + \beta\alpha\alpha). \tag{11-9}$$

A function $|3;\frac{1}{2},\frac{1}{2}\rangle$ can be constructed in two ways, however, as

$$|3;\tfrac{1}{2},\tfrac{1}{2};1\rangle = 1\cdot|2;0,0\rangle\alpha + 0 = \frac{1}{\sqrt{2}}(\alpha\beta - \beta\alpha)\alpha \tag{11-10}$$

or as

$$|3;\tfrac{1}{2},\tfrac{1}{2},2\rangle = -\sqrt{\tfrac{1}{3}}|2;1,0\rangle\alpha + \sqrt{\tfrac{2}{3}}|2;1,1\rangle\beta$$
$$= -\frac{1}{\sqrt{6}}(2\alpha\alpha\beta - \alpha\beta\alpha - \beta\alpha\alpha). \tag{11-11}$$

An additional index has been added to the ket to distinguish these otherwise similarly labeled functions.

It is clear that as the number of electrons increases the number of different functions with the same S and M will increase. The coupling process is conveniently described by a diagram known as the branching diagram. The possible S values are plotted against the number of electrons, N, with an indication of the number of independent functions for each case, as shown in Fig. 11-1. (M_S degeneracy is not included. It is convenient to think of, e.g., $M_S = S$ in each case, with an additional multiplier $2S + 1$ not indicated in the count shown.) The number of independent functions for each given N, S, and M_S is equal to the number of distinct paths on the branching diagram by which the corresponding point can be reached, moving always from left to right. For three electrons the doublet state can be reached in two ways.

For N electrons the possible values of S range from 0 (if N is even) or $\frac{1}{2}$ (if N is odd) to $N/2$ in integer steps. From the method of construction, Eq. (11-6), or from the branching diagram we see that if $f(N, S)$ is the number of independent spin functions for N electrons with quantum number S (and $M_S = S$),

$$f(N,S) = f(N-1, S-\tfrac{1}{2})\bar{\delta}_{S,0} + f(N-1, S+\tfrac{1}{2})\bar{\delta}_{S,N/2}, \tag{11-12}$$

where

$$\bar{\delta}_{jk} = (1-\delta_{jk}) = \begin{cases} 1, & \text{if } j \neq k, \\ 0, & \text{if } j = k, \end{cases} \tag{11-13}$$

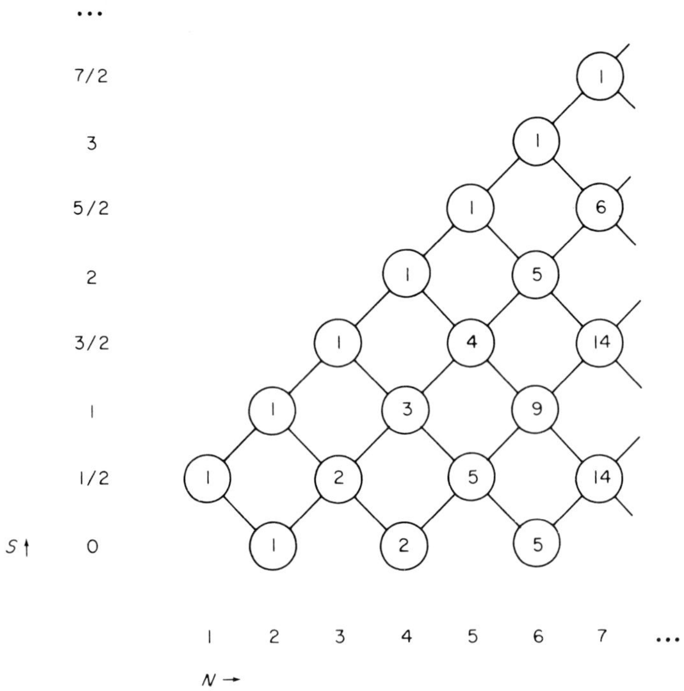

FIG. 11-1. Branching diagram for electron spin coupling. The circled number for each N, S combination is the number of independent spin eigenfunctions with quantum number S (and $M = S$) for N electrons.

has been introduced to take care of the "end point" values of S. The general expression for f is‡

$$f(N, S) = \binom{N}{N/2 - S} - \binom{N}{N/2 - S - 1}\bar{\delta}_{S, N/2}. \qquad (11\text{-}14)$$

The proof is by induction. The expression is readily verified on a case-by-case basis for $N \leq 3$. For $N > 3$, we suppose Eq. (11-14) to be valid for $N - 1$. Then if $S = 0$, (N is then even)

$$f(N, 0) = f(N - 1, \tfrac{1}{2}) = \binom{N-1}{N/2 - 1} - \binom{N-1}{N/2 - 2}$$

$$= \frac{2(N-1)}{(N/2 + 1)!(N/2 - 1)!} = \binom{N}{N/2} - \binom{N}{N/2 - 1}. \qquad (11\text{-}15)$$

‡ The $\bar{\delta}$ is frequently omitted. Compare, e.g., [155, p. 16].

which is the required result. If $S = N/2$,

$$f(N, N/2) = \binom{N-1}{N/2 - N/2} = \binom{N-1}{0} = 1$$
$$= \binom{N}{0} = \binom{N}{N/2 - N/2}, \tag{11-16}$$

which is again the required result. Finally, for $0 < S < N/2$,

$$\begin{aligned} f(N, S) &= f(N-1, S-\tfrac{1}{2}) + f(N-1, S+\tfrac{1}{2}) \\ &= \left[\binom{N-1}{N/2 - S} - \binom{N-1}{N/2 - S - 1}\right] \\ &\quad + \left[\binom{N-1}{N/2 - S - 1} - \binom{N-1}{N/2 - S - 2}\bar{\delta}_{S, N/2-1}\right] \\ &= \binom{N-1}{N/2 - S} - \binom{N-1}{N/2 - S - 2}\bar{\delta}_{S, N/2-1}. \end{aligned} \tag{11-17}$$

For $S = N/2 - 1$, this is

$$f(N, S) = \binom{N-1}{N/2 - (N/2 - 1)} = \binom{N-1}{1} = N - 1, \tag{11-18}$$

which is equal to

$$\binom{N}{N/2 - (N/2 - 1)} - \binom{N}{N/2 - (N/2 - 1) - 1} = \binom{N}{1} - \binom{N}{0} = N - 1, \tag{11-19}$$

and for $0 < S < N/2 - 1$ it is

$$f(N, S) = \binom{N-1}{N/2 - S} - \binom{N-1}{N/2 - S - 2} = \frac{(2S + 1)N!}{(N/2 - S)!(N/2 + S + 1)!}, \tag{11-20}$$

which is again equal to the result given by Eq. (11-14), so the proof is completed.

Projection Operators

Spin eigenfunctions can also be obtained by application of a projection operator to any spin function, e.g., a simple product, which has a nonvanishing component of the desired multiplicity. Two types of spin projection operators can be distinguished. One is defined without reference to any other method of defining spin eigenfunctions and yields simply that component of the function to which it is applied in the full subspace of the given multiplicity. The dimension of this subspace is $f(N, S)$. The other kind of projection operator projects onto a single axis (i.e., a single spin eigenfunction in the subspace) or onto an intermediate subspace of dimension between 1 and $f(N, S)$. It is then necessary that a choice of axes (spin eigenfunctions) be somehow made in advance and contained in the projection operator definition [136]. We will deal at this point only with projection operators of the first type.

Löwdin Spin Projection [108,109,155]

The eigenfunctions of $\mathscr{S}^2$ form a complete set, so any spin function can be expressed as a linear combination of eigenfunctions of $\mathscr{S}^2$. If the function being expanded is an eigenfunction of $\mathscr{S}_z$ with eigenvalue M, then only those spin functions associated with the same value of M will be involved in the expansion. We can thus write

$$|M\rangle = \sum_S \omega_S^{1/2} |S, M\rangle, \tag{11-21}$$

where the form of the coefficient is chosen for later convenience. (The phase of each coefficient depends on the phase chosen for the spin eigenfunctions.) Now consider an operator $A_t = \mathscr{S}^2 - t(t+1)$. When A_t acts on an eigenfunction of $\mathscr{S}^2$ with eigenvalue $S(S+1)$, the result is

$$A_t |S, M\rangle = [S(S+1) - t(t+1)] |S, M\rangle \tag{11-22}$$

which will be zero if $S = t$. A_t is an *annihilation operator*: it destroys any $\mathscr{S}^2$ eigenfunction with $S = t$. Spin eigenfunctions with different eigenvalues will simply be multiplied by a nonzero constant. We are thus led to define an operator

$$\mathscr{O}_S = \prod_{t \neq S} \frac{\mathscr{S}^2 - t(t+1)}{S(S+1) - t(t+1)}. \tag{11-23}$$

What happens when $\mathscr{O}_S$ acts on an eigenfunction of $\mathscr{S}^2$ with quantum number S'? If $S' \neq S$, then there is some factor in the product which will produce 0, but if $S' = S$, each factor is 1. Thus

$$\mathscr{O}_S |S', M\rangle = \delta_{SS'} |S', M\rangle. \tag{11-24}$$

It is clear that from the definition that $\mathscr{O}_S$ is Hermitian. If $\mathscr{O}_S$ acts on any function it will produce either zero or some multiple of the spin eigenfunction with quantum number S. If it is then applied again, it will have no further effect, so $\mathcal{O}_S^2 = \mathcal{O}_S$ and $\mathcal{O}_S$ is a projection operator. For the function $|M\rangle$, for example,

$$\mathcal{O}_S|M\rangle = \sum_{S'} \omega_{S'}^{1/2}\delta_{SS'}|S', M\rangle = \omega_S^{1/2}|S, M\rangle. \tag{11-25}$$

One can start with a simple product function and use the projection operator to obtain a spin eigenfunction. One way is straightforward but messy: just use the definition of $\mathcal{O}_S$ given above and grind away, making use of the known effect of the various terms in $\mathscr{S}^2$ on the product function. This will clearly get so lengthy as to be essentially useless for more than just a very few electrons. Luckily, there is another way of getting the result which is quite practical.

Suppose that we have N electrons and are interested in a state with $\mathscr{S}_z$ quantum number M. Define $\mu = (N/2) + M$ and $\nu = (N/2) - M$. It is only necessary to consider explicitly states with $M \geq 0$, so we can consider $\mu \geq \nu$. We will further consider only one of the possible spin products. Any product for this N and M will have μ factors α and ν factors β. We will consider explicitly only the product in which all the α's come first. Any other product for the same M and N can be obtained by a permutation, and since all permutation operators commute with $\mathcal{O}_S$, we can get the result of projecting other products by permuting the result of projecting this one. To express the result conveniently we need to define some notation. Let $[\alpha^j\beta^k|$ or $|\alpha^j\beta^k]$ denote the sum of all products each of which has j α factors and k β factors. There will be $\binom{j+k}{j}$ terms in the sum. The notation $[\alpha^i\beta^j|\alpha^k\beta^l]$ denotes a product of two such sums; when multiplied out it will be a sum of products each of which has $i + k$ α factors and $j + l$ β factors (but not all such products will be included).

It will be most convenient to first state the results, then show that the form indicated is correct, and finally evaluate the coefficients which occur. Note that, in the notation defined above, the spin product function we will start with can be written $[\alpha^\mu|\beta^\nu]$. Then

$$\mathcal{O}_S[\alpha^\mu|\beta^\nu] = \sum_{k=0}^{\nu} C_k(S, M, n)[\alpha^{\mu-k}\beta^k|\alpha^k\beta^{\nu-k}], \tag{11-26}$$

where $C_k(S, M, n)$ is a coefficient depending on S, M, and $n = N/2$. These coefficients $C_k = C_k(S, M, n)$ are determined from a recursion relationship

$$(\mu - k)(\nu - k)C_{k+1} + [n + 2k(n - k) - S(S + 1) + M^2]C_k + k^2C_{k-1} = 0 \tag{11-27}$$

with $C_0 = (2S + 1)[\mu!\nu!/(n + S + 1)!(n - S)!]$. General solutions for the C_k are known [78,182,193], but are rather complicated and will not be given here. The most useful result is for what is known as the principal case, $M = S$. In this case

$$C_k(S, S, n) = (-1)^k \frac{2S+1}{n+S+1} \binom{n+S}{k}^{-1}. \tag{11-28}$$

The $C_k(S, M, n)$ are known as the "Sanibel coefficients."‡

We first seek to establish that the result of projecting the spin product function can be written in the form above. Since $\mathscr{S}_z$ commutes with $\mathscr{S}^2$, it will commute with $\mathscr{O}_S$. We start with an eigenfunction of $\mathscr{S}_z$, so each term in the expansion of the projected function must be an eigenfunction of $\mathscr{S}_z$ with the same eigenvalue. Each spin product in the expansion must thus contain μ α's and ν β's. Any term in the sum is thus some permutation of $[\alpha^\mu | \beta^\nu]$, so if we introduce coefficients $C(\hat{P})$ depending on the permutation involved and sum over all permutations, we can certainly write

$$\mathscr{O}_S[\alpha^\mu | \beta^\nu] = \sum_{\hat{P}} C(\hat{P}) \hat{P} [\alpha^\mu | \beta^\nu]. \tag{11-29}$$

Let $\hat{Q}$ be any permutation which involves interchanges of the first μ electrons among themselves and/or the last ν electrons among themselves. It follows from this definition that $\hat{Q}$ leaves $[\alpha^\mu | \nu^\beta]$ unchanged. Since $\mathscr{S}^2$ and thus $\mathscr{O}_S$ involve all electrons equivalently, they will commute with all permutations, including $\hat{Q}$. Thus

$$\mathscr{O}_S[\alpha^\mu | \nu^\beta] = \sum_{\hat{P}} C(\hat{P}) \hat{P} [\alpha^\mu | \beta^\nu] = \hat{Q} \mathscr{O}_S [\alpha^\mu | \beta^\nu] = \sum_{\hat{P}} C(\hat{P}) \hat{Q} \hat{P} [\alpha^\mu | \beta^\nu]. \tag{11-30}$$

The result of $\hat{Q}\hat{P}$ acting on the spin product will not in general be the same as that produced by $\hat{P}$, but the equality above must hold for all $\hat{Q}$ of the type defined above. This can be true only if all spin products which can be interrelated in this way have the same coefficient, i.e., $C(\hat{P})$ must be the same for all $\hat{P}$'s that produce the same number of β's among the first μ positions (and thus the same number of α's among the last ν), since they can be intermixed with each other by a $\hat{Q}$. This establishes that the expansion of the projected spin product is of the form given in Eq. (11-26).

We next seek to establish the recursion relation for the coefficients. Let $t_k = [\alpha^{\mu-k}\beta^k | \alpha^k \beta^{\nu-k}]$ to save writing. It is an eigenfunction of $\mathscr{S}_z$, and since $\mathscr{S}_z$ commutes with $\mathscr{S}^2$, $\mathscr{S}^2 t_k$ will also be an eigenfunction of $\mathscr{S}_z$. Noting that permutations commute with $\mathscr{S}^2$ and using a permutation $\hat{Q}$ of the type defined above, we can show by an argument exactly paralleling the one used above that

$$\mathscr{S}^2 t_k = \sum_j D_{kj} t_j. \tag{11-31}$$

‡ The name comes from Sanibel Island, Florida, where many of these properties were first discovered at a series of theoretical chemistry schools and symposia.

The D_{kj} can be evaluated with the help of a relationship among spin operators and permutations acting on spin functions. For a many-electron system

$$\mathscr{S}^2 = \sum_{i,j} \mathscr{s}_i \cdot \mathscr{s}_j = \sum_i \mathscr{s}_i^2 + \sum_{i \neq j} \mathscr{s}_i \cdot \mathscr{s}_j$$
$$= \tfrac{3}{4}N + \sum_{i \neq j} (-\tfrac{1}{4} + \tfrac{1}{2}P_{ij}). \qquad (11\text{-}32)$$

In this expression P_{ij} is the permutation operator which interchanges electrons i and j. The first term in the last expression comes from the fact that $\mathscr{S}_i^2 = \frac{3}{4}$ for any one electron and there are N equal terms in the sum for N electrons. The second term requires that $\mathscr{s}_i \cdot \mathscr{s}_j$ and $(-\frac{1}{4} + \frac{1}{2}P_{ij})$ have the same effect on spin functions. This is readily established. We note that $\mathscr{s}_i \cdot \mathscr{s}_j = \mathscr{s}_{iz}\mathscr{s}_{yz} + \frac{1}{2}(\mathscr{s}_{i+}\mathscr{s}_{j-} + \mathscr{s}_{i-}\mathscr{s}_{j+})$ and let $\alpha\alpha = \alpha(i)\alpha(j)$, etc. Then

$$\begin{aligned} \mathscr{s}_i \cdot \mathscr{s}_j \alpha\alpha &= \tfrac{1}{4}\alpha\alpha \; (= -\tfrac{1}{4}\alpha\alpha + \tfrac{1}{2}\alpha\alpha), \\ \mathscr{s}_i \cdot \mathscr{s}_j \alpha\beta &= -\tfrac{1}{4}\alpha\beta + \tfrac{1}{2}\beta\alpha, \\ \mathscr{s}_i \cdot \mathscr{s}_j \beta\alpha &= -\tfrac{1}{4}\beta\alpha + \tfrac{1}{2}\alpha\beta, \\ \mathscr{s}_i \cdot \mathscr{s}_j \beta\beta &= \tfrac{1}{4}\beta\beta \; (= -\tfrac{1}{4}\beta\beta + \tfrac{1}{2}\beta\beta), \end{aligned} \qquad (11\text{-}33)$$

which is clearly the same as the effect of $(-\frac{1}{4} + \frac{1}{2}P_{ij})$. These are the only possible spin function combinations, so the two operators have the same effect. In addition, $P_{ij} = P_{ji}$ and there are $N(N-1)$ terms in the sum with $i \neq j$, so

$$\mathscr{S}^2 = \tfrac{3}{4}N - \tfrac{1}{4}N(N-1) + \tfrac{1}{2}\sum_{i \neq j} P_{ij} = -n(n-2) + \sum_{i<j} P_{ij}, \qquad (11\text{-}34)$$

where again $n = N/2$. Next consider the effect of P_{ij} on any term in t_k. A term of the type already in t_k will be produced if α is exchanged with α [which can happen in $\mu(\mu-1)/2$ ways], if β is exchanged with β [which can happen in $\nu(\nu-1)/2$ ways], or if α is exchanged with β but both are in either the first μ [$(\mu-k)k$ possibilities] or both are in the last ν [$k(\nu-k)$ possibilities]. A term of the type found in t_{k+1} will be produced if an α from within the first μ is exchanged with a β in the last ν [there are $(\mu-k)(\nu-k)$ possibilities for this]. A term of the type found in t_{k-1} will be produced if a β in the first μ is exchanged with an α in the last ν [k^2 possible ways]. Since we sum over pairwise interchanges, since t_k involves symmetric sums of all spin products of the type considered, and since we know that the result must be expressible in terms of similar symmetric sums, the coefficients must be given just by the relative number of ways in which terms of each type can be produced. The coefficient of t_k will also include a contribution of $-n(n-2)$ from the constant term. Thus

$$\begin{aligned} D_{kk} &= \mu(\mu-1)/2 + \nu(\nu-1)/2 + (\mu-k)k + k(\nu-k) - n(n-1) \\ &= M^2 + n - 2k(n-k). \end{aligned} \qquad (11\text{-}35)$$

The coefficients of t_{k-1} and t_{k+1} are obtained in a similar way, but we must multiply by the number of terms in t_k to get the total number of terms of each type, and then divide by the number of terms in t_{k-1} or t_{k+1} to get the coefficient of that sum. (A similar process is really involved for t_k, but there we are multiplying and dividing by the same thing.) There are $\binom{\mu}{k}\binom{\nu}{k}$ terms in t_k, $\binom{\mu}{k+1}\binom{\nu}{k+1}$ terms in t_{k+1} and $\binom{\mu}{k-1}\binom{\nu}{k-1}$ terms in t_{k-1}. We thus find that

$$D_{k,k+1} = \binom{\mu}{k}\binom{\nu}{k}\binom{\mu}{k+1}^{-1}\binom{\nu}{k+1}^{-1}(\mu - k)(\nu - k) = (k+1)^2,$$

$$D_{k,k-1} = \binom{\mu}{k}\binom{\nu}{k}\binom{\mu}{k-1}^{-1}\binom{\nu}{k-1}^{-1}k^2 = (\mu - k + 1)(\nu - k + 1),$$

$$D_{kj} = 0 \qquad \text{if } j \text{ differs from } k \text{ by more than 1.} \tag{11-36}$$

Our original product function is t_0 in this notation, and its projection is an eigenfunction of $\mathscr{S}^2$ with eigenvalue S, so that

$$\begin{aligned}
0 &= [\mathscr{S}^2 - S(S+1)]\mathscr{O}_S t_0 = \sum_k C_k[\mathscr{S}^2 - S(S+1)]t_k \\
&= \sum_k C_k\{(k+1)^2 t_{k+1} + [M^2 + n - 2k(k-n) \\
&\quad - S(S+1)]t_k + (\mu - k + 1)(\nu - k + 1)t_{k-1}\} \\
&= \sum_k \{k^2 C_{k-1} + [M^2 + n - 2k(k-n) - S(S+1)]C_k \\
&\quad + (\mu - k)(\nu - k)C_{k+1}\}t_k.
\end{aligned} \tag{11-37}$$

Since the t_k for different values of k are orthogonal, the coefficient of each term in this sum must vanish independently. This establishes the recursion formula for the C_k. The overall normalization or the choice of C_0 is determined not by the fact that the projected function is normalized (it isn't) but by the requirement that $\mathscr{O}_S$ be idempotent. For any choice of C_0, the operator corresponding to $\mathscr{O}_S$ but defined by the expansion result will be proportional to its square, but for only one choice will the proportionality constant be 1. The proof that C_0 must have the value specified above will not be given here.

The verification that the special form of C_k when $M = S$ does satisfy the recursion formula is just a matter of substitution and simple algebra.

To illustrate the projection method, we consider the case of the $M = \frac{1}{2}$ states for three electrons. In this case $N = 3$, $n = \frac{3}{2}$, $\mu = 2$, $\nu = 1$, and

$$\mathscr{O}\alpha\alpha\beta = C_0\alpha\alpha\beta + C_1(\alpha\beta + \beta\alpha)\alpha. \tag{11-38}$$

For $S = M = \frac{1}{2}$, the principal case expression above gives $C_0 = \frac{2}{3}$, $C_1 = -\frac{1}{3}$, and

$$\mathscr{O}_{1/2}\alpha\alpha\beta = \tfrac{2}{3}\alpha\alpha\beta - \tfrac{1}{3}(\alpha\beta\alpha + \beta\alpha\alpha). \tag{11-39}$$

For $S = \frac{3}{2}$, we have $C_0 = \frac{1}{3}$ and from the recursion formula with $k = 0$ we get $C_1 = C_0$, so that

$$\mathcal{O}_{3/2}\alpha\alpha\beta = \tfrac{1}{3}(\alpha\alpha\beta + \alpha\beta\alpha + \beta\alpha\alpha). \tag{11-40}$$

Note that

$$\mathcal{O}_{3/2}\alpha\alpha\beta + \mathcal{O}_{1/2}\alpha\alpha\beta = \alpha\alpha\beta. \tag{11-41}$$

This is a special case of the general operator equation

$$\sum_S \mathcal{O}_S = 1. \tag{11-42}$$

A set of projection operators satisfying such an equation is said to be complete.

The effect of projecting the other product functions can be obtained by applying permutation operators.

$$\begin{aligned} \mathcal{O}_{1/2}\alpha\beta\alpha &= P_{23}\mathcal{O}_{1/2}\alpha\alpha\beta = \tfrac{2}{3}\alpha\beta\alpha - \tfrac{1}{3}(\alpha\alpha\beta + \beta\alpha\alpha) \\ \mathcal{O}_{1/2}\beta\alpha\alpha &= P_{13}\mathcal{O}_{1/2}\alpha\alpha\beta = \tfrac{2}{3}\beta\alpha\alpha - \tfrac{1}{3}(\alpha\beta\alpha + \alpha\alpha\beta). \end{aligned} \tag{11-43}$$

Of the three functions obtained in this way, any two are linearly independent but all three are not.

$$\begin{aligned} \mathcal{O}_{1/2}\alpha\alpha\beta + \mathcal{O}_{1/2}\alpha\beta\alpha + \mathcal{O}_{1/2}\beta\alpha\alpha &= \mathcal{O}_{1/2}(\alpha\alpha\beta + \alpha\beta\alpha + \beta\alpha\alpha) \\ &\propto \mathcal{O}_{1/2}|3; \tfrac{3}{2}, \tfrac{1}{2}\rangle = 0. \end{aligned} \tag{11-44}$$

The relationships among the various three-electron $M = \frac{1}{2}$ functions are illustrated in Fig. 11-2.

A complete set of linearly independent S, M eigenfunctions can be obtained by using an appropriately selected subset of permutations. Specifically, it can be shown that for $M_S = S \geq 0$ a complete, independent set will be ob- obtained by applying $\mathcal{O}_S$ to those product functions which satisfy the condition

$$\sum_{j=1}^{k} M_S(j) \geq 0, \qquad \text{all } k, \quad 1 \leq k \leq N, \tag{11-45}$$

i.e., the sum of m_s values for the first k electrons is nonnegative for any choice of k. The proof of this result will not be reproduced here [155]. Functions with $M_S < S$ can be obtained by application of $\mathcal{S}_-$.

The overlap integral between functions obtained in this way and the normalization constant for each function are also of interest, although we will be more concerned with the corresponding quantities after spatial functions are included. An expression is readily obtained for the overlap between projected product spin functions. Let

$$\Psi_j = \hat{P}_j \mathcal{O}_S t_0 = \hat{P}_j \sum_k C_k t_k \tag{11-46}$$

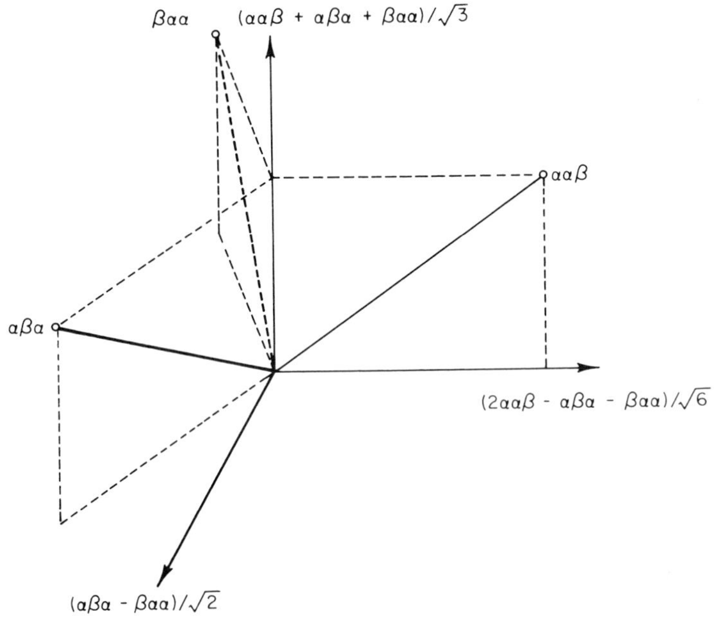

FIG. 11-2. Spin projections in the $M_S = \frac{1}{2}$ space for three electrons.

and

$$S_{ij} = \int \Psi_i^* \Psi_j \, d\tau = \int (\hat{P}_i \mathcal{O}_S t_0)^* (\hat{P}_j \mathcal{O}_S t_0) \, d\tau. \qquad (11\text{-}47)$$

The value of the integral will be unchanged if we apply $\hat{P}_j^{-1}$ to each of the factors in the integrand, since this just amounts to a relabeling of the variables of integration. In addition, all permutation operators commute with $\mathcal{O}_S$ and $\mathcal{O}_S^2 = \mathcal{O}_S = \mathcal{O}_S^\dagger$, so

$$\begin{aligned} S_{ij} &= \int (\mathcal{O}_S \hat{P}_j^{-1} \hat{P}_i t_0)^* (\hat{P}_j^{-1} \hat{P}_j \mathcal{O}_S t_0) \, d\tau \\ &= \int [(\hat{P}_j^{-1} \hat{P}_i) t_0]^* \mathcal{O}_S t_0 \, d\tau \\ &= \int [(P_j^{-1} \hat{P}_i) t_0]^* \sum_k C_k t_k \, d\tau = C_l, \end{aligned} \qquad (11\text{-}48)$$

where l is the number of α, β interchanges produced by $\hat{P}_j^{-1} \hat{P}_i$ acting on t_0. In particular, for any i $S_{ii} = C_0$ and the normalization constant is $C_0^{-1/2}$ for any spin eigenfunction projected from a single product. By using these overlaps, we can construct an orthonormal set of functions from the non-orthogonal but linearly independent set.

Group-Theoretic Projection Operators

Other projection operators which produce spin eigenfunctions can also be defined. They are commonly considered in the context of the spatial and spin behavior of the wave function, rather than of the spin function alone, and are coupled with the overall permutational antisymmetry requirement. They are thus intimately related to the theory of the symmetric group. Different sets of operators can be defined, corresponding to different choices of spin eigenfunctions. Among the possibilities are those corresponding to the genealogical functions or to the valence-bond type functions to be considered next.‡

Rumer-Diagram Methods§

Another method of constructing independent spin eigenfunctions is the Rumer-diagram method used in valence bond (VB) theory. Valence-bond spin eigenfunctions are constructed by coupling the spins of selected pairs of electrons to singlets, until only $2S = 2M_S$ electrons with parallel spin remain. If other M_S values are desired, they can be obtained by application of $\mathscr{S}_-$. The original functions can be expressed as the result of an appropriate permutation operator acting on the function

$$\theta_0 = \prod_{i=1}^{\nu} [(1/\sqrt{2})\{\alpha(2i-1)\beta(2i) - \beta(2i-1)\alpha(2i)\}] \prod_{j=2\nu+1}^{N} \alpha(j). \quad (11\text{-}49)$$

The problem is again to obtain a set of functions which is complete and linearly independent. These VB-type spin eigenfunctions will not be orthogonal.

One way of choosing independent functions is a diagrammatic method, which can be formulated as follows:

1. $N + 2S$ points are located on the circumference of a circle. Of these, N sequential points are marked, e.g., by a dot and are numbered from 1 to N. The remaining $2S$ points are marked in another way, e.g., by x's, and need not be numbered. The N dots correspond to the electrons and the $2S$ x's represent "phantom electrons" which are useful in determining possible pairings. Note that the total number of points, $N + 2S$, is always even.

2. Pairs of points consisting of two dots or a dot and an x are linked by arrows. No links are made between two x's. All points are connected pairwise in this way. To such a diagram is assigned a corresponding spin function

$$\theta_d = \left(\frac{1}{\sqrt{2}}\right)^{\nu} \prod_{i,j(\nu \text{ pairs } ij)} [\alpha(i)\beta(j) - \alpha(j)\beta(i)] \prod_{k(2S \text{ values})} \alpha(k), \quad (11\text{-}50)$$

‡ For a review and references, see Ruedenberg and Poshusta [173].

§ Compare, e.g., [129, Chapter 6].

where i and j are indices of two dots linked by an arrow and k is the index of a dot linked to an x. The only effect of the direction of an arrow will be on the sign of the function, and the direction of an arrow between a dot and an x is not significant. A spin function of the type given in Eq. (11-50) can be put into the form used previously be expanding the product into a sum of terms, each of which is a simple product, and then reordering the factors in such products to put the function for electron 1 first, that for electron 2 second, etc.

3. A complete, linearly independent set of spin eigenfunctions can be obtained by taking only the functions corresponding to diagrams in which no arrows cross. Of sets of diagrams differing only in the direction of arrows, only one member is to be retained.

Consider, for example, the three-electron doublet functions. Possible diagrams include

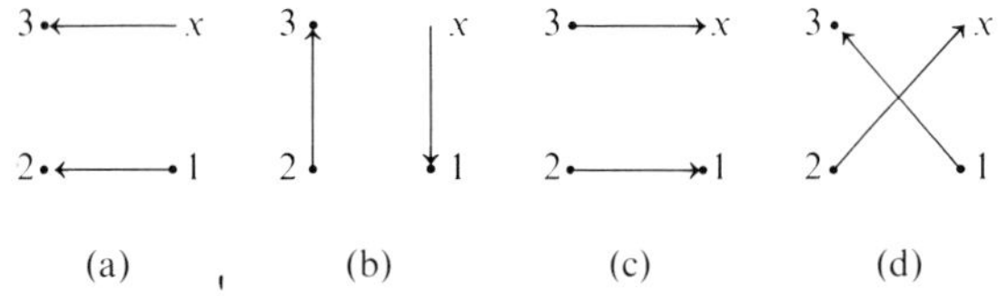

The corresponding functions are

$$\begin{aligned}
\theta_a &= \frac{1}{\sqrt{2}}[\alpha(1)\beta(2) - \beta(1)\alpha(2)]\alpha(3), \\
\theta_b &= \frac{1}{\sqrt{2}}[\alpha(2)\beta(3) - \beta(2)\alpha(3)]\alpha(1), \\
\theta_c &= \frac{1}{\sqrt{2}}[\alpha(2)\beta(1) - \beta(1)\alpha(2)]\alpha(3) = -\theta_a, \\
\theta_d &= \frac{1}{\sqrt{2}}[\alpha(1)\beta(3) - \beta(1)\alpha(3)]\alpha(2) = \theta_a + \theta_b.
\end{aligned} \tag{11-51}$$

The two functions θ_a and θ_b provide a possible choice of independent three-electron doublets. The other two are exluded from consideration, θ_c because diagram (c) differs from diagram (a) only in the direction of arrows, and θ_d because the arrows in diagram (d) cross.

Diagrammatic methods can also be used to obtain the overlap, or other matrix elements, between VB spin functions. A superposition diagram is first constructed for the two functions involved by combining the diagrams corresponding to them. In the superposition diagram, x's and arrows linking them to dots are not included; only dots and arrows between dots are retained. Certain features of the superposition diagram are then noted.

1. An *island* consists of a closed sequence of arrows. The special case of two arrows joining the same pair of points is considered an island. Let n be the number of islands in the superposition diagram.

2. A *chain* is an open sequence of arrows. Two types of chains can be distinguished, even chains involving an even number of points (and thus an odd number of arrows), and odd chains involving an odd number of points (and thus an even number of arrows).

After the superposition diagram has been formed, arrow directions are reversed as necessary to attain a head-to-head or tail-to-tail relationship of all the arrows. Let r be the number of reversals required. This assures that in the product of the corresponding spin functions, the electron associated with each point has the same initial spin in each function. The reversals introduce a factor $(-1)^r$ into the overlap integral.

A consideration of the other spin pairings leads to the conclusion that spins in the two factors cannot be matched completely, so as to give a nonzero overlap, if the superposition diagram contains any even chain. Each of the ν arrows in either Rumer diagram correspond to a factor $2^{-1/2}$ in the spin function, but in the pairing corresponding to an island two products resulting from each such factor have nonvanishing integrals. The resultant expression for the spin overlap integral is

$$\langle \theta_{\mathrm{d}_1} | \theta_{\mathrm{d}_2} \rangle = \begin{cases} 0, & \text{if the superposition of diagrams } \mathrm{d}_1 \text{ and } \mathrm{d}_2 \text{ contains any even chain} \\ (-1)^r 2^{n-\nu}, & \text{if no even chains.} \end{cases} \tag{11-52}$$

In both the valence-bond method, where Rumer-diagram spin functions are used, and in unrestricted or extended Hartree–Fock methods where spin projection operators are employed, nonorthogonal spatial functions are commonly involved. Before going further with a consideration of these methods, we must examine the way in which space and spin functions are combined to give a total wave function.

The Interaction of Space and Spin via Permutational Symmetry

Let us review briefly the consequences of permutational antisymmetry. Consider first the case of two electrons. The wave function including space and spin must be antisymmetric with respect to the interchange of the two electrons.

$$\Psi(x_1, x_2) = -\Psi(x_2, x_1). \tag{11-53}$$

We already know that there are four two-electron spin functions, given by Eqs. (11-7) and (11-8). The three triplet spin functions are symmetric with respect to electron interchange, and must therefore be combined with an antisymmetric spatial function to produce overall antisymmetric behavior:

$$^{3}\Psi(x_1, x_2) = {}^{3}\Phi(\mathbf{r}_1, \mathbf{r}_2)|2; 1, 0\rangle, \tag{11-54}$$

where

$$^{3}\Phi(\mathbf{r}_1, \mathbf{r}_2) = -{}^{3}\Phi(\mathbf{r}_2, \mathbf{r}_1). \tag{11-55}$$

Clearly an expression of the same form can be written involving the other two triplet functions. The singlet spin function, on the other hand, is antisymmetric and must thus be combined with a symmetric spatial function

$$\begin{aligned} ^{1}\Psi(x_1, x_2) &= {}^{1}\Phi(\mathbf{r}_1, \mathbf{r}_2)|2; 0, 0\rangle, \\ ^{1}\Phi(\mathbf{r}_1, \mathbf{r}_2) &= {}^{1}\Phi(\mathbf{r}_2, \mathbf{r}_1). \end{aligned} \tag{11-56}$$

This separation of space and spin factors greatly simplifies the treatment of two-electron systems.

When more than two electrons are involved, it is not in general possible to write a single product function with one spin factor and one spatial factor which is both antisymmetric and a spin eigenfunction. Rather, an antisymmetric function will involve a sum of products of spatial and spin factors. The factors in each term are neither symmetric nor antisymmetric by themselves, but transform according to some other representations of the symmetric group such that the sum of products is antisymmetric.

The construction of antisymmetric spin eigenfunctions by explicit consideration of the properties of the symmetric group will not be considered further here [60,173]. We will depend rather on the use of an antisymmetrizing operator to obtain the desired functions. Two antisymmetrizing operators, differing only in normalization, are commonly used. They are the antisymmetrizer

$$\mathscr{A} = \frac{1}{\sqrt{N!}} \sum_{\hat{P}} (-1)^p \hat{P} \tag{11-57}$$

and the antisymmetric projection operator

$$\mathscr{O}_{\text{as}} = \frac{1}{N!} \sum_{\hat{P}} (-1)^p \hat{P}. \tag{11-58}$$

In each case the sum is over all $N!$ permutations, $\hat{P}$, of the N electrons, and p is the parity of $\hat{P}$. The antisymmetrizer $\mathscr{A}$ is normalized so that when it is applied to a product of N orthonormal spin orbitals it produces a normalized result, while $\mathscr{O}_{\text{as}}$ is normalized as a projection operator, i.e., $\mathscr{O}_{\text{as}}^2 = \mathscr{O}_{\text{as}}$ acting on any function.

It is clear that an antisymmetric spin eigenfunction can be obtained by applying $\mathscr{A}$ or $\mathcal{O}_{\mathrm{as}}$ to any function of the form

$$\Psi = \sum_j \Phi_j \Theta_j, \tag{11-59}$$

where Φ_j is an N-electron spatial function and Θ_j is an N-electron spin eigenfunction obtained by any of the methods considered above. In cases where a spin projection operator of the type defined in Eq. (11-23) is used, it commutes with all permutations and thus with $\mathscr{A}$ or $\mathcal{O}_{\mathrm{as}}$.

If a nonzero result is to be obtained, certain constraints are placed by the choice of spin function on the choice of spatial function, and vice versa.

Comparison of Functions of Different Types

We proceed now to a survey of several of the common types of approximate wave functions. When one attempts to compare different types of wave functions, it is frequently rather difficult to see the significance, for some particular property such as spin density, of the difference. This problem can often be alleviated by considering the reduced density matrices corresponding to the different functions. Reduced density matrices and their spin components are defined in Appendix D and Section 10.

Functions of Hartree–Fock Type

Although the Hartree–Fock method or approximations to it are involved in a majority of practical quantum chemical calculations, there is no agreement as to precisely what a "Hartree–Fock" wave function is. Variations are referred to as restricted, unrestricted, or extended Hartree–Fock, and either of the first two may be called simply "Hartree–Fock". The basic physical idea of the method is that each electron moves in the average field due to the other electrons. This is coupled with the requirement that the wave function be permutationally antisymmetric. After the method is introduced, a distinction will be made between Hartree–Fock (HF) functions, self-consistent field (SCF) functions, and single determinant (SD) or single configuration functions. The distinctions made here are common but not universal.

The mathematically simplest definition of a HF function is as an optimum antisymmetrized single product, i.e., single determinant, of spin orbitals

$$\Psi(x_1, \ldots, x_N) = \mathscr{A}\psi_1(x_1)\psi_2(x_2)\cdots\psi_N(x_N), \tag{11-60}$$

where the argument x_i refers to the space and spin variables of electron i. The spin orbitals $\{\psi_i\}$ are to be chosen so as to minimize the variational energy

$$\tilde{E} = \int \Psi^* \mathscr{H}_0 \Psi \, d\tau \Big/ \left(\int |\Psi|^2 \, d\tau \right). \tag{11-61}$$

It can be shown that the spin orbitals may, without loss of generality, be taken to be orthonormal, in which case Ψ is normalized. The requirement that $\tilde{E}$ be stationary with respect to variations in the $\{\psi_i\}$ which leave them orthonormal leads to a set of equations

$$\mathscr{F}\psi_i = \sum_j \lambda_{ij}\psi_j, \tag{11-62}$$

where $\mathscr{F}$ is the Fock operator

$$\mathscr{F} = -\tfrac{1}{2}\nabla_i^2 + V(\mathbf{r}_i) + \int' dx_2 \, (1 - P_{12})\gamma(x_2, x_2')(1/r_{12}), \tag{11-63}$$

and the λ_{ij} are Lagrange multipliers associated with the orthonormality constraint. They can, again without loss of generality, be taken in the form $\lambda_{ij} = \varepsilon_i \delta_{ij}$ so that

$$\mathscr{F}\psi_i = \varepsilon_i \psi_i. \tag{11-64}$$

This choice defines the canonical Hartree–Fock spin orbitals and the ε_i are by definition the orbital energies. Equation (11-64) will in principle have an infinite number of solutions. The spin orbitals associated with the N lowest energies are used in the construction of Ψ.

The expression for $\mathscr{F}$ is in atomic units $\hbar = m = e = 1$, and $V(\mathbf{r})$ is the potential at $\mathbf{r}$ due to the nuclei. The one-electron density matrix γ is that associated with the function Ψ. It is

$$\gamma(x_1, x_1') = \sum_{k=1}^{N} \psi_k(x_1)\psi_k^*(x_1'). \tag{11-65}$$

Any unitary transformation of $\psi_1, \ldots, \psi_N$ among themselves will leave both Ψ and γ completely unchanged. The action of $\mathscr{F}$ on ψ_i is in keeping with the "primed integral" notation introduced in the previous chapter:

$$\begin{aligned} \mathscr{F}\psi_i(x_1) &= [-\tfrac{1}{2}\nabla_1^2 + V(\mathbf{r}_1)]\psi_i(x_1) \\ &\quad + \int \frac{\gamma(x_2, x_2)}{r_{12}} dx_2 \, \psi_i(x_1) - \int \frac{\gamma(x_1, x_2)}{r_{12}} \psi_i(x_2) \, dx_2. \end{aligned} \tag{11-66}$$

The next to the last term describes the Coulomb interaction between an electron in orbital i and all other electrons. The last term is an exchange interaction. It is, of course, not physically real but is an artifact of the antisymmetric form of the wave function and the forcing of a one-electronlike description. A self-energy contribution implicit in each of these terms cancels out, since they are identical when $x_1 = x_2$. Since $\mathscr{F}$ depends on the ψ_i's through γ, the equation must be solved iteratively until self-consistency is attained.

The simple form of Eq. (11-64), in which only a single Fock operator occurs, is a consequence of the use of spin orbitals rather than orbitals and separate spin functions and of the fact that no symmetry constraints (other than permutational) have been imposed on Ψ. In fact, except in the case of a totally symmetric singlet state, where at least a relative minimum is found in E for a symmetry-adapted Ψ, the Ψ which optimizes the energy will not be an eigenfunction of the symmetry operators which commute with the Hamiltonian, and the orbitals may not be symmetry adapted.

Let us examine this phenomenon for the particular case of spin symmetry. A general spin orbital can be written

$$\psi_i(x_1) = \phi_i^+(\mathbf{r}_1)\alpha(1) + \phi_i^-(\mathbf{r}_1)\beta(1), \tag{11-67}$$

and the one-electron reduced density matrix can be expressed in terms of the components

$$\gamma^{pq}(\mathbf{r}_1, \mathbf{r}_1') = \sum_{k=1}^{N} \phi_k^p(\mathbf{r}_1)\phi_k^{q*}(\mathbf{r}_1'); \qquad p, q = + \text{ or } - \tag{11-68}$$

as

$$\begin{aligned}\gamma(x_1, x_1') = {} & \gamma^{++}(\mathbf{r}_1, \mathbf{r}_1')\alpha(1)\alpha^*(1') + \gamma^{--}(\mathbf{r}_1, \mathbf{r}_1')\beta(1)\beta^*(1') \\ & + \gamma^{+-}(\mathbf{r}_1, \mathbf{r}_1')\alpha(1)\beta^*(1') + \gamma^{-+}(\mathbf{r}_1, \mathbf{r}_1')\beta(1)\alpha^*(1'). \end{aligned} \tag{11-69}$$

For an eigenstate of $\mathscr{S}_z$, γ^{+-} and γ^{-+} do not appear, but we are as yet making no assumptions about the spin properties of Ψ.

Using the notation defined above and letting $f_1 = -\frac{1}{2}\nabla_1^2 + V(\mathbf{r}_1)$, we can write the effect of the Fock operator on the spin orbital ψ as

$$\begin{aligned}\mathscr{F}\psi_i(x_1) & \\ = {} & \left[f_1 + \int \frac{\{\gamma^{++}(\mathbf{r}_2, \mathbf{r}_2) + \gamma^{--}(\mathbf{r}_2, \mathbf{r}_2)\}}{r_{12}}\, d\mathbf{r}_2\right][\phi_i^+(\mathbf{r}_1)\alpha(1) + \phi_i^-(\mathbf{r}_1)\beta(1)] \\ & - \int \frac{\gamma^{++}(\mathbf{r}_1, \mathbf{r}_2)\phi_i^+(\mathbf{r}_2)}{r_{12}}\, d\mathbf{r}_2\, \alpha(1) - \int \frac{\gamma^{--}(\mathbf{r}_1, \mathbf{r}_2)\phi_i^-(\mathbf{r}_2)}{r_{12}}\, d\mathbf{r}_2\, \beta(1) \\ & - \int \frac{\gamma^{-+}(\mathbf{r}_1, \mathbf{r}_2)}{r_{12}}\, \phi_i^-(\mathbf{r}_2)\, d\mathbf{r}_2\, \alpha(1) - \int \frac{\gamma^{+-}(\mathbf{r}_1, \mathbf{r}_2)\phi_i^+(\mathbf{r}_2)}{r_{12}}\, d\mathbf{r}_2\, \beta(1). \end{aligned} \tag{11-70}$$

Equation (11-64) can then be separated into two coupled equations involving only spatial functions by multiplying it by α or β and integrating over the spin coordinate. The result is

$$\begin{aligned}
f_1\phi_i^+(\mathbf{r}_1) &+ \int \frac{\gamma^0(\mathbf{r}_2, \mathbf{r}_2)}{r_{12}}\, d\mathbf{r}_2\, \phi_i^+(\mathbf{r}) - \int \frac{\gamma^{++}(\mathbf{r}_1, \mathbf{r}_2)\phi_i(\mathbf{r}_2)}{r_{12}}\, d\mathbf{r}_2 \\
&= \varepsilon_i\phi_i^+(\mathbf{r}_1) + \int \frac{\gamma^{-+}(\mathbf{r}_1, \mathbf{r}_2)\phi_i^-(\mathbf{r}_2)}{r_{12}}\, d\mathbf{r}_2 \\
f_1\phi_i^-(\mathbf{r}_1) &+ \int \frac{\gamma^0(\mathbf{r}_2, \mathbf{r}_2)}{r_{12}}\, d\mathbf{r}_2\, \phi_i^-(\mathbf{r}_1) - \int \frac{\gamma^{--}(\mathbf{r}_1, \mathbf{r}_2)\phi_i^-(\mathbf{r}_2)}{r_{12}}\, d\mathbf{r}_2 \\
&= \varepsilon_i\phi_i^-(\mathbf{r}_1) + \int \frac{\gamma^{+-}(\mathbf{r}_1, \mathbf{r}_2)\phi_i^+(\mathbf{r}_2)}{r_{12}}\, d\mathbf{r}_2,
\end{aligned} \tag{11-71}$$

where $\gamma^0 = \gamma^{++} + \gamma^{--}$ as is implied by Eq. (10-29).

If we now require that for each i either $\phi_i^+ \equiv 0$ or $\phi_i^- \equiv 0$ it follows that $\gamma^{+-} \equiv \gamma^{-+} \equiv 0$ and the equations are decoupled. It is convenient to renumber the spin orbitals and introduce new notation so that

$$\psi_i(x_1) = \begin{cases} a_i(\mathbf{r}_1)\alpha(1), & i = 1, \ldots, \mu, \\ b_{i-\mu}(\mathbf{r}_1)\beta(1), & i = \mu + 1, \ldots, \mu + \nu = N \end{cases} \tag{11-72}$$

i.e., the ϕ_i^+ which are not zero are denoted by a_i, $1 \leq i \leq \mu$, and the nonzero ϕ_i^- are denoted by b_i, $1 \leq i \leq \nu$. Then

$$\mathscr{F}^+ a_i = \varepsilon_i^+ a_i, \qquad \mathscr{F}^- b_i = \varepsilon_i^- b_i. \tag{11-73}$$

Each of these equations has in principle an infinite number of solutions, but only the μ a's and ν b's associated with the lowest ε's are used in the construction of Ψ. The two Fock operators are given by

$$\mathscr{F}^p\phi(\mathbf{r}_1) = f_1\phi(\mathbf{r}_1) + \int \frac{\gamma^0(\mathbf{r}_2\mathbf{r}_2)}{r_{12}}\, d\mathbf{r}_2\, \phi(\mathbf{r}_1) - \int \frac{\gamma^{pp}(\mathbf{r}_1\mathbf{r}_2)\phi(\mathbf{r}_2)}{r_{12}}\, d\mathbf{r}_2, \qquad p = + \text{ or } -. \tag{11-74}$$

They will differ unless $\gamma^{++} \equiv \gamma^{--}$, which in turn requires that $\gamma^z \equiv 0$.

The assumption about the form of the ψ_i's is a restriction, and we must expect a higher value for the variational energy that if the ϕ_i's were left general, with both ϕ_i^+ and ϕ_i^- nonzero for any i.

The N-electron wave function will now be denoted by a new symbol, for later convenience. It can be written

$$T_0 = \mathscr{A} a_1 \cdots a_\mu b_1 \cdots b_\nu [\alpha^\mu | \beta^\nu]. \tag{11-75}$$

We have chosen to write the N orbitals first, followed by the N spin functions, and the spin function product is in fact just the t_0 considered previously. If the function is to retain this form, implied by the restriction of Eq. (11-72), our freedom to make unitary transformations of the spin orbitals must be limited to transformations of $a_1, \ldots, a_\mu$ among themselves and separately $b_1, \ldots, b_\nu$ among themselves. If the orbitals are chosen to be eigenfunctions of their respective Fock operators [Eq. (11-73)], then each set will be (or can be taken, in the case of degeneracies) orthonormal within itself, but nothing can be said about the overlap of any a with any b. The spin orbitals $a_i\alpha$ and $b_j\beta$ are of course orthogonal, but the orbitals a_i and b_j may be orthogonal, identical, or anything in between. A different choice of the orbitals is possible [4,110], such that

$$\langle a_i | b_j \rangle = d_i \delta_{ij}, \tag{11-76}$$

where d_i is a real number between 0 and 1. This choice defines the corresponding orbitals.

It is obvious that T_0 is an eigenfunction of $\mathscr{S}_z$ with $M_S = \frac{1}{2}(\mu - \nu)$. The $\mathscr{S}^2$ behavior is not so obvious. Because of the antisymmetrizer, T_0 does not involve just a single spin product. However, $\mathscr{S}^2$ commutes with the antisymmetrizer so we can use Eq. (11-31). In this case it becomes

$$\mathscr{S}^2 T_0 = D_{00} T_0 + D_{01} T_1, \tag{11-77}$$

where

$$T_k = \mathscr{A} a_1 \cdots a_\mu b_1 \cdots b_\nu t_k. \tag{11-78}$$

We will consider two cases, in which T_0 is or is not, respectively, an $\mathscr{S}^2$ eigenfunction.

Restricted Hartree–Fock [169]

Suppose that we are dealing with a state having $M_S \geq 0$ so $\mu \geq \nu$. (The other situation can be dealt with by interchanging the roles of μ, a_i, α and ν, b_i, β, respectively.) We now consider the consequences of requiring that

$$b_i \equiv a_i, \qquad 1 \leq i \leq \nu \tag{11-79}$$

keeping all the a_i orthonormal. This is a further restriction on the variational freedom of the trial wave function and will as we shall see, have certain unfortunate consequences. It does, however, guarantee that T_0 be an eigenfunction of $\mathscr{S}^2$.

To see this we must examine T_1. It is in this case

$$T_1 = \mathscr{A} a_1 \cdots a_\mu b_1 \cdots b_\nu [\alpha^{\mu-1}\beta | \alpha\beta^{\nu-1}] \tag{11-80}$$

in terms of the spin function notation introduced earlier. Consider first a term where, before antisymmetrization, β occurs in position j, $1 \leq j \leq \nu$, and α occurs in position $\mu + j$. These two positions correspond to the same spatial function a_j. A permutation $\hat{P}_{j,j+\mu}$ will turn this term back into T_0 and introduce a factor (-1) when commuted with $\mathscr{A}$. Consider next a term in which, before antisymmetrization, the first β occurs in position $j \leq \mu$ and the last α occurs in position $i \neq j + \mu$. In such a term the spin orbitals for electron $i - \mu$ and i are both $a_{i-\mu}\alpha$, and application of $\mathscr{A}$ will give zero. There are ν terms of the first type and all others are of the second type, so we conclude that

$$T_1 = -\nu T_0, \tag{11-81}$$

and thus that T_0 is an eigenfunction of $\mathscr{S}^2$ with eigenvalue

$$\begin{aligned} S(S+1) = D_{00} - \nu D_{01} &= [\tfrac{1}{4}(\mu - \nu)^2 + \tfrac{1}{2}(\mu + \nu)] - \nu \cdot 1 = M + M^2, \\ S = M &= \tfrac{1}{2}(\mu - \nu) \end{aligned} \tag{11-82}$$

from the values previously obtained for the D's [Eqs. (11-35) and (11-36)].

We recognize that in this case T_0 is the usual spin-restricted Hartree–Fock (RHF) function with ν doubly occupied orbitals and $2S$ singly occupied orbitals all associated with the same spin. In addition to a restriction, however, we have introduced an inconsistency. The orbitals $a_i \equiv b_i$ cannot be eigenfunctions of $\mathscr{F}^+$ and $\mathscr{F}^-$ respectively unless $\mu = \nu$, $S = 0$. In other cases the operators differ: $\mathscr{F}^+$ contains an exchange contribution from $a_{\nu+1}, \ldots, a_\mu$ with no corresponding contribution in $\mathscr{F}^-$, and the eigenfunctions of $\mathscr{F}^+$ will thus be different from those of $\mathscr{F}^-$. In the conventional open shell RHF procedure, this difficulty is avoided (concealed) by an averaging process in the definition of the Fock operators, one for the open shell and one for the closed shell orbitals. We will not consider RHF theory further, however, because of another of its aspects which renders it unsuitable for our purposes.

The spin density matrix associated with the RHF function T_0 is

$$\gamma^z(\mathbf{r}, \mathbf{r}') = \sum_{i=\nu+1}^{\mu} a_i(\mathbf{r}) a_i^*(\mathbf{r}'), \tag{11-83}$$

and the spin density is

$$\rho^z(\mathbf{r}) = \sum_{i=\nu+1}^{\mu} |a_i(\mathbf{r})|^2, \tag{11-84}$$

which is nowhere negative. It is known from experiment and from more refined theories that regions of negative spin density exist and are often necessary to give a satisfactory account of ESR phenomena. We will therefore proceed to a more general type of wave function.

It should be noted, nevertheless, that RHF functions are sometimes of value as a starting point for a configuration interaction (CI) or perturbation calculation. These will be discussed later.

Spin-Polarized Hartree–Fock‡

Let us return to the general form of T_0 of Eq. (11-75) with no further restriction on the orbitals. A consistent set of solutions to the Hartree–Fock equations (11-73) can be obtained, and the spin density is

$$\rho^z(\mathbf{r}) = \sum_{i=1}^{\mu} |a_i(\mathbf{r})|^2 - \sum_{j=1}^{\nu} |b_j(\mathbf{r})|^2, \tag{11-85}$$

which can be negative in any region where the b contribution dominates the a contribution.

The problem in this case is that T_1 will include terms involving spin orbitals $a_i\beta$ and $b_j\alpha$ which do not occur in T_0, so Eq. (11-77) shows that T_0 is not an $\mathscr{S}^2$ eigenfunction. Let us follow historical precedent and ignore this problem for the present. The function T_0 is in this case of a form referred to variously as spin-polarized Hartree–Fock (SPHF), (spin) unrestricted Hartree–Fock (UHF), or different orbitals for different spins (DODS). Functions of this type have been extensively used in the calculation of spin properties.

An important concept for the discussion of spin densities has its origin in the difference between SPHF and RHF. We think of starting with a RHF description of a system and then removing the restriction that $a_i \equiv b_i$ for $1 \leq i \leq \nu$. The differing interaction of these orbitals (via the exchange terms in the Fock operators) with the singly occupied orbitals will cause them to become slightly different, or polarized, thereby lowering the total energy. The spin density can then be divided into two parts,

$$\rho^z(\mathbf{r}) = \rho^z_{\text{direct}}(\mathbf{r}) + \rho^z_{\text{spin polarization}}(\mathbf{r}), \tag{11-86}$$

where the direct contribution arises from the singly occupied orbital(s)

$$\rho^z_{\text{direct}}(\mathbf{r}) = \sum_{j=\nu+1}^{\mu} |a_j(\mathbf{r})|^2 \tag{11-87}$$

and is nowhere negative. The spin polarization contribution arises from the "polarized" orbitals

$$\rho^z_{\text{spin polarization}}(\mathbf{r}) = \sum_{i=1}^{\nu} |a_i(\mathbf{r})|^2 - \sum_{i=1}^{\nu} |b_i(\mathbf{r})|^2. \tag{11-88}$$

‡ See, e.g., Refs. [108,161]; also references given for Li atom calculations (Table 11-6).

This contribution can be of either sign. If corresponding orbitals are used [cf. Eq. (11-76)], it is usually found that each d_i is nearly 1 so that a_i and b_i are not "very different." The spin polarization contribution is thus small in magnitude, and it will be qualitatively significant only in regions where the direct contribution is small or zero.

The utility of the spin polarization concept can be extended by redefining it in density matrix terms. We will then be able to apply a very similar definition to non-Hartree–Fock functions. The spin density matrix corresponding to the SPHF function T_0 is

$$\gamma^z(\mathbf{r}, \mathbf{r}') = \sum_{i=1}^{\mu} a_i(\mathbf{r})a_i^*(\mathbf{r}') - \sum_{j=1}^{\nu} b_j(\mathbf{r})b_j^*(\mathbf{r}'). \tag{11-89}$$

It is equivalent to a matrix in some discrete basis, or can be considered as the kernel of an integral operator. Either way, a set of eigenvalues λ_k^z and orthonormal eigenfunctions ϕ_k^z can be found. The set of ϕ_k^z associated with nonzero eigenvalues can be expressed as linear combinations of $a_1, \ldots, a_\mu, b_1, \ldots, b_\nu$ and vice vera. Some care must be exercised, however, because the combined a, b set of orbitals is not orthogonal.

The eigenvalues of the spin density matrix for a spin polarized Hartree–Fock function follow a rather simple pattern [73]. A set of $2M_S = \mu - \nu$ of them are precisely 1. The remainder occur in pairs of equal magnitude and opposite sign. The magnitudes of these paired eigenvalues are found to be small. As the wave function is improved, going beyond the HF level, it remains true that the spin density matrix will have $2M_S$ eigenvalues near 1 and the remainder all small in magnitude. The contribution to the spin density associated with the former is the "direct" contribution, and that associated with the latter is the "spin polarization" contribution. Since some of the eigenvalues are negative, the spin density can be negative in any region where the contribution associated with these eigenvalues is dominant.

Relationship between Spin and Charge Densities

One of the problems associated with the calculation of spin properties is that the Hamiltonian $\mathscr{H}_0$ contains no spin-dependent interactions. It includes one- and two-electron terms so the energy is entirely determined by the two-electron charge density matrix. This also determines the one-electron charge density matrix, but does not in any known way in general determine the spin density matrix or the other components of the two-electron density matrix. It is thus possible in principle to have two wave functions leading to quite different spin densities but corresponding to the same energy and thus equally good by the usual energy variational criterion. (This does not refer to the trivial case of different M_S values, but to a more subtle degeneracy.) In practical calculations this problem does not seem to arise; the ground state is not degenerate except as required by symmetry, and any reasonable variational calculation will reflect this and determine a unique spin density distribution.

In the case of SPHF (or RHF) functions, the spin density and all other properties which can be determined from the wave function can in fact be determined from the one-electron charge density matrix. Proofs are rather lengthy, so only the results will be presented here [73,107,122]. The charge density matrix for an N-electron SPHF function will in general have N nonzero eigenvalues, although in special cases there may be fewer. None are negative and if they are arranged in nonincreasing order they are found to be of the form

$$\begin{aligned} \lambda_i^0 &= 1 + d_i, & i &= i, \ldots, \nu; \\ \lambda_j^0 &= 1, & j &= \nu + 1, \ldots, \mu; \\ \lambda_{\bar{i}}^0 &= 1 - d_i, & \bar{i} &= N - i + 1. \end{aligned} \tag{11-90}$$

The d_i are just the corresponding orbital overlaps of Eq. (11-76), and are normally found to be close to 1. The corresponding orbitals themselves, in terms of which the wave function is given by Eq. (11-75), are related to the natural orbitals (NO's, i.e., the charge density eigenfunctions ϕ_k^0) by

$$a_i = \cos \chi_i\, \phi_i^0 + \sin \chi_i\, \phi_{\bar{i}}^0, \qquad b_i = \cos \chi_i\, \phi_i^0 - \sin \chi_i\, \phi_{\bar{i}}^0, \qquad i = 1, \ldots, \nu;$$
$$a_j = \phi_j^0, \qquad j = \nu + 1, \ldots, \mu; \tag{11-91}$$

where

$$\cos 2\chi_i = d_i = \tfrac{1}{2}(\lambda^0 - \lambda_{\bar{i}}^0). \tag{11-92}$$

If the wave function were expressed in terms of the orthogonal set $\{\phi_k^0\}$ it would be found to have ν orbitals almost doubly occupied, $2M_S = \mu - \nu$ singly occupied orbitals, and ν orbitals only slightly occupied in a configuration interaction expansion.

The spin density eigenvalues and eigenfunctions are simply related to the NO's and the d_i as well. They are

$$\lambda_i^z = -\lambda_{\bar{i}}^z = e_i = \sqrt{1 - d_i^2} = \sin 2\chi_i, \qquad \lambda_j = 1, \tag{11-93}$$

and

$$\phi_i^z = \frac{1}{\sqrt{2}}(\phi_i^0 + \phi_{\bar{i}}^0), \qquad \phi_{\bar{i}}^z = \frac{1}{\sqrt{2}}(\phi_i^0 - \phi_{\bar{i}}^0), \qquad \phi_j^z = \phi_j^0, \tag{11-94}$$

where i, $\bar{i}$, and j have the same ranges as in Eqs. (11-91). The various components of the two-electron density matrix can also be expressed in terms of the ϕ_k^0 and d_i.‡ Rather than considering these results here, let us look at a relationship among the density matrix components themselves.

It is true generally for functions of HF type that the wave function and all density matrix components are determined by the one-electron density matrix [107,122]. In particular

$$\Gamma(x_1, x_2; x_1', x_2') = \tfrac{1}{2}[\gamma(x_1; x_1')\gamma(x_2; x_2') - \gamma(x_1; x_2')\gamma(x_2; x_1')]. \quad (11\text{-}95)$$

If we insert the form of γ for an $\mathscr{S}_z$ eigenfunction

$$\gamma(x_1; x_1') = \tfrac{1}{2}[\gamma^0(\mathbf{r}_1; \mathbf{r}_1') + \gamma^z(\mathbf{r}_1, \mathbf{r}_1')]\alpha(1)\alpha^*(1') + \tfrac{1}{2}[\gamma^0(\mathbf{r}_1; \mathbf{r}_1') - \gamma^z(\mathbf{r}_1; \mathbf{r}_1')]\beta(1)\beta^*(1') \quad (11\text{-}96)$$

and separate spin components [126] of Γ we obtain

$$\Gamma^0(\mathbf{r}_1, \mathbf{r}_2; \mathbf{r}_1', \mathbf{r}_2') = \tfrac{1}{4}[2\gamma^0(\mathbf{r}_1; \mathbf{r}_1')\gamma^0(\mathbf{r}_2; \mathbf{r}_2') - \gamma^0(\mathbf{r}_1, \mathbf{r}_2')\gamma^0(\mathbf{r}_2; \mathbf{r}_1') - \gamma^z(\mathbf{r}_1; \mathbf{r}_2')\gamma^z(\mathbf{r}_2; \mathbf{r}_1')]. \quad (11\text{-}97)$$

We recognize the usual closed shell RHF "twice Coulomb minus exchange" form, with an additional correction term depending on the spin density. The other components of Γ are

$$\Gamma^z(\mathbf{r}_1, \mathbf{r}_2; \mathbf{r}_1', \mathbf{r}_2') = \tfrac{1}{4}[2\gamma^z(\mathbf{r}_1; \mathbf{r}_1')\gamma^0(\mathbf{r}_2; \mathbf{r}_2') - \gamma^z(\mathbf{r}_1; \mathbf{r}_2')\gamma^0(\mathbf{r}_2; \mathbf{r}_1') - \gamma^z(\mathbf{r}_2; \mathbf{r}_1')\gamma^0(\mathbf{r}_1; \mathbf{r}_2')], \quad (11\text{-}98)$$

which is reasonable for the conditional spin density with an exchange correction, and

$$\Gamma^{SS}(\mathbf{r}_1, \mathbf{r}_2; \mathbf{r}_1', \mathbf{r}_2') = \tfrac{1}{4}[\gamma^z(\mathbf{r}_1; \mathbf{r}_1')\gamma^z(\mathbf{r}_2; \mathbf{r}_2') - \gamma^z(\mathbf{r}_1, \mathbf{r}_2')\gamma^z(\mathbf{r}_2; \mathbf{r}_1')], \quad (11\text{-}99)$$

which involves only the spin density matrix.

We have seen that a SPHF wave function gives a qualitatively reasonable description of the spin properties of a system. Such functions are also reasonably easy to obtain within the limits of any fixed basis set (to be discussed later). In fact, SPHF functions are obtained as easily as or more easily than RHF functions for open shell systems. Within the general framework of the HF approximation, then, they would be quite satisfactory were they $\mathscr{S}^2$ eigenfunctions. For the simple calculation of spin distributions, this objection may be more aesthetic than practical. For more complicated properties, like spin–spin coupling, it is probably quite significant. We will return to this point after a discussion of what can be done to obtain $\mathscr{S}^2$ eigenfunctions within the general framework of DODS Hartree–Fock theory.

‡ These results are given by Hardisson and Harriman [72] and Sando and Harriman [181]. The coefficient of the two-electron charge density component $itt\bar{i}$ before projection is given in these references as having a coefficient 0, which should be $\frac{1}{2}$. See also Phillips and Schug [157].

Spin-Projected Hartree–Fock [73]

The spin projection technique discussed earlier can be used to obtain an $\mathscr{S}^2$ eigenfunction from a DODS single-determinant function

$$\Psi_S = \omega_S^{-1/2} \mathscr{O}_S T_0 = \omega_S^{-1/2} \sum_{k=0}^{\nu} C_k(S, M, n) T_k, \tag{11-100}$$

where

$$\omega_S = \langle \mathscr{O}_S T_0 | \mathscr{O}_S T_0 \rangle = \langle T_0 | \mathscr{O}_S T_0 \rangle \tag{11-101}$$

is a normalization constant and the C_k are the Sanibel coefficients discussed earlier. The normalization constant and density matrix components corresponding to Ψ_S can be expressed in a reasonably straightforward way. Again, only the results will be presented here.

We begin by defining some symmetric functions A_k of the parameters d_i

$$\prod_{i=1}^{\nu} (1 + d_i^2 x) = \sum_{k=0}^{\nu} A_k x^k \tag{11-102}$$

or equivalently

$$A_k = \sum_{\substack{\text{all choices of} \\ k \text{ distinct } i\text{'s}}} \prod_{k \text{ factors}} d_i^2. \tag{11-103}$$

Then

$$\omega_S = \sum_{k=0}^{\nu} (-1)^k C_k(S, M, n) A_k. \tag{11-104}$$

We can define in a similar way functions $A_k(i)$

$$\prod_{i'=1\,(i' \neq i)}^{\nu} (1 + d_{i'}^2 x) = \sum_{k=0}^{\nu-1} A_k(i) x^k. \tag{11-105}$$

The $A_k(i)$ are the equivalent of the A_k defined on a set of $\nu - 1$ d's excluding d_i. The quantity corresponding to ω_S is

$$\omega_S(i) = \sum_{k=0}^{\nu-1} (-1)^k C_k(S, M, n-1) A_k(i). \tag{11-106}$$

It is the normalization constant for the function projected from an $N - 2$ electron function in which the corresponding orbitals a_i and b_i do not appear.

The eigenfunctions of the charge density matrix (NO's) and those of the spin density matrix are the same, respectively, after projection as before. The eigenvalues are changed. For the charge density they are

$$\begin{aligned} \xi_i^0 &= 1 + \frac{\omega_S(i)}{\omega_S} d_i, \qquad 1 \leq i \leq \nu, \\ \xi_j^0 &= 1, \qquad \nu + 1 \leq j \leq \mu, \qquad (11\text{-}107) \\ \xi_{\bar{i}}^0 &= 1 - \frac{\omega_S(i)}{\omega_S} d_i, \qquad \bar{i} = N - i + 1. \end{aligned}$$

They still have the property that $\xi_i^0 + \xi_{\bar{i}}^0 = \lambda_i^0 + \lambda_{\bar{i}}^0 = 2$, $\xi_j^0 = \lambda_j^0 = 1$. It is found that $\omega_S(i)/\omega_S \geq 1$, but $d_i \omega_S(i)/\omega_S \leq 1$, so the eigenvalues lie between 0 and 2, as they must. The expressions for the projected-state spin density eigenvalues are somewhat complicated in general, but are reasonably simple in the principal case $M_S = S$. In that case they can be written

$$\begin{aligned} \xi_i^z &= \frac{S}{S+1}\left[\frac{\omega_S(i)}{\omega_S} e_i + \delta_i\right], \qquad \xi_{\bar{i}}^z = \frac{S}{S+1}\left[-\frac{\omega_S(i)}{\omega_S} e_i + \delta_i\right], \\ \xi_j^z &= 1 - \frac{1}{S+1}\sum_{i=1}^{\nu} \delta_i, \qquad (11\text{-}108) \end{aligned}$$

where

$$\delta_i = \frac{\omega_S(i)}{\omega_S} - 1. \qquad (11\text{-}109)$$

Because of the δ_i's these eigenvalues do not occur as pairs of equal magnitude but opposite sign as do the corresponding eigenvalues for the unprojected state. If the δ_i are small, so that $\omega_S(i)/\omega_S \sim 1$, the principal effect of projection on the spin density will be to reduce the spin polarization contribution by a factor $S/(S+1)$, which is $\frac{1}{3}$ for a doublet and $\frac{1}{2}$ for a triplet.

In the principal case [cf. Eq. (11-28)] ω_S and $\omega_S(i)$ can be conveniently expressed in terms of the e_i rather than the d_i. With B_k and $B_k(i)$ defined analogously to A_k and $A_k(i)$ but with e_i replacing d_i,

$$\prod_{i=1}^{\nu}(1 + e_i^2 x) = \sum_{k=0}^{\nu} B_k x^k, \qquad \prod_{i'=1\,(i' \neq i)}^{\nu}(1 + e_{i'}^2 x) = \sum_{k=0}^{\nu-1} B_k(i) x^k, \quad (11\text{-}110)$$

these expressions are

$$\begin{aligned} \omega_S &= \sum_{k=0}^{\nu} (-1)^k \binom{2S+k+1}{k}^{-1} B_k, \\ \omega_S(i) &= \sum_{k=0}^{\nu-1} (-1)^k \binom{2S+k+1}{k}^{-1} B_k(i). \end{aligned} \qquad (11\text{-}111)$$

This form is convenient because in practice $e_i \ll 1$ and expansions converge rapidly. To lowest order

$$\frac{\omega_S(i)}{\omega_S} = 1 + \frac{1}{2(S+1)} e_i^2 + \cdots, \tag{11-112}$$

and δ_i is thus of order e_i^2.

As in Eq. (11-21), T_0 can be expanded in terms of the $\mathscr{S}^2$ eigenfunction components it contains

$$T_0 = \sum_{S=M_S}^{N/2} \omega_S^{1/2} \Psi_S. \tag{11-113}$$

It is found that for normal SPHF functions the principal component with $S = M_S$ is dominant and the next component, with $S = M_S + 1$, is smaller but still significant while components with $S > M_S + 1$ are frequently almost negligible. This explains the success of the single annihilation method developed by Amos, Hall, and Snyder [4,5,194]. This is an approximate projection in which $\mathscr{O}_S$ is replaced by

$$\mathscr{A}_{M+1} = \frac{\mathscr{S}^2 - (M+1)(M+2)}{M(M+1) - (M+1)(M+2)}. \tag{11-114}$$

The function $\mathscr{A}_{M+1} T_0$ is not an $\mathscr{S}^2$ eigenfunction but is nearly so with $S = M$. The spin density matrix after single annihilation (aa) is expressed in terms of $\mathbf{P} = \gamma^{++} = \frac{1}{2}(\gamma^0 + \gamma^z)$ and $\mathbf{Q} = \gamma^{--} = \frac{1}{2}(\gamma^0 - \gamma^z)$ before annihilation as

$$\begin{aligned} \gamma_{\text{aa}}^2 = {} & C_1(\mathbf{P} - \mathbf{Q}) + \mathbf{C}_2\mathbf{P} + C_3\mathbf{Q} + C_4(\mathbf{QP} + \mathbf{PQ}) \\ & + C_5(\mathbf{PQP} - \mathbf{QPQ}) + C_6(\mathbf{PQPQP} - \mathbf{QPQPQ}), \end{aligned} \tag{11-115}$$

where the expansion coefficients are

$$\begin{gathered} C_1 = [A^2 + \mu\nu - (2A + N - 4) \operatorname{tr} \mathbf{PQ} + 2(\operatorname{tr} \mathbf{PQ})^2 - 2 \operatorname{tr} \mathbf{PQPQ}]C_0, \\ C_2 = -2\nu C_0, \qquad C_3 = 2\mu C_0, \qquad C_4 = -SC_0, \\ C_5 = (2A + N - 4 - \operatorname{tr} \mathbf{PQ})C_0, \qquad C_6 = 4C_0, \\ \mu = \operatorname{tr} \mathbf{P}, \qquad \nu = \operatorname{tr} \mathbf{Q}, \qquad N = \mu + \nu, \\ A = \nu - 2(S+1), \\ C_0 = [A^2 + \mu\nu - (2A + N - 2) \operatorname{tr} \mathbf{PQ} + 2(\operatorname{tr} \mathbf{PQ})^2 - 2 \operatorname{tr} \mathbf{PQPQ}]^{-1}. \end{gathered} \tag{11-116}$$

It can be shown that the spin density after single annihilation agrees with the fully projected spin density through order e_i^2 [75].

Given a SPHF function, either single annihilation or full projection is readily carried out. It is not clear, however, that this should be done. In order to obtain an $\mathscr{S}^2$ eigenfunction we have made a sacrifice. The projected function is no longer a variational minimum for functions of its type. As a consequence it no longer has the desirable features of variationally optimized functions. What should be done is to take a function of the form of Ψ_S but with the orbitals a_k and b_l, or equivalently the NO's ϕ_k^0 and the parameters d_i or e_i, chosen so as to minimize the energy after projection. This possibility will be examined shortly. Such a function will be referred to here as spin-extended Hartree-Fock (SEHF).

Prior to the attainment of SEHF functions, it was argued that the spin density of a SPHF function would be closer to the SEHF result than would a projected but not reoptimized result [130]. These arguments were lent credibility by the quite good agreement between the SPHF and *experimental* values for the Fermi contact term in the Li atom. (A large number of calculations for atomic Li will be considered later in this section. See especially Table 11-6.) When the SEHF result was obtained, it was found to be farther from the experimental value than was the SPHF result. In other systems, projected SPHF is sometimes better and sometimes worse than the corresponding unprojected result. It is clear that the agreement between SPHF and experiment in atomic Li is fortuitous.

Spin-Extended Hartree–Fock

As was remarked earlier, another possible treatment is to take a wave function of spin-projected single determinant form and use it in a variational calculation with optimization after projection. Energy expressions are available which make such SEHF calculations possible, but not easy.

One approach is to consider variations in the orbital parts of the Hartree–Fock spin orbitals [62,91]. The result is a set of coupled equations of HF-like form. They cannot be uncoupled and complications arise from the nonorthogonal nature of the orbitals, but in at least some cases they can be solved. An alternative approach based on a density matrix analysis yields an energy expression in terms of the orthogonal NO's and the d_i or e_i parameters [76,181]. A direct minimization of the energy is then sought in the parameter space of the e_i and parameters characterizing the NO's. This is difficult because of the highly nonlinear dependencies involved. Both methods have yielded results, but it appears in retrospect that comparable computational effort would have yielded better results if applied to more general configuration interaction or optimized multiconfiguration calculations, which will be discussed later in this section.

Insofar as a formal analysis is concerned, apart from particular choice of orbitals or parameter values, SEHF functions and density matrices are indistinguishable from those for the SPHF case already considered.

Spin-Optimized Hartree–Fock

One further generalization is possible without abandoning the general Hartree–Fock framework of a function involving at most N orbitals for N electrons. Let $\eta_1(\mathbf{r}), \ldots, \eta_N(\mathbf{r})$ be a set of nonorthogonal orbitals which may even be linearly dependent, and let $\Theta_1, \ldots, \Theta_f$ be a complete set of N-electron S, M eigenfunctions. An N-electron wave function can be constructed as

$$\Psi_{\text{SOHF}} = \mathscr{A}\left[\eta_1(\mathbf{r}_1)\cdots\eta_N(\mathbf{r}_N)\sum_{k=1}^{f} C_k\Theta_k(1, \ldots, N)\right], \qquad (11\text{-}117)$$

and in principle the orbitals and the coefficients can be chosen so as to minimize the energy associated with this function, subject to the constraint that it remain normalized. The result is a spin-optimized Hartree–Fock (SOHF) function [92]. It differs from SEFH by allowing adjustments in the spin coupling scheme. The particular choice of spin coupling in SEHF, as a projected single spin product, will not in general be the optimum choice.

The SOHF method can be formulated in various ways, depending on how the spin functions are obtained and on how energy minimization is carried out. Some calculations of this type have been reported. A density matrix analysis and formulation in terms of orthogonal oribitals (e.g., NO's) has not been reported. Such an analysis can be related to a valence bond approach, and will be briefly discussed in that context later.

Basis Set Considerations

The Hartree–Fock equations which arise in the types of calculations we have been considering were presented as partial differential equations. In practice, in nearly all molecular calculations and many atomic calculations, they are converted to matrix equations. In this Hartree–Fock–Roothaan procedure [168,169], a finite set of basis functions $\{\chi_t\}$ is introduced and the orbitals being sought are expressed as linear combinations of the basis functions

$$\phi_j = \sum_t C_{jt}\chi_t. \qquad (11\text{-}118)$$

The expansion coefficients are treated as variational parameters with the result that Eqs. (11-73), for example, are replaced by

$$\mathbf{F}^{\pm}\mathbf{C}_j^{\pm} = \varepsilon_j^{\pm}\mathbf{S}\mathbf{C}_j^{\pm}, \qquad (11\text{-}119)$$

where **S** is the overlap matrix of the basis orbitals. (It is absent, i.e., a unit matrix, if an orthonormal basis is used.) A significant part of the effort in a calculation is that devoted to the evaluation of integrals involving functions of the basis set and operators from the Hamiltonian. A discussion of the evaluation of such integrals is beyond the scope of this book.[‡] If a complete basis set were used, no further approximation would be introduced by this procedure. In practice the size of the basis set is necessarily finite and sometimes quite small. The quality of the results may thus depend critically on the choice of the basis functions used.

In atomic calculations this problem can be eliminated within the framework of the central field approximation. The HF orbitals are required to be of the form

$$\phi_{nlm}(\mathbf{r}) = R_{nl}(\mathbf{r})Y_l^m(\theta, \phi). \tag{11-120}$$

The orbital index j is replaced by a composite index nlm, where l and m are quantum numbers associated with the (one-electron) orbital angular momentum. It is assumed that the radial part of the orbital is the same for all $2l + 1$ functions associated with a given n and l. This restriction is comparable in spirit to that of Eq. (11-72) and has similar consequences. A consistent theory results for orbitally closed shell (S-state) atoms but must be forced by a spherical averaging of the Fock operator for open shell states. Angular momentum theory can then be used to eliminate all θ and ϕ dependence, leaving "HF" equations for the radial functions. These are now ordinary differential equations which can be dealt with numerically. The radial functions R_{nl} and the potential terms in the Fock operator are given in numerical (tabular) form, and it is not necessary to introduce basis functions. It is of course possible to express the R_{nl} in terms of basis functions and proceed via matrix calculations.

The results of numerical HF and Hartree–Fock–Roothaan (basis set) calculations can be compared for atoms in either restricted or spin-polarized formulations (cf., e.g., Ref. [8]). It is found that insofar as energies are concerned it is not difficult to systematically select basis sets so as to give results equivalent to those obtained numerically. Spin properties, especially the spin density at the nucleus, are much more sensitive to basis set choice. It is in fact possible to use two different basis sets which yield essentially equivalent results for the energy, but quite different spin densities.

With the exception of some diatomic molecules, where basis functions can conveniently be expressed in terms of elliptic coordinates, basis sets are nearly always taken to consist of "atomic orbitals" (AO's) of the form given

‡ Specific integrals not appearing in the zero-order calculation but required for the evaluation of spin Hamiltonian parameters will be discussed in Section 12.

by Eq. (11-20), centered at various points in the system. The radial functions involve either exponentials, leading to Slater-type orbitals (STO's)

$$\chi^{\mu}_{nlm}(\mathbf{r}_i) = C r_{i\mu}^{n-1} e^{-\zeta r_{i\mu}} Y_l^m(\theta_{i\mu}, \phi_{i\mu}) \tag{11-121}$$

or Gaussians, leading to Gaussian orbitals (GO's)

$$\chi^{\mu}_{nlm}(\mathbf{r}_i) = C r_{i\mu}^{n-1} e^{-\gamma r_{i\mu}^2} Y_l^m(\theta_{i\mu}, \phi_{i\mu}) \tag{11-122}$$

The index μ identifies the origin of the coordinate system with respect to which r, θ, and ϕ are defined and C is a normalization constant which is frequently omitted. In the case of Gaussian orbitals the alternative choice of Cartesian coordinates is sometimes made, with

$$\chi^{\mu}_{n_x n_y n_z}(\mathbf{r}_i) = C x_{i\mu}^{n_x} e^{-\gamma_x x_{i\mu}^2} y_{i\mu}^{n_y} e^{-\gamma_y y_{i\mu}^2} z_{i\mu}^{n_z} e^{-\gamma_z z_{i\mu}^2}. \tag{11-123}$$

Fixed linear combinations of GO's, or sometimes of STO's, are also used as basis functions. Most commonly it is combinations of GO's approximating an STO which are chosen.

Exponential STO's are "better" than GO's in the sense that a given variational energy can be attained with a smaller basis set if well chosen STO's are used. On the other hand, integrals involving GO's are much more easily evaluated than those involving STO's. Of course the exact hydrogenic atomic orbitals can be expressed as finite linear combinations of STO's or even a single STO. Gaussian orbitals are at their worst in describing the long-range behavior of electronic wave functions and their behavior in the immediate vicinity of nuclei. It is the latter we are particularly interested in.

As an indication of what can be expected it is instructive to consider a Gaussian approximation to the 1s ground state wave function for the hydrogen atom,

$$\psi_{1s} = (1/2\pi)^{3/2} e^{-r} \simeq \sum_{k=1}^{N} C_k e^{-\gamma_k r^2} = \psi_N. \tag{11-124}$$

For each value of N the coefficients C_k and parameters γ_k can be chosen so as to best approximate ψ_{1s} [203]. The errors in the energy and in the spin density at the nucleus, $|\psi_{1s}(0)|^2$, are shown in Table 11-2. It is clear that a good energy is much easier to obtain than a good spin density.

It is not clear at present how a "good" basis set is to be chosen. The smallest basis set which can be expected to given fairly good energies and molecular geometries is an STO set of the type referred to as "double zeta plus polarization." A minimal basis includes one STO with well chosen parameter ζ for each orbital which would be occupied (doubly or singly) in a HF description of the atoms in the system, plus enough STO's to complete any partially filled l subshell on each atom but not including orbitals which

TABLE 11-2

Energies and Spin Densities for Gaussian Approximations to H Atom Ground State[a]

N	$-E_N$	$\lvert\psi_N(0)\rvert^2$	$\frac{\Delta E}{E} \times 100\%$	$\frac{\Delta\lvert\psi\rvert^2}{\lvert\psi\rvert^2} \times 100\%$
4	0.499277	0.269285	0.145	−15.40
5	0.499805	0.285393	0.039	−10.34
6	0.499936	0.294501	0.013	−7.48
7	0.499968	0.300657	0.006	−5.55
8	0.499976	0.301169	0.005	−5.38
9	0.499979	0.300092	0.005	−5.72
9[b]	0.499999	0.315653	0.000	−0.83
Exact	0.500000	0.318309		

[a] From Tortorelli and Harriman [203].
[b] Three of the γ_k were set initially to large values.

cannot contribute because of symmetry. A double zeta basis uses two STO's with well chosen, different ζ values for each STO of a minimal basis, and for molecules polarization functions are added by including one each of those orbitals of the next higher l value on each atom which can by symmetry be involved in the expansion of occupied molecular orbitals. Consider for example the methyl radical. A minimal basis consists of 1s STO's on each H and 1s, 2s, and three 2p STO's on C. A double zeta plus polarization basis consists of two 1s STO's and a 2p STO (directed toward C) on each H, and two 1s, two 2s, six 2p, and three 3d orbitals on C. Larger basis sets are required to give energies to within experimental accuracy, and still larger basis sets are required to give good spin densities at the nuclei. Compact functions, concentrated near the nuclei, must be included.

A common although not universal usage refers to the HF–Roothaan result within a fixed, finite basis as a self-consistent (SCF) result, while the term HF is reserved for those cases where the basis set is effectively complete—i.e., it is sufficiently large and flexible that no practical advantage can be gained by expanding it. Differences between SCF and HF results, in this sense, are sometimes referred to as expansion error. They are not inherent in the HF method itself.

The results of an SCF calculation with a given number of basis functions can be improved, sometimes dramatically, by optimizing not only the expansion coefficients but also the nonlinear parameters occurring in the basis functions. This optimization should be carried out for the specific system of interest, but this is an extremely time consuming and expensive process for molecular calculations. It is common to use basis functions which have been optimized in atomic calculations without further optimization in molecular calculations. As the size of the basis set increases for a given number of electrons, the importance of optimizing the individual basis functions decreases.

Configuration Interaction Functions

The differences between HF results and exact (nonrelativistic, Born–Oppenheimer) results are known as correlation errors. The term arises from the fact that the behaviors of the various electrons are in fact correlated, while HF theory treats only the influence on any electron of the average behavior of the other electrons. The most common way of improving on HF results is by the introduction of configuration interaction. A configuration interaction (CI) wave function is a linear combination of N-electron functions

$$\Psi(1, \ldots, N) = \sum_K C_K \Phi_K(1, \ldots, N). \tag{11-125}$$

The coefficients C_K are variational parameters. The configurations Φ_K are either single determinants or linear combinations of small numbers of determinants with fixed relative coefficients chosen to provide the appropriate symmetry. That is, each Φ_K has the same symmetry as Ψ.

A complete CI calculation is one in which all possible configurations are included. If R basis functions are available, there are $2R$ spin orbitals and $\binom{2R}{N}$ possible independent, antisymmetric N-electron functions. Symmetry reduces the number which need be considered. If Ψ is an $\mathscr{S}_z$ eigenfunction with quantum number M_S, each determinant to be included in the wave function must contain $\mu = N/2 + M_S$ α spin–spin orbitals and $\nu = N/2 - M_S$ β spin–spin orbitals. The maximum number of configurations would then be $\binom{R}{\mu}\binom{R}{\nu}$, and the actual number is further reduced by $\mathscr{S}^2$ and point group symmetry. Nevertheless, unless the number of electrons is very small or the basis set severely restricted and the number of electrons moderate, a complete CI calculation is not a practical possibility. In a complete CI calculation the result is independent of any symmetry preserving unitary transformation of the set of orbitals used, since this can be offset by a change in the CI coefficients. When the CI expansion is less than complete the choice of configurations to be included and of the orbitals from which they are constructed become critical.

In most CI calculations, the basis orbitals are orthonormal, so that the configurations are orthogonal and can be easily normalized. Valence bond functions, which are of the same form given by Eq. (11-125), are normally constructed from nonorthogonal orbitals and the N-electron functions are then also nonorthogonal. They will be considered very briefly later. A CI calculation requires the construction of the matrix of the Hamiltonian $\mathscr{H}_0$ with respect to the configurations, and the determination of at least its lowest eigenvalue and eigenvector. The construction of the Hamiltonian matrix from integrals involving one- or two-electron operators and basis functions is a major part of the computational effort in a CI calculation. Essentially the same process is required for this as for the determination of the density matrix from the CI function, which will be discussed below.

In a CI calculation one normally starts with the HF function, since it is by definition the best single configuration. Although the RHF function is of higher energy that a SPHF or otherwise unrestricted function, it is convenient to use the RHF function as a starting point because it is symmetry adapted while the others are not. Other configurations and the orbitals from which they are constructed should be chosen to maximize the quality of the result while minimizing the number of configurations required. This remains something of an art. Various choices have been used, but criteria have often been such that spin densities and other properties of interest to us are not necessarily optimal.

It is frequently useful to define a reference configuration, most often although not necessarily the HF function, and categorize other configurations relative to it. A singly excited configuration is one which differs from the reference configuration in only one spin orbital.[‡] A doubly excited configuration differs in two spin orbitals, etc. In a very rough sense, the more highly excited a configuration is with respect to the HF configuration, the smaller will be its coefficient in the CI expansion. Brillouin's theorem shows that matrix elements between the HF determinant and any singly excited determinant is zero. The use of "determinant" rather than "configuration" is deliberate. The theorem applies only to unrestricted HF. Perturbation theory then suggests that singly excited determinants will appear only in "higher order" so their coefficients will be small. On the basis of these considerations, one common limited CI approach includes HF plus all doubly excited configurations. This is not a useful approximation for open-shell systems starting from RHF, and a SPHF starting point leads to spin symmetry problems, so both single and double excitations from RHF are usually included for open-shell systems.

An alternative approach is based on a useful property of the natural spin orbitals (NSO's). If the wave function were known, the NSO's could be determined. It can be shown that a CI expansion in which the configurations are built up from NSO's (the "natural expansion") will have certain optimal properties [44,106]. The lack of knowledge, initially, of the wave function

[‡] To avoid ambiguity, this spin orbital must be orthogonal to all the spin orbitals occupied in the reference configuration.

need not prohibit the use of this approach. In the iterative natural orbital method,‡ approximate NSO's are obtained from a reasonable but fairly small CI wave function. They are used in a new CI calculation and better approximate NSO's obtained. The cycle is repeated until convergence is attained to the required accuracy. Perturbation-theoretic estimates of the CI expansion coefficients can be used to select the configurations to be included. Open-shell systems also provide problems for this approach, since determinants made up of NSO's will not be symmetry adapted [18]. To avoid the loss of the advantages associated with symmetry, the NSO's can be replaced by NO's.§ The price is the loss of the most optimal convergence, but the NO's still provide a very good basis.

When a transformation is made from one orbital basis to another, considerable computing time must be devoted to the transformation of integrals. Convergence advantages may be more than offset by this requirement.

Just as spin properties are more sensitive to the choice of AO basis functions than is energy, so too the selection of configurations required to give good spin properties is more critical than that required for good energies. The severity of the requirements for the choice of configurations will to some extent be alleviated if sufficient flexibility is allowed in the choice of spin coupling schemes.¶

We wish to construct configurations which are $\mathscr{S}^2$, $\mathscr{S}_z$ eigenfunctions. (Other symmetries will not be considered explicitly.) We therefore take configurations of the type

$$\Phi_{KLj} = \mathscr{A}\Upsilon_{KL}\Theta_j^{[\kappa,\lambda]}, \tag{11-126}$$

where Υ_{KL} is a product of orthonormal orbitals

$$\Upsilon_{KL} = \phi_{k_1}\phi_{k_1}\cdots\phi_{k_\kappa}\phi_{k_\kappa}\phi_{l_1}\cdots\phi_{l_\lambda}, \tag{11-127}$$

with K standing for the set of indices $k_1, \ldots, k_\kappa$ of orbitals which are doubly occupied and L for the set of indices $l_1, \ldots, l_\lambda$ of orbitals which are singly occupied. The spin function

$$\Theta_j^{[\kappa,\lambda]} = (\alpha\beta)^\kappa\theta_j^{(\lambda)} \tag{11-128}$$

is the product of κ $\alpha\beta$ factors, corresponding to the doubly occupied orbitals and $\theta_j^{(\lambda)}$, the jth spin eigenfunction for λ electrons with the desired S and M_S values. (These quantum numbers will not be written as explicit labels, but are implicit throughout the discussion.) Antisymmetrization produces singlet coupling in the doubly occupied orbitals, so Φ_{KLj} is a spin eigenfunction with the same S, M_S values as $\theta_j^{(\lambda)}$. Alternatively, one could replace $(\alpha\beta)^\kappa$ by $[(1/\sqrt{2})(\alpha\beta - \beta\alpha)]^\kappa$ in which case $\Theta_j^{[\kappa,\lambda]}$ is itself a spin eigen-

‡ For survey and references, see Davidson [43].

§ If symmetries other than spin are significant, eigenfunctions of the totally symmetric component of the charge density matrix provide the most satisfactory basis set [125].

¶ Salmon and Ruedenberg [179] include many references.

function. The dominant configuration in an expansion of the type expressed in Eq. (11-126) is normally either the RHF function or the function made up of the first $\kappa + \lambda$ NO's (when ordered by decreasing eigenvalues of γ^0). For a doublet state, such a function will have one singly occupied orbital with $(N - 1)/2$ doubly occupied orbitals.

To consider the reduced density matrices associated with CI functions, we look first at the case where no symmetry other than permutational is imposed. The wave function is of the form given in Eq. (11-125) when the Φ_K are single determinants of orthonormal spin orbitals

$$\Phi_K(1, \ldots, N) = \mathscr{A}\psi_{k_1}(1)\psi_{k_2}(2) \cdots \psi_{k_N}(N), \qquad (11\text{-}129)$$

and we let K stand for the set of indices $k_1, \ldots, k_N$. We assume that each set is ordered so that $k_{i+1} > k_i$. A prime on a set label means that each index in the set has a prime on it.

The contribution from Φ_K, $\Phi_{K'}$ cross terms to reduced density matrices are summarized in Table 11-3. The expressions there are equivalent to

TABLE 11-3

Single-Determinant Contributions to Reduced Density Matrices

Relationship between K and K'	Contribution to $\gamma(KK'\vert 1;1') = \int \Phi_K(1, 2, \ldots, N)\Phi_{K'}^* \times (1', 2, \ldots, N)\, dx_2 \cdots dx_N$	Contribution to $\Gamma(KK'\vert 1, 2; 1', 2') = \int \Phi_K(1, 2, 3, \ldots, N)\Phi_K^* \times (1', 2', 3, \ldots, N)\, dx_3 \cdots dx_N$
$K = K'$	$\sum_{i=1}^{N} \psi_{k_i}(1)\psi_{k_i}^*(1')$	$\sum_{i,j=1}^{N}{}' [\psi_{k_i}(1)\psi_{k_j}(2)\psi_{k_i}^*(1')\psi_{k_j}^*(2') - \psi_{k_i}(1)\psi_{k_j}(2)\psi_{k_j}^*(1')\psi_{k_i}^*(2')]$
K and K' differ only in that k_i does not occur in K' and $k'_{i'}$ does not occur in K	$(-1)^{i-i'}\psi_{k_i}(1)\psi_{k'_{i'}}^*(1')$	$(-1)^{i-i'} \sum_{j=1\,(\neq i)}^{N} [\psi_{k_i}(1)\psi_{k_j}(2)\psi_{k'_{i'}}^*(1')\psi_{k_j}^*(2') + \psi_{k_j}(1)\psi_{k_i}(2)\psi_{k_j}^*(1')\psi_{k'_{i'}}^*(2') - \psi_{k_i}(1)\psi_{k_j}(2)\psi_{k_j}^*(1')\psi_{k'_{i'}}^*(2') - \psi_{k_j}(1)\psi_{k_i}(2)\psi_{k'_{i'}}^*(1')\psi_{k_j}^*(2')]$
K and K' differ only in that k_i and k_j do not occur in K' while $k'_{i'}$ and $k'_{j'}$ do not occur in K	0	$(-1)^{i+j-i'-j'}[\psi_{k_i}(1)\psi_{k_j}(2)\psi_{k'_{i'}}^*(1')\psi_{k'_{j'}}^*(2') + \psi_{k_j}(1)\psi_{k_i}(2)\psi_{k'_{j'}}^*(1')\psi_{k'_{i'}}^*(2') - \psi_{k_i}(1)\psi_{k_j}(2)\psi_{k'_{j'}}^*(1')\psi_{k'_{i'}}^*(2') - \psi_{k_j}(1)\psi_{k_i}(2)\psi_{k'_{i'}}^*(1')\psi_{k'_{j'}}^*(2')]$
K and K' differ in more than two spin orbital indices	0	0

"Slater's rules" for calculating matrix elements. It follows that the density matrices are of the form

$$\gamma(1, 1') = \sum_{i,i'} \left(\sum_{K,K'} p_{ii';KK'} C_K C^*_{K'} \right) \psi_i(1)\psi^*_{i'}(1'),$$
$$\Gamma(1, 2; 1', 2') = \sum_{ii'} \sum_{jj'} \left(\sum_{KK'} P_{ii'jj';KK'} C_K C^*_{K'} \right) \psi_i(1)\psi_j(2)\psi^*_{i'}(1')\psi^*_{j'}(2'), \tag{11-130}$$

where the coupling arrays **p** and **P** are given by

$$p_{ii';KK'} = \begin{cases} \delta_{ii'}, & \text{if } K = K' \text{ and } i \text{ is in } K. \\ (-1)^{t-t'}, & \text{if } K \text{ and } K' \text{ differ only in that } i = k_t \text{ in } K \text{ is not in } K' \text{ and } i' = k'_{t'} \text{ in } K' \text{ is not in } K. \\ 0, & \text{if } K \text{ and } K' \text{ differ in more than one index or } i, i' \text{ are not in the sets } K, K', \text{ respectively.} \end{cases}$$

$$P_{ii'jj';KK'} = \begin{cases} \delta_{ii'}\delta_{jj'} - \delta_{ij'}\delta_{ji'}, & \text{if } K = K' \text{ and } i \text{ and } j \text{ are in } K. \\ (-1)^{t-t'}[\delta_{ik_t}\delta_{jk}(\delta_{i'k'_{t'}}\delta_{j'j} - \delta_{i'j}\delta_{j'k'_{t'}}) + \delta_{ik}\delta_{jk_t}(\delta_{i'i}\delta_{j'k'_{t'}} - \delta_{i'k'_{t'}}\delta_{j'i})], & \text{if } K \text{ and } K' \text{ differ only in that } k_t \text{ in } K \text{ is not in } K' \text{ and that } k'_{t'} \text{ in } K' \text{ is not in } K;\ k \neq k_t,\ k'_{t'} \text{ is any index in } K \text{ and } K'. \\ (\delta_{ik_t}\delta_{jk_u} - \delta_{ik_u}\delta_{jk_t}) \times (\delta_{i'k'_{t'}}\delta_{j'k'_{u'}} - \delta_{i'k'_{u'}}\delta_{j'k'_{t'}}), & \text{if } K \text{ and } K' \text{ differ only in that } k_t \text{ and } k_u \text{ in } K \text{ are not in } K', \text{ and } k'_{t'} \text{ and } k'_{u'} \text{ in } K' \text{ are not in } K. \\ 0, & \text{if } K \text{ and } K' \text{ differ in more than two indices, or } i, j \text{ not in } K, \text{ or } i'j' \text{ not in } K'. \end{cases} \tag{11-131}$$

This essentially trivial result can be extended to give expressions for spin components of the reduced density matrices in terms of the orbitals occurring in the Υ_{KL} of Eq. (11-127). The form of each expression will be

$$\gamma^a(\mathbf{r}_1; \mathbf{r}'_1) = \sum_{t,t'} \left(\sum_{KLj} \sum_{KL'j'} C_{KLj} C^*_{K'L'j'} p^a_{KLj,K'L'j';tt'} \right) \phi_t(\mathbf{r}_1)\phi^*_{t'}(\mathbf{r}'_1)$$

$$\Gamma^b(\mathbf{r}_1, \mathbf{r}_2; \mathbf{r}'_1, \mathbf{r}'_2) = \sum_{tu} \sum_{t'u'} \left(\sum_{KLj} \sum_{K'L'j} C_{KLj} C^*_{K'L'j'} P^b_{KLj,K'L'j';tt'uu'} \right) \times \phi_t(\mathbf{r}_1)\phi_u(\mathbf{r}_2)\phi^*_{t'}(\mathbf{r}'_1)\phi^*_{u'}(\mathbf{r}'_2). \tag{11-132}$$

The superscripts $a = 0$ or z and $b = 0$, z, or SS identify density matrix components, since different components will have different coupling arrays $\mathbf{p}^a$ or $\mathbf{P}^b$. The elements of these arrays will depend not only on combinatorial information, as in Eq. (11-131), but also on the spin coupling scheme used to define the $\theta_j^{(\lambda)}$. Efficient computation normally requires the integration of combinatorial and spin coupling schemes. We will consider here a less efficient but straightforward scheme that is of general applicability for formal discussions.

We must have $\lambda \geq 2M$, and $\theta_j^{(\lambda)}$ can be expressed as a linear combination of simple spin products, each with $\lambda/2 + M$ α factors and $\lambda/2 - M$ β factors. Denote these product functions by Π_i and let

$$\theta_j^{(\lambda)} = \sum_{i=1}^{\binom{\lambda}{\lambda/2 - M}} B_{ji}^{(\lambda)} \Pi_i, \qquad j = 1, \ldots, f(\lambda, S). \tag{11-133}$$

There are fewer possible j values than i values because we are considering only one of the possible S values associated with λ and $M = M_S$. The coefficients $B_{ji}^{(\lambda)}$ are determined by and characterize the spin coupling scheme. We can then express each configuration as a sum of single determinants

$$\begin{aligned} \Phi_{KLj} &= \sum_i B_{ji}^{(\lambda)} \Delta_{KLi} \\ \Delta_{KLi} &= \mathscr{A} \Upsilon_{KL} (\alpha\beta)^{\kappa} \Pi_i \\ &= \mathscr{A}(\phi_{k_1}\alpha)(\phi_{k_1}\beta) \cdots (\phi_{k_\kappa}\alpha)(\phi_{k_\kappa}\beta)(\phi_{l_1}\pi_i^1) \cdots (\phi_{l_\lambda}\pi_i^\lambda) \end{aligned} \tag{11-134}$$

where π_i^t is the spin function (α or β) in position t of the product Π_i. The single determinant results can be used to obtain γ and Γ, and the spin components are then separated and expressed in terms of the B's.

The coupling arrays for the charge and spin density matrices are given in Table 11-4. The notation $I(u, u'; i)$ used there is defined as follows: spin product Π_i is produced from spin product $\Pi_{I(u,u';i)}$ by a permutation which moves π_I^u to position u', moving spin functions between u and u' over, e.g., if $u < u'$,

$$\begin{aligned} \pi_I^t &= \pi_i^t, & t < u \quad &\text{or} \quad t > u', \\ \pi_I^t &= \pi_i^{t+1}, & u \leq t < u', & \\ \pi_I^{u'} &= \pi_i^t. & & \end{aligned} \tag{11-135}$$

Such a permutation can be used to bring L and L' into maximum coincidence if they differ in one index. Also used is

$$e_i^t = \begin{cases} +1, & \text{if} \quad \pi_i^t = \alpha, \\ -1, & \text{if} \quad \pi_i^t = \beta. \end{cases} \tag{11-136}$$

TABLE 11-4

Coupling Arrays $\mathbf{p}^0$ and $\mathbf{p}^z$

Relationship between K, L and K', L'	Contribution to $p^0_{KLjK'L'j',tt'}$	Contribution to $p^z_{KLjK'L'j',tt'}$
$K = K'$, $L = L'$	$2\delta_{jj'}\delta_{tt'}$, if $t \in K$	$\delta_{jj'} \sum_i e_i^t B_{ji}^{(\lambda)} B_{ji}^{(\lambda)*}$,
	$\delta_{jj'}\delta_{tt'}$, if $t \in L$	if $t \in L$
$K = K'$, L and L' differ only in that l_u does not occur in L' and $l'_{u'}$ does not occur in L.	$(-1)^{u-u'} \sum_i B_{ji}^{(\lambda)} B_{j\,I(u,u',i)}^{(\lambda)*} \times \delta_{tl_u} \delta_{t'l'_{u'}}$	$(-1)^{u-u'} \delta_{tl_u} \delta_{t'l'_{u'}} \times \sum_i e_i^u B_{ji}^{(\lambda)} B_{j'I(uu'i)}^{(\lambda)*}$
K, L and K', L' differ only in that $k_u = l'_{v'}$ and $k'_{u'} = l_v$ with k_u not in K', $k'_{u'}$ not in K, l_v not in L', $l'_{v'}$ not in L. (A net result of one orbital difference.)	$(-1)^{u-u'+1} \delta_{t,k_u} \delta_{t',k'_{u'}} \times \sum_i B_{ji}^{(\lambda)} B_{j'I(vv'i)}^{(\lambda)*}$	$(-1)^{u-u'+1} \delta_{tku} \delta_{t'k'_{v'}} \times \sum_i e_i^v B_{ji}^{(\lambda)} B_{j'I(vv'i)}^{(\lambda)*}$
K, L and K', L' differ in more than one orbital overall.	0	0

We note that the diagonal elements of $\boldsymbol{\gamma}^0$ are independent of the spin coupling scheme. This is a consequence of the orthonormality of the $\theta_j^{(\lambda)}$. If the expansion is in terms of NO's so that $\boldsymbol{\gamma}^0$ is diagonal, the charge density is entirely independent of spin coupling. Since the conditions on K and L are independent of j, $\boldsymbol{\gamma}^0$ will in this case depend only on the quantities $\sum_j |C_{KLj}|^2$. Even in this case, $\boldsymbol{\gamma}^z$ retains a dependence on spin coupling, as do the components of $\boldsymbol{\Gamma}$.

Various discussions of CI calculations include the equivalent of expressions for $\mathbf{P}^0$. The spin-dependent components of $\boldsymbol{\Gamma}$ are much less commonly discussed, and unfortunately many treatments are limited to closed-shell states. The method used here could provide them, but to do so would occupy more space than is justified.

It is difficult to proceed in a general, algebraic way to useful conclusions. We will therefore consider what is essentially the simplest possible nontrivial example of a CI calculation for an open-shell system. Suppose we have three electrons and three orbitals: a, b, and c. We further suppose that the problem has at least one element of spatial symmetry, under which a and c are symmetric and b is antisymmetric, and that the three-electron wave function for the state of interest is also antisymmetric. The most general doublet-state wave function with the appropriate symmetry can then be written

$$\Psi = C_1[a\bar{a}b] + C_2[c\bar{c}b] + \frac{C_3}{\sqrt{2}}\{[a\bar{c}b] - [\bar{a}cb]\}$$

$$+ \frac{C_4}{\sqrt{6}}\{[a\bar{c}b] + [\bar{a}cb] - 2[ac\bar{b}]\} \qquad (11\text{-}137)$$

or, in terms of single determinants,

$$\Psi = C_1[a\bar{a}b] + C_2[c\bar{c}b] + \left(\frac{C_3}{\sqrt{2}} + \frac{C_4}{\sqrt{6}}\right)[a\bar{c}b]$$

$$+ \left(-\frac{C_3}{\sqrt{2}} + \frac{C_4}{\sqrt{6}}\right)[\bar{a}cb] - 2\frac{C_4}{\sqrt{6}}[ac\bar{b}]. \qquad (11\text{-}138)$$

Here a implies $a(\mathbf{r})\alpha$ and $\bar{a}$ implies $a(\mathbf{r})\beta$, and

$$[a\bar{a}b] = \mathscr{A}a(1)\bar{a}(2)b(3).$$

The normalization condition, assuming all C's are real, is $\sum_{i=1}^{4} C_i^2 = 1$. The charge and spin density matrices corresponding to this function are given in Table 11-5.

Since this is a complete CI calculation within the (very limited!) basis, a symmetry-preserving transformation of the orbitals can be offset by a change in the CI expansion coefficients. We could, e.g., use this freedom to require that the orbitals be NO's, so that $\boldsymbol{\gamma}^0$ is diagonal. In that case the coefficients will be such that $C_3 = 0$, and the density matrix components have a somewhat simpler form.

The spin function choice in the last terms of Eq. (11-137) is such that a and c are singlet coupled in the third term, while the fourth term is the only one for which b is occupied with β spin. In consequence, if C_4 is zero the spin density matrix reduces to the "direct" contribution from orbital b. Thus any correlation obtained by allowing C_2 and C_3 to be nonzero but keeping $C_4 = 0$ does not introduce spin polarization.

Valence Bond Functions

It is appropriate to consider valence bond (VB) functions at this point because of their similarity to other functions of CI type. In the conventional, lowest-order VB description, one orbital is available for each electron being considered explicitly. (Doubly occupied "core" orbitals are often neglected or relegated to implicit recognition only.) The VB function is thus a special

TABLE 11-5

Charge and Spin Density Matrices Associated with Three-Electron, Three-Orbital CI Functions

Charge density

$$\gamma_{aa}^{0} = 2C_1^2 + \tfrac{2}{3}C_4^2 + C_3^2 + \tfrac{1}{3}C_4^2 = 1 + (C_1^2 - C_2^2)$$

$$\gamma_{bb}^{0} = C_1^2 + C_2^2 + C_3^2 + \tfrac{1}{3}C_4^2 + \tfrac{2}{3}C_4^2 = 1$$

$$\gamma_{cc}^{0} = 2C_2^2 + \tfrac{2}{3}C_4^2 + C_3^2 + \tfrac{1}{3}C_4^2 = 1 - (C_1^2 - C_2^2)$$

$$\gamma_{ac}^{0} = \gamma_{ca}^{0} = C_1C_3\frac{1}{\sqrt{2}} - C_2C_3\frac{1}{\sqrt{2}} = \frac{1}{\sqrt{2}}(C_1 - C_2)C_3$$

$$\gamma_{ab}^{0} = \gamma_{ba}^{0} = \gamma_{bc}^{0} = \gamma_{cb}^{0} = 0$$

Spin density

$$\gamma_{aa}^{z} = \frac{2}{3}C_4^2 + \frac{4}{\sqrt{12}}C_3C_4 = \frac{2}{\sqrt{3}}C_4\left(\frac{C_4}{\sqrt{3}} + C_3\right)$$

$$\gamma_{bb}^{z} = C_1^2 + C_2^2 + \left(\frac{C_3}{\sqrt{2}} - \frac{C_4}{\sqrt{6}}\right)^2 - \frac{2}{3}C_4^2 + \left(\frac{C_3}{\sqrt{2}} + \frac{C_4}{\sqrt{6}}\right)^2 = 1 - \frac{4}{3}C_4^2$$

$$\gamma_{cc}^{z} = \frac{2}{3}C_4^2 - \frac{4}{\sqrt{12}}C_3C_4 = \frac{2}{\sqrt{3}}C_4\left(\frac{C_4}{\sqrt{3}} - C_3\right)$$

$$\gamma_{ac}^{z} = \gamma_{ca}^{z} = -C_1\frac{2}{\sqrt{6}}C_4 - C_2\frac{2}{\sqrt{6}}C_4 = \sqrt{\frac{2}{3}}C_4(C_1 + C_2)$$

$$\gamma_{ab}^{z} = \gamma_{ba}^{z} = \gamma_{bc}^{z} = \gamma_{cb}^{z} = 0$$

case of the general CI function in which only one orbital product is involved, but with $\lambda \simeq N$ a large number of spin functions are possible. An additional characteristic is that the orbitals in the VB function are typically AO's, and are nonorthogonal. They could be replaced by an orthogonalized set of orbitals, but "ionic terms" involving doubly occupied orbitals, must then be included and many orbital products considered to obtain satisfactory results. The simplest VB models will be considered briefly in Section 13.

If a large enough basis set is used and many orbital products, including those with doubly occupied orbitals, are included in the expansion the VB method can give excellent results. Even when the number of doubly occupied orbitals is increased at the expense of the singly occupied orbitals, there are still a large number of spin functions possible for each orbital product. The nonorthogonality of the basis greatly increases the difficulty of any calculation [106]. Several workers have considered the problem of systematically calculating the expectation value of any operator with respect to valence bond functions [39,59,199]. This is equivalent to obtaining expressions for elements of the density matrix components. General expressions for matrix elements involving antisymmetrized products of nonorthogonal spin orbitals have been given by Löwdin [106].

Optimum Multiconfiguration Functions

In the CI and VB functions considered above, it is assumed that the orbital set involved is fixed in advance and only the expansion coefficients are treated as variational parameters. In the case of SCF-type functions, the opposite is true, in that the orbitals are varied but only one configuration is involved so there are no CI expansion coefficients to vary. The spin optimized functions involve both types of variability, however, and are an example of the more general optimized multiconfiguration (OMC) type of function, also known as multiconfiguration SCF or extended Hartree–Fock. (A somewhat different use of this term from the spin extended HF discussed previously.) The SEHF can be considered as a special case of OMC as well, in which the orbitals to be varied are the orthonormal NO's, and the expansion coefficients are definite functions of the parameters d_i.

An OMC function is one of the general CI type in which both orbitals and expansion coefficients are varied. Typically, the number of configurations included is rather small, and some of the orbitals may be "frozen" or required to be the same in all configurations. Calculations with functions of this type can give useful results for comparative energies in which core contributions cancel out. Clearly many more terms must be included if spin polarization of the core is to be adequately described.

Other Methods of Calculation

We have dealt thus far in this section with various types of wave functions, which are optimized by varying parameters so as to minimize the expectation value for the Hamiltonian of the system. We will now consider briefly several methods of calculating energies and other molecular electronic properties which do not explicitly involve a wave function. In general they do not produce an energy which is certain to be an upper bound to that of the true ground state of the problem, as do wave function variational methods. It is hoped that if the calculations are well done, results will be good approximations to corresponding true properties. In the case of properties like the spin density at the nucleus, even wave function variational methods do not produce a bounding result for the property, so this distinction is possibly less important. A number of these methods are surveyed in Volume XIV of *Advances in Chemical Physics* [104].

PERTURBATION THEORY

Since correlation energy, defined as the difference between Hartree–Fock energy and the true, nonrelativistic energy, is usually a small part of the total energy it is reasonable to hope that correlation effects can be treated by perturbation theory. If the true nonrelativistic Hamiltonian is

$$\mathscr{H}_0 = \sum_i f(i) + \sum_{i<j} g(ij), \tag{11-139}$$

where $f(i)$ includes the kinetic energy and nuclear attraction terms for electron i and $g(i, j) = 1/r_{ij}$ (in atomic units), then we define

$$\begin{aligned} H_0 &= \sum_i [f(i) + v(i)], \\ V &= \sum_{i<j} \left[g(i, j) - \frac{1}{N-1} \{v(i) + v(j)\} \right], \end{aligned} \tag{11-140}$$

so that

$$\mathscr{H}_0 = H_0 + V. \tag{11-141}$$

The one-electron effective potential $v(i)$ is chosen for convenience and is often taken to be the Coulomb and exchange parts of the Fock operator so that H_0 is the sum over all electrons of the Fock operator for each electron.

It is assumed that a set of one-electron eigenfunctions of $f + v$ is known

$$(f + v)\phi_i = \varepsilon_i \phi_i, \tag{11-142}$$

e.g., the HF spin orbitals. The eigenfunctions of H_0 are then antisymmetrized products of the ϕ_i. These provide the zero-order functions for a perturbation treatment in which the perturbation is V. Although conventional Rayleigh–Schrödinger perturbation theory could be used, a formulation in the language of many-body perturbation theory is more common. The use of second-quantized notation and diagrammatic methods greatly facilitates such a treatment. The direct result is a perturbation series for the energy of the system, but expressions for the expectation values of operators other than the Hamiltonian have also been obtained. It is beyond the scope of this treatment to present them here.

The application of these methods to open-shell atoms and molecules has been developed primarily by Kelly and by Das and their co-workers.

SUBSET CORRELATION METHODS

Another approach to the correlation problem is based on the fact that correlations for only a few (e.g., two) electrons can be well treated with a reasonable investment of effort. Various methods making use of this idea have been developed, including Nesbit's Bethe–Goldstone heirarchy, Sinanoglu's many-electron theory, and several correlated pair approaches.‡ Details vary, but the common, fundamental idea is to treat the correlations of two (or sometimes more) electrons moving in a potential due to nuclei and the remainder of the electrons treated in an average, SCF-like way.

In some approaches a cluster-expansion analysis is used. In other cases the decomposition is different, but often the correlation energy or other property of interest is expressed as a sum of contribution from pairs, triples, etc. The contributions are defined so that, hopefully, the sequence of partial sums will converge rapidly. Some caution must be used in comparing results of such calculations, even for the energy, with experiment. They do not provide bounds in a variational sense and a significant expansion error may be offset by an overestimate of the correlation correction, leading to fortuitous agreement.

In other approaches, an initial transformation of the HF functions to one in terms of localized orbitals is used to improve the pair correlation approximation. This method has been applied primarily to closed-shell systems, and would not be effective in treating spin polarization or delocalized spin densities.

Density and Density Matrix Methods

Several methods of calculation based on reduced density matrices or their equivalent, or even on just the one-electron density, are gaining acceptance. These methods do not provide variationally bounding energies, and the approximations leading to them are of a nature such that *a priori* error estimates are diffcult to obtain. It is found, however, that they give reasonably satisfactory results. Application to spin density calculations on open-shell systems is sometimes possible but in other cases difficult.

The most common of what will be referred to here as density techniques is the $X\alpha$ method [191]. An energy expression is employed in which, based upon statistical analogies, the exchange contribution to the energy of an antisymmetrized spin orbital product is approximated by a term proportional to the four-thirds power of the electron density. Hartree–Fock-like one-electron equations can be obtained from this energy expression and solved iteratively to give the energy. Additional approximations which make rapid numerical solution possible are often made. The formalism is readily extended to allow different densities for different spins, leading to something analogous to SPHF. It is not clear how the $X\alpha$ method is to be extended to give better

‡ See, e.g., McWeeny and Steiner [127] for discussion and references.

results, or even whether $X\alpha$ is a useful starting point if highly accurate results are required.

A somewhat different density formalism is based on the work of Kohn and co-workers.[‡] A rather remarkable theorem shows that *formally*, the nondegenerate ground state energy of a system is a functional of the density for that state. The functional does not depend, apart from one term easily dealt with, on the nature of the system. It is thus "universal." Unfortunately, it is also unknown, even as to its form, but approximate functionals based on the model of a nearly uniform electron gas have been suggested. The restriction to nondegenerate states excludes almost everything of interest to us, but some work has been done assuming again different densities for different spins, in the presence of a magnetic field which removes the degeneracy.

The energy of a system can be expressed exactly in terms of its two-electron reduced density matrix. It is not appropriate to insert a trial density matrix and vary it so as to obtain an energy minimum unless proper auxiliary conditions are imposed. These must be constraints which guarantee that the reduced density matrix is obtainable, in principle, from an antisymmetric, N-electron wave function or density matrix. The determination of these constraints is the unsolved N-representability problem of reduced density matrix theory; a reduced density matrix satisfying them would be said to be "N-representable." A number of calculations have been reported in which constraints known to be necessary, although not sufficient, to guarantee N-representability have been imposed. When the constraints are properly chosen, the results seem to be usefully good [44].

At this point, however, another problems arises. Here as elsewhere we are discussing the zero-order energy, associated with $\mathscr{H}_0$. This is determined by Γ^0, the spin-free component of the two-electron density matrix Γ. In fact, a variational calculation will be totally insensitive to Γ^z and Γ^{SS}. How then can they be determined? The spin density γ^z is determined from Γ^z but not in general from Γ^0 or γ^0. Even if the N-representability problem were solved, it is not clear how spin densities and other spin-dependent properties could be determined from a direct density-matrix calculation.

At the HF level there is no problem. All density matrix components and the wave function itself can be determined from γ^0. This is straightforward for SPHF, and possible in principle even for SEHF.[§] For more general wave functions it seems that in practice we do not have two functions with the same Γ^0 but different γ^z, for example, apart from the trivial M_S degeneracy, but it is not known how γ^z can be determined from Γ^0.

‡ A number of appropriate references are given by Davidson [44].

§ We note, however, that given only γ^0 we could not determine whether it came from a SPHF or SEHF function.

An Example: Lithium Atom

It would be beyond the scope of this book, and is not its intent, to attempt to survey all the spin density and other open-shell calculations which have been reported. It is useful, however, to include at least one specific example. Atomic lithium is not of great interest in experimental free-radical ESR. It is, nevertheless, a reasonable example system for three reasons: a large number of calculations have been done on Li atom, it is a three-electron system so comparison can be made with some of our formal examples, and for the best calculations complete agreement with experiment has been obtained. This last point is particularly important, since it is true of few atoms and essentially no molecules other than H_2^+. Spin densities are hard to get right! Some Li atom calculations are summarized in Table 11-6.

A number of points are illustrated by the entries in this table. For each type of function, as the basis set is increased or the flexibility of the function within its general type otherwise improved, the energy decreases until a limiting value for functions of the type is approached. Spin densities at the nucleus do not settle down even as the energy limit is approached, except for the best functions. Extreme cases are calculation ll, with an energy error of about 0.01 % but a spin density error of more than 10 %, and calculation qq, having energy within 0.001 % but spin density off by nearly 4 %.

The RHF results have an error, the correlation energy, of only about 0.6 % of the total, but are obviously unsatisfactory for spin density, even in this system where the RHF spin density at the nucleus is not zero by symmetry.

TABLE 11-6

Atomic Lithium Calculations

Description of calculation	$-E(au)$	$\frac{\Delta E}{E} \times 100\%^a$	$f(a_0^{-3})^b$	$\frac{\Delta f}{f} \times 100\%^c$
		Restricted Hartree–Fock		
a. 3 1s & 1 2s basis fcns., partial optimization of exponent [146]	7.428 771	0.659	2.549	−12.29
b. 4 basis fcns. [37]	7.428 974	0.657	2.133	−26.61
c. 5 1s & 1 2s basis fcns. [146]	7.431 765	0.619	2.268	−21.95
d. Numerical [70]	7.432 72	0.606	2.097	−27.84
e. 3 exponents, 1s & 2s for each [91,170]	7.432 722	0.606	2.094	−27.94
f. 3 exponents, 1s, 2s, 3s, & 4s for each [170,176]	7.432 727	0.606	2.095	−27.91

(*continued*)

TABLE 11-6 (*continued*)

Description of calculation	$-E(au)$	$\frac{\Delta E}{E} \times 100\%$[a]	$f(a_0^{-3})$[b]	$\frac{\Delta f}{f} \times 100\%$[c]
		Spin-Polarized Hartree–Fock		
g. 1s, 1s′, & 2s STO's [189]	7.417 95	0.804	2.233	−11.24
h. 4 basis fcns. [195]	7.432 744	0.606	2.961 49	1.90
i. 2 1s & 3 2s basis fcns. [7]	7.432 748	0.606	2.920	0.47
j. 5 basis fcns. [195]	7.432 749	0.606	2.868 22	−1.30
k. 6 basis fcns. [195]	7.432 750	0.606	2.822 11	−2.89
l. 3 exponents, 1s to 4s for each [176]	7.432 751	0.606	2.825	−2.79
m. Numerical [8]	7.432 751	0.606	2.823	−2.86
		Projected Spin–Polarized Hartree–Fock		
n. Proj. of h [195]	7.432 759	0.606	2.394 48	−17.61
o. Proj. of i [180]	7.432 766	0.606	2.382	−18.04
p. Proj. of j [195]	7.432 766	0.606	2.367 45	−18.54
q. Proj. of k [195]	7.432 768	0.606	2.344 99	−19.31
r. Proj. of l [176]	Not given		2.337	−19.59
		Spin-Extended Hartree–Fock (SEHF)[d]		
s. Approx. EHF Gaussians [139]	7.432 59	0.608	2.766 5	−4.81
t. Double zeta basis [91]	7.432 805	0.605	3.135	7.87
u. 5 basis fcns. [180]	7.432 809	0.605	3.106	7.22
v. "Large basis" [91]	7.432 813	0.605	3.013	3.62
w. GF, 3 1s & 2s [62]	7.432 813	0.605	3.020	3.62
		Spin-Optimized Hartree–Fock (SOHF)[d]		
x. 3 STO's, ^1S core [86]	7.417 92	0.804	2.093	−27.98
y. 3 determ. 1s, 1s′, & 2s STO's [30, 95]	7.443 6	0.461	3.038 1	4.54
z. G1, 1s, 1s′, & 2s [63]	7.446 137	0.427	2.704	−6.96
aa. 2 determ. numerical [71]	7.447 48	0.409	2.424	−16.59
bb. 2 determ. numerical [70]	7.447 48	0.409	2.400	−17.42
cc. 2 determ. numerical [29]	7.447 532	0.408	2.842	−2.21
dd. G1, 7 basis fcns. [63]	7.447 560	0.408	2.633	−9.40
ee. 6 basis fcns. [92]	7.447 565	0.408	2.846	−2.07
		Configuration Interaction (CI) & Multiconfiguration Self-Consistent Field (MCSCF)		
ff. CI, all single & double excitations from restricted SCF, minimal basis + large exponent 2s [98]	7.418 33	0.799	2.741	−5.68

TABLE 11-6 (*continued*)

Description of calculation	$-E(au)$	$\frac{\Delta E}{E} \times 100\%$ [a]	$f(a_0^{-3})$ [b]	$\frac{\Delta f}{f} \times 100\%$ [c]
gg. As ff except double zeta + large exponent 2s [98]	7.429 01	0.656	2.912	0.20
hh. 6-term CI, 3 basis fcns. [146]	7.431 849	0.618	2.869 96	−1.25
ii. 7-term MCSCF, 3 orbitals from 7 basis fcns. [94]	7.447 565 4	0.408	2.846	−2.07
jj. 35-term CI, ^1S core 6 basis fcns. [131,208]	7.474 02	0.054	3.989	37.26
kk. 41-term CI, ^1S core 10 basis fcns. [131,208]	7.476 22	0.025	2.580	−11.22
ll. 45 term CI, ^1S & ^3S cores 10 basis fcns. [131,208]	7.477 10	0.013	2.595	−10.71
	r_{ij}-Containing			
mm. Closed-shell core, r_{ij} core only, 8 terms [16]	7.474 76	0.044	2.648	−8.88
nn. Closed-shell core, 11 terms [16]	7.476 30	0.024	2.872	−1.18
oo. Open-shell core, 14 terms [16]	7.476 31	0.024	2.883	−0.88
pp. Open-shell core, 13 terms [27, 28]	7.477 9	0.002	2.826	−2.76
qq. 1 doublet fcn., 60 terms [101]	7.478 010	0.001	3.091	3.88
rr. 2 doublet fcns., 100 terms [101]	7.478 025	0.001	2.906	0.00
	Other			
ss. Bruchner–Goldstone many-body perturbation theory, based on numerical HF [34]	7.478	0.001	2.887	−0.66
tt. Bethe–Goldstone, 5 s orbitals [148]	Not given		2.858	−1.66
uu. Bethe–Goldstone, double zeta + polarization [147]	Not given		2.896	−0.35

[a] The experimental value, adjusted for relativistic corrections, is 7.478 069.

[b] $f = 4\pi\gamma^z(0)$.

[c] The experimental value is 2.906.

[d] SEHF and SOHF are not necessarily as described here. An attempt has been made to classify calculations according to the most similar of the methods discussed.

The SPHF results are not significantly better energetically, but the spin density is dramatically improved, to within 2 or 3% of the correct result. This excellent agreement is, unfortunately, an accident of the Li atom. Spin-polarized Hartree–Fock results for other systems are usually not nearly so good. Projection improves the energy slightly but makes the spin density much worse. Reoptimization in the SEHF and SOHF calculations makes more difference, reducing the energy error to about 0.4%. In favorable cases the spin density is good to a few percent, but in other energetically-as-good calculations it is off by 9–17%. As often happens, the SEHF spin densities lie between the SPHF and projected SPHF values, and are not significantly closer to one than to the other.

The contributions to the spin density for SEHF calculation *u* are summarized in Table 11-7. It is seen that the spin polarization contribution to f is about $\frac{1}{3}$ of the total in this case.

TABLE 11-7

Some SEHF Results for Lithium Atom[a]

	k		
Spin density $\gamma^z(0)$[b]	1	2	3
Eigenvalue, ξ_k^z	0.999 954 8	0.004 778 5	−0.004 733 3
$4\pi\|\phi_k^z(0)\|^2$	2.139	205.4	3.040
Contribution to f	2.139	0.981	−0.014
		Direct contribution	2.139
		Spin polarization contribution	0.967
		Total f	3.106

[a] From K. M. Sando [180].
[b] $\gamma^z(0) = \sum_{k=1}^{3} \xi_k^z |\phi_k^z(0)|^2$.

The large CI calculations can, if carried far enough, reduce the energy error to a negligible amount. The spin density error can still be quite substantial, however. The functions containing r_{ij} do even better energetically, and ultimately do very well on spin density as well. It is of interest to compare the two Larsson results quoted here, calculations qq and rr. The function in qq contains 60 terms, expressed as antisymmetrized products of spatial functions and a doublet spin function. When the second three-electron doublet function is introduced, only 40 of the terms survive antisymmetrization, giving a 100-term total for function rr. The energy difference is essentially negligible, but the effect on the spin density is significant. The r_{ij} approach is unfortunately not extendable to systems with more than a few electrons.

The Larsson functions have been reexpressed in natural orbital CI form. Larsson and Smith have also determined NO's, NSO's, natural geminals, and eigenfunctions of the spin density matrix for the 100-term function, which appears to provide essentially the exact, nonrelativistic description of the lithium atom. The eigenvalues of the spin density matrix are given in Table 11-8. They are not very different from those which occur in the SPHF calculation. Changes in the spin density at the nucleus occur from changes in the values of the spin density eigenfunctions at the nucleus as well as from changes in the eigenvalues.

TABLE 11-8

Eigenvalues of the Spin Density Matrix for the Lithium Atom[a]

Eigenvalues		
100-term function	SPHF	Symmetry of eigenfunction
0.999 362	1.000 000	s
0.003 994	0.003 960	s
−0.003 682	−0.003 960	s
0.000 119		p
−0.000 021		p
0.000 010		s
0.000 002		p
0.000 000 4		d
−0.000 000 4		d

* Eigenvalues for normalization tr $\gamma^z = 1$ are ordered according to decreasing magnitude. Each p eigenvalue occurs 3 times and each d eigenvalue 5 times, associated with symmetry-related eigenfunctions. (From Larsson and Smith [102,103].)

The nonvariational results presented provide very good spin densities. The Bethe–Goldstone calculations, in particular, must be viewed with some reservation, however, because of the small size of the basis set used. An examination of other calculations with basis sets of comparable size suggests that in such cases the spin density at the nucleus is quite sensitive to the choice of basis functions, and thus that the good agreement with experiment may be fortuitous.

Many of the methods which have been discussed in general have been illustrated in these calculations for the lithium atom. It is clear that very good, *a priori* calculations of spin density with a large basis set are probably necessary to assure reasonable accuracy. Both the basis set and the choice of configurations must be particularly suited to the problem of interest.

Summary of Section 11

In this section we have reviewed the theory of electronic wave functions with emphasis on spin properties. The construction of spin eigenfunctions by angular momentum coupling and the branching diagram, by Löwdin projection operators, and by Rumer diagrams have been considered, and it was recalled that the choice of spin coupling can have a significant effect on spin-independent properties because the overall permutational antisymmetry requirement couples space and spin variables.

Common types of wave functions were reviewed. A restricted Hartree–Fock function, or other approximate description involving mostly doubly occupied orbitals in the same way, leads to a spin density which is nowhere negative and is thus often unsatisfactory. (It may provide a good starting point for a more sophisticated calculation, however.) Spin polarization improves the description of spin density but gives a function which is not an $\mathscr{S}^2$ *eigenfunction. Spin projection is possible but the resultant function is no longer variationally optimized. Reoptimization to give spin extended or spin optimized Hartree–Fock functions is possible but involves considerable effort. Configuration interaction functions were also discussed, and brief reference made to valence bond functions. In many cases an examination of reduced density matrices in general or for examples has contributed to our understanding of a method, its potentials, and limitations.*

Nonvariational methods involving perturbation theory, subset correlation methods, or density functionals were considered briefly.

As an example, the three-electron Li *atom has been reviewed in detail. Results of nearly* 50 *calculations were summarized. It was seen that although rather simple methods may fortuitously give quite good results, good values of the spin density at the nucleus are dependably available only from the very best calculations.*

12. Evaluation of Spin Hamiltonian Parameters

When a wave function has been obtained for the system and state of interest, and possibly some description of other states as well, the problem of extracting values of spin Hamiltonian parameters from this information remains. It can be divided into two parts, neither of which is trivial. The first step which must be dealt with is the transformation of expressions involving spin-dependent operators and many-electron wave functions into expressions involving spin-independent operators and one-electron basis functions. It is equivalent to the problem of obtaining, for a given wave function, the various spin components of the one- and two-electron reduced density matrices and has been considered to some extent in preceding sections. The second step involves the evaluation of integrals (matrix elements) involving operator–basis function combinations. In this section we will consider the integrals which are specifically characteristic of the theoretical evaluation of spin Hamiltonian parameters.‡

Operators Involved

Certain types of integrals over basis functions are required in the zero-order calculation. In addition to overlap integrals, these are matrix elements of the operators ∇_1^2, $1/r_{1\nu}$, and $1/r_{12}$. Because they occur in all quantum-chemical molecular electronic calculations, integrals involving these operators have been extensively discussed. They will not be considered explicitly here.

We assume that spin has been dealt with and for the moment ignore constants. There remain a set of spatial operators whose matrix elements we want to evaluate. They are given in Table 12-1, with an indication of the spin Hamiltonian parameters to which each contributes. Second-order corrections to the hyperfine interaction are nearly always neglected in free radical work, so the operators arising in the hyperfine gauge correction terms have been omitted. The kinetic energy term in $\Delta\mathbf{g}$ involves as its spatial part the standard operator ∇^2, and thus is also not treated here. It is clear that the number of distinct spatial operators which need be considered is reasonable small.

‡ Many papers consider one or two of these integrals. One systematic treatment is the series of papers by Matcha and co-workers [132–135,140].

TABLE 12-1

Spatial Operators Whose Matrix Elements Appear in Spin Hamiltonian Parameters[a]

Operator: Cartesian form[b]	Operator: spherical form[c]	Parameters contributed to[d]
One-electron operators		
$f_{\text{contact}} = \delta(\mathbf{r}_\nu)$	$f^{0}_{\text{contact}} = \delta(\mathbf{r}_\nu)$	$A^{\nu'}$ (contact)
$f^{ab}_{\text{dipolar}} = \dfrac{k_0(\mathbf{r}_\nu)}{r_\nu^3}\left[\delta_{ab} - 3\dfrac{(\mathbf{r}_\nu)_a(\mathbf{r}_\nu)_b}{r_\nu^2}\right]$	$f^{2,m}_{\text{dipolar}} = \dfrac{k_0(\mathbf{r}_\nu)}{r_\nu^3} P_2^m(\cos\theta)e^{im\phi}$	$\mathbf{A}^{\nu'}$ (dipolar), $\mathbf{q}^{\nu\nu}$ (quadrupole)
$f^{a}_{\text{spin-orbit}} = \dfrac{k_0^2(\mathbf{r}_\nu)}{r_\nu^3} L_{\nu a}$	$f^{1,m}_{\text{spin-orbit}} = \dfrac{k_0^2(\mathbf{r}_\nu)}{r_\nu^3} L_\nu^{(m)}$	$\mathbf{D}''$, $\Delta\mathbf{g}''(SO)$, $\boldsymbol{\sigma}^{\nu''}$
$f^{a}_{\text{orbit}} = L_{\nu a}$	$f^{1,m}_{\text{orbit}} = L_\nu^{(m)}$	$\Delta\mathbf{g}''(SO)$, $\Delta\mathbf{g}''(2e1)$, $\boldsymbol{\sigma}^{\nu''}$
$f^{ab}_{\text{shielding}} = \dfrac{1}{r_\nu}\left[\delta_{ab} - \dfrac{(\mathbf{r}_\nu)_a(\mathbf{r}_\nu)_b}{r_\nu^2}\right]$	$\begin{cases} f^{2,m}_{\text{shielding}} = \dfrac{1}{r_\nu} P^m(\cos\theta)e^{im\phi} \\ f_{\text{shielding}} = -\dfrac{2}{r_\nu} \end{cases}$	$\Delta\mathbf{g}'(SO)$, $\boldsymbol{\sigma}^{\nu'}$
Two-electron operators		
$g^{ab}_{\text{dipolar}} = \dfrac{1}{r_{12}^3}\left[\delta_{ab} - 3\dfrac{(\mathbf{r}_{12})_a(\mathbf{r}_{12})_b}{r_{12}^2}\right]$	$g^{2,m}_{\text{dipolar}} = \dfrac{1}{r_{12}^3} P_2^m(\cos\theta_{12})e^{im\phi_{12}}$	$\mathbf{D}'$
$g^{a}_{\text{spin-orbit}} = \dfrac{1}{r_{12}^3}(\mathbf{r}_{12} \times \nabla_1)_a$	(See text.)	$\mathbf{D}''$, $\Delta\mathbf{g}''(2e1)$
$g^{ab}_{\text{shielding}} = \dfrac{1}{r_{12}^3}[(\mathbf{r}_1 \cdot \mathbf{r}_{12})\delta_{ab} - (\mathbf{r}_1)_a(\mathbf{r}_{12})_b]$	(See text.)	$\Delta\mathbf{g}'(2e1)$

[a] Except those appearing in the zero-order problem and some others—see text.
[b] a and b label Cartesian components x, y, or z; ν labels a nucleus.
[c] Spherical and Cartesian forms may differ by a constant.
[d] The notation is that of Section 9.

Many of the one-electron operators are defined with respect to the position of nucleus ν. If the functions occurring in an integral with such an operator are defined with respect to different centers, the evaluation of the integral is often facilitated by expanding operators and functions about a common center.

It is convenient to rotate the coordinate systems on the two centers so that the vector joining them lies along their z axes, and so that their x and y axes are also parallel.‡ The distance between them will be denoted by R.

‡ The z axes here are parallel. Frequently they are taken to be antiparallel, so that one coordinate system is left handed. This has the effect of changing some signs. (See Fig. 12-5.)

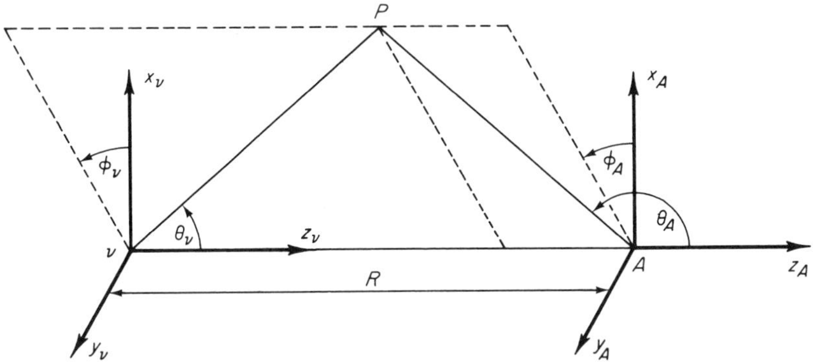

FIG. 12-1. Relationships between coordinate systems on different centers.

We then consider a field point P as shown in Fig. 12-1. Note that $\phi_\nu = \phi_A$. Making use of elementary trigonometry, including the fact that $\cos(\pi - \theta) = -\cos\theta$, and $\sin(\pi - \theta) = \sin\theta$, we find that

$$r_\nu \sin\theta_\nu = r_A \sin\theta_A, \qquad r_\nu \cos\theta_\nu = R + r_A \cos\theta_A, \qquad r_\nu^2 = r_A^2 + R^2 + 2r_A R\cos\theta_A. \tag{12-1}$$

Functions or multiplicative operators which are of the form of solid spherical harmonics can be expressed in terms of associated Legendre functions and functions of ϕ. The ϕ dependence is the same in terms of ϕ_ν or $\phi_A = \phi_\nu$, and [82,158,196]

$$\frac{P_n^M(\cos\theta_\nu)}{r_\nu^{n+1}} = \begin{cases} \dfrac{1}{R^n}\displaystyle\sum_{l=M}^{\infty}\binom{l+M}{n-M}\frac{r_A^l}{R^{l+1}}P_l^M(-\cos\theta_A), & r_A < R, \\ \dfrac{(-1)^{n-M}}{R^n}\displaystyle\sum_{l=n}^{\infty}\binom{l-M}{n-M}\frac{R^l}{r_A^{l+1}}P_l^M(-\cos\theta_A), & r_A > R. \end{cases} \tag{12-2}$$

Other relationships will be considered in connection with particular operators.

Basis Functions

We have considered the choice of basis functions in the previous section. With a few exceptions, usually for small atoms or molecules where explicit r_{ij} dependence is included, basis functions are Slater-type or Gaussian orbitals centered at various positions in the molecule. Integrals are commonly classified according to the number of electrons (one or two) and the number of centers (one to four) involved in the operator and basis functions. Evaluation of an integral often involves the expansion of an operator or function defined with respect to one center about some other center.

Slater-Type Orbitals

The most effective basis functions, although not necessarily the easiest to use, are Slater-type orbitals (STO's). Each STO is characterized by the position about which it is centered, an orbital exponent, and three integers. Complex or real forms are possible.

$$\chi_{nlm}^{A}(\zeta:\mathbf{r}) = r_A^{n-1} e^{-\zeta r_A} Y_l^m(\theta_A, \phi_A) \tag{12-3}$$

or

$$\chi_{nlk_{k'}}^{A}(\zeta:r) = r_A^{n-1} e^{-\zeta r_A} \mathscr{P}_l^{|m|}(\cos\theta_A)\begin{cases}(1/\sqrt{2\pi})\sin k\phi_A,\\(1/\sqrt{2\pi})\cos k'\phi_A.\end{cases} \tag{12-4}$$

Here Y_l^m is a normalized spherical harmonic and $\mathscr{P}$ is the normalized associated Legendre function. In these functions r_A, θ_A, and ϕ_A are the polar coordinates of the point $\mathbf{r}$ with respect to center A.

We note that, in addition to specifying the location of the center, we must specify the orientation of the axis system. In a polyatomic molecule it is usually most convenient to take all axis systems on the various centers to be parallel. In the evaluation of specific integrals it is often more convenient to have, e.g., z axes pointing along a particular internuclear vector. Rotations of the basis functions are readily accomplished for the complex, spherical harmonic forms and involve linear combinations over m-type indices. In other cases the real forms may be more convenient.

The functions have been written here with normalized angular parts but unnormalized radial parts. If completely normalized functions are required, the STO's χ_{nlm}^{A} must be multiplied by a normalized constant

$$C_n(\zeta) = \left[\frac{\zeta^{2n+1}}{(2n)!}\right]^{1/2}. \tag{12-5}$$

An orbital on one center can be expressed in terms of functions on another center. Consider for example an STO centered at v as shown in Fig. 12-1. The ϕ dependence is the same in terms of ϕ_A or ϕ_v, and the rest of the angular part can be expressed in terms of powers of $r_v \sin\theta_v$ and $r_v \cos\theta_v$. (If $n > l$, as is normally the case, there will be at least as many r_v's as $\sin\theta_v$'s and $\cos\theta_v$'s.) These can be related to functions of r_A and θ_A by Eqs. (12-1). It is then necessary to expand the exponential and any remaining powers of r_v in terms of functions centered at A.

One approach is to use the molecular zeta function expansion method developed by Coulson and Barnett [12]:

$$r_\nu^{m-1}e^{-\beta r_\nu} = \beta^{-m+1}\sum_{n=0}^{\infty}[(2n+1)/(t\tau)^{1/2}]P_n(-\cos\theta_A)\zeta_{mn}(1, t:\tau), \qquad (12\text{-}6)$$

where $t = \beta r_A$, $\tau = \beta R$, and ζ_{mn} is a function which can be related to Bessel functions. Recursion formulas and series expansions for the ζ_{mn} are known and make the evaluation of radial integrals involving them possible by analytic or numerical methods.

Alternative methods exist, including the use of Fourier and Gaussian transforms. A recent, general treatment leading to an expansion in terms of exponentials is that of Sharma, who also gives references to a number of previous results [188].

Gaussian Orbitals

The use of Gaussian basis functions is motivated primarily by the ease with which integrals involving them can be evaluated. This ease is a consequence of two factors: that the product of two Gaussians is itself a Gaussian, and that recursion formulas can be obtained, by differentiation with respect to parameters, which relate integrals involving more complicated functions to those involving only simple functions [21,40].

We write an unnormalized Gaussian orbital (GO) centered at position **A** as

$$\eta_{\mathbf{a}}^{\mathbf{A}}(\alpha:\mathbf{r}) = (x - A_x)^{a_1}(y - A_y)^{a_2}(z - A_z)^{a_3}(\mathbf{r} - \mathbf{A})^{2a_4}e^{-\alpha(\mathbf{r}-\mathbf{A})^2} \qquad (12\text{-}7)$$

We will in general suppress labels on η which are constant throughout a series of equations.

To obtain expressions relating different functions, we consider derivatives of η. From Eq. (12-7) with $a_4 = 0$ we obtain

$$\frac{\partial}{\partial A_x}\eta_{a_1, a_4=0} = -a_1\eta_{a_1-1, a_4=0} + 2\alpha\eta_{a_1+1, a_4=0} \qquad (12\text{-}8)$$

or

$$\eta_{a_1+1, a_4=0} = \frac{a}{2\alpha}\eta_{a_1-1, a_4=0} + \frac{1}{2\alpha}\eta_{a_1, a_4=0} \qquad (12\text{-}9)$$

and corresponding expressions for 2 and 3 in place of 1. For general a_4,

$$\frac{\partial}{\partial\alpha}\eta_{a_4} = -\eta_{a_4+1}. \qquad (12\text{-}10)$$

The quantities α, **a**, and **A** occur as parameters in integrals involving η and thus, by a combination of recursion and differentiation, expressions for an integral over any Gaussian can be obtained from the integral involving only 1s Gaussians.

We next consider two 1s-type Gaussians on different centers

$$\eta_A = \eta_{\mathbf{0}}^{\mathbf{A}}(\alpha; \mathbf{r}) = e^{-\alpha(\mathbf{r}-\mathbf{A})^2}, \qquad \eta_B = \eta_{\mathbf{0}}^{\mathbf{B}}(\beta; \mathbf{r}) = e^{-\beta(\mathbf{r}-\mathbf{B})^2} \tag{12-11}$$

The product of these will be

$$\eta_A \eta_B = e^{-(\alpha r_A^2 + \beta r_B^2)}, \tag{12-12}$$

where $r_A = |\mathbf{r} - \mathbf{A}|$ and $r_B = |\mathbf{r} - \mathbf{B}|$. We define a point **P** by the relation

$$\mathbf{P} = \frac{\alpha}{\alpha+\beta}\mathbf{A} + \frac{\beta}{\alpha+\beta}\mathbf{B} \tag{12-13}$$

and let $R_{AB} = |\mathbf{A} - \mathbf{B}|$. Then

$$\begin{aligned} |\mathbf{A} - \mathbf{P}| &= \left|\frac{\beta}{\alpha+\beta}\mathbf{A} - \frac{\beta}{\alpha+\beta}\mathbf{B}\right| = \frac{\beta}{\alpha+\beta}R_{AB}, \\ |\mathbf{B} - \mathbf{P}| &= \left|\frac{\alpha}{\alpha+\beta}\mathbf{A} - \frac{\alpha}{\alpha+\beta}\mathbf{B}\right| = \frac{\alpha}{\alpha+\beta}R_{AB}. \end{aligned} \tag{12-14}$$

The relationships among these distances are shown in Fig. 12-2, with θ the angle between $(\mathbf{A} - \mathbf{B})$ and $(\mathbf{r} - \mathbf{P})$. From the law of cosines and the fact that $\cos(\pi - \theta) = -\cos\theta$,

$$\begin{aligned} r_A^2 &= r_P^2 + \frac{\beta^2}{(\alpha+\beta)^2}R_{AB}^2 + 2r_P\left(\frac{\beta}{\alpha+\beta}\right)R_{AB}\cos\theta, \\ r_B^2 &= r_P^2 + \frac{\alpha^2}{(\alpha+\beta)^2}R_{AB}^2 - 2r_P\left(\frac{\alpha}{\alpha+\beta}\right)R_{AB}\cos\theta, \end{aligned} \tag{12-15}$$

where $r_P = |\mathbf{r} - \mathbf{P}|$. Thus

$$\alpha r_A^2 + \beta r_B^2 = (\alpha+\beta)r_P^2 + \frac{\alpha\beta}{\alpha+\beta}R_{AB}^2. \tag{12-16}$$

(The same result can be obtained without trigonometry by expansion and completion of the square.) It follows that

$$\begin{aligned} \eta_{\mathbf{0}}^{\mathbf{A}}(\alpha; \mathbf{r})\eta_{\mathbf{0}}^{\mathbf{B}}(\beta; \mathbf{r}) &= e^{-(\alpha\beta/\alpha+\beta)R_{AB}^2}e^{-(\alpha+\beta)r_P^2} \\ &= e^{-(\alpha\beta/\alpha+\beta)R_{AB}^2}\eta_{\mathbf{0}}^{\mathbf{P}}(\alpha+\beta; \mathbf{r}). \end{aligned} \tag{12-17}$$

The GO's considered here are of the form

$$\eta_{\mathbf{a}}^{\mathbf{A}}(\alpha; \mathbf{r}) = \eta_{a_1 a_4}^{A_x}(\alpha; x)\eta_{a_2 a_4}^{A_y}(\alpha; y)\eta_{a_3 a_4}^{A_z}(\alpha; z). \tag{12-18}$$

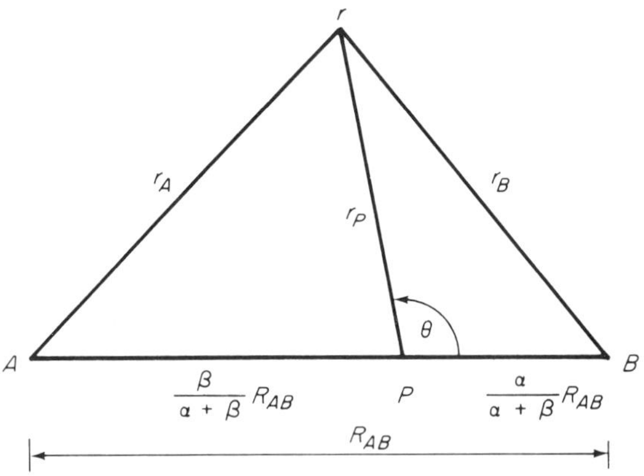

FIG. 12-2. Relationship among Gaussian orbitals.

Linear combinations could be constructed to give functions of the form

$$\eta_{nlm}^{\mathbf{A}}(\alpha; \mathbf{r}) = r_A^{n-1} e^{-\alpha r^2} Y_l^m(\theta_A, \phi_A) \tag{12-19}$$

or equivalent real functions. They could also be normalized. For example, $\eta_{a_1 a_4}^{A_x}(\alpha; x)$ could be multiplied by a normalization constant

$$C'_{n_x}(\alpha) = \left[\frac{\alpha^{n_x+1/2} 2^{3n_x+1/2}}{(2n_x)!\sqrt{\pi}}\right]^{1/2}, \tag{12-20}$$

where $n_x = a_1 + 2a_4$, and similar normalization constants applied to $\eta_{a_2 a_4}^{A_y}(\alpha; y)$ and $\eta_{a_3 a_4}^{A_z}(\alpha; z)$.

Integrals

It would not be possible to give explicit expressions here for all operator-basis function combinations, nor would it be particularly useful. Evaluation of integrals must be closely coordinated with other computational techniques to make efficient use of computing time and programming effort. An attempt will be made to provide explicit results in a few particularly interesting cases and to discuss methods and give references in other cases.

CONTACT HYPERFINE INTERACTION

The delta function operator leads to the simplest possible integrals to evaluate, since

$$\int \rho(\mathbf{r})\delta(\mathbf{r}_\nu)\, d\mathbf{r} = \rho(\mathbf{r}_\nu). \tag{12-21}$$

The delta function is centered on a nucleus labeled by ν and ρ will be a product of two basis functions. If either (or both) of the orbitals is centered on nucleus ν, then for that orbital, either $n = 1$ (STO's) or $\mathbf{a} = \mathbf{0}$ (GO's) or the integral will be zero. When neither function is centered on ν, the integral will in general be nonzero but is likely to be small. It should be emphasized that the $n = 1$ restriction is characteristic of STO's. For hydrogenic orbitals or atomic HF orbitals, in general all s orbitals will contribute nonzero values. These orbitals can be expressed as linear combinations of STO's or GO's, however, and contributions evaluated term by term.

The one-center integrals are

$$\langle nlm, \zeta | f_{\text{contact}} | n'l'm', \zeta' \rangle = \delta_{n,1}\delta_{n',1} \begin{cases} (\zeta\zeta')^{3/2}/2, & \text{normalized STO's,} \\ 1, & \text{unnormalized STO's,} \end{cases} \tag{12-22}$$

and

$$\langle \mathbf{a}\alpha | f_{\text{contact}} | \mathbf{a}'\alpha' \rangle = \delta_{\mathbf{a},\mathbf{0}}\delta_{\mathbf{a}'\mathbf{0}} \begin{cases} \pi/2\sqrt{\alpha\alpha'}, & \text{normalized GO's,} \\ 1, & \text{unnormalized GO's.} \end{cases} \tag{12-23}$$

($\delta_{\mathbf{a},\mathbf{0}} = 1$ if each of $a_1, \ldots, a_4$ is zero, $\delta_{\mathbf{a},\mathbf{0}} = 0$ otherwise.)

The general two- and three-center integrals are also readily evaluated in this case. For STO's they are

$$\begin{aligned} \langle \mathbf{A}, nlm, \zeta | f^{\nu}_{\text{contact}} | \mathbf{B}, n'l'm', \zeta \rangle = {} & C_n(\zeta)C_{n'}(\zeta')r_{A\nu}^{n-1}r_{B\nu}^{n'-1}e^{-\zeta r_{A\nu}-\zeta' r_{B\nu}} \\ & \times Y_l^{-m}(\theta_{A\nu}, \phi_{A\nu})Y_{l'}^{m'}(\theta_{B\nu}, \phi_{B\nu}), \end{aligned} \tag{12-24}$$

where $r_{A\nu}$, $\theta_{A\nu}$, $\phi_{A\nu}$ are the polar coordinates of the nuclear position with respect to center **A**, etc. The normalization constants C_n and $C_{n'}$ would of course be omitted for unnormalized functions. For GO's

$$\begin{aligned} \langle \mathbf{A}, \mathbf{a}, \alpha | f^{\nu}_{\text{contact}} | \mathbf{B}, \mathbf{b}, \beta \rangle = {} & C_{\mathbf{a}}(\alpha)C_{\mathbf{b}}(\beta)x_{A\nu}^{a_1+2a_4}y_{A\nu}^{a_2+2a_4}z_{A\nu}^{a_3+2a_4} \\ & \times x_{B\nu}^{b_1+2b_4}y_{B\nu}^{b_2+2b_4}z_{B\nu}^{b_3+2b_4}e^{-\alpha r_{A\nu}^2-\beta r_{B\nu}^2}, \end{aligned} \tag{12-25}$$

where $x_{A\nu}$ is the x component of $\mathbf{r}_A$, etc., and each normalization constant is a product of three factors of the form given in Eq. (12-20). For the simple case of 1s Gaussians, the result can also be written

$$\langle \mathbf{A}, \mathbf{0}, \alpha | f^{\nu}_{\text{contact}} | \mathbf{B}, \mathbf{0}, \beta \rangle = e^{-(\alpha\beta/\alpha+\beta)R_{AB}^2}e^{-(\alpha+\beta)r_{P\nu}^2} \tag{12-26}$$

(for unnormalized functions).

In a minimal basis calculation, two- and three-center contributions to the contact hyperfine interaction are likely to be negligible (at least relative to other error sources). As more diffuse functions are included in the basis this is no longer necessarily true, and they cannot be dismissed without at least an estimate of their effect.

Dipolar Hyperfine Interaction

The one-center integrals involving the dipolar hyperfine interaction are readily evaluated for STO's and for GO's in the polar coordinate form. It is also convenient to use the spherical form of the operator. The integrals then factor into products of angular parts, depending only on quantum numbers, and radial parts. The angular integrals are of the form

$$I\begin{pmatrix} l & 2 & l' \\ -m & M & m' \end{pmatrix} = \int_0^{2\pi}\int_0^{\pi} Y_l^{m*}(\theta, \phi) Y_2^M(\theta, \phi) Y_{l'}^{m'}(\theta, \phi) \sin\theta \, d\theta \, d\phi. \quad (12\text{-}27)$$

The general expression for I is given in Eq. (C-79) of Appendix C. We note in particular that this integral will be zero unless $m + m' = M$ and $|l - 2| \leq l' \leq l + 2$. It is thus necessarily zero if two s orbitals are involved.

The radial integrals for STO's are of the form

$$\int_0^\infty r^{n-1} e^{-\zeta r} \frac{k_0(r)}{r^3} r^{n'-1} e^{-\zeta' r} r^2 \, dr = \int_0^\infty k_0(r) e^{n+n'-3} e^{-(\zeta+\zeta')r} \, dr$$

$$\simeq \frac{(n + n' - 3)!}{(\zeta + \zeta')^{n+n'-2}} \qquad \text{for} \qquad n + n' > 2.$$

(12-28)

This follows from the properties of k_0 (cf. Section 2), which are such that it can be replaced by 1 in the integrand with only negligible change in the integral value provided $n + n' > 2$ so there is no singularity at the origin. When $n = n' = 1$, however, we must retain

$$k_0(r) = \frac{r}{r + r_0}, \quad (12\text{-}29)$$

where r_0 is the square of the fine structure constant times the Bohr radius and is thus much less than 1 in atomic units. The integral in this case is

$$\int_0^\infty \frac{k_0(r)}{r} e^{-(\zeta+\zeta')r} \, dr = \int_0^\infty \frac{e^{-(\zeta+\zeta')r}}{r + r_0} \, dr = -e^{(\zeta+\zeta')r_0} \, \mathrm{Ei}(-(\zeta + \zeta')r_0), \quad (12\text{-}30)$$

where Ei is the exponential integral function, which can be expanded for negative arguments as

$$\mathrm{Ei}(-(\zeta + \zeta')r_0) = \gamma + \ln(\zeta + \zeta')r_0 + \sum_{k=1}^{\infty} \frac{[(\zeta + \zeta')r_0]^k}{k \cdot k!}. \quad (12\text{-}31)$$

($\gamma = 0.5772157\ldots$ is Euler's constant.) Since $(\zeta + \zeta')r_0 \ll 1$ this gives

$$\int_0^\infty \frac{k_0(r)}{r} e^{-(\zeta+\zeta')r} \, dr \simeq -\ln(\zeta + \zeta')r_0 - \gamma. \quad (12\text{-}32)$$

For $\zeta + \zeta' = 2\ \text{bohr}^{-1}$, for example, this is 9.72.... In any case, basis functions are normally restricted to have $n > l$ so this finite integral will be multiplied by a zero angular integral in those cases where it occurs.

The one-center radial integrals for GO's can be similarly evaluated, with

$$\int_0^\infty r^{n-1}e^{-\alpha r^2}\frac{k_0(r)}{r^3}r^{n'-1}e^{-\beta r^2}r^2\,dr$$

$$= \int_0^\infty k_0(r)r^{n+n'-3}e^{-(\alpha+\beta)r^2}\,dr$$

$$\simeq \begin{cases} \dfrac{1\cdot 3\cdot 5\cdots(2N-1)}{2^{N+1}(\alpha+\beta)^N}\sqrt{\pi/\alpha+\beta}, & \text{if } 2N = n+n'-3 \geq 0 \text{ is even,} \\[2ex] \dfrac{N!}{2(\alpha+\beta)^N} & \text{if } 2N+1 = n+n'-3 \geq 0 \text{ is odd.} \end{cases} \tag{12-33}$$

This is again neglecting the effect of k_0. For $n = n' = 1$, with k_0 included, the integral of interest is

$$\int_0^\infty \frac{k_0(r)}{r}e^{-(\alpha+\beta)r^2}\,dr = \int_0^\infty \frac{e^{-(\alpha+\beta)r^2}}{r+r_0}\,dr. \tag{12-34}$$

This integral is not readily evaluated analytically, but is clearly finite and will normally occur only multiplying a zero angular factor. If required, it could be evaluated numerically.

When the nucleus ν, with respect to which $\mathbf{f}_{\text{dipolar}}$ is being computed, does not coincide with the point(s) at which the orbitals are centered, the integrals can be simplified by an expansion of $\mathbf{f}_{\text{dipolar}}$ about another point. We make use of the expansion of Eq. (12-2) with $n = 2$, but it is necessary to give special attention to what happens when $r = R$ [158]. We are interested in the integral

$$I = \int \rho(\mathbf{r})k_0(\mathbf{r}_\nu)\frac{P_2^M(\cos\theta_\nu)}{r_\nu^3}e^{iM\phi_\nu}\,d\mathbf{r}, \tag{12-35}$$

where $\rho(\mathbf{r})$ is a distribution corresponding to the product of two orbitals and the remainder of the integrand differs from f^M_{dipolar} only by a constant. We divide the integral into three contributions, $I = I_1 + I_2 + I_3$, corresponding to $r \leq R - \varepsilon < R$ (I_1), $r \geq R + \varepsilon > R$ (I_2), and $R - \varepsilon < r < R + \varepsilon$ (I_3). From Eqs. (12-2), then

$$I_1 = \sum_{l=M}^{\infty}\binom{l+2}{2-M}\frac{1}{R^{l+3}}\int d\Omega\int_0^{R-\varepsilon}dr\,P_l^M(-\cos\theta)e^{iM\phi}r^{l+2}\rho(\mathbf{r}) \tag{12-36}$$

and

$$I_2 = \sum_{l=2}^{\infty} \binom{l-M}{2-M} (-1)^M R^{l-2} \int d\Omega \int_{R+\varepsilon}^{\infty} P_l^M(-\cos\theta) e^{iM\phi} r^{-l+1} \rho(\mathbf{r}). \quad (12\text{-}37)$$

The subscript A on the variables of integration has been dropped, it being understood that $\rho(\mathbf{r}) = \rho(\mathbf{r}_A)$. We will ultimately be interested in the limit $\varepsilon \to 0$, but the contribution I_3 does not necessarily vanish in that limit. It must be carefully treated.

In order to deal with I_3 we further subdivide the region of integration as shown in Fig. 12-3. All of region 3 lies between two spheres centered at the origin, with radii $R - \varepsilon$ and $R + \varepsilon$, respectively. Two more spheres are centered at v. Their radii are ε and δ, where δ is thus far arbitrary except that $\varepsilon < \delta < R$. Then region $3a$ is that part of region 3 which lies outside the sphere of radius δ, region $3c$ is that part of region 3 which lies inside the sphere of radius ε, and region $3b$ is that part of region 3 which lies between these two spheres. The integral I_3 is expressed as a sum of three parts, $I_3 = I_{3a} + I_{3b} + I_{3c}$, corresponding to this division of the integration region.

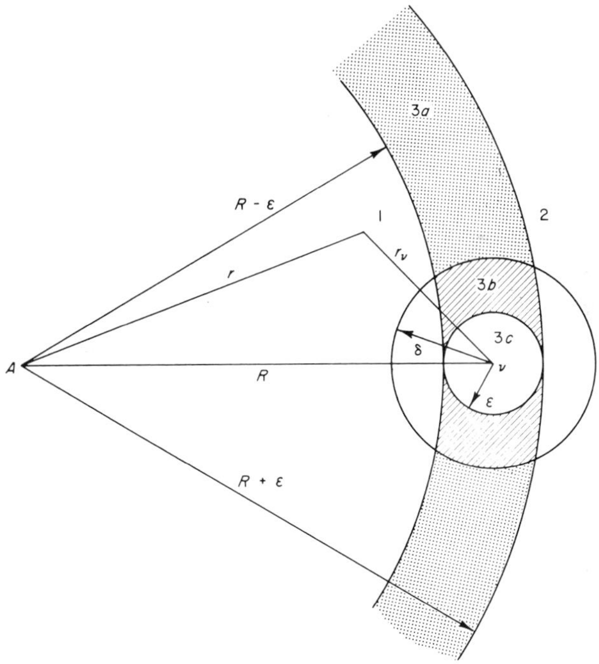

FIG. 12-3. Regions of integration. The origin of the coordinate system with respect to which $\rho(\mathbf{r})$ is defined is at A. The nucleus of interest is at v, and the vector from A to v is $\mathbf{R}$.

In region $3a$, the integrand is finite everywhere and as $\varepsilon \to 0$ the volume of integration goes to zero, so

$$\lim_{\varepsilon \to 0} I_{3a} = 0. \tag{12-38}$$

In order to treat regions $3b$ and $3c$, we will find it convenient to expand the distribution $\rho(\mathbf{r})$ about the point ν. This can be done in two ways:

$$\rho(\mathbf{r}) = \rho(\mathbf{R}) + (\nabla\rho)_{\mathbf{R}} \cdot \mathbf{r}_\nu + \tfrac{1}{2}(\nabla\nabla\rho)_{\mathbf{R}} : \mathbf{r}_\nu \mathbf{r}_\nu + \cdots \tag{12-39}$$

or

$$\rho(\mathbf{r}) = \sum_{l=0}^{\infty} \sum_{m=-l}^{l} \sum_{k=0}^{\infty} C_{klm} r_\nu^{l+2k} P_l^{|m|}(\cos\theta_\nu) e^{im\phi_\nu}. \tag{12-40}$$

The expansion coefficients C_{klm} are clearly related to the values of ρ and its derivatives at $\mathbf{R}$, the position of nucleus ν, and we can choose δ small enough (with ε still less than δ) so that the first expansion is convergent in the region of interest.

We consider I_{3c} in terms of a coordinate system centered at ν. The region of integration is spherical, so only the term with $l = 2$ and $m = -M$ will survive the angular integration. The angular integration produces a constant, finite factor multiplying the radial integral

$$I'_{3c} = \sum_{k=0}^{\infty} C_{k,2,-M} \int_0^{\varepsilon} k_0(r_\nu) r_\nu^{2k+1}\, dr_\nu, \tag{12-41}$$

which goes to zero as $\varepsilon \to 0$. We note that if k_0 were omitted, the radial integral for the term with $l = 0$ would be divergent, leading to an ambiguous $\infty \cdot 0$ for the product of radial and angular parts. When k_0 is included, however, the radial integral is finite even for $l = 0$ and we conclude that $I_{3c} \equiv 0$.

The remaining contribution, I_{3b}, must be treated carefully to determine its limiting behavior as $\varepsilon \to 0$. We consider this contribution also in terms of a spherical polar coordinate system centered on ν. The limits on r_ν and ϕ_ν are clearly $\varepsilon \le r_\nu \le \delta$ and $0 \le \phi_\nu \le 2\pi$, but the limits on θ_ν are not so clear. The relationships shown in Fig. 12-4 will help to clarify the situation. The original origin, e.g., of ρ, the point ν, and the field point form a triangle as shown. By the law of cosines

$$r^2 = R^2 + r_\nu^2 - 2r_\nu R\cos\theta_\nu. \tag{12-42}$$

If the field point is in region 3,

$$R - \varepsilon < r < R + \varepsilon, \tag{12-43}$$

and since all of the quantities are positive

$$(R - \varepsilon)^2 < r^2 < (R + \varepsilon)^2. \tag{12-44}$$

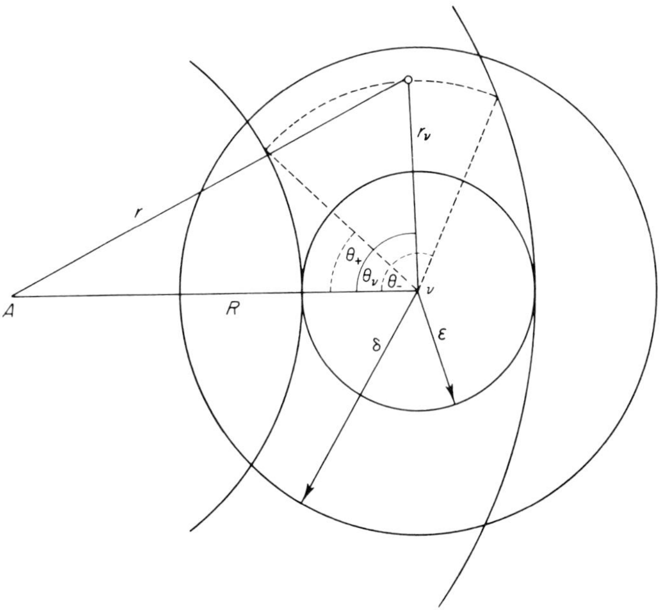

FIG.12-4. Limits on θ_ν in region 3*b*. For fixed r_ν, $\mu_\pm = \cos\theta_\pm$, and $\mu = \cos\theta$ lies between μ_+ and μ_- for points in region 3. (The coordinate system on ν has its z axis pointing toward A. The magnitudes of ε and δ are large so the figure will be more clear.)

We substitute the expression for r_ν, subtract $r_\nu^2 + R^2$ from each term, divide by the negative quantity $-2r_\nu R$ (thus changing the sense of the inequalities), and define $\mu = \cos\theta_\nu$. The inequality can then be written

$$\mu_- \equiv \frac{r_\nu^2 - \varepsilon^2 - 2\varepsilon R}{2r_\nu R} < \mu < \frac{r_\nu^2 - \varepsilon^2 + 2\varepsilon R}{2r_\nu R} \equiv \mu_+, \qquad (12\text{-}45)$$

and the integral becomes

$$I_{3b} = \int_0^{2\pi} d\phi_\nu \int_\varepsilon^\delta dr_\nu\, r_\nu^2 \int_{\mu_-(r_\nu)}^{\mu_+(r_\nu)} d\mu\, \frac{P_2^M(\mu)}{r_\nu^3}\, e^{im\phi}\rho(r_\nu, \mu, \phi_\nu). \qquad (12\text{-}46)$$

We insert the expansion for ρ, but note that the orthogonality properties of the P_M^l cannot be used because the range of the μ integration is incomplete. The ϕ integration does give $2\pi\delta_{m,-M}$.

To treat the μ integration we note that $P_l^{|m|}(\mu)$ is the product of $(1 - \mu^2)^{|m|/2}$ and a polynomial of degree $l - |m|$. In this polynomial, only odd or only even powers of μ occur, as $l - |m|$ is odd or even. We can thus write

$$P_2^M(\mu)P_l^M(\mu) = \sum_j p_{lj}\mu^j \qquad (12\text{-}47)$$

since $(1-\mu^2)^{M/2}(1-\mu^2)^{M/2}=(1-\mu^2)^M$ is also a polynomial. The maximum value of j is $2-M+l-M+2M=l+2$, and each p_{lj} is zero unless j is the same parity (odd or even) as l. The nonzero values are defined by Eq. (12-47).

The integration is then readily performed to give

$$\int_{\mu_-}^{\mu_+} d\mu\Big\{\sum_j p_{lj}\mu^j\Big\} = \sum_j \frac{p_{lj}}{j+1}\{(\mu_+)^{j+1}-(\mu_-)^{j+1}\}, \tag{12-48}$$

and (writing now r for r_ν)

$$\begin{aligned}(\mu_\pm)^{j+1} &= \left(\frac{r^2-\varepsilon^2\pm 2\varepsilon R}{2rR}\right)^{j+1} = \sum_{t=0}^{j+1}\binom{j+1}{t}\frac{(r^2-\varepsilon^2)^{j+1-t}(\pm 2\varepsilon R)^t}{(2rR)^{j+1}}\\ &= \sum_{t=0}^{j+1}\sum_{u=0}^{j+1-t}\binom{j+1}{t}\binom{j+1-t}{u}\frac{(r^2)^u(-\varepsilon^2)^{j+1-t-u}(\pm 2\varepsilon R)^t}{(2rR)^{j+1}}.\end{aligned} \tag{12-49}$$

The terms with t even will be the same for μ_+ and μ_-, so we find after some cancellation

$$\begin{aligned}(\mu_+)^{j+1}-(\mu_-)^{j+1} &= \sum_{t=1\,(t\text{ odd})}^{j+1}\ \sum_{u=0}^{j+1-t} 2\binom{j+1}{t}\binom{j+1-t}{u}(2R)^{t-j-1}\\ &\quad\times(-1)^{j-u}\varepsilon^{2j-2u-t+2}r^{2u-j-1}.\end{aligned} \tag{12-50}$$

With the insertion of this result, the r $(=r_\nu)$ integration can be done to give

$$\begin{aligned}I_{3b} &= \sum_{l=M}^{\infty}\sum_{k=0}^{\infty}\sum_{j=0}^{l+2}\ \sum_{t=1\,(t\text{ odd})}^{j+1}\ \sum_{u=0}^{j+1-t} 4\pi C_{k,l,-M}\\ &\quad\times\frac{p_{lj}}{j+1}\binom{j+1}{t}\binom{j+1-t}{u}(2R)^{t-j-1}\frac{(-1)^{j-u}}{l+2k+2u-j-1}\\ &\quad\times[\varepsilon^{2j-2u-t+2}\delta^{l+2k+2u-j-1}-\varepsilon^{2j-2u-t+2+l+2k+2u-j-1}].\end{aligned} \tag{12-51}$$

The denominator which comes from the integration is odd (since l and j have the same parity) so it cannot be zero. Equivalently, we could note that the exponent of r in the integrand is even, so there can be no log term in the integral.

The exponent of ε in the term involving δ is

$$2j-2u-t+2\geq 2j+2-t-2(j+1-t)=t>0, \tag{12-52}$$

since $u \leq j + 1 - t$. Thus in the limit $\varepsilon \to 0$ this term will go to zero. The term arising from the lower limit of the r integration has as the exponent of ε

$$l + 2k + j - t + 1 \geq l + 2k \geq 0, \tag{12-53}$$

since $t \leq j + 1$. This term will also go to zero as $\varepsilon \to 0$ unless the exponent is in fact equal to zero. Such equality can be attained if and only if $t = j + 1$, which implies $u = 0$ and $l = k = 0$. This in turn is possible only if $M = 0$ and restricts j to 0 or 2. With these restrictions we find

$$\lim_{\varepsilon \to 0} I_{3b} = -4\pi\delta_{M.0} C_{000}[-p_{00} - \tfrac{1}{9}p_{02}]. \tag{12-54}$$

Since for $l = 0$ we are considering

$$P_2(\mu)P_0(\mu) = \tfrac{1}{2}(3\mu^2 - 1) \cdot 1, \tag{12-55}$$

we have $p_{00} = -\frac{1}{2}$, $p_{02} = \frac{3}{2}$, and

$$\lim_{\varepsilon \to 0} I_{3b} = -(4\pi/3)C_{000}\delta_{M.0}. \tag{12-56}$$

Finally, from an examination of the expansions of ρ we can identify C_{000} with $\rho(\mathbf{R})$, so, combining terms in the limit as $\varepsilon \to 0$, we find

$$\begin{aligned} I = {} & \sum_{l=M}^{\infty} \binom{l+2}{2-M} \frac{1}{R^{l+3}} \int d\Omega \int_0^R dr\, r^{l+2} P_l^M(-\cos\theta) e^{iM\phi} \rho(\mathbf{r}) \\ & + \sum_{l=2}^{\infty} \binom{l-M}{2-M} (-1)^M R^{l+2} \int d\Omega \int_R^{\infty} dr\, r^{-l+1} P_l^M(-\cos\theta) e^{iM\phi} \rho(\mathbf{r}) \\ & - \frac{4\pi}{3} \rho(\mathbf{R}) \delta_{M,0}. \end{aligned} \tag{12-57}$$

At this point the question may well arise as to what happened to k_0. So long as $\varepsilon \gg r_0$, k_0 can be ignored in all regions except $3c$, where it provides a useful convergence factor. It is in region $3b$ where k_0 becomes troublesome, since if k_0 is thought of as part of ρ, $\rho(\mathbf{R})$ becomes $k_0(0)\rho(\mathbf{R})$ which is zero. On the other hand, it is possible to have ε small enough so that terms involving ε or its powers are negligible compared with the term in I_{3b} independent of ε, and also that $\rho(r_v = \varepsilon) \sim \rho(\mathbf{R})$, while still ε is large enough that $k_0(\varepsilon) \sim 1$. The "contact" term in Eq. (12-56) thus seems to be present. We will see that in fact it must be retained if I is to behave correctly as $R \to 0$. It may be recalled that in Section 2 the inclusion of k_0 caused some terms to be zero, but derivatives of k_0 then produced contributions from other terms that were essentially equivalent to those k_0 caused to drop out (Fermi contact and Darwin terms).

Consider the case where $\rho(\mathbf{r})$ is a 1s Gaussian distribution centered at the origin. (That is, start with arbitrary 1s GO's and take the origin to be at **P**.)

$$\rho(\mathbf{r}) = e^{-\gamma r^2}. \tag{12-58}$$

In this case

$$\int d\Omega\, P_l^M(-\cos\theta) e^{iM\phi} e^{-\gamma r^2} = 4\pi e^{-\gamma r^2} \delta_{l,0}\delta_{M,0} \tag{12-59}$$

and

$$\begin{aligned} I &= \frac{4\pi}{R^3}\int_0^R r^2 e^{-\gamma r^2}\, dr + 0 - \frac{4\pi}{3} e^{-\gamma R^2} \\ &= \frac{2\pi}{\gamma R^3}\int_0^R e^{-\gamma r^2}\, dr - \frac{2\pi}{\gamma R^2} e^{-\gamma R^2} - \frac{4\pi}{3} e^{-\gamma R^2}, \end{aligned} \tag{12-60}$$

by integration by parts in the first term.

To consider the behavior for small R, we note that for R sufficiently small we can make expansions

$$\begin{aligned} R^{-3}\int_0^R e^{-\gamma r^2}\, dr &= R^{-3}\int_0^R (1 - \gamma r^2 + \tfrac{1}{2}\gamma^2 r^4 - \cdots)\, dr \\ &= R^{-3}(R - \tfrac{1}{3}\gamma R^2 + \tfrac{1}{10}\gamma^2 R^4 - \cdots) \\ &= \frac{1}{R^2} - \tfrac{1}{3}\gamma + \tfrac{1}{10}\gamma^2 R^2 - \cdots \end{aligned} \tag{12-61}$$

and

$$R^{-2} e^{-\gamma R^2} = \frac{1}{R^2} - \gamma + \tfrac{1}{2}\gamma^{2R^2} - \cdots, \tag{12-62}$$

so

$$I = \frac{2\pi}{\gamma}[\tfrac{2}{3}\gamma - \tfrac{2}{5}\gamma^2 R^2 + \cdots] - \frac{4\pi}{3}[1 - \gamma^2 R^2 + \cdots], \tag{12-63}$$

which goes to zero as $R \to 0$, as we know it must. Without the region $3b$ "contact" contribution, the $R \to 0$ limit would be the incorrect value $4\pi/3$.

The result expressed in Eq. (12-60) in fact allows us to obtain any anisotropic hyperfine integrals over Gaussian functions. As has previously been indicated, any integral for Gaussian functions can be obtained from those for 1s GO's. Two 1s GO's, wherever centered, give a ρ proportional to the form given in Eq. (12-58).

If ρ arises from two STO's on the same center, which we take to be center A, we can still use the expansion of Eqs. (12-2) and obtain the result in Eq.

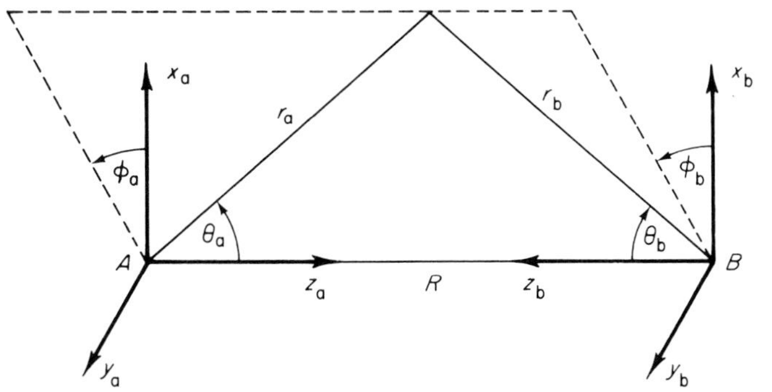

FIG. 12-5. Two-center coordinate systems. Note: a change to a right-handed coordinate system on B would have the effect $z_b \to -z_b$, $\theta_b \to \pi - \theta_b$, $\phi_b \to -\phi_b$.

(12-57).[‡] The angular integration will give zero for all but a few terms in the form given in Eq. (12-28) and radial integrals which can be obtained from the sums over l, so only a few radial integrals need be evaluated. If the operator is used in spherical form and

$$\rho(\mathbf{r}) = r^{n+n'-2}e^{-(\zeta+\zeta')r}Y_l^{m*}(\theta, \phi)Y_{l'}^{m'}(\theta, \phi), \qquad (12\text{-}64)$$

then the integrals in Eqs. (12-57) involve products of angular integrals of the form given in Eq. (12-28) and radial integrals which can be obtained from the indefinite integral

$$\int r^k e^{-ar}\,dr = -k!\left(\sum_{j=0}^{k} \frac{r^{k-j}}{(k-j)!\,a^{j+1}}\right)e^{-ar}. \qquad (12\text{-}65)$$

If ρ arises from STO's on different centers, the expansion of Eq. (12-6) or some other expansion can be used to reduce the integral to a sum of one-center integrals. If one of the STO's is on ν, the expansion is made about ν and the angular integration reduces the sum to one or a few terms. If neither STO is on ν, one orbital and the operator are both expanded about the center with respect to which the remaining orbital are defined. A double summation results, but is reduced by the orthogonality in the angular integrations to a single, infinite sum. Enough terms, each involving radial integrals, will need to be evaluated so that an essentially converged partial sum is obtained. Convergence and the methods of evaluating radial integrals are discussed by Barnett [12].

Alternative methods of evaluating integrals involving STO's on two centers depend on the introduction of elliptic coordinates. We consider two centers, A and B, but now take a left-handed coordinate system at B, with its z axis pointed toward A. The z axis at A points toward B, and the x and y

[‡] For explicit results for simple STO's, see McConnell and Strathdee [117]. See also Ref. [158] for corrections.

TABLE 12-2

Relationship of Elliptic Coordinates to Coordinates on Two Centers

A. Definition of elliptic coordinates

$$\xi = \frac{r_a + r_b}{R} \qquad \eta = \frac{r_a - r_b}{R} \qquad \phi = \phi_a = \phi_b$$

Range of variables

$$1 \le \xi \le \infty \qquad -1 \le \eta \le 1 \qquad 0 \le \phi < 2\pi$$

Volume element

$$d\tau = (R/2)^3(\xi^2 - \eta^2)$$

B. Coordinates on centers A and B in terms of elliptic coordinates

$$r_a = \frac{R}{2}(\xi + \eta) \qquad r_b = \frac{R}{2}(\xi - \eta)$$

$$\cos\theta_a = \frac{(1 + \xi\eta)}{(\xi + \eta)} \qquad \cos\theta_b = \frac{(1 - \xi\eta)}{(\xi - \eta)}$$

$$\sin\theta_a = \frac{[(\xi - 1)(1 - \eta)]^{1/2}}{(\xi + \eta)} \qquad \sin\theta_b = \frac{[(\xi - 1)(1 - \eta)]^{1/2}}{(\xi - \eta)}$$

$$\phi_a = \phi \qquad \phi_b = \phi$$

axes on the two centers are parallel. The relationships are shown in Fig. 12-5, and expressions relating the various coordinate systems are given in Table 12-2.

If the operator is defined with respect to a third center, i.e., v does not coincide with either A or B, it is expanded onto one of these centers by means of Eq. (12-2). The orbitals and operator(s) are then expressed in terms of elliptic coordinates. The ϕ integration can, as usual, be performed immediately. The remaining two-dimensional integral can be evaluated numerically [134] or expressed in terms of auxiliary functions [174]

$$C_{\alpha\beta}^{\gamma\delta\varepsilon}(\zeta_a R, \zeta_b R) = (\tfrac{1}{2}\zeta_b R)^{\alpha+\beta+\gamma+\delta+2\varepsilon+1} \times \int_1^\infty d\xi \int_{-1}^1 d\eta\, e^{-1/2(\zeta_a+\zeta_b)R\xi - 1/2(\zeta_a-\zeta_b)R\eta} \times (\xi + \eta)^\alpha(\xi - \eta)^\beta(1 + \eta\xi)^\gamma(1 - \eta\xi)^\delta(\xi^2 - 1)^\varepsilon(1 - \eta)^\varepsilon. \tag{12-66}$$

These auxiliary functions can in turn be evaluated by means of recursion relationships.

SPIN–ORBIT INTERACTION

One-center integrals involving the spin–orbit operator are readily evaluated. They factor into products of an angular integral, which is trivial if the basis functions are expressed in terms of spherical harmonics and the spherical components of **L** are used, and a radial factor. If the sum of the two n-quantum numbers is greater than 2, k_0 can be ignored and the radial integral is readily evaluated. If both n's are 1, k_0 provides a convergence factor so that the radial integral is finite. Since one normally has both l's $= 0$ in this case, the angular integral is zero and the product of radial and angular factors in unambiguously zero.

The angular momentum about one center can be expressed in terms of angular momenta about another center [158]. Suppose that $\mathbf{r}_\nu = \mathbf{r}_A + \mathbf{R}$. Then in atomic units where $\hbar = 1$,

$$\mathbf{L}_\nu = -i(\mathbf{r}_\nu \times \mathbf{R}) = -i[(\mathbf{r}_A + \mathbf{R}) \times \nabla] = \mathbf{L}_A - i(\mathbf{R} \times \nabla). \qquad (12\text{-}67)$$

The components of $(\mathbf{R} \times \nabla)$ can be expressed in terms of spherical polar coordinates centered on A, and further

$$-i\frac{\partial}{\partial\phi} = L_z,$$

$$i\frac{\partial}{\partial\theta} = \cot\theta\cot\phi\, L_z + \frac{1}{\sin\phi}L_x = -\cot\theta\tan\phi\, L_z - \frac{1}{\cos\phi}L_y. \qquad (12\text{-}68)$$

The nonuniqueness of the expression for $\partial/\partial\theta$ results from the "linear dependence" of the components of **L** implied by the fact that $\mathbf{r}\cdot\mathbf{L} = 0$. In particular, when $\mathbf{R} = (0, 0, R)$, it is found that

$$L_{x\nu} = R\sin\theta\sin\phi\, i\frac{\partial}{\partial r} + \frac{R}{r}\sin\theta\cos\phi\, L_{zA} + \left(1 + \frac{R}{r}\cos\theta\right)L_{xA},$$

$$L_{y\nu} = -R\sin\theta\cos\phi\, i\frac{\partial}{\partial r} + \frac{R}{r}\sin\theta\sin\phi\, L_{zA} + \left(1 + \frac{R}{r}\cos\theta\right)L_{yA},$$

$$L_{z\nu} = L_{zA}, \qquad (12\text{-}69)$$

where r, θ, and ϕ are defined with respect to center A. Making use of Eqs. (12-1), we can show that

$$\frac{L_{\nu z}}{r_\nu^3} = \left\{\frac{P_1^1(\cos\theta_\nu)}{r_\nu^2}\right\}\frac{L_{zA}}{r_A\sin\theta_A}. \qquad (12\text{-}70)$$

It is convenient to combine L_x and L_y in $L_\pm = L_x \pm iL_y$, and we note that

$$r_A^2 + r_A R\cos\theta_A = r_\nu^2 + R^2 - 2r_\nu R\cos\theta_\nu + R(r_\nu\cos\theta_\nu - R) \qquad (12\text{-}71)$$

from which we find

$$\frac{L_{\pm,\nu}}{r_\nu^3} = \left\{\frac{P_1^1(\cos\theta_\nu)}{r_\nu^2}\right\}\frac{R}{r_A^2}e^{\pm i\phi}\left(L_{zA} \mp r_A\frac{\partial}{\partial r_A}\right)$$
$$+\left\{\frac{P_0^0(\cos\theta_\nu)}{r_\nu} + R\frac{P_1^0(\cos\theta_\nu)}{r_\nu^2}\right\}\frac{1}{r_A^2}L_{\pm,A}. \tag{12-72}$$

The functions in braces { } in Eqs. (12-70) and (12-72) are of the form to which Eq. (12-2) can be applied, giving a result entirely in terms of coordinates and angular momenta defined with respect to center A.

Using this result we can evaluate the general, three-center integral involving 1s GO's

$$\mathbf{I} = \int e^{-\beta r_B^2}\frac{\mathbf{L}_\nu}{r_\nu^3}e^{-\alpha r_A^2}\,d\mathbf{r}. \tag{12-73}$$

The three centers A, B, and ν will not in the general case be colinear, but we can choose a coordinate system on ν and A as in the previous discussions. Then

$$\frac{L_{z\nu}}{r_\nu}e^{-\alpha r_A^2} = 0$$
$$\frac{L_{\pm\nu}}{r_\nu^3}e^{-\alpha r_A^2} = \left\{\frac{P_1^1(\cos\theta_\nu)}{r_\nu^2}\right\}\frac{R}{r_A^2}e^{\pm i\phi}\left(\mp r_A\frac{\partial}{\partial r_A}\right)e^{-\alpha r_A^2}, \tag{12-74}$$
$$= \pm 2\alpha R\frac{P_1^1(\cos\theta_\nu)e^{\pm i\phi}}{r_\nu^2}e^{-\alpha r_A^2},$$

since $L_A e^{-\alpha r_A^2} \equiv 0$. We now associate the $e^{\pm i\phi}$ with the operator rather than with the function, i.e., take $\phi = \phi_\nu$ and write

$$I_\pm = \pm 2\alpha R_{A\nu}e^{-(\alpha\beta/\alpha+\beta)R_{AB}^2}I'_\pm,$$
$$I'_\pm = \int\frac{P_1^1(\cos\theta_\nu)e^{\pm i\phi_\nu}}{r_\nu^2}e^{-\gamma r_P^2}, \tag{12-75}$$

where $\mathbf{P}$ is defined as in Eq. (12-13), $\gamma = \alpha + \beta$, and $R_{A\nu} = R$. The coordinate system on center ν is then rotated so that the new z axis points toward center P, and the expansion of P_1^M/r^2 is inserted. Only the part with $M = 0$ survives ϕ integration, and only the term in the expansion with $l = 0$ survives θ integration. The result is that

$$I'_\pm \propto \frac{4\pi}{R_{P\nu}^2}\int_0^{R_{P\nu}} e^{-\gamma r^2}\,dr, \tag{12-76}$$

where the proportionality constant depends on the rotation, i.e., the geometry of the A, B, ν system.

If STO's on different centers are involved, methods of evaluation similar to those used for the dipolar hyperfine interaction can be used. If the operator is defined with respect to a third center it is transferred to one of the orbital centers by means of Eqs. (12-70), (12-72), and (12-2). Then either one orbital is expanded about the center of the other or the two-center expression is evaluated in elliptic coordinates.

SHIELDING

The shielding operator does not correspond to a single, irreducible tensor. In spherical form it is thus convenient to express it as the sum of two operators as indicated in Table 12-1. The isotropic part, $f^{0}_{\text{shielding}}$, is just proportional to $1/r_\nu$, and matrix elements of this operator have been thoroughly studied in connection with the zero-order calculation. We will consider here the remaining part, $f^{2,m}_{\text{shielding}}$. It should be noted that this is not of the form of an irregular, solid spherical harmonic because r^{-1} is involved, rather than r^{-3}, together with $l = 2$. Equation (12-2) is thus not directly applicable.

As usual, the one-center integrals present no problem. They can be directly evaluated and the lower power of $1/r$ results in k_0 not being needed as a convergence factor. Integrals involving STO's on two centers, one of which is ν, can also be directly evaluated in elliptic coordinates. These integrals will be expressible as a sum of products which can be separated so that only simple integrals over ξ only or η only need be evaluated. This can be done in terms of the simpler auxiliary functions

$$A_n(\alpha) = \int_0^\infty e^{-\alpha\xi}\xi^n \, d\xi, \qquad B_n(\alpha) = \int_{-1}^{1} e^{-\alpha\eta}\eta^n \, d\eta, \tag{12-77}$$

which can be evaluated from simple recursion relations [99].

If it is necessary to expand the operator about some other center, this can be done by first writing it as

$$f^{2,m}_{\text{shielding}} = (r_\nu^2)((1/r_\nu^3)P_l^m(\cos\theta_\nu)e^{im\phi_\nu}). \tag{12-78}$$

Equations (12-2) can be applied to the second factor, and the third of Eqs. (12-1) applied to the first factor, r_ν^2. The result is an expansion about some other center, A, as required. Since no essentially new features arise, these integrals will not be considered further.

TWO-ELECTRON DIPOLAR INTERACTION

The two-electron operators do not include dependence on any nuclear position. The number of centers involved in any integral is thus determined entirely by the orbitals. Involvement of the coordinates of two electrons rather than just one makes these integrals more difficult to evaluate, however. One way of seeking to simplify the calculation is to try to separate the dependence of $\mathbf{r}_1$ and $\mathbf{r}_2$. It is also helpful to relate these integrals to those involving $1/r_{12}$, which have been extensively studied.

As a first step, we express the elements of $\mathbf{g}_{\text{dipolar}}$ in terms of derivatives of $1/r_{12}$ [184]. For Cartesian indices $a, b = x, y, z$, and $(\mathbf{r}_i)_a$ being the a component of $\mathbf{r}_i$, etc., we find

$$\begin{aligned} g^{ab}_{\text{dipolar}} &= \frac{1}{r_{12}^3}\left[\delta_{ab} - \frac{3(\mathbf{r}_{12})_a(\mathbf{r}_{12})_b}{r_{12}^2}\right] \\ &= \frac{\partial^2}{\partial(\mathbf{r}_1)_a\,\partial(\mathbf{r}_2)_b}\frac{1}{r_{12}} - \frac{4\pi}{3}\delta(\mathbf{r}_{12})\delta_{ab}. \end{aligned} \tag{12-79}$$

The derivative term is straightforward; direct evaluation just gives the previous expression. One then wonders why the delta-function term appears. In the case of a three-dimensional potential problem it is reasonably well known (see, e.g., Panofsky and Phillips [152, p.3]) that

$$\nabla^2(1/r) = -4\pi\delta(\mathbf{r}).$$

Symmetry requires that $\frac{1}{3}$ of this term be associated with each of the three second derivatives. The corresponding correction occurs as the last term in Eq. (12-79).

We next consider an integral involving $\mathbf{g}_{\text{dipolar}}$. Since the operator is purely multiplicative, the product of two orbitals for either electron can be expressed simply as a density distribution for that electron. Then

$$I_{ab} = \iint g^{ab}_{\text{dipolar}}\,\rho(\mathbf{r}_1)\rho'(\mathbf{r}_2)\,d\mathbf{r}_1\,d\mathbf{r}_2. \tag{12-80}$$

Inserting the expression for g^{ab}_{dipolar}, integrating the first term by parts and the second term over the coordinates of electron 2, we find

$$I_{ab} = \iint \frac{1}{r_{12}}\left[\frac{\partial}{\partial(\mathbf{r}_1)_a}\rho(\mathbf{r}_1)\right]\left[\frac{\partial}{\partial(\mathbf{r}_2)_b}\rho'(\mathbf{r}_2)\right]d\mathbf{r}_1\,d\mathbf{r}_2 - \frac{4\pi}{3}\delta_{ab}\int\rho(\mathbf{r}_1)\rho'(\mathbf{r}_1)\,d\mathbf{r}_1. \tag{12-81}$$

The surface terms arising from the integration by parts vanish for quadratically integrable functions, which we would invariably be using.

Let us next consider the evaluation of I_{ab} for 1s GO's. We take

$$\begin{aligned} \rho(\mathbf{r}_1) &= \eta_{\mathbf{0}}^{\mathbf{A}}(\mathbf{r}_1)\eta_{\mathbf{0}}^{\mathbf{B}}(\mathbf{r}_1) = e^{-(\alpha\beta/\alpha+\beta)R_{A}^2}e^{-(\alpha+\beta)(\mathbf{r}_1-\mathbf{P})^2}, \\ \rho'(\mathbf{r}_2) &= \eta_{\mathbf{0}}^{\mathbf{C}}(\mathbf{r}_2)\eta_{\mathbf{0}}^{\mathbf{D}}(\mathbf{r}_2) = e^{-(\gamma\delta/\gamma+\delta)R_{CD}^2}e^{-(\gamma+\delta)(\mathbf{r}_2-\mathbf{Q})^2}, \end{aligned} \tag{12-82}$$

with **P** defined by Eq. (12-13) and **Q** defined analogously in terms of positions **C** and **D** and corresponding exponents γ and δ. It is readily shown that

$$\begin{aligned} \frac{\partial}{\partial(\mathbf{r}_1)_a}\rho(\mathbf{r}_1) &= -\frac{\partial}{\partial P_a}\rho(\mathbf{r}_1), \\ \frac{\partial}{\partial(\mathbf{r}_2)_b}\rho'(\mathbf{r}_2) &= -\frac{\partial}{\partial Q_b}\rho'(\mathbf{r}_2), \end{aligned} \tag{12-83}$$

and thus

$$I_{ab} = e^{-(\alpha\beta/\alpha+\beta)R_{AB}^2} e^{-(\gamma\delta/\gamma+\delta)R_{CD}^2}\left[\frac{\partial^2}{\partial P_a\,\partial Q_b} I - \frac{4\pi}{3}\delta_{ab} I'\right], \tag{12-84}$$

where

$$\begin{aligned} I &= \iint e^{-(\alpha+\beta)(\mathbf{r}_1-\mathbf{P})^2}\frac{1}{r_{12}}e^{-(\gamma+\delta)(\mathbf{r}_2-\mathbf{Q})^2}\,d\mathbf{r}_1\,d\mathbf{r}_2, \\ I' &= \int e^{-(\alpha+\beta)(\mathbf{r}_1-\mathbf{P})^2} e^{-(\gamma+\delta)(\mathbf{r}_1-\mathbf{Q})^2}\,d\mathbf{r}_1. \end{aligned} \tag{12-85}$$

The integral I is well known. It can be evaluated, e.g., by using the multipole (Neumann) expansion for $1/r_{12}$

$$\frac{1}{r_{12}} = \sum_{k=0}^{\infty}\sum_{m=-k}^{k}\frac{4\pi}{2k+1}\frac{r_<^k}{r_>^{k+1}} Y_k^m(\theta_1,\phi_1)Y_k^{-m}(\theta_2,\phi_2) \tag{12-86}$$

($r_>$ is the larger of r_1 and r_2, $r_<$ the smaller). The result is

$$I = \frac{2\pi^{5/2}}{(\alpha+\beta)(\gamma+\delta)(\alpha+\beta+\gamma+\delta)^{1/2}} f\left(\frac{[(\alpha+\beta)(\gamma+\delta)]^{1/2}}{\alpha+\beta+\gamma+\delta} R_{PQ}\right), \tag{12-87}$$

where

$$f(x) = \frac{1}{x}\int_0^x e^{-y^2}\,dy. \tag{12-88}$$

The integral I', arising from the delta-function contribution, is of the form of a simple GO overlap. It is

$$\begin{aligned} I' &= e^{-[(\alpha+\beta)(\gamma+\delta)/\alpha+\beta+\gamma+\delta]R_{PQ}^2}\int e^{-(\alpha+\beta+\gamma+\delta)r^2}\,d\mathbf{r} \\ &= \frac{\pi^{3/2}}{(\alpha+\beta+\gamma+\delta)^{3/2}} e^{-[(\alpha+\beta)(\gamma+\delta)/(\alpha+\beta+\gamma+\delta)]R_{PQ}^2}. \end{aligned} \tag{12-89}$$

It is convenient to define $x = [(\alpha + \beta)(\gamma + \delta)/(\alpha + \beta + \gamma + \delta)]^{1/2} R_{PQ}$. The expressions above can then be combined to give, after some manipulations involving f and its derivatives (which can be expressed in terms of f and e^{-x^2}),

$$I_{ab} = \frac{2\pi^{5/2}}{3(\alpha + \beta + \gamma + \delta)^{3/2}} e^{-(\alpha\beta/\alpha+\beta)R_{AB}^2} e^{-(\gamma\delta/\gamma+\delta)R_{CD}^2} \times \left[3\frac{(P_a - Q_a)(P_b - Q_b)}{R_{PQ}} - \delta_{ab}\right]\left[\frac{1}{x^2}\{(2x^2 + 3)e^{-x^2} - 3f(x)\}\right]. \tag{12-90}$$

For $x \ll 1$,

$$(1/x^2)\{(2x^2 + 3)e^{-x^2} - 3f(x)\} = -\tfrac{4}{5}x^2 + O(x^4), \tag{12-91}$$

and thus $I_{ab} \to 0$ as $R_{PQ} \to 0$. This is the correct behavior, and it would not be found for $a = b$ if the delta-function correction was absent. Asymptotically, as $x \to \infty$, this term is proportional to $1/x^3$ since $f \sim 1/x$.

When STO's are involved, Eq. (12-81) can still be used, together with an expansion of the form [133]

$$\frac{\partial}{\partial(r)_\mu} \chi_{nlm}(\zeta : \mathbf{r}) = \sum_{n'l'} C^a(nlm|n'l'm + \mu)\chi_{n'l'm+\mu}(\zeta : \mathbf{r}). \tag{12-92}$$

(Here $(r)_\mu$ is a spherical component of $\mathbf{r}$, $\mu = 0, \pm 1$. The expansion coefficient values are given in Ref. [133].) The two-electron dipolar interaction can then be expressed in terms of $1/r_{12}$ integrals and generalized "overlap" integrals which can be evaluated, e.g., by use of an orbital expansion if different centers are involved.

An alternative approach involves the use of an operator expansion [158]. For the zz component, for example,

$$\frac{3z_{12}^2 - r_{12}^2}{r_{12}^5} = \sum_{l=1}^{\infty} \sum_{m=-l+1}^{l-1} \frac{(l - m - 1)!\, r_j^{l-1}}{(l + m + 1)!\, r_k^{l+1}} \times P_{l-1}^m(\cos\theta_j)P_{l+1}^m(\cos\theta_k)e^{im(\phi j - \phi k)} - \frac{4\pi}{3} P_2(\cos\theta_j)\delta(\mathbf{r}_1 - \mathbf{r}_2), \tag{12-93}$$

where $j, k = 1, 2$, or $2, 1$ such that $r_j < r_k$. The dipolar interaction integral can then be expressed as a sum of products of one-electron integrals. The details of evaluating these integrals for STO's will not be presented here. Other treatments are also available [120,162].

Two-Electron Spin–Orbit Interaction

As a first step in treating integrals involving $\mathbf{g}_{SO}$ (where SO refers to spin–orbit interaction), we express it as

$$\mathbf{g}_{SO} = \nabla_2(1/r_{12}) \times \nabla_1. \qquad (12\text{-}94)$$

Integration by parts can be used to express the integral in terms of $1/r_{12}$ integrals. If GO's are used, ∇_1 and ∇_2 can be replaced by deriviatives with respect to orbital position parameters. [Compare Eqs. (12-83).] If STO's are involved, Eq. (12-94) can be used. The details will not be given here [162].

Two-Electron Shielding

The two-electron shielding operator is treated in a simpler way, starting from

$$g^{ab}_{\text{shielding}} = \mathbf{r}_1 \cdot \nabla_2\left(\frac{1}{r_{12}}\right)\delta_{ab} - (\mathbf{r}_1)_a \frac{\partial}{\partial(\mathbf{r}_2)_b}\left(\frac{1}{r_{12}}\right). \qquad (12\text{-}95)$$

No essential new features appear, so details will not be given.

Summary of Section 12

In this section the integrals required in the evaluation of spin Hamiltonian parameters have been considered. When spin properties have been taken care of, by the methods of the previous sections, only a reasonably small number of distinct spatial operators need be treated. Those which arise in the zero-order calculation have been discussed by others in many places and were thus not included here. Rather, attention was concentrated on those integrals which are of particular interest to ESR.

Basis functions of both Gaussian and Slater type have been considered. The former are easier to deal with, and all integrals for a given operator can be obtained from that involving 1s *orbitals on general centers. Explicit expressions for such integrals have been given for most of the operators. Some of the simpler results for Slater type orbitals were also given, and methods were presented and references given for others.*

In treating multicenter integrals we often find it convenient or necessary to expand functions, operators, or both about a common center. Some of the methods for making such expansions have been presented.

13. Semiempirical Methods

In the preceding sections of this chapter we have been concerned with the *a priori* calculation of wave functions for open-shell systems and of spin Hamiltonian parameters. Really good calculations have been done only on small systems. Extension to larger systems, including most of those of experimental interest, is limited by considerations of computing technology and finance. It is therefore essential that alternative, more tractable methods be available. In this section we will consider some of the semiempirical methods which have been developed.

Semiempirical methods involve the use of experimental data, or occasionally the results of *a priori* calculations, to evaluate certain integrals or other parameters. In the problems of interest to us, this can be done in two rather different ways. An approximate, typically minimal-basis self-consistent field (SCF) calculation can be done rigorously, but hyperfine coupling constants may then be evaluated with the introduction of adjustable proportionality constants. Secondly, empirically adjusted parameters may enter into the determination of the wave function itself.

Atomic Orbital Spin Density

A concept which is important in many semiempirical calculations is that of atomic orbital spin density [113]. Suppose that a basis set of atomic orbitals $\{\chi_\mu\}$ has been introduced. The spin density matrix can then be expressed as

$$\gamma^z(\mathbf{r}_1:\mathbf{r}_1') = \sum_{\mu,\nu} \gamma^z_{\mu\nu}\chi_\mu(\mathbf{r}_1)\chi^*_\nu(\mathbf{r}_1'). \tag{13-1}$$

The coefficient matrix $(\gamma^z_{\mu\nu})$ might be referred to as the atomic orbital spin density matrix. It is particularly easy to deal with in a minimal basis case. In a pi-electron calculation, for example, there is commonly only one atomic orbital basis function per atom. In that case $\gamma^z_{\mu\mu}$ is the (atomic orbital) spin density "on atom μ," and $\gamma^z_{\mu\nu}$ represents a bond spin density. A similar expansion of the charge density matrix yields coefficients $\gamma^0_{\mu\nu}$ which make up the "charge and bond order" matrix.

The way in which these matrices are to be interpreted depends on the size of the basis set and whether or not nonorthogonality of the basis functions is taken into account. In situations where only one basis function per atom is considered, it is common to take the hyperfine coupling constant to be proportional to the atomic orbital spin density on the atom involved. The special case of pi-electron calculations will be considered in more detail later.

All-Valence-Electron Semiempirical Methods

Semiempirical methods were developed first for conjugated, planar molecules in which only the "pi electrons" were considered explicitly. This approach will be considered later in this section. We wish now to consider the more recently developed methods in which all electrons except those associated with the inner cores of the constituent atoms are considered explicitly. Two fundamental approaches of this type exist: SCF methods such as CNDO/INDO (complete (intermediate) neglect of differential overlap) or spherical Gaussian, and the extended Hückel method. The latter has not been extensively used in ESR calculations, where it has little to recommend it, and will not be considered here. The pi-electron Hückel method will be considered later.

INDO Methods

Of the all-valence-electron methods, those most extensively applied to spin density calculations are the INDO model and its variations. The method was developed by Pople, Beveridge, and co-workers, and extensive discussions are readily available [160] so details will not be repeated here. The essential features of this SCF-like model are these:

1. Core orbitals are not included. The inner electrons are collapsed into the nucleus, reducing the effective values of the number of electrons, N, and the nuclear charge, Z.
2. A minimal basis set is used for the valence electrons.
3. Integrals over basis functions are approximated by comparison with experimental data in some cases, and by mathematical models or actual calculation in others.

Most commonly, a spin-polarized SCF calculation is performed. The isotropic hyperfine coupling constants are taken to be proportional to appropriate atomic orbital spin densities, but rather than the proportionality constants being determined from the AO values at the nuclei, they are adjusted to give the best fit between calculated AO spin densities and experimental coupling constants.

Gaussian Methods

If a small basis of GO's (usually 1s, floating) is used, all integrals can be easily evaluated and an *a priori* calculation done. The introduction of empirically adjusted proportionality constants relating "AO" spin densities to coupling constants allows some of the shortcomings of the basis set to be corrected for.

Pi-Electron Methods

With the advent of INDO, Gaussian and other all-electron, small-basis methods and the increasing availability of substantial computing facilities, the importance of pi-electron-only calculations is reduced. Such calculations retain at least a significant historical interest, however. The sigma–pi separation and pi-electron methods in general will not be extensively discussed here, but some aspects of interest to ESR will be presented.

In the simplest cases, pi-electron theories apply to completely planar molecules. When all nuclei of a molecule have their equilibrium positions in a plane, reflection in that plane is a symmetry operation for the molecule. In such a case molecular orbitals, natural orbitals, and in most cases basis functions as well, can be divided into two groups: those which are symmetric with respect to reflection in the molecular plane are called sigma orbitals; those which change sign on reflection are called pi orbitals. Among the occupied Hartree–Fock orbitals or the strongly occupied natural orbitals will be found some sigma orbitals and some pi orbitals. As a consequence not so much of the planar structure as of the bonding which leads to that structure, sigma and pi orbitals tend to contribute rather differently to molecular properties.

The pi-electron approximation consists of treating only electrons in pi oribitals explicitly. The electrons in sigma orbitals are relegated to an implicit treatment as part of the background against which the pi system is considered. Many properties of these systems can be treated to a useful degree of accuracy within the pi-electron approximation. Two pi-electron methods will be discussed here: Hückel theory and the semiempirical SCF Pariser–Parr–Pople (PPP) theory.

Hückel and McLachlan Theories

The oldest and crudest of pi-electron models is the simple Hückel theory (see, e.g., Salem [177]). Hückel theory is a molecular orbital method, but in modern quantum chemistry it is usually considered to involve a model Hamiltonian best described by second quantization and propagator or

Green's function techniques, rather than as an approximation to an SCF treatment.

Hückel theory involves the use of an unspecified, effective one-electron Hamiltonian. The basis set consists of one p-pi orbital centered on each atom participating in the pi structure. (Thus not including H atoms, even though they lie in the molecular plane.) These basis orbitals are implicitly assumed to be orthonormal but are otherwise unspecified. The theory provides a prescription for the construction of the matrix of the effective Hamiltonian in this basis, and its eigenvalues and eigenvectors provide the orbital energies and molecular orbital (MO) expansion coefficients, respectively. It is a peculiarity of Hückel theory that the total energy is given simply as the sum of orbital energies of the occupied orbitals. Of more interest to us are the MO expansion coefficients.

The effective Hamiltonian matrix elements do not depend (in simple Hückel theory) on the number of electrons in the system. After they are determined, the molecular orbitals are assumed to be filled by the available pi electrons in order of increasing orbital energy. (It should be noted that in most treatments a negative unit of energy is used, so the energy ordering appears to be reversed.) Each MO can accommodate two electrons with opposite spin, these being effectively singlet coupled. If the available number of electrons is odd, as in a doublet radical, the occupied orbital of highest energy will contain only one electron, and the AO spin density matrix is (for the $M_S = +\frac{1}{2}$ state)

$$\gamma^{z}_{\mu\nu} = C_{i\mu} C_{i\nu}, \tag{13-2}$$

where $\mathbf{C}_i$ is the column eigenvector of coefficients for the singly occupied MO.

In view of the extreme simplicity of the Hückel method, it is remarkable how well it works in predicting spin density distributions. The pi AO spin densities can be related to hyperfine coupling constants via the McConnell equation, which will be considered shortly. Although more sophisticated rationalizations of the success of the method are possible, it seems apparent that any theory which correctly treats molecular symmetry and topology has dealt with the most important aspects of the calculation.

The use of doubly occupied orbitals except for "the unpaired electron" means that Hückel theory cannot give any negative spin densities. These are known to be necessary for a qualitatively correct description in some cases. A solution to this problem is provided by the McLachlan modification of the Hückel method, giving it a spin-polarized character.

McLachlan [118] developed expressions for the spin density by making a first-order perturbation approximation to the effect of spin polarization within the Pariser–Parr theory. He then further approximated the results in terms of Hückel theory, and it is in this form that the method is normally used. A Hückel calculation is done and the expansion coefficients C_{or} for the singly occupied MO obtained. The Hückel parameters are then modified by adding to the rth diagonal matrix element $2\lambda C_{or}^2\beta$, where β is the usual Hückel parameter (the off-diagonal matrix element between bonded carbon atoms) and λ is a new parameter usually taken to have the value 1.2.

A "spin-polarized" function is then constructed by using the original Hückel MO's for the β-spin electrons but those obtained with the modified parameters for the α-spin electrons. Spin densities of either sign can then result.

Pariser–Parr–Pople Theory

A considerable advance over Hückel theory can be made by considering electron–electron interactions explicitly, although approximately. Such a treatment for pi electrons was developed by Pariser and Parr and modified by Pople.‡ The result is the PPP method, which is an approximate SCF method.

The basis set in the PPP method consists of one p-pi orbital on each atom participating in the pi system. Only pi electrons are considered explicitly. Their interaction with electrons of the sigma system as well as kinetic energy and nuclear attraction terms are included in an effective, one-electron operator. The matrix elements of this operator are treated as parameters to be evaluated from experimental data. As in Hückel theory, off-diagonal one-electron matrix elements between orbitals on atoms not bonded to each other are taken to be zero. Two-electron integrals involving pi orbitals are considered explicitly in a zero-differential-overlap approximation. Any integral in which a charge distribution for one electron is on two centers is set to zero. Only one- and two-center Coulomb integrals remain. These are evaluated by a variety of methods leading to a smoothly varying value as a function of internuclear distance.

Since the PPP method is an SCF method with explicit consideration of electron–electron interactions, spin polarized [5,194], spin-extended [76], or CI calculations can be done.

McConnell and Related Equations

One of the problems for pi-electron theories is to explain contact hyperfine interactions with nuclei in the molecular plane. In an all-electron treatment this is provided by spin polarization of sigma orbitals. When sigma orbitals

‡ Many of the relevant papers are preprinted, and a discussion presented, in Ref. [153].

are not explicitly considered, it must be treated separately. A very important relationship in the theory of pi-electron radicals has been the McConnell equation [114–116,119].‡ In its simplest form this is

$$a_{\mathrm{H}}^{i} = Q\rho_i^{\pi} \tag{13-3}$$

where a_{H}^{i} is the isotropic hyperfine coupling constant of proton i, ρ_i^{π} is the atomic orbital spin density in the 2p orbital on the carbon to which H_i is bonded, and Q is a constant with a value of about -22 to -27 G. (An energy unit should be used but the field strength unit is more common.) Similar equations relate isotropic coupling constants of other nuclei in the plane, e.g., ^{13}C, ^{14}N, to pi-electron spin densities [93,137]. In general, the form is

$$a_{\nu} = \mathrm{tr}\, \mathbf{Q}^{\nu}\boldsymbol{\rho}^{\pi}, \tag{13-4}$$

where $\boldsymbol{\rho}^{\pi}$ is a pi-electron AO spin density matrix. Only terms in $\mathbf{Q}^{\nu}$ whose indices label atoms in the immediate vicinity of nucleus ν make a significant contribution. We will consider here the form and origin of such relationships. A simple example will be followed by a more general treatment. Evaluation of parameters will not be done, however, for reasons to be discussed later.

Let us first consider a system of three electrons and three orbitals. We denote the orbitals by σ, σ', and π, and suppose that the ground state wave function is reasonably well approximated by a function of restricted SCF form

$$\Phi_1 = \mathscr{A}\sigma(q)\bar{\sigma}(2)\pi(3). \tag{13-5}$$

(A bar over the orbital indicates β spin, no bar indicates α spin.) If a CI calculation is done, the function will be of the form given in Eq. (11-137) or (11-138), where we identify σ with a, π with b, and σ' with c. We expect that $C_1 \sim 1$ and $C_2, C_3, C_4 \ll 1$. The spin density will have a pi part, $\gamma_{\pi\pi}^{z}$, and a sigma part $\gamma_{\sigma\sigma}^{z}$, $\gamma_{\sigma\sigma'}^{z}$, $\gamma_{\sigma'\sigma}^{z}$, and $\gamma_{\sigma'\sigma'}^{z}$. The matrix elements are related to the CI expansion coefficients in Table 11-5. Only the sigma part of $\boldsymbol{\gamma}^{z}$ can contribute to the contact hyperfine interactions of nuclei in the molecular plane, and since $C_4^2, C_3C_4, C_2C_4 \ll C_1C_4$, the dominant part of $\boldsymbol{\gamma}^{z}$ (sigma) is

$$\gamma_{\sigma\sigma'}^{z} = \gamma_{\sigma'\sigma}^{z} \simeq (\sqrt{6}/3)C_1C_4. \tag{13-5}$$

The value of C_4 can be estimated by perturbation theory, using, e.g., the definitions of H_0 and V of Eqs. (11-140). To first order

$$C_4 \simeq \frac{\langle\Phi_4|V|\Phi_1\rangle}{E_1^{(0)} - E_4^{(0)}}, \tag{13-6}$$

‡ For additional references, see [119,137].

where

$$\Phi_4 = (1/\sqrt{6})\mathscr{A}[\sigma\bar{\sigma}'\pi + \bar{\sigma}\sigma'\pi - 2\sigma\sigma'\bar{\pi}] \tag{13-7}$$

and

$$\begin{aligned} H_0\Phi_1 &= E_1^{(0)}\Phi_1, \qquad E_1^{(0)} = 2\varepsilon_\sigma + \varepsilon_\pi, \\ H^0\Phi_4 &= E_4^{(0)}\Phi_4, \qquad E_4^{(0)} = \varepsilon_\sigma + \varepsilon_\pi + \varepsilon_{\sigma'}. \end{aligned} \tag{13-8}$$

The matrix element $\langle\Phi_4|V|\Phi_1\rangle$ can be evaluated in a completely straightforward way. All the one-electron terms cancel out and there remains

$$\langle\Phi_4|V|\Phi_1\rangle = (3/\sqrt{6})\langle\sigma(1)\pi(2)|(1/r_{12})|\pi(1)\sigma'(2)\rangle. \tag{13-9}$$

If the pi orbital is expanded in terms of $2p_z$ AO's on various centers, denoted by p_i,

$$\pi = \sum_i A_i p_i, \tag{13-10}$$

one finds for positions in the plane

$$\gamma^z(\mathbf{r}) \sim \frac{1}{2}\frac{\sigma(\mathbf{r})\sigma'(\mathbf{r})}{\varepsilon_\sigma - \varepsilon_{\sigma'}} \sum_{i,j} \langle\sigma(1)p_i(2)|\frac{1}{r_{12}}|p_j(1)\sigma'(2)\rangle A_i A_j. \tag{13-11}$$

But A_iA_j is just the i, j element of the zero order, pi-electron spin density matrix. If σ and σ' are localized orbitals in the same region of space, e.g., a CH bond, it can be seen that the two electron "exchange" integral will be small unless $i = j$ and p_i is in that same region. A relationship of the simple McConnell form results. The presence of additional, doubly occupied sigma or pi orbitals will not affect the essential features of this argument. Rather than pursuing it farther on this basis, however, let us move on to a more general treatment. (A similar but not quite as rigorous approach is used by McLachlan, Dearman, and Lefebvre [119].)

In order for the problem to be well defined, we must have some form of zero-order description in which there is no spin density in the sigma system. We thus take [96,121,122,128,129]

$$\Psi^{(0)}(1,\ldots,N) = \mathscr{A}^{(N,n)}\Sigma_0(1,\ldots,n)\Pi_0(n+1,\ldots,N). \tag{13-12}$$

Here Σ_0 is a normalized, antisymmetric singlet function for an even number, n, of electrons and Π_0 is a normalized, antisymmetric function for $N - n$ electrons that is either an eigenfunction of $\mathscr{S}^2$ and $\mathscr{S}_z$ with the same quantum numbers S and M which characterize the overall state, or not an $\mathscr{S}^2$ eigenfunction (e.g., spin polarized) in which case $\Psi^{(0)}$ is also not an $\mathscr{S}^2$ eigenfunction. The operator $\mathscr{A}^{(N,n)}$ antisymmetrizes and renormalizes the product in a way to be considered shortly. We think of Σ_0 and Π_0 as being the first members of two sets of orthonormal functions $\{\Sigma_i\}$ and $\{\Pi_j\}$,

$$\langle\Sigma_i|\Sigma_k\rangle = \delta_{ik}, \qquad \langle\Pi_j|\Pi_l\rangle = \delta_{jl}. \tag{13-13}$$

Each Σ_i is expressible as a single configuration or a linear combination of configurations made up entirely of sigma spin orbitals. Each Π_j is similarly expressible in terms of pi spin orbitals. Because of this Σ_i and Π_j are strongly orthogonal

$$\int \Sigma_i(\ldots, x_p, \ldots)\Pi_j(\ldots, x_p, \ldots)\, dx_p \equiv 0, \tag{13-14}$$

where x_p stands for the space and spin coordinates of any one electron appearing in both Σ_i and Π_j.

The "true" wave function (i.e., the best function available within the given basis) is expressed as

$$\Psi = \sum_{i,j,\kappa} C_{ij}^{(\kappa)}\Phi_{ij}^{(\kappa)}, \tag{13-15}$$

where

$$\Phi_{ij}^{(\kappa)} = \mathscr{A}^{(N,n-2\kappa)}\Sigma_i^{(\kappa)}\Pi_j^{(\kappa)} \tag{13-16}$$

with $\Sigma_i^{(\kappa)}$ a function for $n - 2\kappa$ electrons and $\Pi_j^{(\kappa)}$ a function for $N - n + 2\kappa$ electrons. If $\mathscr{S}^2$ eigenfunctions are involved

$$\Phi_{ij}^{(\kappa)} = \mathscr{A}^{(N,n-2\kappa)}\left[\sum_{\mu} (S_i S_j SM \mid S_1 \mu S_2 M - \mu)\Sigma_i^{(\kappa)}(S_i, \mu)\Pi_j^{(\kappa)}(S_j, M - \mu)\right]. \tag{13-17}$$

In this expansion S_i is the spin quantum number for $\Sigma_i^{(\kappa)}$, and S_j that for $\Pi_j^{(\kappa)}$; the sum is over m-type quantum numbers; and the quantities in parentheses are Clebsch–Gordan coefficients. In a typical situation Σ_0 and Π_0 might be single-configuration SCF functions and the $\Sigma_i^{(\kappa)}$ and $\Pi_j^{(\kappa)}$ other configurations built up from a set of orthonormal orbitals, but either Σ_0 or Π_0 or both could be of CI type, with $\Sigma_i^{(\kappa)}$ and $\Pi_j^{(\kappa)}$ other orthonormal linear combinations of configurations. The only necessary restrictions are that Σ_0 be a singlet and that Eqs. (13-13) and (13-14) are satisfied.

The index κ can assume both positive and negative values, such that $n - 2\kappa$ and $N - n + 2\kappa$ are both nonnegative. The number of electrons in the pi part (or sigma part) can change only by an even number 2κ, because the overall function Ψ has a definite symmetry with respect to reflection in the molecular plane. If $N - n$ is odd, $\Psi \to -\Psi$ on reflection; if $N - n$ is even, $\Psi \to \Psi$. Each term in the expansion must have the same behavior, which is determined by the number of electrons in the pi part. The superscript κ gives the number of electron pairs transferred between the sigma and pi parts relative to the numbers occurring in the dominant term $\Psi^{(0)}$. When $\kappa = 0$ it is suppressed, as in Σ_0 and Π_0.

In considering the one-electron reduced density matrix associated with Ψ, we will find that cross contributions between terms with different values of κ do not occur, because of the strong orthogonality of the sigma and pi functions. We will also use a perturbation estimate of the expansion coefficients and consider only the first-order corrections in the spin density. It follows that terms involving $\kappa \neq 0$, which can contribute to the spin density only in second or higher order, will be neglected. We will thus treat explicitly only terms with n electrons in the sigma part and $N - n$ electrons in the pi part of the wave function.

We consider next the operator $\mathscr{A}^{(N,n)}$, looking first at the antisymmetric projection operator

$$\mathscr{O}^N = (N!)^{-1} \sum_{\hat{P}} (-1)^p \hat{P}, \tag{13-18}$$

where P is a permutation of N indices, p its parity, and the sum extends over all $N!$ possible permutations. It is readily shown that $(\mathscr{O}^N)^2 = \mathscr{O}^N$ and $(\mathscr{O}^N)^\dagger = \mathscr{O}^N$. For any $\hat{P}$

$$\hat{P} = \hat{T}\hat{Q}\hat{R} \tag{13-19}$$

where $\hat{Q}$ is a permutation on the first n indices, $\hat{R}$ is a permutation on the last $N - n$ indices, and $\hat{T}$ is of the form

$$\hat{T} = (q_1, r_1)(q_2, r_2)\cdots, \tag{13-20}$$

where (q_i, r_i) transposes indices q_i and r_i and

$$1 \leq q_1 < q_2 < \cdots \leq n, \qquad n + 1 \leq r_1 < r_2 < \cdots \leq N. \tag{13-21}$$

The sum over all $\hat{P}$ is equivalent to independent sums over all $\hat{T}$, $\hat{Q}$, and $\hat{R}$ of the specified form (including any or all of these being the identity "do nothing" operation), and p is the sum of the parities t, q, and r of $\hat{T}$, $\hat{Q}$, and $\hat{R}$, respectively, so

$$\begin{aligned}\mathscr{O}^N &= (N!)^{-1} \sum_{\hat{Q}\hat{R}\hat{T}} (-1)^{q+r+t} \hat{T}\hat{Q}\hat{R} \\ &= (N!)^{-1} n!\,(N-n)! \left(\sum_{\hat{T}} (-1)^t \hat{T}\right)\left(\frac{1}{n!}\sum_{\hat{Q}} (-1)^q \hat{Q}\right)\left(\frac{1}{(N-n)!}\sum_{\hat{R}} (-1)^r \hat{R}\right) \\ &= \binom{N}{n}^{-1} \sum_{\hat{T}} (-1)^t \hat{T} \mathscr{O}^n \mathscr{O}^{N-n},\end{aligned} \tag{13-22}$$

it being understood that $\mathscr{O}^n$ acts on indices $1, \ldots, n$ while $\mathscr{O}^{N-n}$ acts on $n + 1, \ldots, N$. Since Σ_i and Π_j are already antisymmetric

$$\begin{aligned}&\mathscr{O}^N \Sigma_i(1, \ldots, N)\Pi_j(n + 1, \ldots, N) \\ &\qquad = \binom{N}{n}^{-1} \sum_{\hat{T}} (-1)^t \hat{T} \Sigma_i(1, \ldots, n)\Pi_j(n + 1, \ldots, N).\end{aligned} \tag{13-23}$$

Finally, let

$$\mathscr{A}^{(N,n)} = \binom{N}{n}^{1/2} \mathscr{O}^N. \tag{13-24}$$

Then

$$\begin{aligned}
&\langle \mathscr{A}^{(N,n)}\Sigma_i \Pi_j | \mathscr{A}^{(N,n)}\Sigma_i \Pi_j\rangle \\
&= \binom{N}{n}\langle \mathscr{O}^N\Sigma_i\Pi_j|\mathscr{O}^N\Sigma_i\Pi_j\rangle \\
&= \binom{N}{n}\langle \Sigma_i\Pi_j|(\mathscr{O}^N)^2\Sigma_i\Pi_j\rangle = \binom{N}{n}\langle\Sigma_i\Pi_j|\mathscr{O}^N\Sigma_i\Pi_j\rangle \\
&= \sum_{\hat{T}} (-1)^t \langle \Sigma_i\Pi_j|\hat{T}\Sigma_i\Pi_j\rangle \\
&= \langle\Sigma_i|\Sigma_i\rangle\langle\Pi_j|\Pi_j\rangle = 1.
\end{aligned} \tag{13-25}$$

The only term in the sum over $\hat{T}$ which contributes is the identity $\hat{T} = 1$, since all other terms give zero because of the strong orthogonality. The operator $\mathscr{A}^{(N,n)}$ thus provides normalized, antisymmetrized functions when acting on $\Sigma_i \Pi_j$ products, as required.

In the evaluation of the spin density associated with Ψ and the estimation of the coefficients C_{ij}, we will make use of one- and two-electron reduced transition density matrices

$$\gamma(ij, kl|1; 1') = N \int \Phi_{ij}(1, 2, \ldots, N)\Phi_{kl}^*(1', 2, \ldots, N)\, dx_2 \cdots dx_N,$$

$$\Gamma(ij, kl|1, 2; 1', 2') = \binom{N}{2} \int \Phi_{ij}(1, 2, 3, \ldots, N)\Phi_{kl}^*(1', 2', 3, \ldots, N)\, dx_3 \cdots dx_N. \tag{13-26}$$

We will consider explicitly only Φ's which are single products. If angular momentum coupling schemes are involved the required density matrices will be linear combinations of density matrices involving single products, and density matrix components differing only in the m quantum numbers of the states involved are proportional to each other. (See Tables 10-1 and 10-2.)

Before evaluating the transition density matrices we will find it convenient to divide the possible $\hat{T}$'s into various types and determine the number of terms of each type. The total number of $\hat{T}$'s is

$$\# = \sum_{u=0}^{\min(n, N-n)} \binom{n}{u}\binom{N-n}{u} = \binom{N}{n}. \tag{13-27}$$

The number of transpositions, u, can vary between 0 ($\hat{T} = 1$) and the maximum number possible, which is the smaller of n and $N - n$. The sum is of the form of a standard relationship among binomial coefficients (cf., e.g., Gradshteyn and Ryzhik [65, p.4]).

If we consider those $\hat{T}$ which do not involve the index 1, the number of possibilities is reduced to

$$\#(\text{not } 1) = \sum_{u=0}^{\min(n-1,N-n)} \binom{n-1}{u}\binom{N-n}{u} = \binom{N-1}{n-1} \tag{13-28}$$

with the same number, #(not 2), which do not involve the index 2 (but may involve 1). The number of $\hat{T}$'s not involving 1 or 2 is

$$\#(\text{not 1 or 2}) = \sum_{u=0}^{\min(n-2,N-n)} \binom{n-2}{u}\binom{N-n}{u} = \binom{N-2}{n-2}. \tag{13-29}$$

The number of $\hat{T}$'s involving 1 is the total number minus the number not involving 1

$$\#(\text{incl } 1) = \# - \#(\text{not } 1) = \binom{N}{n} - \binom{N-1}{n-1} = \binom{N-1}{n}, \tag{13-30}$$

and there are the same number, #(incl 2), involving 2. The number involving 1 but not 2 (or 2 but not 1) is

$$\begin{aligned}\#(\text{incl 1, not 2}) &= \#(\text{not } 2) - \#(\text{not 1 or 2})\\ &= \binom{N-1}{n-1} - \binom{N-2}{n-2} = \binom{N-2}{n-1}.\end{aligned} \tag{13-31}$$

Finally, the number of $\hat{T}$'s involving both 1 and 2 is

$$\begin{aligned}\#(\text{incl 1 and 2}) &= \#(\text{incl } 1) - \#(\text{incl 1, not 2})\\ &= \binom{N-1}{n} - \binom{N-2}{n-1} = \binom{N-2}{n}.\end{aligned} \tag{13-32}$$

We can now consider the one-electron reduced density matrix between any two functions of the form Φ_{ij}

$$\begin{aligned}\gamma(ij, kl|1, 1') &= N \int [\mathscr{A}^{(N,n)}\Sigma_i(1, 2, \ldots, n)\Pi_j(n+1, \ldots, N)]\\ &\quad \times [\mathscr{A}^{(N,n)}\Sigma_k(1', 2, \ldots, n)\Pi_l(n+1, \ldots, N)]^* dx_2 \cdots dx_N\\ &= N\binom{N}{n}^{-1} \int\left[\sum_{\hat{T}} (-1)^t \hat{T}\Sigma_i \Pi_j\right]\left[\sum_{\hat{T}'} (-1)^{t'} \hat{T}'\Sigma_k \Pi_l\right]^* dx_2 \cdots dx_N.\end{aligned} \tag{13-33}$$

We cannot make use of the Hermiticity and idempotency of $\mathcal{O}^N$ to get a single sum as in the normalization calculation because the integration here is incomplete. We note, however, that for terms with $\hat{T}' \neq \hat{T}$, at least two variables will be interchanged between Σ_k and Π_l relative to Σ_i and Π_j. At least one of these will be integrated over and the result will be zero. Only terms with $\hat{T}' = \hat{T}$ will contribute to γ.

Each term where $\hat{T}$ does not include 1 (and $\hat{T}' = \hat{T}$ does not include 1′) will lead to a contribution $n^{-1}\gamma^\sigma(ik|1;1')\delta_{kl}$, where

$$\gamma^\sigma(ik|1;1') = n\int \Sigma_i(1, 2, \ldots, n)\Sigma_k^*(1', 2, \ldots, n)\, dx_2 \cdots dx_N. \quad (13\text{-}34)$$

Those $\hat{T}' = \hat{T}$ which do include 1 (and 1′) contribute $\delta_{ik}(N-n)^{-1}\gamma^\pi(jl|1;1')$, where

$$\gamma^\pi(jl|1;1') = (N-n)\int \Pi_j(1, 2, \ldots, N-n) \times \Pi_l^*(1', 2, \ldots, N-n)\, dx_2 \cdots dx_{N-n}. \quad (13\text{-}35)$$

These contributions are to be multiplied by the common coefficient $N\binom{N}{n}^{-1}$, and each is multiplied by the number of times it appears, which is the relevant number of appropriate transpositions $\hat{T}$. We note that

$$N\binom{N}{n}^{-1}\binom{N-1}{n-1}n^{-1} = 1, \qquad N\binom{N}{n}^{-1}\binom{N-1}{n}(N-n)^{-1} = 1, \quad (13\text{-}36)$$

and thus

$$\gamma(ij, kl|1;1') = \gamma^\sigma(ik|1;1')\delta_{jl} + \delta_{ik}\gamma^\pi(jl|1;1'). \quad (13\text{-}37)$$

Exactly equivalent equations apply to the charge and spin density components of these density matrices, and only the first, or γ^σ, term will be of interest to us. (In general, $\gamma = \sum_\kappa \gamma^{(\kappa)}$, but we are considering only the lowest order, $\kappa = 0$ contribution.)

The evaluation of two-electron density matrices is more involved, since some terms with $\hat{T}' \neq \hat{T}$ do contribute. We will consider first the $\hat{T}' = \hat{T}$ part, however. The starting point is

$$\Gamma(ij, kl|1, 2; 1', 2') = \binom{N}{2}\binom{N}{n}^{-1}\int\left[\sum_{\hat{T}}(-1)^t\hat{T}\Sigma_i\Pi_j\right] \times \left[\sum_{\hat{T}'}(-1)^{t'}\hat{T}'\Sigma_k\Pi_l\right]^* dx_3 \cdots dx_N. \quad (13\text{-}38)$$

When $\hat{T}' = \hat{T}$ and neither 1 nor 2 (1′ nor 2′) is involved in the transposition, the contribution of the integral is $\binom{n}{2}^{-1}\Gamma^{\sigma}(ik|1, 2; 1', 2')\delta_{jl'}$, where

$$\Gamma^{\sigma}(ik|1, 2; 1', 2') = \binom{n}{2}\int \Sigma_i(1, 2, 3, \ldots, n)\Sigma_k^*(1', 2', 3, \ldots, n)\, dx_3 \cdots dx_n. \tag{13-39a}$$

Similarly, when $\hat{T}' = \hat{T}$ and both 1 and 2 (1′ and 2′) are involved, the contribution is $\delta_{ik}\binom{N-n}{2}^{-1}\Gamma^{\pi}(jl|1, 2; 1', 2')$, where

$$\Gamma^{\pi}(jl|1, 2; 1', 2') = \binom{N-n}{2}\int \Pi_j(1, 2, 3, \ldots, N-n)$$
$$\times\, \Pi_l^*(1', 2', 3, \ldots, N-n)\, dx_3 \cdots dx_{N-n}. \tag{13-39b}$$

It is also possible to have $\hat{T}' = \hat{T}$ with each transposition involving only one of the pair 1, 2 (or 1′, 2′). The contribution then is

$$n^{-1}(N-n)^{-1}\gamma^{\sigma}(ik|1, 1')\gamma^{\pi}(jl|2, 2')$$

or

$$n^{-1}(N-n)^{-1}\gamma^{\sigma}(ik|2; 2')\gamma^{\pi}(jl|1; 1').$$

The number of times each of these $\hat{T}' = \hat{T}$ combinations occur is just the relevant number of transpositions possible.

A few terms with $\hat{T}' \neq \hat{T}$ must also be considered. In particular, if $\hat{T}$ includes the transposition $(1, r)$ where $n + 1 \leq r \leq N$ and does not include any transposition involving 2, and if $\hat{T}'$ is the same as $\hat{T}$ except that in place of $(1, r)$ it includes $(2', r)$, then there will be a contribution $-n^{-1}(N-n)^{-1} \times \gamma^{\sigma}(ik|2; 1')\gamma^{\pi}(jl|1; 2')$. The minus sign occurs because the overall permutations involved differ by the (odd-parity) single interchange (1, 2). Similarly, the roles of 1 and 2 can be interchanged to get contributions $-n^{-1}(N-n)^{-1} \times \gamma^{\sigma}(ik|1; 2')\gamma^{\pi}(jl|2; 1')$. The transpositions $\hat{T}'$ and $\hat{T}$ are the same except in the one transposition specified, for a nonzero contribution, and the number of occurrences of a contribution of either type is thus again $\binom{N-2}{n-1}$.

If $\hat{T}'$ and $\hat{T}$ differ other than in the way just discussed, variables to be integrated over will occur in Σ in one product and in Π in the other, so strong orthogonality will give zero. It might seem that $\hat{T}'$ and $\hat{T}$ could differ only in that one includes $(1, r)(2, r')$ where the other includes $(1, r')(2, r)$. Integration would not give zero in such a case, but in fact it cannot occur since $r < r'$ and $r' < r$ would be simultaneously required [cf. Eqs. (13-21)].

When the contributions to Γ are added together, each multiplied by the number of times it occurs and by the common factor $\binom{N}{2}\binom{N}{n}^{-1}$, the result is

$$\begin{aligned}\Gamma(ij, kl|1, 2; 1', 2') = {} & \Gamma^{\sigma}(ik|1, 2; 1', 2')\delta_{jl} + \delta_{ik}\Gamma^{\pi}(jl|1, 2; 1', 2') \\ & + \tfrac{1}{2}[\gamma^{\sigma}(ik|1, 1')\gamma^{\pi}(jl|2, 2') \\ & + \gamma^{\sigma}(ik|2, 2')\gamma^{\pi}(jl|1, 1') \\ & - \gamma^{\sigma}(ik|1; 2')\gamma^{\pi}(jl|2, 1') \\ & - \gamma^{\sigma}(ik|2; 1')\gamma^{\pi}(jl|1, 2')]. \end{aligned} \tag{13-40}$$

This result is valid for $\kappa = 0$. Exactly similar terms would arise for other values of κ. In additon, Γ (but not γ) can include contributions from cross terms where the two factors are associated with different values of κ. Because these terms do not enter the treatment of the first-order spin density, they will not be considered in detail. We will make use of the expression above shortly, in our evaluation of the expansion coefficients C_{ij}.

The best wave function available within the given basis set would be determined by constructing a matrix $\mathbf{H}$ with elements

$$H_{ij,kl} = \int \Phi_{ij}^{*} \mathscr{H}_0 \Phi_{kl} \, d\tau \tag{13-41}$$

(recall that $\mathscr{H}_0$ is a spin-free operator) and taking the $\{C_{ij}\}$ that form the eigenvector of H_0 associated with the lowest eigenvalue. To avoid the necessity of carrying the additional index κ, we now assume it to be implicit in the indices i and j, i.e., different sets of i's and j's apply for each κ. In order to define a perturbation problem without specifying the precise form of the Σ_i and Π_j, we simply define matrices $\mathbf{H}^{(0)}$ and $\mathbf{V}$ as the diagonal and off-diagonal parts, respectively, of $\mathbf{H}$:

$$H_{ij,kl}^{(0)} = H_{ij,ij}\delta_{ik}\delta_{jl}, \qquad \mathbf{V} = \mathbf{H} - \mathbf{H}^{(0)} \qquad (V_{ij,ij} = 0). \tag{13-42}$$

Each coefficient C_{ij} is assumed to have a perturbation expansion

$$C_{ij} = C_{ij}^{(0)} + C_{ij}^{(1)} + C_{ij}^{(2)} + \cdots. \tag{13-43}$$

We are assuming that the single term $\Psi^{(0)}$ of Eq. (13-12) is a good approximation, and thus take

$$C_{ij}^{(0)} = \delta_{i0}\delta_{j0}. \tag{13-44}$$

The zero-order energies consistent with Eq. (13-42) are

$$E_{ij}^{(0)} = H_{ij,ij} \tag{13-45}$$

and we define

$$\Delta E_{ij} = E_{00}^{(0)} - E_{ij}^{(0)}. \tag{13-46}$$

From conventional perturbation theory

$$C_{ij}^{(1)} = V_{ij,00}/\Delta E_{ij}$$
$$C_{ij}^{(2)} = \sum_{k,l(\neq i,j)} \frac{V_{ij,kl} V_{kl,00}}{\Delta E_{kl}\, \Delta E_{ij}} - \frac{1}{2} \sum_{k,l(\neq i,j)} \frac{|V_{00,kl}|^2}{(\Delta E_{kl})^2} \delta_{i0} \delta_{j0} \tag{13-47}$$
$$\vdots$$

The total, one-electron reduced density matrix can be divided into spin and charge density components and each of these separated into sigma and pi parts. Finally, each part of each component is given as a sum of contributions of various orders.

$$\begin{aligned} \gamma(1;1') &= \sum_{i,j} \sum_{k,l} C_{ij} C_{kl}^* \gamma(ij, kl \,|\, 1;1') \\ &= \gamma_\sigma(1;1') + \gamma_\pi(1;1'), \end{aligned} \tag{13-48}$$

$$\begin{aligned} \gamma^\sigma(1;1') &= \sum_{ij} \sum_{kl} C_{ij} C_{kl}^* \gamma^\sigma(ik \,|\, 1;1') \delta_{jl} \\ &= \sum_{ik} \left(\sum_j C_{ij} C_{kj}^* \right) \gamma^\sigma(ik \,|\, 1;1'), \end{aligned} \tag{13-49}$$

and of particular interest to us the spin density component $\gamma_\sigma^{\mathrm{z}}$, with

$$\gamma_\sigma^{\mathrm{z}} = \gamma_\sigma^{\mathrm{z}(0)} + \gamma_\sigma^{\mathrm{z}(1)} + \gamma_\sigma^{\mathrm{z}(2)} + \cdots. \tag{13-50}$$

Substituting the expansion of C_{ij} and collecting terms by order we find

$$\begin{aligned} \gamma_\sigma^{\mathrm{z}(0)}(\mathbf{r}_1;\mathbf{r}_1') &= \sum_{ik} \left(\sum_j C_{ij}^{(0)} C_{kj}^{(0)*} \right) \gamma^{\sigma \mathrm{z}}(ik \,|\, \mathbf{r}_1;\mathbf{r}_1') \\ \gamma_\sigma^{\mathrm{z}(1)}(\mathbf{r}_1;\mathbf{r}_1') &= \sum_{ik} \left(\sum_j [C_{ij}^{(0)} C_{kj}^{(1)*} + C_{ij}^{(1)} C_{kj}^{(0)*}] \right) \gamma^{\sigma \mathrm{z}}(ik \,|\, \mathbf{r}_1;\mathbf{r}_1') \\ \gamma_\sigma^{\mathrm{z}(2)}(\mathbf{r}_1;\mathbf{r}_1') &= \sum_{ik} \left(\sum_j [C_{ij}^{(0)} C_{kj}^{(2)*} + C_{ij}^{(1)} C_{kj}^{(1)*} + C_{ij}^{(2)} C_{kj}^{(0)*}] \right) \gamma^{\sigma \mathrm{z}}(ik \,|\, \mathbf{r}_1;\mathbf{r}_1') \\ &\vdots \end{aligned} \tag{13-51}$$

Substitution of the form of the $C_{ij}^{(0)}$ from Eq. (13-44) then gives

$$\gamma_\sigma^{\mathrm{z}(0)}(\mathbf{r}_1, \mathbf{r}_1') = \gamma^{\sigma \mathrm{z}}(00 \,|\, \mathbf{r}_1, \mathbf{r}_1') = 0. \tag{13-52}$$

The zero results from the fact that, by assumption, Σ_0 is a singlet state and thus its spin density vanishes identically.

Similarly, the first-order contribution becomes

$$\gamma_\sigma^{\mathrm{z}(1)}(\mathbf{r}_1;\mathbf{r}_1') = \sum_{i(\text{triplet}, \kappa=0)} \{C_{i0}^{(1)*} \gamma^{\sigma \mathrm{z}}(0i \,|\, \mathbf{r}_1;\mathbf{r}_1') + C_{i0}^{(1)} \gamma^{\sigma \mathrm{z}}(i0 \,|\, \mathbf{r}_1;\mathbf{r}_1')\}. \tag{13-53}$$

We note that only the zero-order pi state ($j = 0$) is involved, and that only triplet sigma states with $\kappa = 0$ can have $\gamma^{\sigma z}(0i|\mathbf{r}_1;\mathbf{r}'_1)$ different from zero. (See Table 10-1 and Ref. [126].) The coefficients $C_{i0}^{(1)}$ are given in terms of matrix elements, and these can in turn be evaluated from the two-electron density matrices and reduced Hamiltonian $\mathscr{K}$ related to $\mathscr{H}_0$. Since $\mathscr{H}_0$ and $\mathscr{K}$ are spin free, only the spinless or charge density components are required. We are interested in $i \neq 0$ so the Γ^{π} term in Eq. (13-40) drops out, and Σ_i is a triplet state while Σ_0 is a singlet, so $\Gamma^{\sigma,0}(i0|\mathbf{r}_1, \mathbf{r}_2;\mathbf{r}'_1, \mathbf{r}'_2) = 0$. The γ's can be expressed in terms of γ^0 and γ^z and the Γ^0 component extracted. The result is that the $\gamma^{\pi 0}$ contributions cancel out, with $\gamma^{\sigma 0}(i0|\mathbf{r}_1;\mathbf{r}'_1) \equiv 0$, and

$$\Gamma^0(ij00|\mathbf{r}_1\mathbf{r}_2;\mathbf{r}'_1\mathbf{r}'_2) = -\tfrac{1}{4}[\gamma^{\sigma z}(i0|\mathbf{r}_1;\mathbf{r}'_2)\gamma^{\pi z}(j0|\mathbf{r}_2;\mathbf{r}'_1) + \gamma^{\sigma z}(i0|\mathbf{r}_2;\mathbf{r}'_1)\gamma^{\pi z}(j0|\mathbf{r}_1;\mathbf{r}'_2)], \qquad (13\text{-}54)$$

i.e., only the exchangelike terms survive. Because of the strong orthogonality

$$\int \gamma^{\sigma z}(\mathbf{r}_1;\mathbf{r}_2)\gamma^{\pi z}(\mathbf{r}_2,\mathbf{r}'_1)\,d\mathbf{r}_1 = \int \gamma^{\sigma z}(\mathbf{r}_2;\mathbf{r}'_1)\gamma^{\pi z}(\mathbf{r}_1,\mathbf{r}_2)\,d\mathbf{r}_2 = 0, \qquad (13\text{-}55)$$

and the one-electron part of $\mathscr{K}$ drops out. The two-electron part of $\mathscr{K}$ is just the multiplicative operator $1/r_{12}$, and thus

$$\begin{aligned} C_{i0}^{(1)} &= -\frac{1}{4\Delta E_{i0}}\int [\gamma^{\sigma z}(i0|\mathbf{r}_1;\mathbf{r}_2)\gamma^{\pi z}(00|\mathbf{r}_2,\mathbf{r}_1) \\ &\quad + \gamma^{\sigma z}(i0|\mathbf{r}_2;\mathbf{r}_1)\gamma^{\pi z}(00|\mathbf{r}_1;\mathbf{r}_2)]\frac{1}{r_{12}}\,d\mathbf{r}_1\,d\mathbf{r}_2 \\ &= -\frac{1}{2\Delta E_{i0}}\int \gamma^{\sigma z}(i0|\mathbf{r}_1;\mathbf{r}_2)\gamma^{\pi z}(00|\mathbf{r}_2;\mathbf{r}_1)\frac{1}{r_{12}}\,d\mathbf{r}_1\,d\mathbf{r}_2. \end{aligned} \qquad (13\text{-}56)$$

We can freely relabel variables of integration in any one term, since $r_{21} = r_{12}$, and use the fact that $\gamma(ij|1;1') = \gamma(ji|1';1)^*$. It follows that, finally,

$$\begin{aligned} \gamma_\sigma^{z(1)}(\mathbf{r};\mathbf{r}') &= -\tfrac{1}{2}\sum_{i\,(\text{triplet},\,\kappa=0)} (\Delta E_{i0})^{-1}[\gamma^{\sigma z}(0i|\mathbf{r},\mathbf{r}')\int d\mathbf{r}_1\,d\mathbf{r}_2\frac{1}{r_{12}} \\ &\quad \times \gamma^{\sigma z}(0i|\mathbf{r}_1;\mathbf{r}_2)\gamma^{\pi z}(00|\mathbf{r}_2;\mathbf{r}_1) \\ &\quad + \gamma^{\sigma z}(i0|\mathbf{r},\mathbf{r}')\int d\mathbf{r}_1\,d\mathbf{r}_2\frac{1}{r_{12}}\gamma^{\sigma z}(i0|\mathbf{r}_1;\mathbf{r}_2)\gamma^{\pi z}(00|\mathbf{r}_2;\mathbf{r}_1)] \\ &= \int \mathscr{Q}(\mathbf{r},\mathbf{r}';\mathbf{r}_1,\mathbf{r}_2)\gamma^{\pi z}(00|\mathbf{r}_2;\mathbf{r}_1)\,d\mathbf{r}_1\,d\mathbf{r}_2, \end{aligned} \qquad (13\text{-}57)$$

where

$$\mathcal{Q}(\mathbf{r}, \mathbf{r}'; \mathbf{r}_1, \mathbf{r}_2) = -\frac{1}{2r_{12}} \sum_{i\,(\text{triplet}, \kappa=0)} (\Delta E_{i0})^{-1}$$

$$\times [\gamma^{\sigma z}(0i|\mathbf{r}, \mathbf{r}')\gamma^{\sigma z}(0i|\mathbf{r}_1, \mathbf{r}_2) + \gamma^{\sigma z}(i0|\mathbf{r}, \mathbf{r}')\gamma^{\sigma z}(i0|\mathbf{r}_1, \mathbf{r}_2)]. \tag{13-58}$$

This is a generalized form of the McConnell relationship, giving the first-order sigma spin density matrix as an integral transform of the zero-order, pi spin density matrix.

We look next at

$$a_\nu = \frac{8\pi}{3} g_e' \beta g_\nu \beta_N \frac{1}{2S} \gamma^z(\mathbf{r}_\nu; \mathbf{r}_\nu) \tag{13-59}$$

and note that for a nucleus lying in the molecular plane $\gamma^z(\mathbf{r}_\nu; \mathbf{r}_\nu) = \gamma^{\sigma z}(\mathbf{r}_\nu; \mathbf{r}_\nu)$. The pi orbital basis set $\{p_i\}$ is introduced and $\gamma^{\pi z}$ expanded as

$$\gamma^{\pi z}(00|\mathbf{r}, \mathbf{r}') = \sum_{j,k} \rho_{jk}^\pi p_j(\mathbf{r}) p_k^*(\mathbf{r}'). \tag{13-60}$$

We then find that, to first order, we can write

$$a_\nu = \sum_{j,k} Q_{kj}^\nu \rho_{jk}^\pi = \operatorname{tr} \mathbf{Q}^\nu \boldsymbol{\rho}^\pi, \tag{13-61}$$

where

$$Q_{kj}^\nu = -\frac{2\pi g_e' \beta g_\nu \beta_N}{S} \sum_{i\,(\text{triplet}, \kappa=0)} \left\{ \frac{1}{\Delta E_{i0}} \right.$$

$$\times [\gamma^{\sigma z}(0i|\mathbf{r}_\nu; \mathbf{r}_\nu) \int d\mathbf{r}_1\, d\mathbf{r}_2 \frac{1}{r_{12}} \gamma^{\sigma z}(0i|\mathbf{r}_1; \mathbf{r}_2) p_j(\mathbf{r}_2) p_k^*(\mathbf{r}_1)$$

$$\left. + \gamma^{\sigma z}(i0|\mathbf{r}_\nu; \mathbf{r}_\nu) \int d\mathbf{r}_1\, d\mathbf{r}_2 \frac{1}{r_{12}} \gamma^{\sigma z}(i0|\mathbf{r}_1; \mathbf{r}_2) p_j(\mathbf{r}_2) p_k^*(\mathbf{r}_1)] \right\}. \tag{13-62}$$

This is the standard, general form of the McConnell equation. It should be noted that the expansion coefficients ρ_{jk}^π are equal to the matrix elements

$$\gamma_{jk}^{\pi z} = \int p_j^*(\mathbf{r}_1) \gamma^{\pi z}(00|\mathbf{r}_1; \mathbf{r}_1') p_k(\mathbf{r}_1')\, d\mathbf{r}_1\, d\mathbf{r}_1' \tag{13-63}$$

only if the basis set $\{p_j\}$ is orthonormal.

An extension of this treatment to second and higher order would be possible. It is found, however, that the higher-order terms in $\gamma^{\sigma z}$ are no longer proportional to $\gamma^{\pi z}$ for the initial state; terms involving $\gamma^{\pi z}(j0|\mathbf{r}; \mathbf{r}')$ or $\gamma^{\sigma z}(jl|\mathbf{r}; \mathbf{r}')$ for $j, l \neq 0$ appear, products of $\gamma^{\pi z}$'s are involved, and other terms do not contain $\gamma^{\pi z}$. The conclusion is that the McConnell form is not valid beyond first order. The first-order approximation will be good, however, if $\Psi^{(0)}$ provides a good enough description of the system.

To relate the result obtained here to the simple form of the McConnell equation, we must show that the Q_{kj}^{ν} are small unless j and k label p function(s) on the atom(s) nearest ν. This requires further assumptions about the form of Σ_0 and Σ_i. A quantitative treatment will not be given here, but a qualitative argument suffices to make the point. Suppose that Σ_0 and Σ_i are single configuration functions expressed in terms of localized orbitals $\sigma_1, \sigma_2, \ldots$. Such localized orbitals will look much like inner core orbitals, bond orbitals, or possibly lone pair orbitals. The ground state function Σ_0 will contain $n/2$ orbitals, each doubly occupied. To obtain an excited, triplet state we transfer an electron from one occupied orbital σ_i to an excited (not occupied in Σ_0) orbital σ_i' and take the triplet coupling

$$\sigma_i\sigma_i'(1/\sqrt{2})(\alpha\beta - \beta\alpha) \rightarrow (1/\sqrt{2})(\sigma_i\sigma_i' + \sigma_i'\sigma)\begin{cases}\alpha\alpha,\\ (1/\sqrt{2})(\alpha\beta + \beta\alpha),\\ \beta\beta.\end{cases}$$

In such a case the transition spin density matrix will involve only σ_i and σ_i'

$$\gamma^{\sigma z}(i0\,|\,\mathbf{r}, \mathbf{r}'),\ \gamma^{\sigma z}(0i\,|\,\mathbf{r}, \mathbf{r}') \propto \sigma_i(\mathbf{r})\sigma_i'(\mathbf{r}'),\ \sigma_i(\mathbf{r}')\sigma_i'(\mathbf{r}).$$

Since these orbitals are localized, $\gamma^{\sigma z}(i0\,|\,\mathbf{r}_\nu; \mathbf{r}_\nu)$ will be very small unless σ_i and σ_i' are localized in the vicinity of nucleus ν. The integrals, on the other hand, become things like

$$\int p_k^*(\mathbf{r})\sigma_i^*(\mathbf{r}_1)\frac{1}{r_{12}}\sigma_i'(\mathbf{r}_1)p_j(\mathbf{r}_2)\,d\mathbf{r}_1\,d\mathbf{r}_2,$$

which is very small unless σ_i is localized near p_j and σ_i' is localized near p_k. It thus follows that Q_{jk}^{ν} will be very small unless p_j and p_k are near nucleus ν. Numerical estimates suggest that "near" means centered on nucleus ν or on a nearest neighbor.

The simplest form of the equation occurs in Eq. (13-62) when ν labels a hydrogen nucleus, p_j is a p-pi orbital on the carbon atom to which this atom is bonded, and $Q_{kl}^{\nu} = Q_{jj}^{\nu}\delta_{jk}\delta_{jl} = Q$. To the extent that "all CH bonds are alike," σ_i in the previous treatment can be taken as the CH bonding orbital, σ_i' the corresponding antibonding orbital, and ΔE_{i0} a "bond excitation energy," all approximately the same for any CH bond where C is part of the pi system. Then Q would be a universal constant. This is found to be not quite the case, and Q is a variable constant.

A major problem underlying any discussion of these phenomena is the inadequacy of the minimal-basis description of the pi system. Additional approximations may also be made in the determination of π_0. These can be avoided by considering symmetric, R-membered ring molecules in which (for orthonormal p_j) $\rho^{\pi}_{jj} = 1/R$ by symmetry. One can also appeal to pairing theorems for even-alternant hydrocarbons, which show that for quite general Π_0, corresponding ρ^{π}_{jj} should be the same for anion and cation radicals in these systems. It is found experimentally that corresponding anion and cation coupling constants differ, and that Q varies with R in symmetry-determined ring cases.

Two corrections have been proposed, either of which is capable of "explaining" the anion–cation result. The bond spin densities ρ^{π}_{jk} (carbon atoms j and k bonded) are equal in magnitude but opposite in sign for anions and cations for even-alternant hydrocarbons. An expression [61]

$$a^j_{\mathrm{H}} = Q\rho^{\pi}_{jj} + Q' \sum_{k\,(\text{bonded to } j)} \rho^{\pi}_{jk} \qquad (13\text{-}64)$$

will thus give different a values for anion and cation radicals. It is a first step toward the more complete expression of Eq. (13-61). Alternatively, a first correction can be made for the inadequacy of the basis set. The orbital exponents of the p-pi orbitals should be optimized, and the optimum values will differ for different cases. An estimate of this effect suggests a correction proportional to the pi-electron excess charge density

$$q_j = \gamma^{\pi 0}_{jj} - 1, \qquad (13\text{-}65)$$

where $\boldsymbol{\gamma}^{\pi 0}$ is the matrix of expansion coefficients for the pi-electron charge density. The McConnell relationship is then generalized to [38,183]

$$a^j_{\mathrm{H}} = (Q + Kq_j)\rho^{\pi}_{jj}. \qquad (13\text{-}66)$$

Either of Eqs. (13-64) or (13-66) leads to a better correlation between calculated $\boldsymbol{\rho}^{\pi}$ and experimentally determined a_{H} values. In a similar way, hybrid orbitals used in the sigma basis will change with bond angles, and the ring results can be "understood."

For nuclei such as ^{13}C and ^{14}N, nearest neighbor effects must definitely be included; and arguments could be made for bond spin density, charge density, and hybridization corrections. Restrictive assumptions about wave function form, neglect of nonorthogonality, etc., become more important because there are often large terms with opposite signs, which tend to cancel.

In order to obtain theoretical values for the elements of $\mathbf{Q}^{\mathrm{v}}$, it is necessary to take explicit forms for Σ_0 and for the choice of both sigma and pi basis sets. The results, encouragingly, are in reasonable qualitative or semiquantitative agreement with parameters estimated from pi-electron calculations and experimental hyperfine coupling constants. Precise values depend on the model chosen [137]. Such calculations will not be presented here. If one is to work within the pi approximation at all, it seems more appropriate to use theory as a guide to the form of the relationship between a_v and $\boldsymbol{\rho}^{\pi}$, and then to choose parameters by fitting experimental data. In doing so, one is able to compensate in part for the inadequacies of the model. Estimates of the reliability of results must be based on experience rather than on any rigorous but approximate calculation. Any rigorously calculated, theoretical error bounds would surely be so widely spaced as to make the McConnell equation itself appear useless, which it is not.

Nuclei Not in the Plane

The discussion thus far has assumed a rigorous separability, based on symmetry, of sigma and pi functions. This is possible only if all nuclei lie in a plane. Often basically planar molecules have nonplanar substituents, one of the simplest being a methyl group, for example. Out-of-plane vibrations must also be considered even when the equilibrium positions of all nuclei do lie in a plane. Spin density at out-of-plane nuclei in pi radicals will be nonzero for several reasons.

Orbitals centered on hydrogen, or even on other nuclei with "saturated" bonds (e.g., the methyl C's in a *t*-butyle group) are not normally included in the expansion of "pi" orbitals even though these nuclei do not lie in the pi orbital nodal plane. Such exclusion is arbitrary, and nonzero coefficients will occur in a calculation when permitted. The result is the possibility of a direct spin density contribution at the nucleus in question. Such an effect is, for historical reasons, known as hyperconjugation. These same orbitals also participate in "sigma" functions since in fact there is no clear-cut sigma–pi separation. A spin polarization mechanism similar to that leading to the McConnell equation can also lead to nonzero spin densities.

In more complicated cases, the "conjugated" system itself may not be entirely planar. It is then most appropriate to use an all-electron (or at least all-valence-electron) method, rather than trying to force a "sigma–pi" separation and then introducing substantial corrections. In any case, in a discussion seeking to distinguish different "mechanisms" of spin density propagation, care must be taken to deal with concepts which can have model-independent definitions. A distinction between direct and spin polarization contributions based on eigenvalues of the spin density matrix is always possible and is not dependent on molecular symmetry.

Simple Valence Bond Treatments

We saw in Section 11 that the valence bond (VB) method provides an alternative approach to *a priori* calculations. It can also be used as the basis for semiempirical calculations. The principal advantage of the VB method is that VB functions can be identified with molecular "structures" involving electron pair bonds, and chemical intuition or experience invoked to suggest which terms will be the most important.

In simple cases, especially with saturated molecules, only one structure can be written without charge separation, long bonds, or other features that suggest the corresponding functions will make relatively small contributions. In slightly more complicated cases, more than one such structure is possible but only one linear combination of the appropriate symmetry is possible. In general, for a conjugated molecule, several symmetry-adapted structures that appear to be of reasonably comparable likelihood can be written, and a calculation must be performed to determine relative coefficients. Semiempirical methods for doing this exist,[‡] but they will not be considered here. *A priori* calculations show that ionic contributions may in fact be significant, and that semiempirical results may be misleading [149].

Despite the limitations involved in excluding ionic and other presumably important structures, the simplest VB approach provides a useful way to obtain a "back of an envelope," qualitative estimate of spin density distributions. Let us consider a few examples.

The methyl radical has only one simple structure

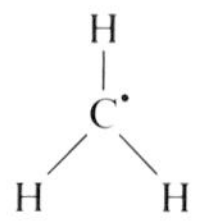

A corresponding VB function might be written

$$\Psi = C\mathscr{A}(1s)^2(\alpha\beta - \beta\alpha)h_a\sigma_a(\alpha\beta - \beta\alpha)h_b\sigma_b(\alpha\beta - \beta\alpha)h_c\sigma_c(\alpha\beta - \beta\alpha)p_z\alpha. \tag{13-67}$$

The orbitals are 1s on C, h_x a 1s on hydrogen x, σ_x an sp^2 hybrid on C pointed toward hydrogen x, and p_z a $2p_z$ on C. These orbitals are not all orthogonal, and their overlaps will appear in the normalization constant C. Of the other functions which might be written, the most important for us are those in which

$$h_x\sigma_x(\alpha\beta - \beta\alpha)p_z\alpha \rightarrow h_x\sigma_x p_z(\alpha\beta\alpha + \beta\alpha\alpha - 2\alpha\alpha\beta).$$

These are "spin polarization" terms which account for the hyperfine interaction with the protons.

Consider next the pi electrons of the allyl radical. The sigma system would be described by singlet-coupled electron pairs in the C atomic cores, and in C–C and C–H bonds made up of sp^2 orbitals on C's and 1s orbitals on H's.

[‡] For application to radical ions, see Schug, Brown, and Karplus [185].

Small contributions from triplet coupling in these cases describe spin polarization, but will not be explicitly considered. The pi system consists of three electrons. The two spin functions θ_a and θ_b of Eq. (11-51) correspond to the structures

(a) (b)

which are clearly appropriate but are not symmetry adapted. The sum $\theta_a + \theta_b = 1/\sqrt{2}(\alpha\alpha\beta - \beta\alpha\beta)$ corresponds to the long-bond structure

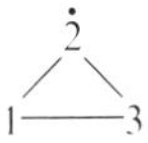

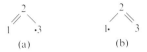

and is found to describe a higher energy state that is antisymmetric with respect to the symmetry operation of reflection in a plane perpendicular to the molecular plane and bisecting the 1–2–3 angle. The other linear combination

$$\theta_a - \theta_b = (1/\sqrt{2})(\alpha\alpha\beta + \beta\alpha\alpha - 2\alpha\beta\alpha) \tag{13-68}$$

describes the ground state which is symmetric with respect to this reflection.

We denote the normalized p-pi orbital on atom i by χ_i and write the VB wave function

$$\Psi = C\mathscr{A}\chi_1\chi_2\chi_3(\alpha\alpha\beta + \beta\alpha\alpha - 2\alpha\beta\alpha) \tag{13-69}$$

with C a normalization constant. The spin density matrix can then be expanded as

$$\gamma^z(\mathbf{r}, \mathbf{r}') = \sum_{i,j=1}^{3} \rho_{ij}\chi_i(\mathbf{r})\chi_j(\mathbf{r}'), \tag{13-70}$$

and it is found that

$$\rho_{1,1} = \rho_{3,3} = C^2(4 + 5S_{1,2}^2), \qquad \rho_{2,2} = -2C^2(1 - S_{1,3}^2), \tag{13-71}$$

where, for the nonorthogonal p orbitals,

$$\int \chi_i\chi_j \, d\mathbf{r} = S_{ij}. \tag{13-72}$$

We note that atoms 1 and 3, where the unpaired electron appears in the contributing structures, have larger spin density than atom 2, and in fact the spin density on atom 2 is negative. This is a common qualitative feature.

As a final and completely qualitative example we consider the pi system of the nitrobenzene anion radical. Many structures can be written. To avoid duplication of effort, we will consider the ring and the nitro group separately. The nitro group structure

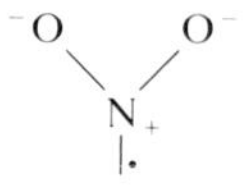

or the symmetrical combination of

and

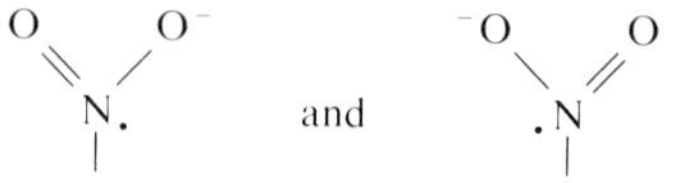

can combine with any of the ordinary benzene structures

etc.,   or   . etc.

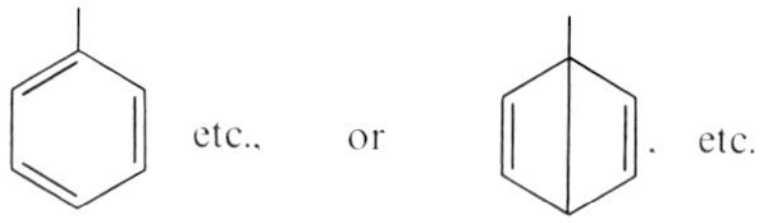

Other nitro structures

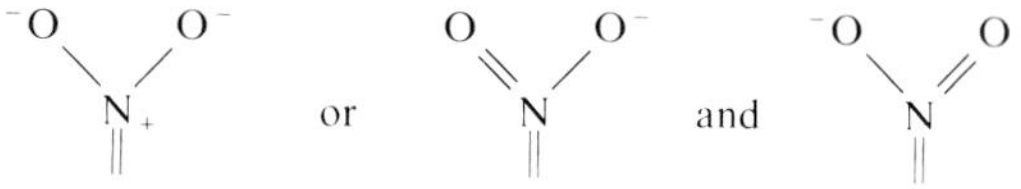

or   and

can combine with

or   and

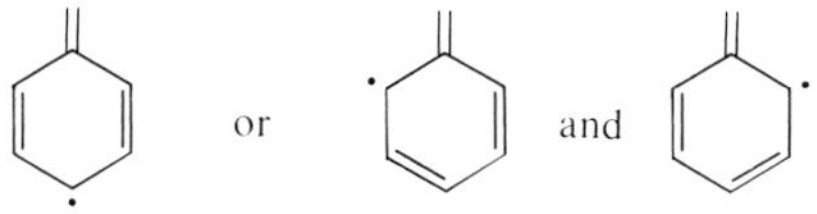

Other structures are expected to be less likely and thus we predict that the charge remains predominantly on the nitro group, that there is large spin density on nitrogen, and that in the ring the *ortho* and *para* spin densities are much larger in magnitude that the *meta* spin density, which may well be negative. These conclusions are borne out by experiment and by calculations.

These methods of obtaining qualitative estimates of spin density distributions are not really "calculations," but are useful as a starting point.

Summary of Section 13

The extreme difficulty and expense of a priori calculations of a quality sufficient to assure usefully good spin properties for large systems require that semiempirical methods be used at least most of the time. This section has briefly considered INDO and spherical Gaussian all-valence-electron methods and Hückel, Hückel–McLachlan, and Pariser–Parr–Pople pi-electron methods. Not only the wave function but also the relationship between an atomic orbital spin density and a hyperfine coupling constant can be treated with empirically adjusted parameters.

A generalized McConnell-type equation was derived and it was shown that very generally the spin density in a "closed-shell" sigma system is given to first order by an integral transform of the pi system spin density. With suitable approximations the result reduced to the usual McConnell equation. Effects of bond angle and charge density, and extension to nonplanar molecules were briefly considered.

The use of very simple valence bond theory for qualitative estimates of spin density distribution was illustrated.

14. External Perturbations

We have thus far implicitly assumed that the molecular radicals we are attempting to describe exist in an otherwise empty, field-free region of space. This would be appropriate if our calculation was to correlate with the results of an experiment carried out for a low-pressure gas. Such is not usually the case; most free-radical ESR work investigates radicals in condensed phases. Interaction of a radical with its surroundings will affect the electronic wave function and thus the values of spin Hamiltonian parameters. Distinctions among interactions can be made on a number of bases: magnitude of the effect, nature of the perturbation. lifetime of the perturbed state, etc. In this section we will briefly consider some of these effects. The presentation consists primarily of a warning that something must be done, rather than a prescription for how to do it.

Surveys of experimental (and some theoretical) results are included in several review articles. [20,58,198].

Static and Dynamic Effects

Interactions between molecules in a fluid are dynamic, and even in crystals relative motions may occur. In some cases a species such as an ion pair may persist for a time that is long on the ESR time scale, so the problem can be treated as static. At the other extreme, very rapid processes can be treated by simple averaging. Processes of intermediate rate require special treatment and such processes, along with other dynamic effects, are not discussed in this book. We note, however, that a description of instantaneous states is usually required, and the "static" situation which is only an instantaneous state of some dynamic process is treated just like a situation which is physically static (at least in the sense of a Born–Oppenheimer electronic calculation).

Nature of the Interaction

We next distinguish between two fundamentally different kinds of radical-environment interactions, although there is in fact essentially a continuum of intermediate cases. At one extreme we have the situation in which a tight ion pair or other complex is formed, with even the possibility of resolvable hyperfine interactions with nuclei of the addend. In such a case the appropriate procedure is clearly to redefine the system under consideration so as to include the addend as part of the radical. Any of the methods of the previous sections could be applied, although occasionally a perturbation treatment will be useful. At the other extreme are the cases where the effect of a radical's environment can be described by an electric field it experiences, by immersing it in a dielectric medium, etc. The environment itself is then not explicitly considered. (An approach of this type to solvent effects in electronic spectroscopy is discussed, e.g., by Amos and Burrows [3].)

A criterion clearly demanding explicit consideration of an addend is overlapped between radical and addend wave functions. In such a case the electronic wave function must be permutationally antisymmetric for all the electrons involved. In an independent particle model this implies an exchange interaction between radical and addend. In a more sophisticated treatment, electronic motions in one will be correlated with those in the other. Some of the most complete treatments of "environmental" effects have dealt with the shift in the hyperfine interaction of H atoms interacting with rare gases at various pressures.

Perturbation Treatments

If the effect on the radical of its environment is reasonably small, it may be convenient to describe that effect by perturbation theory. At least the first-order wave function will be required, however, and it may prove preferable to do a variational calculation including the perturbation. A significant advantage of perturbation theory is that many perturbations can sometimes be treated essentially together. This will be helpful if, for example, a series of intermediate states in a dynamic process must be considered.

Semiempirical Methods

In a semiempirical theory, especially the simple pi-electron theories, it is often possible to treat external perturbations, or even chemical substitution or additions, by simply changing a few parameter values. It may then be possible to treat the effect of these changes by perturbation theory. As with other semiempirical treatments, the advantage of readily attainable, qualitatively useful results may outweigh the disadvantages of the approximations involved.

Summary of Section 14

This section was intended to call attention to the existence of potential problems rather than to go into detail as to how they should be treated. It is clear that the spin distribution and other properties of a radical will be influenced by its surroundings. In some cases, such as tight ion pairs, it is appropriate to extend the system being considered explicitly. In other cases environmental effects can be dealt with approximately by the introduction of external fields or polarizabilities, etc.

APPENDICES

Appendix A
Classical Mechanics and Fields including Relativistic Forms; Units

We will begin with a very brief review of nonrelativistic mechanics, then consider electromagnetic fields, four-vectors, and Lorentz transformations, and finally relativistic mechanics.

Classical Mechanics of Particles [64]

The basis of classical mechanics is Newton's law

$$\mathbf{F} = \frac{d\mathbf{p}}{dt} = m\mathbf{a} = m\frac{d^2\mathbf{r}}{dt^2}. \tag{A-1}$$

Here $\mathbf{p}$ is the momentum, $\mathbf{a}$ the acceleration, and $\mathbf{r}$ the position of a body of mass m. An applied force $\mathbf{F}$ produces an acceleration proportional to the force. Rather than the Cartesian coordinates implicit in $\mathbf{r}$, etc., generalized coordinates q_i can be introduced. In addition, there may be several particles in the system, labeled by indices k. The q_i may be interparticle coordinates, etc. For N particles a total of $3N$ coordinates is necessary. The generalized forces can be defined as

$$Q_j = \sum_k \mathbf{F}^{(k)} \cdot \frac{\partial \mathbf{r}^{(k)}}{\partial q_i}. \tag{A-2}$$

If the system is conservative (does not exchange mass, energy, or momentum with its "surroundings"), then the Q_j can be obtained from a potential $V(q_1, q_2, \ldots, q_{3N})$

$$Q_j = -\frac{\partial V}{\partial q_j}. \tag{A-3}$$

In other cases it may still be possible to define a generalized potential $U(q, \dot{q})$‡ which may depend on the velocities as well as positions such that

$$Q_j = -\frac{\partial U}{\partial q_j} + \frac{d}{dt}\left(\frac{\partial U}{\partial \dot{q}_j}\right). \tag{A-4}$$

The Lagrangian function $L(q, \dot{q}, t)$ is

$$L = T - U, \tag{A-5}$$

where T is the kinetic energy

$$T = \frac{1}{2}\sum_k m_k(\dot{r}_k)^2 \tag{A-6}$$

and for generalized coordinates will usually depend on q as well as $\dot{q}$. The Lagrange equations of motion are

$$\frac{d}{dt}\left(\frac{\partial L}{\partial \dot{q}_j}\right) - \frac{\partial L}{\partial q_j} = 0, \tag{A-7}$$

and the essential test of a correct Lagrangian L is that these equations be correct, i.e., equivalent to Newton's law, Eq. (A-1). Lagrangians can be obtained from a variation principle but this approach will not be treated here.

A generalized momentum p_j conjugate to coordinate q_j is defined as

$$p_j = \frac{\partial L(q, \dot{q}, t)}{\partial \dot{q}_j}, \tag{A-8}$$

and the Hamiltonian function is§

$$H(p, q, t) = \sum_j \dot{q}_j p_j - L(q, \dot{q}, t). \tag{A-9}$$

The Hamiltonian form of the equations of motion can be obtained, but they will not be considered here.

Electromagnetic Fields and Potentials [100,152]

The electric field $\mathbf{E}$ and the magnetic field $\mathbf{B}$ are governed by Maxwell's equations *

$$\nabla \cdot \mathbf{B} = 0, \qquad \nabla \cdot \mathbf{E} = 4\pi\rho,$$
$$\nabla \times \mathbf{B} = \frac{1}{c}\frac{\partial \mathbf{E}}{\partial t} + \frac{4\pi\mathbf{j}}{c}, \qquad \nabla \times \mathbf{E} = -\frac{1}{c}\frac{\partial \mathbf{B}}{\partial t}. \tag{A-10}$$

‡ The symbol q stands for the set $\{q_i\}$, $\dot{q}_i = dq_i/dt$, and thus $\dot{q}$ represents the set $\{dq_i/dt\}$.

§ p stands for the set $\{p_j\}$. Expressions can always be obtained for the $\dot{q}_j$ in terms of p and q, and by definition H is to be expressed in terms of p and q with no explicit dependence on $\dot{q}$.

* This is in free space and expressed in Gaussian units. See end of this appendix and Table A-2 for a discussion of units.

Here ρ is the charge density and $\mathbf{j}$ the current density. For a system of point particles

$$\rho(\mathbf{r}) = \sum_k \varepsilon_k \delta(\mathbf{r} - \mathbf{r}_k), \qquad \mathbf{j}(\mathbf{r}) = \sum_k \varepsilon_k \delta(\mathbf{r} - \mathbf{r}_k)\dot{\mathbf{r}}_k, \tag{A-11}$$

where $\mathbf{r}_k$ is the position of the $\mathbf{k}$th particle, having charge ε_k. A scalar potential ϕ and a vector potential $\mathbf{A}$ can be introduced in terms of which $\mathbf{E}$ and $\mathbf{B}$ are given by

$$\mathbf{E} = -\frac{1}{c}\frac{\partial \mathbf{A}}{\partial t} - \nabla\phi, \qquad \mathbf{B} = \nabla \times \mathbf{A}. \tag{A-12}$$

Only the fields are physically meaningful: a *gauge transformation*

$$\mathbf{A} \to \mathbf{A}' + \nabla f(\mathbf{r}, t), \qquad \phi \to \phi' - \frac{1}{c}\frac{\partial f(\mathbf{r}, t)}{\partial t} \tag{A-13}$$

changes the potentials but can have no physical consequences.

Charged Particles in Fields

A particle of charge ε at position $\mathbf{r}$ in given fields $\mathbf{E}$ and $\mathbf{B}$ will experience a force (the Lorentz force)

$$\begin{aligned} \mathbf{F} &= \varepsilon\left[\mathbf{E}(\mathbf{r}) + \frac{1}{c}\dot{\mathbf{r}} \times \mathbf{B}(\mathbf{r})\right] \\ &= \varepsilon\left[-\nabla\phi(\mathbf{r}) - \frac{1}{c}\frac{\partial \mathbf{A}(r)}{\partial t} + \frac{1}{c}\dot{\mathbf{r}} \times (\nabla \times \mathbf{A}(\mathbf{r}))\right]. \end{aligned} \tag{A-14}$$

This is obtainable from a generalized potential

$$U = \varepsilon\left[\phi(\mathbf{r}) - \frac{1}{c}\mathbf{A}(\mathbf{r})\cdot\dot{\mathbf{r}}\right]. \tag{A-15}$$

The Lagrangian is

$$L = \frac{1}{2}m\dot{r}^2 - \varepsilon\left[\phi(\mathbf{r}) - \frac{1}{c}\mathbf{A}(\mathbf{r})\cdot\dot{\mathbf{r}}\right] \tag{A-16}$$

and the generalized momentum conjugate to r_j ($=x$, y, or z) becomes

$$p_j = \frac{\partial L}{\partial \dot{r}_j} = m\dot{r}_j + \frac{\varepsilon}{c}A_j(\mathbf{r}). \tag{A-17}$$

The Hamiltonian is

$$H = \mathbf{r}\cdot\mathbf{p} - L = \frac{1}{2}m\dot{r}^2 + \varepsilon\phi(\mathbf{r}) = \frac{1}{2m}\left[\mathbf{p} - \frac{\varepsilon}{c}\mathbf{A}(\mathbf{r})\right]^2 + \varepsilon\phi(\mathbf{r}). \tag{A-18}$$

Four-Vectors and Lorentz Transformations [166]

The principle of relativity requires that the form of equations governing physical systems be the same in any two coordinate systems moving relative to one another with constant velocity. Maxwell's equations are already of this form, but the equations of Newtonian mechanics must be modified. The transformation from one coordinate system to another moving uniformly with respect to the first requires that the time variable be considered explicitly on a basis comparable to that of the three spatial coordinates of any point.

We introduce the four-vector of position, x_μ, with

$$x_1 = x, \qquad x_2 = y, \qquad x_3 = z, \qquad x_4 = ict. \tag{A-19}$$

The transformation to another coordinate system is accomplished by a Lorentz transformation‡

$$x'_\mu = \sum_{\nu=1}^{4} L_{\mu\nu} x_\nu. \tag{A-20}$$

Lorentz transformations are orthogonal and preserve "intervals" or four-dimensional distances, the squares of which are

$$\sum_\mu (x'_\mu - \bar{x}'_\mu)^2 = \sum_\mu (x_\mu - \bar{x}_\mu)^2. \tag{A-21}$$

The matrix $(L_{\mu\nu})$ is a 4×4 orthogonal matrix subject to the constraint that L_{ij}, $1 \le i, j \le 3$, and L_{44} are real while L_{i4} and L_{4j} are pure imaginary so that the form of x_μ is preserved.

It would also be possible to introduce the real variable $x_0 = ct$ in place of $x_4 = ict$. A metric tensor would then have to be introduced. This formulation is preferable when it is useful to distinguish between covariant and contravariant indices, but is not required here.

A general Lorentz transformation includes the possibility of ordinary, three-dimensional rotations. It can be considered as the product of such a rotation and a "pure" Lorentz transformation involving only uniformly moving coordinate systems whose axes are parallel. Spatial rotations are considered in Appendix C. For a pure Lorentz transformation corresponding to relative velocity v along the z axes of the coordinate systems

$$\mathbf{L} = \begin{pmatrix} 1 & 0 & 0 & 0 \\ 0 & 1 & 0 & 0 \\ 0 & 0 & \dfrac{1}{(1-\beta^2)^{1/2}} & \dfrac{i\beta}{(1-\beta^2)^{1/2}} \\ 0 & 0 & \dfrac{-i\beta}{(1-\beta^2)^{1/2}} & \dfrac{1}{(1-\beta^2)^{1/2}} \end{pmatrix}, \qquad \beta = \frac{v}{c}. \tag{A-22}$$

‡ A convention is commonly introduced in which summation is assumed over any repeated index. Summations will be explicitly indicated here, however.

Corresponding to the four-vector x_μ we define the four-gradient

$$\partial_\mu = \partial/\partial x_\mu. \tag{A-23}$$

The vector and scalar potentials can be combined in (see, e.g., Ref. [100, Chapter 4])

$$(A_\mu) = (\mathbf{A}, i\phi), \tag{A-24}$$

and the fields make up an antisymmetric electromagnetic field tensor

$$(F_{\mu\nu}) = \begin{pmatrix} 0 & B_z & -B_y & -iE_x \\ -B_z & 0 & B_x & -iE_y \\ B_y & -B_x & 0 & -iE_z \\ iE_x & iE_y & iE_z & 0 \end{pmatrix} \tag{A-25}$$

Equations (A-12) are then replaced by

$$F_{\mu\nu} = \partial_\mu A_\nu - \partial_\nu A_\mu. \tag{A-26}$$

The gauge transformation (A-13) becomes

$$A_\mu \to A'_\mu = A_\mu + \partial_\mu f, \tag{A-27}$$

and $F_{\mu\nu}$ is clearly unchanged since $\partial_\mu \partial_\nu f = \partial_\nu \partial_\mu f$.

The homogeneous Maxwell equations $\nabla \cdot \mathbf{B} = 0$ and $\nabla \times \mathbf{E} = (-1/c)(\partial \mathbf{B}/\partial t)$ become

$$\partial_\mu F_{\nu\lambda} + \partial_\nu F_{\lambda\mu} + \partial_\lambda F_{\mu\nu} = 0. \tag{A-28}$$

These equations are automatically satisfied when the $F_{\mu\nu}$ are given by (A-26). The remaining, inhomogeneous Maxwell equations become

$$\sum_\mu \partial_\mu F_{\nu\mu} = \frac{4\pi}{c} j_\nu, \tag{A-29}$$

where (j_ν) is the current four-vector

$$(j_\nu) = (\mathbf{j}, ic\rho). \tag{A-30}$$

It satisfies a conservation equation

$$\sum_\mu \partial_\mu j_\mu = 0. \tag{A-31}$$

These equations have been written in explicitly covariant form. They relate quantities which transform as scalars, vectors, or tensors under a Lorentz transformation. We must now consider equations governing the motions of particles and try to express them in comparable form. Explicitly covariant Lagrangian and Hamiltonian functions can be obtained, but it is sufficient to have functions which, although not themselves covariant, lead to relativistically correct equations of motion.

The four-vector of position for a particle can be differentiated with respect to the "proper time," τ, associated with the particle to give a four-velocity u_μ. The proper time is defined by

$$(d\tau)^2 = -\frac{1}{c^2}\sum_\mu (dx_\mu)^2 = -\frac{1}{c^2}[dx^2 + dy^2 + dz^2 - c^2\,dt^2] \qquad \text{(A-32)}$$

and is the time measured by a clock traveling with the particle. The four-velocity is thus

$$u_\mu = \frac{dx_\mu}{d\tau} = \left(\frac{\mathbf{v}}{(1-\beta^2)^{1/2}}, \frac{ic}{(1-\beta^2)^{1/2}}\right), \qquad \text{(A-33)}$$

since $d\tau = dt(1-\beta^2)^{1/2}$ with $\beta = v/c$.

The desired form of the equation of motion, to correspond to Newton's law, is [64]

$$d(mu_\nu)/d\tau = K_\nu, \qquad \text{(A-34)}$$

where K_ν is an appropriate force four-vector. The ordinary (three-component) force acting on a charged particle moving in an electromagnetic field, given in Eq. (A-14), can be written as‡

$$F_j = -\varepsilon\left[\frac{\partial}{\partial x_j}\left(\phi - \frac{1}{c}\mathbf{v}\cdot\mathbf{A}\right) + \frac{1}{c}\frac{\partial A_j}{\partial t}\right], \qquad \text{(A-35)}$$

where $\mathbf{v}$ is the ordinary (three-component) velocity $\dot{\mathbf{r}}$. If we recall that $(A_\mu) = (\mathbf{A}, i\phi)$ then we will see that

$$\phi - \frac{1}{c}\mathbf{v}\cdot\mathbf{A} = -\frac{(1-\beta^2)^{1/2}}{c}\sum_\nu u_\nu A_\nu$$

and

$$F_j = -\frac{\varepsilon}{c}(1-\beta^2)^{1/2}\left[-\frac{\partial}{\partial x_j}\left(\sum_\nu u_\nu A_\nu\right) + \frac{\partial A_j}{\partial \tau}\right]. \qquad \text{(A-36)}$$

We are thus led to consider

$$F_j = K_j(1-\beta^2)^{1/2} \qquad \text{(A-37)}$$

with

$$K_j = \frac{\varepsilon}{c}\left[\frac{\partial}{\partial x_\mu}\left(\sum_\nu u_\nu A_\nu\right) - \frac{\partial A_\mu}{\partial \tau}\right]. \qquad \text{(A-38)}$$

‡ Indices $j, k, \ldots$ are in the range 1–3. Indices $\mu, \nu, \ldots$ have the range 1–4.

The fourth component of K_μ can be found by multiplying the equation of motion (A-34) by u_ν and summing:

$$\sum_\nu u_\nu \frac{d}{d\tau}(mu_\nu) = \sum_\nu u_\nu K_\nu = \frac{1}{2}\frac{d}{d\tau}\left[m\left(\sum_\nu u_\nu u_\nu\right)\right] = 0. \qquad \text{(A-39)}$$

The equality to zero follows from the fact that

$$\sum_\nu u_\nu u_\nu = \frac{v^2}{(1-\beta^2)} - \frac{c^2}{(1-\beta^2)} = -c^2$$

is a constant. Thus

$$0 = \sum_\nu K_\nu u_\nu = \frac{\mathbf{F}\cdot\mathbf{v}}{(1-\beta^2)} + \frac{icK_4}{(1-\beta^2)^{1/2}},$$

so

$$K_4 = \frac{i}{c}\frac{\mathbf{F}\cdot\mathbf{v}}{(1-\beta^2)^{1/2}}. \qquad \text{(A-40)}$$

We now consider a Lagrangian

$$L = -mc^2(1-\beta^2)^{1/2} - \varepsilon\phi + \frac{\varepsilon}{c}\mathbf{A}\cdot\mathbf{v}. \qquad \text{(A-41)}$$

The equation of motion obtained from L is

$$0 = \frac{d}{dt}\left(\frac{\partial L}{\partial v_j}\right) - \frac{\partial L}{\partial x_j} = \frac{d}{dt}\left(mu_j + \frac{\varepsilon}{c}A_j\right) + \varepsilon\frac{\partial\phi}{\partial x_j} - \frac{\varepsilon}{c}\frac{\partial}{\partial x_j}(\mathbf{A}\cdot\mathbf{v}), \qquad \text{(A-42)}$$

which can be written

$$\begin{aligned}(1-\beta^2)^{1/2}\frac{d}{d\tau}(mu_j) &= -\varepsilon\frac{\partial\phi}{\partial x_j} - \frac{\varepsilon}{c}\frac{\partial A_j}{\partial t} + \frac{\varepsilon}{c}\frac{\partial}{\partial x_j}(\mathbf{A}\cdot\mathbf{v}) \\ &= -\varepsilon\left[\frac{\partial}{\partial x_j}\left(\phi - \frac{1}{c}\mathbf{v}\cdot\mathbf{A}\right) + \frac{1}{c}\frac{\partial \mathbf{A}_j}{\partial t}\right] \\ &= F_j = (1-\beta^2)^{1/2}K_j \qquad \text{(A-43)}\end{aligned}$$

so the proposed L does lead to the desired equation of motion.

The momentum conjugate to x_j is

$$p_j = \frac{\partial L}{\partial v_j} = \frac{mv_j}{(1-\beta^2)^{1/2}} + \frac{\varepsilon}{c}A_j = mu_j + \frac{\varepsilon}{c}A_j \qquad \text{(A-44)}$$

and a Hamiltonian can be determined according to the usual prescription

$$H = \mathbf{v} \cdot \mathbf{p} - L = \frac{mc^2}{(1 - \beta^2)^{1/2}} + \varepsilon\phi. \qquad \text{(A-45)}$$

However, β contains v, and H should be expressed in terms of p. From Eq. (A-44) we find

$$\begin{aligned} \left(\mathbf{p} - \frac{\varepsilon}{c}\mathbf{A}\right)^2 &= \frac{m^2c^2\beta^2}{1 - \beta^2} = mc^2\left(\frac{1}{1 - \beta^2} - 1\right) \\ \frac{1}{1 - \beta^2} &= 1 + \frac{1}{m^2c^2}\left(\mathbf{p} - \frac{\varepsilon}{c}\mathbf{A}\right)^2 \end{aligned} \qquad \text{(A-46)}$$

so that

$$\begin{aligned} (H - \varepsilon\phi)^2 &= \frac{(mc^2)^2}{1 - \beta^2} = (mc^2)^2 + c^2\left(\mathbf{p} - \frac{\varepsilon}{c}\mathbf{A}\right)^2 \\ H &= \varepsilon\phi + \left[(mc^2)^2 + c^2\left(\mathbf{p} - \frac{\varepsilon}{c}\mathbf{A}\right)^2\right]^{1/2}. \end{aligned} \qquad \text{(A-47)}$$

In obtaining this result we have treated time and spatial variables inequivalently, and it must thus be used with caution.

If we extend Eq. (A-44) to define p_4 by simply inserting u_4 and A_4 we find

$$p_4 = \frac{imc}{(1 - \beta^2)^{1/2}} + \frac{\varepsilon}{c} i\phi = \frac{i}{c}\left(\frac{mc^2}{(1 - \beta^2)^{1/2}} + \varepsilon\phi\right) = \frac{i}{c} H. \qquad \text{(A-48)}$$

An equivalent result can be obtained in other ways, identifying p_4 with iE/c, where E is the energy of the particle. The p_μ so obtained does transform as a four-vector.

Units

As indicated in the introduction, and as the perceptive reader will have noted independently, this book has used a mixture of Gaussian and atomic units. The use of atomic units is clearly appropriate, especially in connection with actual molecular calculations, but why should Gaussian units be used now that we are well into the Systèm International (SI) era? This subsection of the appendix will address that question and will present a comparison of different systems of units. It is assumed that the reader already has some familiarity with the various systems.

Comparison of Gaussian and SI Units [187]

In the context of mechanical units (mass, length, energy, etc.) the distinction between different systems of units is of relatively minor significance. Conversions are readily made and both cgs and MKS units are much too large for molecular quantities. The standard definitions now are those of the international system (SI). The SI units of length, mass, and time are

Meter (m) The meter is the length equal to 1,650,763.73 wavelengths in vacuum of the radiation corresponding to the transition between levels $2p_{10}$ and $5d_5$ of the krypton-86 atom.

Kilogram (kg) The unit of mass (kilogram) is equal to the mass of the international prototype of the kilogram (a carefully maintained, specific chunk of metal).

Second (sec) The second is the duration of 9,192,631,770 periods of the radiation corresponding to the transition between the two hyperfine levels of the ground state of the cesium-133 atom.

Other mechanical units can be obtained from these in the usual MKS system—e.g., a newton (N) is that force which will accelerate a mass of 1 kg by 1 m sec^{-2}. The cgs mechanical units are simply related to SI units: the centimeter (cm) is defined as 10^{-2} m and the gram (g) as 10^{-3} kg. The second is common to the two systems. Then, e.g., 1 dyne = 1 g cm sec^{-2} = 10^{-5} N.

Electromagnetic units can be based on two simple relationships, Coulomb's law

$$F \propto q_1 q_2 / r^2, \tag{A-49}$$

which relates the force of interaction of two charges q_1 and q_2 to the distance r between them, and the law of Biot and Savart

$$F \propto 2(i_1 i_2 / r)L, \tag{A-50}$$

which relates the force F per length L between long, parallel conductors to the currents i_1 and i_2 they carry and the distance r between them. (The 2 is present for essentially geometric reasons.) The most straightforward approach would be to take the proportionality constant to be dimensionless and of magnitude 1 in each case. Thus Coulomb's law is written in the cgs electrostatic system as

$$F = q_1 q_2 / r^2, \tag{A-51}$$

and the electrostatic unit of charge (esu or statcoulomb) is defined so that (1 dyne) = (1 esu)^2/(1 cm)^2. In the cgs electromagnetic system of units, the unit of current is the abampere, defined by (1 dyne) = 2(1 abamp)^2(1 cm)/(1 cm).

Another possible definition of the unit of current is the statampere, defined as one statcoulomb per second. The statampere and abampere are not equal, and the constant relating them must be determined by experiment or by theory relating it to other fundamental constants. In fact, 1 abamp/1 statamp $= c$, the velocity of light.

The Gaussian system of units mixes cgs electrostatic and electromagnetic units, and in consequence includes the constant c explicitly. In this system Coulomb's law is expressed as in Eq. (A-51) and the definition of the esu is the same. However, Eq. (A-50) is replaced by

$$F = 2i_1 i_2 L/c^2 r. \tag{A-52}$$

Units of electric and magnetic field strength are then defined in terms of the forces produced on test charges. Equation (A-14) can be used, although it simplifies matters to think of either **E** or **B** being zero. In an electric field of unit strength, a charge of 1 esu (statcoulomb) will experience a force of 1 dyne. The electric field strength unit is not commonly given a name, but it can be expressed as a potential gradient of 1 statvolt per centimeter, thereby providing one possible definition of the statvolt. The unit of magnetic field strength is the gauss (G): a charge of 1 esu moving in a field of 1 G at a velocity of 1 cm sec^{-1} will experience a force of $\cong 3.336 \times 10^{-11}$ $(=1/c)$ dynes. Alternatively, if the charge could move with the velocity of light, it would experience a force of 1 dyne.

When field strengths are so defined, in the Gaussian system, factors of 4π occur in Maxwell's equations (Eqs. (A-10)] and in the equation relating **D** to **E** or **H** to **B**. This is inconvenient when these equations are of primary importance. A system of "rationalized" units (Lorentz–Heaviside units) can be introduced by putting factors of 4π into Coulomb's law and the law of Biot and Savart, or its equivalent

$$F = \frac{q_1 q_2}{4\pi r^2}, \qquad F = \frac{i_1 i_2}{2\pi r} L. \tag{A-53}$$

For our purposes, however, this is a step backward. We have not had occasion to use Maxwell's equations, and are dealing with charged particles in empty space, so **D** and **H** are of little interest. On the other hand, Coulombic forces between charged particles are of primary importance so it is desirable to keep Coulomb's law in the simplest possible form.

The SI electromagnetic units are defined in a rationalized MKS scheme. Proportionality constants carrying dimensions are introduced into *both* of Eqs. (A-49) and (A-50)

$$F = \frac{q_1 q_2}{4\pi\varepsilon_0 r^2}, \tag{A-54}$$

$$F = \frac{\mu_0}{2\pi} \frac{i_1 i_2}{r} L. \tag{A-55}$$

The constants ε_0 and μ_0 are not independent

$$\varepsilon_0 \mu_0 = 1/c^2, \qquad \text{(A-56)}$$

but one degree of freedom remains. In order to produce units of convenient size, μ_0 is taken to have the value $4\pi \times 10^{-7}$ newton ampere^{-2} (exactly). The fundamental electromagnetic SI unit is the *ampere* (A) defined as that constant current which, if maintained in two straight parallel conductors of infinite length, of negligible circular cross section, and placed 1 meter apart, would produce between these conductors a force of 2×10^{-7} newton per meter of length. The unit of charge, the coulomb (C), is then defined as 1 ampere second, and for consistency $\varepsilon_0 = 10^7/4\pi c^2 \cong 8.854185 \times 10^{-12}$ C^2 N^{-1} m^{-2}.

The MKS-SI form of the Lorentz force expression is

$$\mathbf{F} = q(\mathbf{E} + \mathbf{v} \times \mathbf{B}). \qquad \text{(A-57)}$$

The unit of **E** is newton/coulomb = volt/meter, and that of **B** is 1 tesla (T) = 1 newton/(coulomb centimeter per second). In consequence 1 tesla = 10^4 gauss.

The use of SI units, in addition to being the officially recognized norm, is very convenient in practical macroscopic calculations, especially those involving fields in material media. These units are not appropriate for our purposes, however, because of the more complicated form of Coulomb's law and the related fact that fundamental equations are not as readily reduced to "dimensionless" form when SI units are used as when Gaussian units are used.

Atomic Units

In the (zero-order) quantum mechanical problems we are interested in, the electronic Hamiltonian is expressed as a sum of electronic kinetic energy terms, $-(\hbar^2/2m)\nabla_i^2$ and potential energy terms $Z_\nu e/r_{i\nu}$ or e^2/r_{ij} (in Gaussian units!). These obviously will assume a very simple form if it is possible to use units in which $\hbar$, m and e are all numerically unity. In the Gaussian system electromagnetic units are not independent of mechanical units—e.g., 1 esu = 1 dyne$^{1/2}$ cm—so three quantities must be specified to define units. Normally these are mass (gram), length (cm), and time (sec). It is possible, however, to take mass (m = electronic mass = 1 thomson), charge (e = magnitude of electronic charge = 1 millikan), and action or angular momentum ($\hbar$ = Planck's constant divided by 2π = 1 planck). Names have been assigned to these basic quantities, and will be assigned later to derived units, to facilitate discussion and comparison. *These names are not standard.* In fact, except for the bohr (length) and hartree (energy) to be defined later, names have not generally been given to the atomic units of various quantities. It becomes tedious to continue referring to "the atomic unit of..." so names with obvious connotations have been introduced here.

Other quantities in the atomic system of units can be defined in the usual way from fundamental equations.[‡] The most important are the unit of length

$$a_0 = \hbar^2/me^2 \tag{A-58}$$

(1 bohr = 1 planck^2 thomson^{-1} millikan^{-2}) and of energy

$$\mathscr{E}_0 = e^2/a_0 = \alpha^2 mc^2 \tag{A-59}$$

(1 hartree = 1 millikan^2 bohr^{-1}). The atomic unit of time is

$$t_0 = \hbar a_0/e^2 \tag{A-60}$$

(1 jiffy = 1 planck bohr millikan^{-2}). Other mechanical units in the atomic system are given in Table A-2 (page 342) with their cgs and SI equivalents.

The atomic units of field strength are defined in terms of forces acting on a charge of magnitude e. The atomic unit of force is $ma_0/t_0^2 = e^2/a_0^2$ and the atomic unit of electric field strength is thus e/a_0^2 (1 stark = 1 millikan bohr^{-2}). Definition of the magnetic field strength unit requires the introduction of the velocity of light, c. This is best done via the fine structure constant $\alpha = e^2/\hbar c$. In fact, the atomic unit of velocity is $a_0/t_0 = e^2/\hbar$, so the velocity of light is $\alpha^{-1} \cong 137$ bohr jiffy^{-1}. The unit of magnetic field strength is thus $\alpha^{-1}e/a_0^2$ (1 zeeman = α^{-1} millikan bohr^{-2}). Whereas atomic units for mechanical quantities tend to be small compared with macroscopic units, atomic field strength units are large. A typical x-band ESR field strength of 3400 G (0.34 T), for example, is only 1.4×10^{-6} zeeman.

Magnetic moments in atomic units are usually given in Bohr magnetons, $\beta = e\hbar/2mc = \alpha a_0 e/2$, i.e., 1 Bohr magneton = $\frac{1}{2}$ hartree/zeeman.[§] Magnetic interactions between particles commonly involve $\beta^2 = \alpha^2 a_0^2 e^2/4 = (\alpha^2/4)\mathscr{E}_0 a_0^3$. The β^2 is multiplied by a factor having units of volume^{-1}, and is thus conveniently expressed as (1 Bohr magneton)^2 = $(\alpha^2/4)$ hartree bohr^{-3}. The convenient unit for nuclear moments is the nuclear magneton $\beta_N = e\hbar/2M_P c$. It differs from the Bohr magneton by the ratio of electronic and proton masses, $M_P/m \cong 1836.11$.

Natural Units

Before leaving this topic we should mention another possible choice of units. It has not been used here, but is frequently used in relativistic quantum mechanics. This is the system of so-called "natural units," chosen so that $\hbar = c = 1$. It is possible to require in addition that $m = 1$. The unit of energy is then mc^2, the rest mass energy of the electron. It is not possible to take $e = 1$

‡ Equations appropriate to the Gaussian system are used. Some MKS equivalents are included in Table A-2.

§ The unit $\alpha a_0 e$, 1 hartree/zeeman, might be more straightforward, but the Bohr magneton is well established and is the quantity which most often arises. (Compare Chapter I.)

as well as $\hbar = c = 1$, because $\alpha = e^2/\hbar c$ is a dimensionless constant.‡ In fact, in this system e^2 plays the role of "smallness parameter" otherwise played by α or $1/c$. The values of other units in this system will not be pursued here.

TABLES

We conclude the discussion of units with two tables. Values of physical constants are given in Table A-1 and atomic units are presented in Table A-2.

TABLE A-1

Some Physical Constants

Symbol	Quantity	Value[a] Gaussian units	SI units
e	Electronic charge	4.80325×10^{-10} esu	1.602192×10^{-19} C
m	Electronic mass	9.10956×10^{-28} g	9.10956×10^{-31} kg
$\hbar$	Planck's constant divided by 2π	1.054592×10^{-27} erg sec	1.054592×10^{-34} J sec
c	Velocity of light	2.997925×10^{10} cm sec^{-1}	2.997925×10^{8} msec^{-1}
α	Fine structure constant	$\dfrac{e^2}{\hbar c} = 7.29735 \times 10^{-3}$	$\dfrac{\mu_0 c^2}{4\pi}\dfrac{e^2}{\hbar c} = \dfrac{e^2}{4\pi\varepsilon_0 \hbar c} = 7.29735 \times 10^{-3}$
M_p/m	Ratio of proton and electron masses	1836.11	1836.11
r_0 $(= \alpha^2 a_0)$	Classical radius of electron	$\dfrac{e^2}{mc^2} = 2.81794 \times 10^{-13}$ cm	$\dfrac{\mu_0 c^2}{4\pi}\dfrac{e^2}{mc^2} = \dfrac{e^2}{4\pi\varepsilon_0 mc^2} = 2.81794 \times 10^{-15}$ m
μ_0	Permeability of free space		$4\pi \times 10^{-7}$ NA^{-2}
ε_0	Permittivity of free space		8.854185×10^{-12} C^{2}N^{-1}m^{-2}
g	Electronic g factor (Zeeman)	2.00231929	2.00231929
g'	Electronic g factor (spin-orbit)	2.00463858	2.00463858

[a] Adapted from the final recommended values of Taylor, Parker, and Langenberg [200] and Section 3.

‡ In SI units $\alpha = e^2/4\pi\varepsilon_0 \hbar c$.

TABLE A-2

Atomic Units

			Gaussian		SI	
Quantity	Symbol	Name[a]	Expression	Value	Expression	Value
Length	a_0	bohr	$\hbar^2/me^2$	5.291772×10^{-9} cm	$\hbar^2/4\pi\varepsilon_0 me^2$	5.291772×10^{-11} m
Mass	m	thomson	m	9.10956×10^{-28} g	m	9.10956×10^{-31} g
Time	t_0	jiffy	$\hbar a_0/e^2 = \hbar/\alpha^2 mc^2$	2.418885×10^{-17} sec	$4\pi\varepsilon_0 \hbar a_0/e^2 = \hbar/\alpha^2 mc^2$	2.418885×10^{-17} sec
Charge	e	millikan	e	4.80325×10^{-10} esu	e	1.602192×10^{-19}C
Energy	$\mathscr{E}_0$	hartree	$e^2/a_0 = \alpha^2 mc^2$	4.359827×10^{-11} erg	$e^2/4\pi\varepsilon_0 a_0 = \alpha^2 mc^2$	4.359828×10^{-18} J
Force			e^2/a_0^2	8.238879×10^{-3} dyne	$e^2/4\pi\varepsilon_0 a_0^2$	8.238879×10^{-8} N
Velocity			$a_0/t_0 = \alpha c$	2.187691×10^{8} cm sec^{-1}	$a_0/t_0 = \alpha c$	2.187691×10^{6} M sec^{-1}
Scalar potential			e/a_0	9.076828×10^{-2} esu cm^{-1} (statvolt)	$e/4\pi\varepsilon_0 a_0$	27.21165 volt
Electric field strength		stark	e/a_0^2	1.715272×10^{7} esu cm^{-2} (statvolt cm^{-1})	$e/4\pi\varepsilon_0 a_0^2$	5.142257×10^{11} V m^{-1}
Magnetic field strength		zeeman	$\alpha^{-1}e/a_0^2$	2.350540×10^{9} G	$\hbar/a_0^2 e$	2.350540×10^{5} T
Magnetic moment	β	Bohr magneton	$e\hbar/2mc$	9.27410×10^{-21} erg G^{-1}	$e\hbar/2m$	9.27410×10^{-24} J T^{-1}

[a] Except for the Bohr magneton and possibly for bohr and hartree, these are not in common use. See text.

Appendix B
Gauge Transformations in Nonrelativistic Quantum Mechanics

The time-dependent Schrödinger equation for a particle of charge $-e$ in electric and magnetic fields characterized by potentials ϕ and $\mathbf{A}$ can be written

$$\left[\frac{1}{2m}\left(\mathbf{p} + \frac{e}{c}\mathbf{A}\right)^2 - e\phi - i\hbar\frac{\partial}{\partial t}\right]\psi = 0. \qquad \text{(B-1)}$$

We know that if a gauge transformation

$$\phi \to \phi' = \phi - \frac{1}{c}\frac{\partial f}{\partial t}, \qquad \mathbf{A} \to \mathbf{A}' = \mathbf{A} + \nabla f \qquad \text{(B-2)}$$

is made with $f(\mathbf{r}, t)$ an arbitrary function, the fields $\mathbf{E}$ and $\mathbf{B}$, and thus the physical situation, are unchanged. The Hamiltonian operator

$$\mathscr{H} = \frac{1}{2m}\left(\mathbf{p} + \frac{e}{c}\mathbf{A}\right)^2 - e\phi \qquad \text{(B-3)}$$

is changed, however, and the change must be offset by some change in the wave function ψ.

Suppose that $\psi(\mathbf{r}, t)$ is a solution of Eq. (B-1). Let

$$\psi' = e^{-(ie/\hbar c)f}\psi. \qquad \text{(B-4)}$$

We note that

$$\begin{aligned}\left(-e\phi' - i\hbar\frac{\partial}{\partial t}\right)\psi' &= -e\phi e^{-(ie/\hbar c)f}\psi + \frac{e}{c}\frac{\partial f}{\partial t}e^{-(ie/\hbar c)f}\psi \\ &\quad - i\hbar\left(-\frac{ie}{\hbar c}\right)\frac{\partial f}{\partial t}\psi - i\hbar e^{-(ie/\hbar c)f}\frac{\partial \psi}{\partial t} \\ &= e^{-(ie/\hbar c)f}\left(-e\phi - i\hbar\frac{\partial}{\partial t}\right)\psi.\end{aligned} \qquad \text{(B-5)}$$

Similarly,

$$\left(\mathbf{p} + \frac{e}{c}\mathbf{A}'\right)\psi' = e^{-(ie/\hbar c)f}\left(\mathbf{p} + \frac{e}{c}\mathbf{A}\right)\psi,$$
$$\left(\mathbf{p} + \frac{e}{c}\mathbf{A}'\right)^2\psi' = e^{-(ie/\hbar c)f}\left(\mathbf{p} + \frac{e}{c}\mathbf{A}\right)^2\psi, \tag{B-6}$$

and

$$\left[\frac{1}{2m}\left(\mathbf{p} + \frac{e}{c}\mathbf{A}'\right)^2 - e\phi' - i\hbar\frac{\partial}{\partial t}\right]\psi'$$
$$= e^{-(ie/\hbar c)f}\left[\frac{1}{2m}\left(\mathbf{p} + \frac{e}{c}\mathbf{A}\right)^2 - e\phi - i\hbar\frac{\partial}{\partial t}\right]\psi = 0, \tag{B-7}$$

so that ψ' is a solution of the Schrödinger equation with the transformed potentials.

A many-electron wave function can be expressed as a linear combination of antisymmetrized products of one-electron functions. Each one-electron function experiences the same gauge transformation so for the N-electron function

$$\Psi \rightarrow \Psi' = e^{-i(Ne/\hbar c)f}\Psi. \tag{B-8}$$

It would be possible to choose a different gauge function f_i for each electron [69], but the potentials would then be defined in $3N$-dimensional space rather than 3-dimensional space.

If the gauge function f is in fact time independent, ϕ is unchanged. If the original Hamiltonian does not depend explicitly on time we are likely to be interested in stationary state solutions. A gauge transformation affecting only **A** does not change their stationary character. For

$$\psi(\mathbf{r}, t) = \chi(\mathbf{r})e^{iEt/\hbar} \tag{B-9}$$

with $f = f(\mathbf{r})$,

$$\psi'(\mathbf{r}, t) = e^{-(ie/\hbar c)f(\mathbf{r})}\chi(\mathbf{r})e^{iEt/\hbar}$$
$$= \chi'(\mathbf{r})e^{iEt/\hbar}. \tag{B-10}$$

Suppose that $\mathscr{F}$ is any operator which does not contain derivatives, or contains them only as powers of $\mathbf{p} + (e/c)\mathbf{A}$. The derivation of Eq. (B-6) can be extended to arbitrary powers of $(\mathbf{p} + (e/c)\mathbf{A})$, so that

$$\mathscr{F}'\chi' = \mathscr{F}\left[\mathbf{p} + \frac{e}{c}\mathbf{A}'\right]\chi' = e^{-(ie/\hbar c)f}\mathscr{F}\left[\mathbf{p} + \frac{e}{c}\mathbf{A}\right]\chi$$
$$= e^{-(ie/\hbar c)f}\mathscr{F}\chi, \tag{B-11}$$

and a matrix element is unchanged by the gauge transformation if functions are transformed and the operator expressed in terms of the new potential:

$$\int \chi_1'(\mathbf{r})^* \mathscr{F}' \chi_2'(\mathbf{r})\, d\mathbf{r} = \int e^{(ie/\hbar c)f} \chi_1(\mathbf{r})^* e^{-(ie/\hbar c)f} \mathscr{F} \chi_2(\mathbf{r})\, d\mathbf{r}$$

$$= \int \chi_1(\mathbf{r})^* \mathscr{F} \chi_2(\mathbf{r})\, d\mathbf{r}. \tag{B-12}$$

Among the consequences of this is the fact that if $\mathscr{F}$ and $\mathscr{G}$ are any two operators containing $\mathbf{A}$ only in the combination $\mathbf{p} + (e/c)\mathbf{A}$, and they commute in one gauge, they also commute for any other gauge related by a time-independent f.

Appendix C
Rotations, Tensors, Angular Momentum, and Related Topics

The purpose of this appendix is to summarize, without proof, a number of useful results pertaining to angular momentum, rotations, tensors, and related topics. Many sources are available for more extensive treatments [25,49,52,138,171,210]. Unfortunately, there are several conventions in common use as to notation and choice of phases. Another function of this appendix, thus, is to establish the conventions used here.

Angular Momentum Operators

The classical angular momentum of a particle moving with momentum $\mathbf{p}$ at position $\mathbf{r}$ is $\mathbf{L} = \mathbf{r} \times \mathbf{p}$. When quantum mechanical operators are substituted for the classical quantities, it is found that the components of $\mathbf{L}$ do not commute with each other. All of the essentials of the quantum theory of angular momentum can be obtained from these commutation relationships.

Alternatively, one can consider angular momentum operators as the infinitesimal generators of the continuous group whose elements are rotations in three dimensions. In either way, one is led to the definition that a set of three Hermitian operators J_x, J_y, and J_z are the components of an angular momentum if they have the commutation relationship

$$[J_a, J_b] = iJ_c. \tag{C-1}$$

Here and in what follows a, b, c are any cyclic permutation of x, y, z and units are chosen so that $\hbar = 1$. (That is, angular momenta are measured in units of $\hbar$.)

The square of the total angular momentum is the product of $\mathbf{J}$ with itself. The operator is Hermitian and commutes with any component:

$$J^2 = \mathbf{J} \cdot \mathbf{J} = J_x^2 + J_y^2 + J_z^2, \qquad [J^2, J_a] = 0. \tag{C-2}$$

It is also convenient to define two non-Hermitian operators

$$J_\pm = J_x \pm iJ_y, \qquad (J_\pm)^\dagger = J_\mp. \tag{C-3}$$

Angular Momentum Eigenfunctions

It is possible to find simultaneous eigenfunctions of J^2 and any one component of $\mathbf{J}$: J_z is customarily chosen.[‡] It follows from the commutation relationships of Eq. (C-1) that if $|j, m\rangle$ is an eigenfunction of J^2 and J_z,

$$J^2|j, m\rangle = j(j+1)|j, m\rangle, \qquad J_z|j, m\rangle = m|j, m\rangle, \tag{C-4}$$

then j and m are either both integers or both half-odd-integers, also $j \geq 0$ and $-j \leq m \leq j$.

We reserve the notation $|j, m\rangle$ for a normalized eigenfunction satisfying Eqs. (C-4). The effect of $J_\pm$ is then

$$J_\pm|j, m\rangle = [j(j+1) - m(m \pm 1)]^{1/2}|j, m \pm 1\rangle. \tag{C-5}$$

The magnitude of the coefficient is determined by the previous definitions, including the normalization constraint; its phase must be specified by convention. The choice here, that it be real and nonnegative, is by far the most common.

When $\mathbf{J}$ is the orbital angular momentum of a particle it is usually denoted by $\mathbf{L}$ and the quantum number j by l. In such a case l must be an integer and the eigenfunctions are spherical harmonics of the angular polar coordinates of the particle

$$|l, m\rangle = Y_l^m(\theta, \phi) = (-1)^m \left[\frac{(2l+1)(l-m)!}{4\pi(l+m)!}\right]^{1/2} P_l^m(\cos\theta)e^{im\phi}, \tag{C-6}$$

where P_l^m is the associated Legendre function generalized to either sign of m

$$P_l^m(u) = \frac{(1-u^2)^{m/2}}{2^l l!}\left(\frac{d}{du}\right)^{l+m}(u^2-1)^l. \tag{C-7}$$

This equation is valid for $-l \leq m \leq l$. It follows from this definition that

$$P_l^{-m} = (-1)^m \frac{(l-m)!}{(l+m)!} P_l^m,$$

and thus the complex conjugate of a spherical harmonic is

$$[Y_l^m(\theta, \phi)]^* = (-1)^m Y_l^{-m}(\theta, \phi). \tag{C-8}$$

Under inversion, for which $\theta \to \pi - \theta$, $\phi \to \phi + \pi \pmod{2\pi}$[§]

$$Y_l^m(\theta, \phi) \to Y_l^m(\pi - \theta, \phi + \pi) = (-1)^l Y_l^m(\theta, \phi). \tag{C-9}$$

[‡] In polar coordinates L_z assumes a simpler form than L_x or L_y, and θ and ϕ dependence is separable for L^2, L_z eigenfunctions (the spherical harmonics).

[§] Since ϕ is normally defined for $0 \leq \phi \leq 2\pi$, it can be taken modulo 2π, i.e., multiples of 2π are added or subtracted as necessary to bring ϕ into the desired range. The range of θ, $0 \leq \theta \leq \pi$ remains unchanged.

It is occasionally convenient to use a different phase convention or even a different normalization. Related functions are

$$\mathscr{Y}_l^m(\theta, \phi) = (i)^l Y_l^m(\theta, \phi), \qquad C_l^m(\theta, \phi) = \left(\frac{4\pi}{2l + 1}\right)^{1/2} Y_l^m(\theta, \phi). \tag{C-10}$$

It should be noted that

$$[\mathscr{Y}_l^m(\theta, \phi)]^* = (-1)^{l+m}\mathscr{Y}_l^{-m}(\theta, \phi). \tag{C-11}$$

The harmonic polynomials

$$\Upsilon_l^m(\mathbf{r}) = r^l Y_l^m(\theta, \phi) \tag{C-12}$$

for $-l \leq m \leq l$ form a set of $2l + 1$ linearly independent homogeneous polynomials of degree l. They satisfy Laplace's equation

$$\nabla^2 \Upsilon_l^m(\mathbf{r}) = 0. \tag{C-13}$$

When j is half-odd-integer, $|j, m\rangle$ cannot be expressed as a function of physical coordinates. For $j = \frac{1}{2}$, $\mathbf{J}$ is usually written $\mathbf{s}$ and a basis of two-component spinors introduced

$$|\tfrac{1}{2}, \tfrac{1}{2}\rangle = \alpha = \begin{pmatrix}1\\0\end{pmatrix}, \qquad |\tfrac{1}{2}, -\tfrac{1}{2}\rangle = \beta = \begin{pmatrix}0\\1\end{pmatrix}. \tag{C-14}$$

In this basis the components of the matrix corresponding to $\mathbf{s}$ are proportional to the Pauli spin matrices, $\mathbf{s} = \frac{1}{2}\boldsymbol{\sigma}$, where

$$\sigma_x = \begin{pmatrix}0 & 1\\1 & 0\end{pmatrix}, \qquad \sigma_y = \begin{pmatrix}0 & -i\\i & 0\end{pmatrix}, \qquad \sigma_z = \begin{pmatrix}1 & 0\\0 & -1\end{pmatrix}. \tag{C-15}$$

Spin functions for systems of electrons are constructed in a basis of products of the one-electron bases.

Matrices of Angular Momentum Operators

The $|j, m\rangle$ eigenfunctions provide a basis in terms of which any of the angular momentum operators can be expressed as matrices. With the phase convention implicit in Eq. (C-5) the nonzero matrix elements of J_x are real and positive while those of J_y are pure imaginary. Of course the matrix elements of J^2 and J_z are real (only diagonal elements are nonzero) and those of J^2 are nonnegative. Specifically,

$$\langle j', m'|J^2|j, m\rangle = j(j + 1)\delta_{jj'}\delta_{mm'}, \qquad \langle j', m'|J_z|j, m\rangle = m\delta_{jj'}\delta_{mm'}, \tag{C-16}$$

and

$$\langle j', m'|J_x|j, m\rangle = \frac{\delta_{jj'}}{2}$$

$$\times \{[j(j+1) - m(m+1)]^{1/2}\delta_{m',m+1} + [j(j+1) - m(m-1)]^{1/2}\delta_{m',m-1}\},$$

$$\langle j', m'|J_y|j, m\rangle = -i\frac{\delta_{jj'}}{2}$$

$$\times \{[j(j+1) - m(m+1)]^{1/2}\delta_{m',m+1} - [j(j+1) - m(m-1)]^{1/2}\delta_{m',m-1}\}. \quad \text{(C-17)}$$

Coupling of Angular Momenta

Situations frequently arise in which it is desirable to combine two (or more) angular momenta into a single, total angular momentum

$$\mathbf{J} = \mathbf{J}_1 + \mathbf{J}_2, \quad \text{(C-18)}$$

for example $\mathbf{J}_1 = \mathbf{L}$ and $\mathbf{J}_2 = \mathbf{s}$ for an electron, or $\mathbf{J}_1$ and $\mathbf{J}_2$ referring to different electrons in a two-electron system. If $\mathbf{J}_1$ and $\mathbf{J}_2$ are angular momenta in the sense that their components satisfy (C-1), and the components of one commute with those of the other,

$$[J_{1a}, J_{2b}] = 0 \quad \text{(C-19)}$$

then the components of $\mathbf{J}$ will satisfy Eq. (C-1), so $\mathbf{J}$ is an angular momentum.

It follows from Eq. (C-19) and earlier results that

$$[J^2, J_1^2] = [J^2, J_2^2] = 0 \quad \text{(C-20)}$$

and, with $J_z = J_{1z} + J_{2z}$,

$$[J^2, J_z] = 0 \quad \text{(C-21)}$$

but

$$[J^2, J_{1a}] \neq 0, \qquad [J^2, J_{2a}] \neq 0. \quad \text{(C-22)}$$

It is thus possible to find simultaneous eigenfunctions $|j_1, j_2, j, m\rangle$ of J_1^2, J_2^2, J^2, and J_z. These functions will not in general be eigenfunctions of J_{1z} and J_{2z}. Alternatively, we can take simple product functions which are simultaneous eigenfunctions of J_1^2, J_{1z}, J_2^2, and J_{2z}:

$$|j_1 m_1 j_2 m_2\rangle = |j_1, m_1\rangle|j_2, m_2\rangle$$

$$J_i^2|j_1 m_1 j_2 m_2\rangle = j_i(j_i+1)|j_1 m_1 j_2 m_2\rangle, \qquad i = 1, 2, \quad \text{(C-23)}$$

$$J_{iz}|j_1 m_1 j_2 m_2\rangle = m_i|j_1 m_1 j_2 m_2\rangle, \qquad i = 1, 2.$$

These product functions are in fact eigenfunctions of J_z as well, with $m = m_1 + m_2$, but they are not in general eigenfunctions of J^2. A transformation to J^2 eigenfunctions can be made in various ways.

Since both sets of functions are eigenfunctions of J_1^2 and J_2^2, we will take j_1 and j_2 to be fixed. It is then found that

$$|j_1 j_2 jm\rangle = \sum_{m_1, m_2} |j_1 m_1 j_2 m_2\rangle\langle j_1 m_1 j_2 m_2 | jm\rangle. \tag{C-24}$$

The coefficients $\langle j_1 m_1 j_2 m_2 | jm\rangle = C(jm; j_1 m_1 j_2 m_2) =$ etc. are the Clebsch–Gordan coefficients. They vanish unless $m = m_1 + m_2$, so the double summation reduces to a single sum. In addition, for the coefficients to be nonzero, j_1, j_2, and j must be able to form a triangle, i.e., $|j_1 - j_2| \le j \le j_1 + j_2$. This restricts the possible values of j, corresponding to the classical limits of $\mathbf{J}_1$ and $\mathbf{J}_2$ antiparallel or parallel.

The Clebsch–Gordan coefficients $\langle j_1 m_1 j_2 m_2 | jm\rangle$ for fixed j_1 and j_2 are the elements of a $(2j_1 + 1)(2j_2 + 1)$-dimensional unitary matrix. Thus, with $\langle jm | j_1 m_1 j_2 m_2\rangle \equiv \langle j_1 m_1 j_2 m_2 | jm\rangle^*$,

$$\begin{aligned} \sum_{j, m} \langle j_1 m_1 j_2 m_2 | jm\rangle\langle jm | j_1 m_1' j_2 m_2'\rangle &= \delta_{m_1 m_1'}\delta_{m_2 m_2'}, \\ \sum_{m_1, m_2} \langle jm | j_1 m_1 j_2 m_2\rangle\langle j_1 m_1 j_2 m_2 | j'm'\rangle &= \delta_{jj'}\delta_{mm'}. \end{aligned} \tag{C-25}$$

The relative phases of the Clebsch–Gordan coefficients with the same j but differing m can be fixed by requiring the $|j_1 j_1 jm\rangle$ to satisfy Eq. (C-5) (assuming that $|j_1, m_1\rangle$ and $|j_2, m_2\rangle$ already do), but relative phases for different j's remain to be established. This is accomplished by requiring that $\langle j_1 j_2 j\ (m = j) | j_1\ (m_1 = j_1)\ j_2\ (m_2 = j - j_1)\rangle$ be real and positive. All the coefficients are then real, and they are given by

$$\begin{aligned} C(jm; j_1 m_1 j_2 m_2) &= \langle j_1 m_1 j_2 m_2 | jm\rangle = \delta_{m_1 + m_2, m}\Delta(j_1, j_2, j_3) \\ &\times \left[\frac{(2j + 1)(j_1 + j_2 - j)!(j_1 - j_2 + j)!(-j_1 + j_2 + j)!}{(j_1 + j_2 + j + 1)!}\right]^{1/2} \\ &\times [(j_1 + m_1)!(j_1 - m_1)!(j_2 - m_2)!(j + m)!(j - m)!]^{1/2} \\ &\times \sum_s (-1)^s [s!(j_1 + j_2 - j - s)!(j_1 - m_1 - s)!(j_2 + m_2 - s)! \\ &\qquad \times (j - j_2 + m_1 + s)!(j - j_1 - m_2 + s)!]^{-1}. \end{aligned} \tag{C-26}$$

Here $\Delta(j_1, j_2, j) = 1$ if the three j's satisfy the triangle condition and is zero otherwise. The sum over s extends over all s values for which all the factorials are defined.

The Clebsch–Gordan coefficients have a number of symmetry properties.

These can be more readily expressed, however, for the closely related Wigner 3-j symbols

$$\begin{pmatrix} j_1 & j_2 & j_3 \\ m_1 & m_2 & m_3 \end{pmatrix} = \frac{(-1)^{j_1 - j_2 - m_3}}{(2j_3 + 1)^{1/2}} \langle j_1 m_1 j_2 m_2 | j_3 (-m_3) \rangle. \qquad \text{(C-27)}$$

The 3-j symbols have the following symmetries:

1. The value is unchanged by an even permutation of columns.
2. The value is changed by a factor $(-1)^{j_1 + j_2 + j_3}$ when any odd permutation of columns is made.
3. The value is changed by a factor $(-1)^{j_1 + j_2 + j_3}$ when the signs of all three m's are changed.

It should be noted that (for nonzero coefficients) either all of j_1, j_2 and j_3 are integers or two are half-odd-integer and the other is an integer. In either case $j_1 + j_2 + j_3$ is an integer. For integer n, $(-1)^n = (-1)^{-n}$ is real. The 3-j coefficients can be thought of as describing the coupling of three angular momenta to a resultant zero.

When more than two angular momenta are to be coupled, different states of the same total j and m can in general be obtained by choosing different coupling orders and different intermediate angular momenta. These sets of states can be related by unitary transformations. The coefficients of such a transformation can be related to a highly symmetric set of coefficients: the Wigner 6-j symbol. Suppose we have three angular momenta, j_1, j_2, and j_3, which we wish to combine to a total J, M. We can first combine j_1 and j_2 to j_{12} and then combine j_{12} with j_3 to give J. We denote the result by $|(j_1 j_2) j_{12}, j_3; JM\rangle$. Alternatively, we can combine j_2 and j_3 to get j_{23} and combine this with j_1 to get J. We denote this result by $|j_1, (j_2 j_3) j_{23}; JM\rangle$. These two sets of states are related by

$$|(j_1 j_2) j_{12}, j_3; JM\rangle = \sum_{j_{23}} |j_1, (j_2 j_3) j_{23}; JM\rangle [(2j_{12} + 1)(2j_{23} + 1]^{1/2} \times (-1)^{j_1 + j_2 + j_3 + J} \begin{Bmatrix} j_1 & j_2 & j_{12} \\ j_3 & J & j_{23} \end{Bmatrix}, \qquad \text{(C-28)}$$

where braces { } denote the Wigner 6-j symbol.

The 6-j symbols can be expressed in terms of 3-j symbols

$$\begin{Bmatrix} j_1 & j_2 & j_{12} \\ j_3 & J & j_{23} \end{Bmatrix} = (-1)^{2j_2 - j_1 - j_3}(2J + 1) \sum_{m_1, m_3} (-1)^{m_3 - m_1} \times \begin{pmatrix} j_1 & j_2 & j_{12} \\ m_1 & M + m_3 - m_1 & -m_3 - M \end{pmatrix} \begin{pmatrix} j_{12} & j_3 & J \\ -m_3 - M & m_3 & M \end{pmatrix} \times \begin{pmatrix} j_2 & j_3 & j_{23} \\ m_1 - m_3 - M & m_3 & M - m \end{pmatrix} \begin{pmatrix} j_{23} & j_1 & J \\ m_1 - M & -m_1 & M \end{pmatrix}. \qquad \text{(C-29)}$$

A 6-j symbol can be associated with a tetrahedron whose edges are labeled by the j values, as shown in Fig. C-1. The symmetry operations of the tetrahedron are related to those of the 6-j symbol. The 6-j symbol is invariant to

1. any permutation of its columns, or
2. exchange of any two elements in the first row with the corresponding elements of the second row.

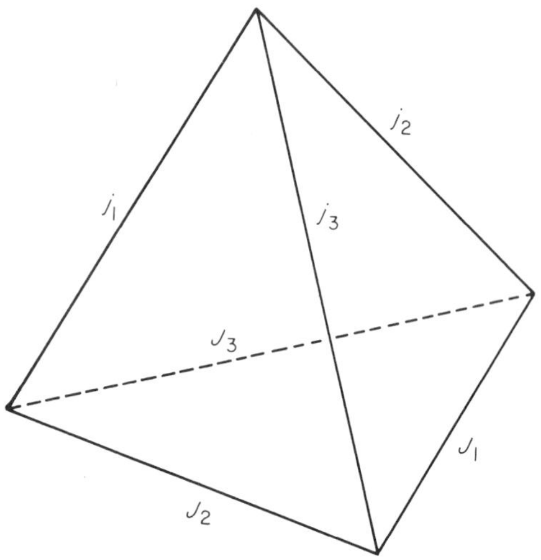

FIG. C-1. Association between regular tetrahedron and 6-j symbol $\begin{Bmatrix} j_1 & j_2 & j_3 \\ J_1 & J_2 & J_3 \end{Bmatrix}$.

A limitation of permissible j's is that the formation of such a tetrahedron be possible, i.e., the j's associated with any face must satisfy the triangle condition. Another relationship between 3-j and 6-j symbols is

$$\sum_M \begin{pmatrix} J_1 & j_2 & J \\ M_1 & m_2 & M \end{pmatrix} \begin{pmatrix} j_1 & J_2 & J \\ m_1 & M_2 & -M \end{pmatrix}$$

$$= \sum_{j,m} (-1)^{-j-J-m_1-M_1}(2j+1) \begin{Bmatrix} j_1 & j_2 & j \\ J_1 & J_2 & J \end{Bmatrix} \begin{pmatrix} j_1 & j_2 & j \\ m_1 & m_2 & m \end{pmatrix} \begin{pmatrix} J_1 & J_2 & j \\ M_1 & M_2 & -m \end{pmatrix}. \tag{C-30}$$

Coefficients relating to the coupling of more than three angular momenta can be defined but will not be required here.

Time Reversal, Complex Conjugation, and Kramers Conjugation [52,210]

For the current discussion it will be convenient to use a scalar product notation. In terms of integrals over wave functions

$$(\phi, \psi) = \int \phi^* \psi \, d\tau, \tag{C-31}$$

and thus $(\phi, \psi) = (\psi, \phi)^*$. The scalar product corresponds to a Dirac bracket $\langle \phi | \psi \rangle = (\phi, \psi)$, but the Dirac notation can be ambiguous when non-Hermitian operators are involved. In what follows, Greek letters will denote state functions, lower case Roman letters will be (complex) numbers, and Roman capitals will be operators.

We recall some fundamental definitions. An operator L is *linear* if, for any a, b, ϕ, and ψ

$$L(a\phi + b\psi) = aL\phi + bL\psi. \tag{C-32}$$

An operator A is *antilinear* if, for any a, b, ϕ, and ψ

$$A(a\phi + b\psi) = a^* A\phi + b^* B\psi. \tag{C-33}$$

The *adjoint* of an operator X is denoted by $X^\dagger$ and is defined by

$$(X^\dagger \phi, \psi) = (\phi, X\psi) \tag{C-34}$$

for all ϕ, ψ. A linear operator H for which $H^\dagger = H$ is *Hermitian*. A linear operator U for which

$$(U\phi, U\psi) = (\phi, \psi) \tag{C-35}$$

for all ϕ and ψ is *unitary*. This is equivalent to

$$U^\dagger U = UU^\dagger = 1. \tag{C-36}$$

An antilinear operator V for which

$$(V\phi, V\psi) = (\phi, \psi)^* = (\psi, \phi) \tag{C-37}$$

for all ϕ and ψ is *antiunitary*. The product of two linear operators or two antilinear operators is linear, while the product of a linear and an antilinear operator is antilinear. The product of two unitary operators or of two antiunitary operators is unitary; the product of an antiunitary operator and a unitary operator is antiunitary. Any operator X with the property that

$$|(\phi, \psi)| = |(X\phi, X\psi)| \tag{C-38}$$

for all ϕ and ψ is either unitary or antiunitary.

Let K_0 be the complex conjugation operator

$$K_0 \psi = \psi^*. \tag{C-39}$$

The operation of complex conjugation depends on the representation chosen: K_0 is defined with respect to the usual coordinate representation in which $p_x = -i(\partial/\partial x)$, etc.‡ By definition, K_0 has no effect on spin functions

$$K_0\alpha = \alpha, \qquad K_0\beta = \beta. \tag{C-40}$$

It is clear that K_0 is an antilinear operator, also that it is antiunitary and in fact $K_0^2 = 1$.

The complex conjugate of an operator $\mathscr{F}$ is

$$\mathscr{F}^* = K_0 \mathscr{F} K_0 \tag{C-41}$$

or equivalently, the effect of $\mathscr{F}^*$ on any function ψ is given by

$$\mathscr{F}^*\psi = (\mathscr{F}\psi^*)^*. \tag{C-42}$$

If a real basis set is introduced, the matrix of $\mathscr{F}^*$ is the complex conjugate of the matrix of $\mathscr{F}$. In the coordinate representation, the operators for position **X**, linear momentum **P**, and angular momentum **L**, have

$$\mathbf{X}^* = \mathbf{X}, \qquad \mathbf{P}^* = -\mathbf{P}, \qquad \mathbf{L}^* = -\mathbf{L}. \tag{C-43}$$

In the usual representation of spin $\mathbf{S} = \frac{1}{2}\boldsymbol{\sigma}$ [cf. eq. (C-15)] and it follows that

$$S_x^* = S_x, \qquad S_y^* = -S_y, \qquad S_z^* = S_z. \tag{C-44}$$

We next consider the unitary operator

$$U = \prod_{k=1}^{N} \sigma_{ky} = 2^N \prod_{k=1}^{N} S_{ky} \tag{C-45}$$

for a system of N electrons.§ Since spin operators for different electrons commute and $\sigma_y^2 = 1$ for each, $U^2 = 1$. The complex conjugate of U is

$$U^* = 2^N \prod_{k=1}^{N} (-S_{ky}) = (-1)^N U. \tag{C-46}$$

The operator U does not affect spatial functions and its effect on any spin function is well defined.

An antilinear operator K can be defined as

$$K = UK_0. \tag{C-47}$$

We note that

$$K^2 = UK_0UK_0 = UU^* = (-1)^N, \tag{C-48}$$

and it follows that

$$K^{-1} = (-1)^N K = K_0^{-1}U^{-1} = K_0U. \tag{C-49}$$

‡ Recall that units with $\hbar = 1$ are assumed.

§ For particles with spin $s > \frac{1}{2}$, the factor for each can be taken to be $\exp(-i\pi S_y)$.

If we define an overbar notation

$$\bar{F} = KFK^{-1} = UK_0FK_0U \tag{C-50}$$

Then $\overline{FG} = \bar{F}\bar{G}$ and

$$\bar{X} = \mathbf{X}^* = \mathbf{X}, \qquad \bar{\mathbf{P}} = \mathbf{P}^* = -\mathbf{P}, \qquad \bar{\mathbf{L}} = \mathbf{L}^* = -\mathbf{L}, \qquad \bar{\mathbf{S}} = -\mathbf{S}, \tag{C-51}$$

since S_y anticommutes with S_x and S_z. It follows that for any angular momentum

$$\bar{\mathbf{J}} = -\mathbf{J}. \tag{C-52}$$

In the usual representation it is clear that

$$\sigma_y\alpha = i\beta, \qquad \sigma_y\beta = -i\alpha. \tag{C-53}$$

Any angular momentum eigenfunction can be expressed as a linear combination of products of basic spin functions and spherical harmonics. From Eqs. (C-8) and (C-53) then, it can be shown that

$$K|j, m\rangle = (-1)^m|j, -m\rangle. \tag{C-54}$$

A number c can be thought of as a special case of an operator (multiplication by c) and $\bar{c} = c^*$.

The operator K will be referred to here as the Kramers conjugation operator. It is the same (apart from possible, irrelevant phase factors) as the time reversal operator of Wigner. The physical operation of time reversal may suggest other attributes than those possessed by K as defined here, however.

It is of some interest to note that, for a system containing an even number of electrons it is possible to take a basis set ψ_j such that

$$K\psi_j = \psi_j, \qquad N \text{ even}. \tag{C-55}$$

This is not possible for odd-electron systems. Rather, the basis functions come in orthogonal pairs, ψ_j and $\bar{\psi}_j$ with

$$\bar{\psi}_j = K\psi_j, (\psi_j, \bar{\psi}_j) = (\psi_j, K\psi_j) = 0, \qquad N \text{ odd}. \tag{C-56}$$

It can be shown that for a system with an odd number of electrons in the absence of any magnetic field (nuclear dipole fields also excluded) all levels are evenly degenerate, and K transforms one member of the degenerate pair into the other. This is Kramers degeneracy.

Rotations

We will be interested in rotations in three-dimensional space, but as a preliminary let us consider a rotation in a plane. We assume a coordinate system OXY and an object, with our attention concentrated on some particular point P, attached to the object and having Cartesian coordinates (x, y) or polar coordinates (r, θ) as shown in Fig. C-2a.

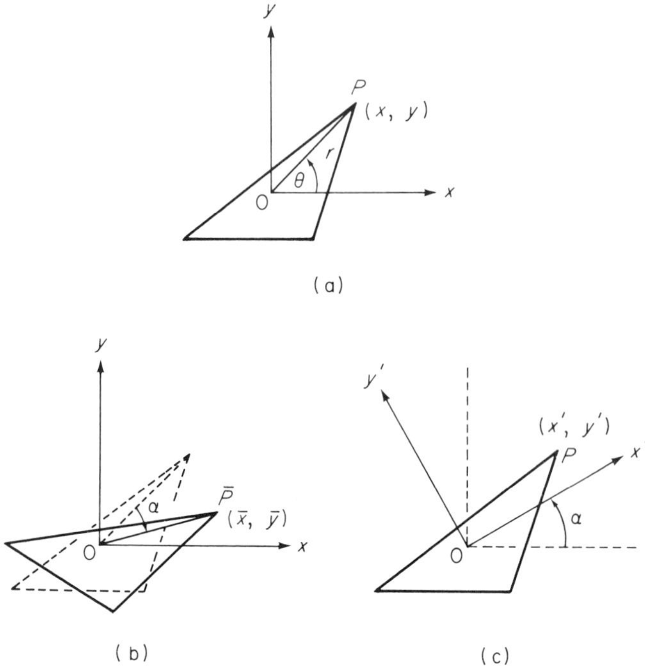

FIG. C-2. Rotations in a plane. In (b) $\bar{r} = r$ and $\bar{\theta} = \theta - \alpha$. In (c) $r' = r$ and $\theta' = \theta' - \alpha$.

We can consider a rotation of the object about the origin of the coordinate system, say by a clockwise angle α. (See Fig. C-2b.) The new coordinates of the point will be given by

$$\bar{r} = r, \qquad \bar{\theta} = \theta - \alpha,$$
$$\bar{x} = \bar{r} \cos \bar{\theta} = x \cos \alpha + y \sin \alpha, \tag{C-57}$$
$$\bar{y} = \bar{r} \sin \bar{\theta} = -x \sin \alpha + y \cos \alpha.$$

In this case the original point P has moved to a new position $\bar{P}$.

Alternatively, we could leave the object in place but rotate the coordinate system by a positive (counterclockwise) angle α (Fig. C-2c). The point P

remains "in the same place" but it has different coordinates with respect to the new coordinate system. They are

$$\begin{gathered} r' = r, \qquad \theta' = \theta - \alpha, \\ x' = x \cos \alpha + y \sin \alpha, \qquad y' = -x \sin \alpha + y \cos \alpha. \end{gathered} \tag{C-58}$$

The two transformations of coordinates are in fact identical. Note, however, that the rotations are in opposite directions.

We can let $\mathbf{r} = (x, y)$ and

$$\mathbf{R}(\alpha) = \begin{pmatrix} \cos \alpha & \sin \alpha \\ -\sin \alpha & \cos \alpha \end{pmatrix}. \tag{C-59}$$

Then

$$\bar{\mathbf{r}} = \mathbf{r}' = \mathbf{R}(\alpha)\mathbf{r}, \tag{C-60}$$

and $\mathbf{R}$ is a matrix describing a rotation of the coordinate system by α or the object by $-\alpha$. It is clear that $\mathbf{R}(-\alpha) = \mathbf{R}^{-1}(\alpha)$: the operations of rotating object and coordinate system are inversely related to each other. One must be careful in any given context to determine whether a rotation is being carried out on the system (the object) or on the coordinate system.

Rotations in a plane form a commutative group

$$\mathbf{R}(\alpha)\mathbf{R}(\beta) = \mathbf{R}(\alpha + \beta) = \mathbf{R}(\beta)\mathbf{R}(\alpha). \tag{C-61}$$

Any rotation in three dimensions can be specified by three angles. These might be, for example, two angles specifying the direction of the axis about which the rotation occurs, and the angle of rotation. This is usually not a convenient choice of angles, however. It is customary to describe a coordinate system rotation in terms of three Euler angles α, β, and γ, defining the rotation in three stages:

1. a rotation by α about the z axis;
2. a rotation by β about the y' axis, i.e., the new y axis after step 1;[‡] and
3. a rotation by γ about the z'' axis, i.e., the new z axis after steps 1 and 2.

These angles and axes are shown in Fig. C-3.

The effect of this rotation is to change the coordinates of a point $\mathbf{r} = (x, y, z)$ to new coordinates $\bar{\mathbf{r}} = (\bar{x}, \bar{y}, \bar{z})$, with

$$\bar{\mathbf{r}} = \mathbf{R}\mathbf{r} \tag{C-62}$$

[‡] Sometimes the second rotation is taken about the x' axis, cf., e.g., Goldstein [64].

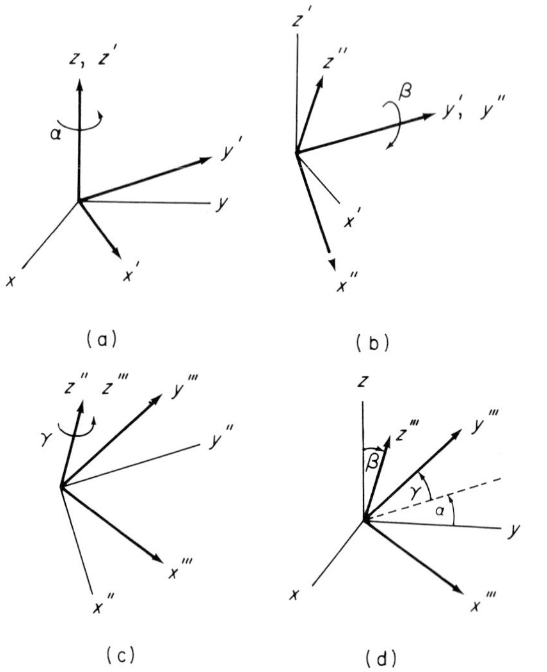

FIG. C-3. Three-dimensional rotations in terms of Euler angles.

where the rotation matrix **R** is given by[‡]

$$\mathbf{R}(\alpha\beta\gamma)$$

$$= \begin{pmatrix} \cos\gamma & \sin\gamma & 0 \\ -\sin\gamma & \cos\gamma & 0 \\ 0 & 0 & 1 \end{pmatrix} \begin{pmatrix} \cos\beta & 0 & -\sin\beta \\ 0 & 1 & 0 \\ \sin\beta & 0 & \cos\beta \end{pmatrix} \begin{pmatrix} \cos\alpha & \sin\alpha & 0 \\ -\sin\alpha & \cos\alpha & 0 \\ 0 & 0 & 1 \end{pmatrix}$$

$$= \begin{pmatrix} \cos\alpha\cos\beta\cos\gamma - \sin\alpha\sin\gamma & \sin\alpha\cos\beta\cos\gamma + \cos\alpha\sin\gamma & -\sin\beta\cos\gamma \\ -\cos\alpha\cos\beta\sin\gamma - \sin\alpha\cos\gamma & -\sin\alpha\cos\beta\sin\gamma + \cos\alpha\cos\gamma & \sin\beta\sin\gamma \\ \cos\alpha\sin\beta & \sin\alpha\sin\beta & \cos\beta \end{pmatrix}. \tag{C-63}$$

Rotations in three dimensions also form a group, but do not in general commute.

The matrix **R** is orthogonal, $\mathbf{R}^{\mathrm{T}} = \mathbf{R}^{-1}$, and in addition we note that

$$\mathbf{R}^{-1}(\alpha\beta\gamma) = \mathbf{R}(-\gamma, -\beta, -\alpha). \tag{C-64}$$

‡ The β rotation *is* correct for a positive rotation (z into x) about y. Compare Fig. C-3.

This follows directly from the definitions. To avoid ambiguity later, however, we will restrict the angles to lie in the ranges $0 \le \alpha \le 2\pi$, $0 \le \beta \le \pi$, $0 \le \gamma \le 2\pi$.

Suppose that we have a function $\psi(\mathbf{r})$ of position (e.g., the position of a particle). A rotation of the coordinate system will clearly affect such a function. We denote by $\mathscr{R}(\alpha\beta\gamma)$ the operator which, when acting on ψ, produces the function in the rotated coordinate system. The value of any observable will be unaffected by a change of coordinate system, however, and

$$\mathscr{R}\psi(\mathbf{r}) = \psi(\mathbf{R}^{-1}\mathbf{r}). \tag{C-65}$$

The operators corresponding to observables are also transformed by $\mathscr{R}$:

$$Q \to \mathscr{R}Q\mathscr{R}^{-1}, \tag{C-66}$$

and since $\mathscr{R}$ is unitary, $\mathscr{R}^{-1} = \mathscr{R}^{\dagger}$.

It can be shown that for a rotation by an angle ξ about an axis determined by a unit vector $\hat{\mathbf{u}}$, the rotation operator is

$$\mathscr{R}_{\hat{u}}(\xi) = e^{-i\xi\hat{\mathbf{u}}\cdot\mathbf{J}}, \tag{C-67}$$

where $\mathbf{J}$ is the total angular momentum of the system described by the functions $\mathscr{R}$ is to act on. For a rotation defined by Euler angles α, β, γ

$$\mathscr{R}(\alpha\beta\gamma) = e^{-i\gamma J_{z''}}e^{-i\beta J_{y'}}e^{-i\alpha J_z}, \tag{C-68}$$

where z is the initial z axis, y' the intermediate y axis, and z'' the final z axis. It will be desirable to have an expression in terms of the initial coordinate system only. This can be shown to be

$$\mathscr{R}(\alpha\beta\gamma) = e^{-i\alpha J_z}e^{-i\beta J_y}e^{-i\gamma J_z}. \tag{C-69}$$

The product of two rotation operators is of course a rotation operator corresponding to the total rotation.

Angular momentum eigenfunctions form a complete set and thus provide a basis for a representation of the group of rotations. They provide a good basis because the representation is irreducible. Let the angular momentum eigenfunctions be denoted by $|qjm\rangle$, where q represents any additional quantum numbers appropriate to the system and can thus distinguish distinct states having the same j and m. Then

$$\langle qjm|\mathscr{R}(\alpha\beta\gamma)|q'j'm'\rangle = \delta_{qq'}\delta_{jj'}D^{(j)}_{mm'}(\alpha\beta\gamma). \tag{C-70}$$

The quantities $D^{(j)}_{mm'}$ are independent of q and of all properties of the system other than angular momentum. They can be thought of as a set of matrices

$\mathbf{D}^{(j)}(\alpha\beta\gamma)$ of dimension $2j + 1$, for each j, which provide a $(2j + 1)$-dimensional, irreducible representation of the rotation group. If θ' and ϕ' are polar coordinates resulting from θ, ϕ after a rotation defined by α, β, γ,

$$Y^l_{m'}(\theta', \phi') = \sum_m D^{(l)}_{m'm}(\alpha\beta\gamma) Y^l_m(\theta, \phi), \tag{C-71}$$

or in general

$$|qjm'\rangle = \sum_m D^{(j)}_{m'm} |qjm\rangle, \tag{C-72}$$

where $|qjm'\rangle$ is defined with respect to the new coordinate system and $|qjm\rangle$ is defined with respect to the old.

We can now drop the label q and consider

$$D^{(j)}_{mm'}(\alpha\beta\gamma) = \langle jm|\mathscr{R}(\alpha\beta\gamma)|jm'\rangle = e^{-i\alpha m - i\gamma m'}\, d^{(j)}_{mm'}(\beta), \tag{C-73a}$$

where

$$d^{(j)}_{mm'}(\beta) = \langle jm|e^{-i\beta J_y}|jm'\rangle. \tag{C-73b}$$

It can be shown that

$$d^{(j)}_{mm'}(\beta) = \sum_t (-1)^t \frac{[(j+m)!(j-m)!(j+m')!(j-m')!]^{1/2}}{(j+m-t)!(j-m'-t)!t!(t-m+m')!} \times (\cos \tfrac{1}{2}\beta)^{2j+m-m'-2t}(\sin \tfrac{1}{2}\beta)^{2t-m+m'}, \tag{C-74}$$

where t ranges over all values for which all the factorials are defined. When either of the m values is zero (this can happen only for j an integer), the D's are simply related to spherical harmonics

$$\begin{aligned} D^{(l)}_{m0}(\alpha\beta\gamma) &= (-1)^m \left(\frac{4\pi}{2l+1}\right)^{1/2} Y_l^{-m}(\beta, \alpha), \\ D^{(l)}_{0m}(\alpha\beta\gamma) &= \left(\frac{4\pi}{2l+1}\right)^{1/2} Y_l^{-m}(\beta, \gamma). \end{aligned} \tag{C-75}$$

Since they form a representation of the rotation group, the $\mathbf{D}$'s have the property that if two successive rotations described by Euler angles α', β', γ' and α, β, γ, respectively, are equivalent to a rotation with Euler angles α'', β'', γ'', then

$$D^{(j)}_{mm'}(\alpha''\beta''\gamma'') = \sum_\mu D^{(j)}_{m\mu}(\alpha\beta\gamma) D^{(j)}_{\mu m'}(\alpha'\beta'\gamma'). \tag{C-76}$$

The symmetries of the $d^{(j)}_{mm'}$ include

$$\begin{aligned} d^{(j)}_{mm'}(\beta) &= d^{(j)}_{m'm}(-\beta) = (-1)^{m-m'}\, d^{(j)}_{m'm}(\beta) \\ &= (-1)^{m-m'}\, d^{(j)}_{-m,-m'}(\beta). \end{aligned} \tag{C-77}$$

Products of two or three D's can be expressed as sums of D's, and integrals of products can also be evaluated. In particular

$$\begin{aligned}\frac{1}{8\pi^2}\int_0^{2\pi}\int_0^{\pi}\int_0^{2\pi}&[D^{(j_1)}_{m_1m_1'}(\alpha\beta\gamma)]^*D^{(j_2)}_{m_2m_2'}(\alpha\beta\gamma)\,d\alpha\,\sin\beta\,d\beta\,d\gamma\\&=\delta_{m_1m_2}\delta_{m_1'm_2'}\delta_{j_1j_2}(2j_1+1)^{-1},\\\frac{1}{8\pi^2}\int_0^{2\pi}\int_0^{\pi}\int_0^{2\pi}&D^{(j_1)}_{m_1m_1'}(\alpha\beta\gamma)D^{(j_2)}_{m_2m_2'}(\alpha\beta\gamma)D^{(j_3)}_{m_3m_3'}(\alpha\beta\gamma)\,d\alpha\,\sin\beta\,d\beta\,d\gamma\\&=\begin{pmatrix}j_1&j_2&j_3\\m_1&m_2&m_3\end{pmatrix}\begin{pmatrix}j_1&j_2&j_3\\m_1'&m_2'&m_3'\end{pmatrix}.\end{aligned}\tag{C-78}$$

This can be specialized to the case of three spherical harmonics [cf. Eq. (C-75)]

$$\begin{aligned}\int_0^{2\pi}\int_0^{\pi}&Y^{m_1}_{l_1}(\theta\phi)Y^{m_2}_{l_2}(\theta\phi)Y^{m_3}_{l_3}(\theta\phi)\sin\theta\,d\theta\,d\phi\\&=\left[\frac{(2l_1+1)(2l_2+1)(2l_3+1)}{4\pi}\right]^{1/2}\begin{pmatrix}l_1&l_2&l_3\\0&0&0\end{pmatrix}\begin{pmatrix}l_1&l_2&l_3\\m_1&m_2&m_3\end{pmatrix}.\end{aligned}\tag{C-79}$$

Tensors and Tensor Operators

Cartesian Tensors

If $\mathbf{v}$ is any ordinary, i.e., three-component, physical vector, it will transform under a rotation the same way that the position vector $\mathbf{r}$ does:

$$v_a' = \sum_b R_{ab} v_b. \tag{C-80}$$

A scalar quantity is invariant under rotations. Other quantities transform like products of coordinates x^2, xy, ... We are lead to the following definition: a tensor $\mathbf{T}$ of degree n is a set of quantities labeled by n indices which transform linearly among themselves under rotations according to

$$T'_{a_1a_2\cdots a_n} = \sum_{b_1b_2\cdots b_n} R_{a_1b_1}R_{a_2b_2}\cdots R_{a_nb_n}T_{b_1b_2\cdots b_n}. \tag{C-81}$$

A scalar is a tensor of degree zero and an ordinary vector is a tensor of degree one. Since each of the indices a_i can assume three values, $\mathbf{T}$ consists of 3^n quantities. We consider the index sets $(a_1, \ldots, a_n) \equiv A$ and $(b_1, \ldots, b_n) \equiv B$ for the moment as single indices and write

$$T_A' = \sum_B \bar{R}_{AB} T_B. \tag{C-82}$$

The matrices

$$\bar{R}_{AB}(\alpha\beta\gamma) = \prod_{i=1}^{n} R_{a_i b_i}(\alpha\beta\gamma) \tag{C-83}$$

provide a representation of the rotation group, but this representation is in general reducible. A reduction can be accomplished by a transformation of the tensor basis. For example, a general tensor of degree 2 has 9 independent quantities. It can be separated into three parts: $\mathbf{T} = \mathbf{T}^{(0)} + \mathbf{T}^{(1)} + \mathbf{T}^{(2)}$. These have the properties that

$$\begin{aligned} T_{ab}^{(0)} &= t\delta_{ab} && \text{(1 quantity)}, \\ T_{ab}^{(1)} &= -T_{ba}^{(1)} && \text{(3 independent quantities)}, \\ T_{ab}^{(2)} &= T_{ba}^{(2)}, \quad \sum_a T_{aa}^{(2)} = 0 && \text{(5 independent quantities)}. \end{aligned} \tag{C-84}$$

These quantities are defined in terms of the elements of $\mathbf{T}$ in Table C-1. Each subset transforms only within itself under rotations. These subsets are irreducible tensors and provide bases for irreducible representations of the rotation group of dimension 1, 3, and 5, respectively. A similar reduction is possible for tensors of higher degree.

TABLE C-1

Cartesian and Spherical Components of a Tensor of Degree 2

Irreducible Cartesian components	Spherical components[a]
$T_{ab}^{(0)} = t\delta_{ab}$ $\left(t = \frac{1}{3}\sum_a T_{aa}\right)$	$T_0^{(0)} = -(1/\sqrt{3})t$
$T_{ab}^{(1)} = \frac{1}{2}(T_{ab} - T_{ba})$	$T_1^{(1)} = -\frac{1}{2}[(T_{xz} - T_{zx}) + i(T_{yz} - T_{zy})]$
	$T_0^{(1)} = (i/\sqrt{2})(T_{xy} - T_{yx})$
	$T_{-1}^{(1)} = -\frac{1}{2}[(T_{xz} - T_{zx}) - i(T_{yz} - T_{zy})]$
$T_{ab}^{(2)} = \frac{1}{2}(T_{ab} + T_{ba}) - t\delta_{ab}$	$T_2^{(2)} = \frac{1}{2}[T_{xx} - T_{yy} + i(T_{xy} + T_{yx})]$
	$T_1^{(2)} = -\frac{1}{2}[T_{xz} + T_{zx} + i(T_{yz} + T_{zy})]$
	$T_0^{(2)} = (1/\sqrt{6})(2T_{zz} - T_{xx} - T_{yy})$
	$T_{-1}^{(2)} = \frac{1}{2}[T_{xz} + T_{zx} - i(T_{yz} + T_{zy})]$
	$T_{-2}^{(2)} = \frac{1}{2}[T_{xx} - T_{yy} - i(T_{xy} + T_{yx})]$

[a] These are chosen to satisfy $[T_m^{(k)}]^* = (-1)^{k+m}T_{-m}^{(k)}$. [Compare Eq. (C-93).]

Spherical Tensors

An alternative choice of components is possible. For the ordinary vector **v** the Cartesian components can be replaced by the spherical components

$$v_1 = -\frac{1}{\sqrt{2}}(v_x + iv_y), \qquad v_0 = v_z, \qquad v_{-1} = \frac{1}{\sqrt{2}}(v_x - iv_y). \quad \text{(C-85)}$$

These components transform under rotations like the comonents of Y_1^m, and a general irreducible spherical tensor $T_m^{(l)}$ transforms like Y_l^m. The spherical components of the tensor of degree 2 considered above are also given in Table C-1.

The product of two irreducible tensors will in general be reducible, but proper linear combinations of such products will again be irreducible. The result is exactly analogous to the coupling of angular momenta. The notation that will be used is $[\mathbf{A}^{(k)} \times \mathbf{B}^{(k')}]_m^{(l)}$ for the m component of the rank l irreducible tensor product of irreducible tensors $A_\alpha^{(k)}$ of rank k and $B_\beta^{(k')}$ of rank k'. It is given by

$$\begin{aligned}[\mathbf{A}^{(k)} \times \mathbf{B}^{(k')}]_m^{(l)} &= \sum_{\alpha,\beta} A_\alpha^{(k)} B_\beta^{(k')} \langle k\alpha k'\beta | lm\rangle \\ &= \sum_{\alpha,\beta} A_\alpha^{(k)} B_\beta^{(k')} (-1)^{k-k'-m}(2l+1)^{1/2} \begin{pmatrix} k & k' & l \\ \alpha & \beta & -m \end{pmatrix} \end{aligned} \quad \text{(C-86)}$$

in terms of the Clebsch–Gordan coefficients or 3-j symbols, respectively. Of particular interest is the scalar product, with $l = 0$. This is conventionally given by

$$(\mathbf{A} \cdot \mathbf{B}) = \sum_\alpha (-1)^\alpha A_\alpha^{(k)} B_{-\alpha}^{(k)}, \quad \text{(C-87)}$$

which differs from the $l = m = 0$ case of Eq. (C-86) by a constant factor.

$$[\mathbf{A}^{(k)} \times \mathbf{B}^{(k)}]^{(0)} = (-1)^k (2k+1)^{-1/2} (\mathbf{A} \cdot \mathbf{B}). \quad \text{(C-88)}$$

It is defined only for the case $k = k'$, as indicated.

A combination of frequent interest is that written in Cartesian form as $\mathbf{A} \cdot \mathbf{T} \cdot \mathbf{B}$, where **A** and **B** are vectors and **T** is a tensor of degree 2. (**A** and **B** are spins, fields, etc.) This can be expressed in terms of irreducible spherical tensor components as

$$\mathbf{A} \cdot \mathbf{T} \cdot \mathbf{B} = \sum_{l=0}^{2} (2l+1)^{1/2} (\mathbf{T}^{(l)} \cdot [\mathbf{A} \times \mathbf{B}]^{(l)}). \quad \text{(C-89)}$$

The components of $\mathbf{T}^{(l)}$ are given in terms of those of **T** in Table C-1. For particular interactions of interest, often only one or two values of l correspond to nonzero components. The expressions in Table C-1 can also be used for $[\mathbf{A} \times \mathbf{B}]^{(l)}$ by taking $[\mathbf{A} \times \mathbf{B}]_{ab} = A_a B_b$.

TENSOR OPERATORS

In the preceding discussion tensors have been treated as arrays of numbers. It is also possible to have tensor operators. An irreducible tensorial operator is a member of a set (or sometimes the term applies to the whole set) of operators which transform among themselves under rotations in the proper tensorial fashion.

$$\mathscr{R}(\alpha\beta\gamma)T_\mu^{(k)}\mathscr{R}^\dagger(\alpha\beta\gamma) = \sum_\nu T_\nu^{(k)}D_{\nu\mu}^{(k)}(\alpha\beta\gamma). \tag{C-90}$$

The adjoint $\mathbf{T}^\dagger$ of a tensorial *set* $\mathbf{T}$ of operators can be defined in terms of the adjoints of the component operators by

$$T_\mu^{\dagger(k)} = (-1)^\mu[T_{-\mu}^{(k)}]^\dagger. \tag{C-91}$$

If k is an integer (rather than half-odd-integer) it is possible to have self-adjoint sets with $\mathbf{T}^\dagger = \mathbf{T}$. The components of such a set are related by

$$[T_\mu^{(k)}]^\dagger = (-1)^\mu T_{-\mu}^{(k)}. \tag{C-92}$$

If v_x, v_y, and v_z are Hermitian operators, the spherical components defined by Eq. (C-85) satisfy this relationship. The tensor product of two such self-adjoint tensor sets is not self-adjoint, but if one requires that, instead of satisfying Eq. (C-92), the members of a self-adjoint set be related by

$$[T_\mu^{(k)}]^\dagger = (-1)^{k+\mu}T_{-\mu}^{(k)} \tag{C-93}$$

[cf. Eq. (C-11)], this property will be preserved in a tensor product of commuting operators.

Matrix elements of tensorial operators taken between angular momentum eigenfunctions are related by the Wigner–Eckart theorem.

$$\langle gjm|\mathbf{T}^{(k)}|g'j'm'\rangle = (-1)^{j-m}\begin{pmatrix} j & k & j' \\ -m & \mu & m' \end{pmatrix}\langle qj\|\mathbf{T}^{(k)}\|q'j'\rangle. \tag{C-94}$$

The reduced matrix element $\langle qj\|\mathbf{T}^{(k)}\|q'j'\rangle$ is independent of all m-type indices. It can be evaluated, e.g., from any one nonzero matrix element. All matrix elements associated with different m, m', and μ are then immediately given by Eq. (C-94).‡

Relationships between matrix elements of a tensor operator and those of its Kramers conjugate are discussed, e.g., by Fano and Racah [52]. Many other relationships can also be obtained, but they are not required here.

‡ Different expressions are sometimes given, e.g., in terms of Clebsch–Gordan coefficients, such that the reduced matrix elements differ from those defined here by a constant factor. So long as the same expression is used consistently, such constants will cancel out of all matrix elements.

Appendix D
Reduced Density Matrices[‡]

Since all electrons are equivalent, meaningful wave functions and operators must treat all electrons equivalently. According to the Pauli principle, an acceptable wave function will be antisymmetric with respect to permutation of electron labels (on spatial and spin coordinates simultaneously)

$$\hat{P}\Psi = (-1)^p\Psi \tag{D-1}$$

where p is the parity of permutation $\hat{P}$. The Hermitian operator corresponding to any physical observable must be symmetric in electron labels, and thus commute with any permutation

$$[\hat{P}, \mathscr{F}] = 0. \tag{D-2}$$

Known physical interactions involve only one or two electrons at a time. A "one-electron" operator is of the form

$$\mathscr{F} = \sum_i f(i), \tag{D-3}$$

where $f(i)$ acts on the coordinates of electron i only and all f's are the same except for the electron label involved. Typical one-electron operators are the kinetic energy, $-(\frac{1}{2})\nabla_i^2$, and the nuclear attraction, $-Z_\nu/r_{i\nu}$, terms in the Hamiltonian. A "two-electron" operator is of the form

$$\mathscr{G} = \sum_{i<j} g(ij), \tag{D-4}$$

where $g(ij)$ involves coordinates of electrons i and j and all g's are the same except for the electron labels involved. The most common example is the electron–electron Coulomb interaction $1/r_{ij}$.

We consider a matrix element of $\mathscr{F}$[§]

$$\langle A|\mathscr{F}|B\rangle = \int \Psi_A^*(x_1, \ldots, x_N)\left[\sum_{i=1}^{N} f(i)\right]\Psi_B(x_1, \ldots, x_N)\, dx_1 \cdots dx_N. \tag{D-5}$$

‡ See Refs. [44,106,122].

§ As usual, x_i stands for the set of space and spin coordinates of electron i.

Since each of the terms in the sum is in fact the same, differing only in the labeling of dummy variables of integration and an equivalent permutation of electrons in Ψ_A and Ψ_B

$$\langle A|\mathscr{F}|B\rangle = N \int \Psi_A^*(x_1, x_2, \ldots, x_N) f(1) \times \Psi_B(x_1, x_2, \ldots, x_N)\, dx_1\, dx_2 \cdots dx_N. \tag{D-6}$$

The $N - 1$ integrations over coordinates $x_2, \ldots, x_N$ can be carried out independent of what $\mathscr{F}$ is, so we define

$$D^{(1)}(BA|x_1; x_1') = \int \Psi_B(x_1, x_2, \ldots, x_N)\Psi_A^*(x_1', x_2, \ldots, x_N)\, dx_2 \cdots dx_N \tag{D-7}$$

and can then write

$$\langle A|\mathscr{F}|B\rangle = N \int' f(1) D^{(1)}(BA|x_1; x_1')\, dx_1, \tag{D-8}$$

where the prime on the integration sign indicates that the following prescription is to be followed: $f(1)$ acts only on the unprimed variables in $D^{(1)}$. Following action of f, primed variables are to be set equal to the corresponding unprimed variables. The integration is then performed.

The function $D^{(1)}$ is a *one-electron, transition reduced density matrix*. If $A = B$ is a single state of interest, the label A is frequently omitted and $D^{(1)}(x_1; x_1')$ is simply the one-electron reduced density matrix (RDM) for the state. The factor N of Eq. (D-8) can be absorbed into the definition of the RDM, in which case we will write

$$\gamma(BA|x_1; x_1') = N D^{(1)}(BA|x_1; x_1'). \tag{D-9}$$

A similar examination of two-electron operators and their matrix elements leads us to define the two-electron RDM's

$$D^{(2)}(BA|x_1, x_2; x_1', x_2') = \int \Psi_B(x_1, x_2, x_3, \ldots, x_N) \times \Psi_A^*(x_1', x_2', x_3, \ldots, x_N)\, dx_3 \cdots dx_N, \tag{D-10}$$

$$\Gamma(BA|x_1, x_2; x_1', x_2') = \binom{N}{2} D^{(2)}(BA|x_1, x_2; x_1', x_2')$$

such that

$$\langle A|\mathscr{G}|B\rangle = \int' g(1, 2)\Gamma(BA|x_1, x_2; x_1', x_2')\, dx_1\, dx_2. \tag{D-11}$$

The Hamiltonian operator combines one- and two-electron operators

$$\mathscr{H} = \sum_{i=1}^{N} f(i) + \sum_{i>j=1}^{N} g(ij). \tag{D-12}$$

It can be rewritten as a "purely two-electron" operator

$$\mathscr{H} = \sum_{i>j=1}^{N} K(ij) \tag{D-13}$$

by using

$$K(ij) = \frac{1}{N-1}[f(i) + f(j)] + g(ij). \tag{D-14}$$

The operator $K(1, 2)$ is known as the *reduced Hamiltonian* of the system for which $\mathscr{H}$ is the Hamiltonian, and

$$\langle A|\mathscr{H}|B\rangle = \int' K(1, 2)\Gamma(BA|x_1, x_2; x_1', x_2')\, dx_1\, dx_2. \tag{D-15}$$

In general we can divide the variables for the N electrons into two groups

$$P = x_1, \ldots, x_p, \qquad Q = x_{p+1}, \ldots, x_N \tag{D-16}$$

and define

$$D^{(p)}(BA|P; P') = \int \Psi_B(P, Q)\Psi_A^*(P', Q)\, dQ, \tag{D-17}$$

the p-electron RDM or p-matrix. The physically interesting cases are $p = 1$ or 2, but it is sometimes convenient to consider them (and others) at the same time.

Let us now specialize to a single state with $A = B$ and suppress the state label. Corresponding to the RDM $D^{(p)}$ we can define an operator $\hat{D}^{(p)}$ which is an integral operator with $D^{(p)}$ as kernel, normally considered to act on p-electron functions

$$\hat{D}^{(p)}\Phi(P) = \int D^{(p)}(P; P')\Phi(P')\, dP'. \tag{D-18}$$

It is readily shown from the definitions that $\hat{D}^{(p)}$ is Hermitian

$$\hat{D}^{(p)\dagger} = \hat{D}^{(p)} \tag{D-19}$$

and positive, i.e.,

$$\int \Phi(P)\hat{D}^{(p)}\Phi(P)\, dP \geq 0 \tag{D-20}$$

for any Φ. If $p > 1$, $D^{(p)}(P; P')$ is antisymmetric with respect to permutation of electron labels within the primed or within the unprimed set of variables. The trace of $\hat{D}^{(p)}$ is

$$\operatorname{tr} \hat{D}^{(p)} = \int D^{(p)}(P; P)\, dP = 1. \tag{D-21}$$

The Hermitian operator $\hat{D}^{(p)}$ has real, nonnegative eigenvalues whose sum is 1.

$$\hat{D}^{(p)}\Phi_k^{(p)} = \lambda_k^{(p)}\Phi_k^{(p)}, \qquad 0 \le \lambda_k^{(p)} \le 1, \quad \sum_k \lambda_k^{(p)} = 1. \tag{D-22}$$

It can be shown that the spectrum of $\hat{D}^{(p)}$ is purely discrete—i.e., there are no eigenvalues lying continuously in some range.

The eigenfunctions of γ are called natural spin orbitals (NSO's) and those of Γ are called natural spin geminals (NSG's). The wave function Ψ from which γ is obtained can be expanded in terms of configurations built up from NSO's (associated with nonzero eigenvalues). This is called the natural expansion of Ψ and has certain optimal properties.

The spinless component of γ obtained by integrating over the spin coordinate is the (one-electron) charge density matrix

$$\gamma^0(\mathbf{r}_1; \mathbf{r}_1') = \int \gamma(\mathbf{r}_1, \xi_1; \mathbf{r}_1', \xi_1)\, d\xi_1. \tag{D-23}$$

Its eigenfunctions are natural orbitals (NO's). For an $\mathcal{S}^2$, $\mathcal{S}_z$ eigenfunction with $M_S = 0$, each NSO can be taken as an NO times a simple α or β spin function. When $M_S \neq 0$, the relationship between NO's and NSO's is complicated.

The two-electron charge density matrix Γ^0, obtained by integration over spin variables in Γ, has eigenfunctions known as natural geminals (NG's). They are permutationally symmetric or antisymmetric. The NSG's are simply related to the NG's only when $M_S = 0$.

Other spin components of RDM's have been thoroughly treated, and other aspects of symmetry have been considered. Many other properties of RDM's are known, but will not be considered here. The aspects of the spin component analysis of use to us have been presented in Section 10.

If a basis set of p-electron functions $\{\chi_k(P)\}$ is introduced, the matrix $\mathbf{D}^{(p)}$ corresponding to the operator $\hat{D}^{(p)}$ will have elements

$$\begin{aligned} D_{kl}^{(p)} &= \int \chi_k^*(P)\hat{D}^{(p)}\chi_l(P)\, dP \\ &= \iint \chi_k^*(P) D^{(p)}(P; P')\chi_l(P')\, dP'\, dP. \end{aligned} \tag{D-24}$$

The function $D^{(p)}(P; P')$ can also be expanded in terms of the basis set as

$$D^{(p)}(P; P') = \sum_{k,l} \bar{D}_{kl}^{(p)} \chi_k(P) \chi_l^*(P'). \tag{D-25}$$

The matrix of expansion coefficients, $\bar{\mathbf{D}}^{(p)}$, is related to the matrix of the operator, $\mathbf{D}^{(p)}$, by

$$\mathbf{D}^{(p)} = \mathbf{S}\bar{\mathbf{D}}^{(p)}\mathbf{S}, \tag{D-26}$$

where $\mathbf{S}$ is the basis set overlap matrix

$$S_{ij} = \int \chi_i^*(P) \chi_j(P)\, dP. \tag{D-27}$$

The matrices $\bar{\mathbf{D}}^{(p)}$ and $\mathbf{D}^{(p)}$ are thus the same only if the basis set is orthonormal. If the eigenfunctions $\Phi_k^{(p)}$ are used as the basis, the expansion is of the form

$$D^{(p)}(P; P') = \sum_k \lambda_k^{(p)} \Phi_k^{(p)}(P) \Phi_k^{(p)*}(P'). \tag{D-28}$$

This is the spectral expansion of the operator $\hat{D}^{(p)}$.

In a typical case $D^{(p)}$ will have been obtained from a wave function which, in turn, will have been calculated using some one-electron basis set. If $p = 1$, the same basis set or some set spanning the same space should be used to expand $D^{(p)}$. If $p > 1$, the complete set of p-electron configurations built up from the one-electron set should be used. If a smaller basis set is used, the expansion of $D^{(p)}$ may be incomplete.

Appendix E
Some Useful Operator Identities and Matrix Relationships

It is the function of this appendix to present, in a somewhat random fashion, a number of operator and matrix results which have been useful in the derivation of results or might be useful in connection with the application of results presented in this book. Proofs (where given) are formal only. In each particular case it may be necessary to investigate convergence, domain, etc., as appropriate.

Inverse of Operator Sum

If A and B are operators such that A^{-1} and $(A - B)^{-1}$ exist, then

$$(A - B)^{-1} = A^{-1} \sum_{k=0}^{\infty} (BA^{-1})^k. \tag{E-1}$$

To verify this expression we multiply from the left by $(A - B)$ to obtain

$$\begin{aligned}(A - B)(A - B)^{-1} &= (A - B)A^{-1} \sum_{k=0}^{\infty} (BA^{-1})^k \\ &= \sum_{k=0}^{\infty} (BA)^{-1})^k - (BA^{-1}) \sum_{k=0}^{\infty} (BA^{-1})^k \\ &= (BA^{-1})^0 = 1.\end{aligned}$$

If the operators are well behaved, then the right inverse will also be a left inverse.

Exponential Operators

The exponential of an operator is defined by its series expansion

$$e^A = \sum_{n=0}^{\infty} \frac{1}{n!} A^n \tag{E-2}$$

or by its effect on eigenfunctions of the operator. Suppose

$$A\phi_n = a_n \phi_n \tag{E-3}$$

and a general function ψ can be expanded as

$$\psi = \sum_n C_n \phi_n. \tag{E-4}$$

Then

$$e^A \psi = \sum_n C_n e^{a_n} \phi_n. \tag{E-5}$$

We now consider an operator $B(\xi)$ which depends on a parameter ξ and is defined by

$$B(\xi) = e^{A\xi} B_0 e^{-A\xi}, \tag{E-6}$$

where A and B_0 do not depend on ξ. The derivative of $B(\xi)$ with respect to ξ, defined as

$$\frac{dB}{d\xi} = \lim_{x \to 0} \frac{B(\xi + x) - B(\xi)}{x} \tag{E-7}$$

is

$$\frac{dB}{d\xi} = Ae^{A\xi} B_0 e^{-A\xi} + e^{A\xi} B_0 e^{-A\xi}(-A) = [A, B]. \tag{E-8}$$

We note that $B_0 = B(0)$ and integrate to obtain

$$B(\xi) = B_0 + \int_0^\xi [A, B(x)]\, dx = B_0 + \left[A, \int_0^\xi B(x)\, dx\right]. \tag{E-9}$$

This equation can be solved by iteration to obtain

$$\begin{aligned}
B(\xi) &= B_0 + \left[A, \int_0^\xi \left\{B_0 + \left[A, \int_0^x B(y)\, dy\right]\right\} dx\right] \\
&= B_0 + \left[A, \int_0^\xi \left\{B_0 + \left[A, \int_0^x \left(B_0 + \left[A, \int_0^y B(z)\, dz\right]\right) dy\right]\right\} dx\right] \\
&= B_0 + [A, B_0] \int_0^\xi dx + [A, [A, B_0]] \int_0^\xi \int_0^x dy\, dx \\
&\quad + [A, [A, [A, B_0]]] \int_0^\xi \int_0^x \int_0^y dz\, dy\, dx + \cdots \\
&= B_0 + \xi[A, B_0] + \tfrac{1}{2}\xi^2[A, [A, B_0]] + \frac{\xi^3}{3!}[A, [A, [A, B_0]]] + \cdots \\
&= \sum_{n=0}^{\infty} \frac{\xi^n}{n!} ([A,)^n\, B_0(])^n.
\end{aligned} \tag{E-10}$$

We now let $\xi = 1$ and substitute from Eq. (E-6) on the left side to obtain

$$e^A B_0 e^{-A} = B_0 + [A, B_0] + \tfrac{1}{2}[A, [A, B_0]] + \cdots$$
$$= \sum_{n=0}^{\infty} \frac{1}{n!} ([A,)^n B_0(])^n. \tag{E-11}$$

Suppose that A depends on some variable t (different from ξ) and let $B_0 = d/dt$. We distinguish between the operator product $(d/dt)\,A$, in which d/dt acts on A and everything following it, and (dA/dt) in which d/dt does not act on what follows. Then

$$e^A \frac{de^{-A}}{dt} = e^A\left[\frac{d}{dt}, e^{-A}\right] = e^A \frac{d}{dt} e^{-A} - e^A e^{-A} \frac{d}{dt} \tag{E-12}$$

The second term is just $d/dt = B_0$, so from Eq. (E-11)

$$e^A \frac{de^{-A}}{dt} = \left[A, \frac{d}{dt}\right] + \frac{1}{2}\left[A, \left[A, \frac{d}{dt}\right]\right] + \frac{1}{3!}\left[A, \left[A, \left[A, \frac{d}{dt}\right]\right]\right] + \cdots$$
$$= -\frac{dA}{dt} - \frac{1}{2}\left[A, \frac{dA}{dt}\right] - \frac{1}{3!}\left[A, \left[A, \frac{dA}{dt}\right]\right] - \cdots$$
$$= -\sum_{n=0}^{\infty} \frac{1}{(n+1)!} ([A,)^n \frac{dA}{dt} (])^n. \tag{E-13}$$

Eigenvalues and Eigenvectors of a Complex Hermitian Matrix

Many of the matrices of interest in quantum chemistry are in principle Hermitian but in actual calculations are real symmetric. Many algorithms and computer programs are available for obtaining eigenvalues and eigenvectors of a real symmetric matrix. In connection with single crystal ESR, matrices arise which actually are complex Hermitian (cf. Section 7). Algorithms and programs to deal with these matrices exist but are less common. An approach will be presented here in which the eigenvalue–eigenvector problem for a complex Hermitian matrix of dimension N is converted into that for a real symmetric matrix of dimension $2N$.

We are interested in obtaining the eigenvalues E and eigenvectors $\mathbf{C}$ of a Hermitian matrix $\mathbf{H}$:

$$(\mathbf{H} - E\mathbf{1})\mathbf{C} = 0. \tag{E-14}$$

Let us separate the real and imaginary parts of $\mathbf{H}$ and $\mathbf{C}$ (E is real),

$$\mathbf{H} = \mathbf{U} + i\mathbf{V}, \qquad \mathbf{C} = \mathbf{X} + i\mathbf{Y}, \tag{E-15}$$

where $\mathbf{U}$, $\mathbf{V}$, $\mathbf{X}$, and $\mathbf{Y}$ are real. The real and imaginary parts of Eq. (E-14) hold separately, and the resultant two equations can be combined into a single equation involving a real, symmetric matrix of double the original size

$$\begin{pmatrix} \mathbf{U} - E\mathbf{1} & -\mathbf{V} \\ \mathbf{V} & \mathbf{U} - E\mathbf{1} \end{pmatrix} \begin{pmatrix} \mathbf{X} \\ \mathbf{Y} \end{pmatrix} = 0. \tag{E-16}$$

It is clear that a solution of Eq. (E-14) provides a solution of Eq. (E-16), but we are interested in going the other way. Since the matrix of Eq. (E-16) is twice the size of that of Eq. (E-14), it will have twice as many eigenvalues and eigenvectors. How can those desired be identified?

The equations are homogeneous and the phases of the eigenvectors are not determined. In particular, if $\mathbf{C}$ is an eigenvector of $\mathbf{H}$ associated with eigenvalue E, then $i\mathbf{C}$ is also an eigenvector, associated with the same eigenvalue. The separation of real and imaginary parts then gives

$$i\mathbf{C} = -\mathbf{Y} + i\mathbf{X}. \tag{E-17}$$

The vector $(-\mathbf{Y}, \mathbf{X})$ is a solution of Eq. (E-16) associated with eigenvalue E as well. The form of the matrix is such that the equations associated with eigenvectors $(\mathbf{X}, \mathbf{Y})$ and $(-\mathbf{Y}, \mathbf{X})$ are in fact equivalent; one of the pair of equations contained in Eq. (E-16) has the sign of each term reversed in one case as compared with the other.

Since (X, Y) and $(-Y, X)$ are degenerate, any linear combination of them will also be an eigenvector with the same eigenvalue. In general

$$[\cos\theta\, \mathbf{X} + \sin\theta\, (-\mathbf{Y})] + i[\cos\theta\, \mathbf{Y} + \sin\theta\, \mathbf{X}] = e^{i\theta}\mathbf{C}. \tag{E-18}$$

We conclude that the solutions of Eq. (E-16) occur in degenerate pairs (or possibly higher, even degeneracy, if $\mathbf{H}$ has degenerate eigenvalues). The eigenvalues are also eigenvalues of $\mathbf{H}$, and any eigenvector can be related to a complex eigenvector of $\mathbf{H}$, with the other degenerate eigenvector corresponding to a different phase choice.

Diagonalization and Inversion of 2×2 Matrices

Because 2×2 matrices can be dealt with analytically, they are of particular interest as sample or special cases. We consider here the diagonalization and inversion of 2×2 matrices.

Let

$$\mathbf{H} = \begin{pmatrix} H_{1,1} & H_{1,2} \\ H_{1,2}^* & H_{2,2} \end{pmatrix} \tag{E-19}$$

be a Hermitian matrix. Its eigenvalues are given by

$$\begin{aligned} 0 = |\mathbf{H} - E\mathbf{1}| &= \begin{vmatrix} H_{1,1} - E & H_{1,2} \\ H_{1,2}^{*} & H_{2,2} - E \end{vmatrix} \\ &= (H_{1,1} - E)(H_{2,2} - E) - |H_{1,2}|^2 \\ &= E^2 - (H_{1,1} + H_{2,2})E + H_{1,1}H_{2,2} - |H_{1,2}|^2 \\ E &= \tfrac{1}{2}(H_{1,1} + H_{2,2}) \pm ([\tfrac{1}{2}(H_{1,1} - H_{2,2})]^2 + |H_{1,2}|^2)^{1/2}. \end{aligned} \tag{E-20}$$

We rewrite $H_{1,2}$ as

$$H_{1,2} = |H_{1,2}|e^{i\theta}. \tag{E-21}$$

The eigenvectors of $\mathbf{H}$ are

$$\mathbf{c}_+ = \begin{pmatrix} \cos\theta \\ \sin\theta\, e^{-i\theta} \end{pmatrix}, \qquad \mathbf{c}_- = \begin{pmatrix} -\sin\theta\, e^{i\theta} \\ \cos\theta \end{pmatrix}, \tag{E-22}$$

where θ is determined so that

$$\tan 2\theta = \frac{2|H_{1,2}|}{H_{1,1} - H_{2,2}}. \tag{E-23}$$

This can be verified by direct calculation. Let $\mathbf{C}$ be the matrix whose columns are $\mathbf{c}_+$ and $\mathbf{c}_-$, and define

$$\Delta = \mathbf{C}^{\dagger}\mathbf{H}\mathbf{C}. \tag{E-24}$$

Then from matrix multiplication and trigonometric identities

$$\Delta_{1,2} = \Delta_{2,1}^{*} = [-\tfrac{1}{2}(H_{1,1} - H_{2,2})\sin 2\theta + |H_{1,2}|\cos 2\theta]e^{i\theta}. \tag{E-25}$$

This will vanish if θ satisfies Eq. (E-23), so $\mathbf{C}$ diagonalizes $\mathbf{H}$. The diagonal elements are

$$\Delta_{1,1} = \tfrac{1}{2}(H_{1,1} + H_{2,2}) + K, \qquad \Delta_{2,2} = \tfrac{1}{2}(H_{1,1} + H_{2,2}) - K, \tag{E-26}$$

where

$$K = \tfrac{1}{2}(H_{1,1} - H_{2,2})\cos 2\theta + |H_{1,2}|\sin 2\theta. \tag{E-27}$$

This is consistent with Eq. (E-20) and by considering the limit $H_{1,2} \to 0$ we see that the eigenvector $\mathbf{c}_+$ is associated with eigenvalue E_+, and $\mathbf{c}_-$ with E_-.

The inverse of any matrix, if it exists, can be expressed as the transposed matrix of cofactors divided by the determinant. In the 2×2 case this is simple because each cofactor is just a single element. Suppose

$$\mathbf{A} = \begin{pmatrix} a & b \\ c & d \end{pmatrix}. \tag{E-28}$$

Then if $ad - bc \neq 0$,

$$\mathbf{A}^{-1} = (ad - bc)^{-1}\begin{pmatrix} d & -b \\ -c & a \end{pmatrix}. \tag{E-29}$$

This is readily verified by direct computation of $\mathbf{AA}^{-1} = 1$.

Commutators of Spin-Dependent Operators with $\mathscr{S}^2$

In a system with N electrons the spin operators are

$$\begin{aligned} \mathscr{S}_a &= \sum_{i=1}^{N} s_a(i), \qquad a = x, y, \text{ or } z, \\ \mathscr{S}^2 &= \sum_a \mathscr{S}_a^2 = \mathscr{S} \cdot \mathscr{S}. \end{aligned} \tag{E-30}$$

Everyone knows that the components of $\mathscr{S}$ commute with $\mathscr{S}^2$, but it is sometimes forgotten that one- and two-electron operators including both spin and spatial parts do not in general commute with $\mathscr{S}^2$. Explicit expressions for the commutators are obtained here.

Certain properties of the one-electron spin operators will be required. Of course they satisfy the usual angular momentum commutation relationships, and operators associated with different electrons commute. In addition, from the fact that $\mathbf{s} = \frac{1}{2}\boldsymbol{\sigma}$ and the properties of the Pauli matrices $\boldsymbol{\sigma}$ [cf. Eq. (C-15)] we obtain additional relationships. It is convenient to introduce the antisymmetric tensor

$$\varepsilon_{abc} = \begin{cases} +1, & \text{if } a, b, c \text{ is an even permutation of } x, y, z, \\ -1, & \text{if } a, b, c \text{ is an odd permutation of } x, y, z, \\ 0, & \text{if any two of } a, b, c \text{ are equal.} \end{cases} \tag{E-31}$$

Indices $a, b, c, \ldots$ will be used to label Cartesian components x, y, and z. Indices $j, k, l, \ldots$ will be used to label electrons. We can then write

$$\begin{aligned} [s_a(j), s_b(k)] &= i\delta_{jk} \sum_c \varepsilon_{abc} s_c(j), \\ s_a(j)s_b(j) &= \frac{i}{2}\sum_c \varepsilon_{abc} s_c(j) + \tfrac{1}{4}\delta_{ab}. \end{aligned} \tag{E-32}$$

We consider first a one-electron spin-dependent operator, which we write as

$$\mathscr{F} = \sum_a \sum_j f_a(j) s_a(j). \tag{E-33}$$

It is convenient to introduce a more general notation

$$F_b^a = \sum_j f_a(j) s_b(j) \tag{E-34}$$

in terms of which $\mathscr{F} = \sum_a F_a^a$. We then consider

$$
\begin{aligned}
[F_a^a, \mathscr{S}^2] &= \sum_{jkl} \sum_b [f_a(j)s_a(j), s_b(k)s_b(l)] \\
&= \sum_{jkl} \sum_b f_a(j)\{s_b(k)[s_a(j), s_b(l)] + [s_a(j), s_b(k)]s_b(l)\} \\
&= i \sum_{j,k} \sum_{b,c} \varepsilon_{abc} f_a(j)\{s_b(k)s_c(j) + s_c(j)s_b(k)\} \\
&= i \sum_{b,c} \varepsilon_{abc}\{\mathscr{S}_b F_c^a + F_c^a \mathscr{S}_b\}.
\end{aligned} \tag{E-35}
$$

The commutator of $\mathscr{F}$ with $\mathscr{S}^2$ can then be written

$$
[\mathscr{F}, \mathscr{S}^2] = \sum_a [F_a^a, \mathscr{S}^2] = -i(\mathscr{S} \cdot \mathscr{F}^\times + \mathscr{F}^\times \cdot \mathscr{S}), \tag{E-36}
$$

where $\mathscr{F}^\times$ is the one-electron vector operator

$$
\mathscr{F}^\times = \sum_j (\mathbf{f}(j) \times \mathbf{s}(j)), \tag{E-37}
$$

since the cross product can be expressed in terms of ε_{abc}. It can be verified that if the components of $\mathbf{f}$ are constants, so that $\mathscr{F}$ is proportional to a pure spin operator, then $[\mathscr{F}, \mathscr{S}^2]$ vanishes. This is essentially because $f_a(j)$ is independent of j in such a case.

A similar result can be obtained for two-electron operators. If the operator involves the spin of only one electron (e.g., the spin–other-orbit operator) it can be treated just like the one-electron operators: for

$$
G_a^a = \sum_{j,k}{}' g_a(j,k)s_a(j), \tag{E-38}
$$

we simply define

$$
f_a(j) = \sum_{k\,(\neq j)} g_a(j,k) \tag{E-39}
$$

and proceed as above. When spins of both electrons are involved we consider

$$
\mathscr{G} = \sum_{a,b} G_{ab}^{ab}, \tag{E-40}
$$

where, in general,

$$
G_{cd}^{ab} = \sum_{j,k} g_{ab}(j,k)s_c(j)s_d(k). \tag{E-41}
$$

A treatment similar to that in Eqs. (E-35) leads to the result

$$
[G_{ab}^{ab}, \mathscr{S}^2] = 2i \sum_{c,d} \{\varepsilon_{bcd} G_{ad}^{ab} \mathscr{S}_c + \varepsilon_{acd} \mathscr{S}_c G_{db}^{ab}\} \tag{E-42}
$$

and

$$[\mathcal{G}, \mathcal{S}^2] = \sum_{a,b} [G_{ab}^{ab}, \mathcal{S}^2] = -2i(\mathcal{G}^{\times} \cdot \mathcal{S} - \mathcal{S} \cdot {}^{\times}\mathcal{G}) \qquad \text{(E-43)}$$

where

$$\begin{aligned} \mathcal{G}_c^{\times} &= \sum_{j,k}{}' \sum_{abd} \varepsilon_{cdb}\, g_{ab}(j,k) s_a(j) s_d(k) \\ {}^{\times}\mathcal{G}_c &= \sum_{j,k}{}' \sum_{abd} \varepsilon_{cad}\, g_{ab}(j,k) s_d(j) s_b(k). \end{aligned} \qquad \text{(E-44)}$$

These could be expressed as cross products in the components relating to one of the electrons in each case.

Appendix F
Summary of Terms in the Hamiltonian

The function of this appendix is to review some features of the approximate (two-component per electron) electronic Hamiltonian. This is done in two tables. Table F-1 lists the various terms in the Hamiltonian, and Table F-2 reviews their origins and indicates how they contribute to spin Hamiltonian parameters.

The Hamiltonian terms in Table F-1 are divided into five basic groups: (0) terms of the zero-order Hamiltonian, (1) relativistic corrections not depending on spins or magnetic field, (2) terms depending on spins but not magnetic field, (3) terms depending on magnetic field but not on spins, and (4) terms depending on spins and field. Terms depending on an external electric field are not included, and the external magnetic field is assumed to be uniform over the dimensions of any system of interest. In the spirit of the Born–Oppenheimer separation, no terms involving derivatives with respect to nuclear coordinates have been included.

Within each group, terms independent of nuclear spins come before any depending on nuclear spin. Within each subgroup, finally, any terms independent of electronic coordinates come first, one-electron operators next, and two-electron operators last. A descriptive name has been given in the second column for each term. In some cases these names are reasonably standard; in other cases they are (probably) used only within this book.

The third column in Table F-1 gives the operators themselves, apart from certain constants. Summation indices j and k label electrons, while ν and ν' label nuclei. The coordinate representation is assumed, so $\mathbf{\nabla}_j$ is written in place of $\mathbf{p}_j$, and $\mathbf{r}_j \times \mathbf{\nabla}_j$ in place of $\boldsymbol{l}_j$, etc. Spin operators are in units of $\hbar$. Explicit signs and numerical coefficients of order of magnitude one are included in this column. The coefficients g and g' are the electronic g factors appropriate to the Zeeman interaction and the spin–orbit interaction, respectively. In terms of the parameter g_1 of Section 3 they are $g = 2(1 + g_1)$ and $g' = 2(1 + 2g_1)$. Although g' is certainly appropriate in term 2.1 and g is correct in term 4.1, the treatment of radiative corrections here has been incomplete so great significance should not be attached to the distinction between g, g', and 2 in higher-order terms. In no case should g or g' be used to higher than first order in perturbation theory. It is of interest to note that if the Fermi contact term is obtained by the Foldy–Wouthuysen (FW) method

TABLE F-1

The Approximate Hamiltonian

Term	Description	Operator	Coefficient: Atomic units	Coefficient: Gaussian units
Zero-order				
0.0	Nuclear–nuclear Coulomb interaction	$\sum_{v<v'} \left(\frac{Z_v Z_{v'}}{R_{vv'}}\right)$	$\mathscr{E}_0 a_0$	e^2
0.1	Kinetic energy	$\sum_j \left(-\frac{1}{2}\nabla_j^2\right)$	$\mathscr{E}_0 a_0^2$	$\frac{\hbar^2}{m}$
0.2	Electron–nuclear Coulomb interaction (nuclear attraction)	$\sum_{j,v} \left(-\frac{Z_v}{r_{jv}}\right)$	$\mathscr{E}_0 a_0$	e^2
0.3	Electron–electron Coulomb interaction (electron repulsion)	$\sum_{j<k} \left(\frac{1}{r_{jk}}\right)$	$\mathscr{E}_0 a_0$	e^2
Relativistic corrections independent of spin and field				
1.1	Kinetic energy mass correction	$\sum_j \left(-\frac{1}{8}\nabla_j^4\right)$	$\alpha^2 \mathscr{E}_0 a_0^4$	$\frac{\hbar^4}{m^3 c^2}$
1.2	(Electron–nuclear) Darwin term	$\sum_{j,v} Z_v \frac{\pi}{2} \delta(\mathbf{r}_{jv})$	$\alpha^2 \mathscr{E}_0 a_0^3$	$4\beta^2$

TABLE F-1 (*continued*)

TABLE F-1 (*continued*)

Term	Description	Operator	Coefficient: Atomic units	Coefficient: Gaussian units
1.3	Electron–electron Darwin term	$\sum_{j<k}(-\pi\delta(\mathbf{r}_{jk}))$	$\alpha^2\mathscr{E}_0 a_0^3$	$4\beta^2$
1.4	Electron–electron orbital interaction	$\sum_{j<k}\left[+\frac{1}{2}\left(\frac{\nabla_j\cdot\nabla_k}{r_{jk}}-\frac{(\mathbf{r}_{jk}\cdot\nabla_j)(\mathbf{r}_{jk}\cdot\nabla_k)}{r_{jk}^3}\right)\right]$	$\alpha^2\mathscr{E}_0 a_0^3$	$4\beta^2$
1.5	Electron–electron orbital interaction	$\sum_{j<k}\left[+\frac{1}{4}\frac{1}{r_{jk}^3}(\mathbf{r}_{jk}\cdot\nabla_k-\mathbf{r}_{jk}\cdot\nabla_j)\right]$	$\alpha^2\mathscr{E}_0 a_0^3$	$4\beta^2$
1.6	Electron–electron orbital interaction	$\sum_{j<k}[\pi\delta(\mathbf{r}_{jk})(\mathbf{r}_{jk}\cdot\nabla_j-\mathbf{r}_{jk}\cdot\nabla_k)]$	$\alpha^2\mathscr{E}_0 a_0^3$	$4\beta^2$
Terms depending on spin but not field				
(Electron spin)				
2.1	Spin–orbit interaction	$\sum_{j,\nu}\left(-\frac{g'}{4}Z_\nu i\frac{k_0^2(\mathbf{r}_{j\nu})}{r_{jk}^3}\mathbf{S}_j\cdot(\mathbf{r}_{j\nu}\times\nabla_j)\right)$	$\alpha^2\mathscr{E}_0 a_0^3$	$4\beta^2$
2.2	Spin–other-orbit interaction	$\sum_{j,k}'\frac{i}{r_{jk}^3}\mathbf{S}_j\cdot[(\mathbf{r}_{kj})\times\nabla_k]$	$\alpha^2\mathscr{E}\,a_0^3$	$4\beta^2$
2.3	Electron–electron spin–orbit interaction	$\sum_{j,k}'\left(\frac{g'}{4}\frac{i}{r_{jk}^3}\mathbf{S}_j\cdot\mathbf{r}_{jk}\times\nabla_j\right)$	$\alpha^2\mathscr{E}_0 a_0^3$	$4\beta^2$
2.4	Spin–spin dipolar interaction	$\sum_{j<k}\left(\frac{\mathbf{S}_j\cdot\mathbf{S}_k}{r_{jk}^3}-\frac{(\mathbf{S}_j\cdot\mathbf{r}_{jk})(\mathbf{S}_k\cdot\mathbf{r}_{jk})}{r_{jk}^5}\right)$	$\alpha^2\mathscr{E}_0 a_0^3$	$4\beta^2$

TABLE F-1 (*continued*)

2.5	Spin–spin contact interaction	$\sum_{j<k}\left(-\frac{8\pi}{3}\mathbf{S}_j\cdot\mathbf{S}_k\,\delta(\mathbf{r}_{jk})\right)$	$\alpha^2\mathscr{E}_0 a_0^3$	$4\beta^2$
(Nuclear spin)				
2.6	Nuclear dipole–dipole interaction	$\sum_{\nu<\nu'}\frac{g_\nu g_{\nu'}}{4}\left[\frac{\mathbf{I}_\nu\cdot\mathbf{I}_{\nu'}}{R_{\nu\nu'}^3}-3\frac{(\mathbf{I}_\nu\cdot\mathbf{R}_{\nu\nu'})(\mathbf{I}_{\nu'}\cdot\mathbf{R}_{\nu\nu'})}{R_{\nu\nu'}^5}\right]$	$\left(\frac{m}{M_\mathrm{P}}\right)^2\alpha^2\mathscr{E}_0 a_0^3$	$4\beta_\mathrm{N}^2$
2.7	Nuclear quadrupole interaction	$\sum_{j,\nu}\left[\frac{Q_\nu}{2I_\nu(2I_\nu-1)}\right]\left[\frac{I_\nu^2}{r_{j\nu}^3}-3\frac{(\mathbf{r}_{j\nu}\cdot\mathbf{I}_\nu)^2}{r_{j\nu}^5}\right]$	$\mathscr{E}a_0$	e^2
2.8	Orbital hyperfine interaction	$\sum_{j,\nu}\frac{-g_\nu}{2}k_0(r_{j\nu})\frac{i}{r_{j\nu}^3}(\mathbf{r}_{j\nu}\times\nabla_j)\cdot\mathbf{I}_\nu$	$\left(\frac{m}{M_\mathrm{P}}\right)\alpha^2\mathscr{E}_0 a_0^3$	$4\beta\beta_\mathrm{N}$
2.9	Orbital hyperfine correction	$\sum_{j,\nu}\frac{g_\nu}{4}k_0^3(r_{j\nu})\nabla_j^2\frac{i}{r_{j\nu}^3}(\mathbf{r}_{j\nu}\times\nabla_j)\cdot\mathbf{I}_\nu$	$\left(\frac{m}{M_\mathrm{P}}\right)\alpha^2\mathscr{E}_0 a_0^5$	$4\left(\frac{\hbar}{mc}\right)^2\beta\beta_\mathrm{N}$
2.10	Electron coupled nuclear spin–spin interaction	$\sum_j\sum_{\nu,\nu'}\frac{g_\nu g_{\nu'}}{8}\frac{k_0(r_{\nu j})}{r_{j\nu}^3 r_{j\nu'}^3}\times[(\mathbf{I}_\nu\cdot\mathbf{I}_{\nu'})(\mathbf{r}_{j\nu}\cdot\mathbf{r}_{j\nu'})-(\mathbf{I}_\nu\cdot\mathbf{r}_{j\nu})(\mathbf{I}_{\nu'}\cdot\mathbf{r}_{j\nu})]$	$\left(\frac{m}{M_\mathrm{P}}\right)^2\alpha^4\mathscr{E}a_0^4$	$\frac{4e^2}{mc^2}\beta_\mathrm{N}^2$
(Electron and nuclear spins)				
2.11	Dipolar hyperfine interaction	$\sum_{j,\nu}\left(-\frac{gg_\nu}{4}k_0(r_{j\nu})\left[\frac{\mathbf{S}_{j\nu}\cdot\mathbf{I}_\nu}{r_{j\nu}^3}-3\frac{(\mathbf{S}_j\cdot\mathbf{r}_{j\nu})(\mathbf{I}_\nu\cdot\mathbf{r}_{j\nu})}{r_{j\nu}^5}\right]\right)$	$\left(\frac{m}{M_\mathrm{P}}\right)\alpha^2\mathscr{E}_0 a_0^3$	$4\beta\beta_\mathrm{N}$
2.12	(Fermi) contact hyperfine interaction	$\sum_{j,\nu}\frac{2\pi}{3}g'g_\nu\mathbf{S}_j\cdot\mathbf{I}_\nu\,\delta(\mathbf{r}_{j\nu})$	$\left(\frac{m}{M_\mathrm{P}}\right)\alpha^2\mathscr{E}_0 a_0^3$	$4\beta\beta_\mathrm{N}$

TABLE F-1 (*continued*)

Term	Description	Operator	Coefficient: Atomic units	Coefficient: Gaussian units
2.13	Spin–orbit hyperfine correction	$\sum_j \sum'_{\nu,\nu'} \frac{g_\nu g'}{8} \frac{Z_{\nu'} k_0^2(r_{j\nu})}{r_{j\nu}^3 r_{j\nu'}^3} \times [(\mathbf{r}_{j\nu} \cdot \mathbf{r}_{j\nu'})(\mathbf{S}_j \cdot \mathbf{I}_\nu) - (\mathbf{S}_j \cdot \mathbf{r}_{j\nu'})(\mathbf{I}_\nu \cdot \mathbf{r}_{j\nu})]$	$\left(\frac{m}{M_P}\right)\alpha^4 \mathscr{E}_0 a_0^4$	$8 \frac{e}{\hbar c} \beta^2 \beta_N$
2.14	Spin–other-orbit hyperfine correction	$\sum'_{j,k} \sum_\nu \frac{g_\nu}{4} \frac{1}{r_{jk}^3} \frac{1}{r_{j\nu}^3} \times [(\mathbf{r}_{kj} \cdot \mathbf{r}_{k\nu})(\mathbf{S}_j \cdot \mathbf{I}_\nu) - (\mathbf{r}_{kj} \cdot \mathbf{I}_\nu)(\mathbf{r}_{k\nu} \cdot \mathbf{S}_j)]$	$\left(\frac{m}{M_P}\right)\alpha^4 \mathscr{E}_0 a_0^4$	$8 \frac{e}{\hbar c} \beta^2 \beta_N$
2.15	Electron–electron spin–orbit hyperfine correction	$\sum'_{j,k} \sum_\nu \frac{g' g_\nu}{8} \frac{1}{r_{jk}^3} \frac{1}{r_{j\nu}^3} \times [(\mathbf{r}_{kj} \cdot \mathbf{r}_{j\nu})(\mathbf{S}_j \cdot \mathbf{I}_\nu) - (\mathbf{S}_j \cdot \mathbf{r}_{j\nu})(\mathbf{I}_\nu \cdot \mathbf{r}_{kj})]$	$\left(\frac{m}{M_P}\right)\alpha^4 \mathscr{E}_0 a_0^4$	$8 \frac{e}{\hbar c} \beta^2 \beta_N$
Terms depending on field but not spin				
3.1	Orbital Zeeman interaction	$\sum_j \left(-\frac{i}{2}(\mathbf{r}_j \times \nabla_j) \cdot \mathbf{B}\right)$	$\alpha a_0 e$	2β
3.2	Orbital Zeeman kinetic energy correction	$\sum_j \left(-\frac{i}{4} k_0^3(r_j) \nabla_j^2 (\mathbf{r}_j \times \nabla_j) \cdot \mathbf{B}\right)$	$\alpha^3 a_0^3 e$	$2\beta\left(\frac{\hbar}{mc}\right)^2$

3.3	Diamagnetic	$\sum_j \frac{1}{8}[B^2 r_j^2 - (\mathbf{B}\cdot\mathbf{r}_j)^2]$	$\alpha^2\varepsilon_0/a_0$	$\frac{e^2}{mc^2}$
Terms depending on spins and field (electron spin)				
4.1	(Electron spin) Zeeman	$\sum_j \frac{g}{2}\mathbf{S}_j\cdot\mathbf{B}$	$\alpha a_0 e$	2β
4.2	(Electron spin) Zeeman kinetic energy correction	$\sum_j -\frac{g}{2}\nabla_j^2\mathbf{S}_j\cdot\mathbf{B}$	$\alpha^3 a_0^3 e$	$2\beta\left(\frac{\hbar}{mc}\right)^2$
4.3	Spin–orbit Zeeman gauge correction	$\sum_{j,\nu} g'\frac{k_0^2}{8}\frac{Z_\nu}{r_{j\nu}^3}[(\mathbf{r}_{j\nu}\cdot\mathbf{r}_j)(\mathbf{S}_j\cdot\mathbf{B}) - (\mathbf{S}_j\cdot\mathbf{r}_j)(\mathbf{r}_j\cdot\mathbf{B})]$	$\alpha^3 a_0^2 e$	$2\beta\frac{e^2}{mc^2}$
4.4	Electron–electron spin–orbit Zeeman gauge correction	$\sum_{j,k}{}' \frac{g'}{8}\frac{1}{r_{jk}^3}[(\mathbf{r}_{kj}\cdot\mathbf{r}_j)(\mathbf{S}_j\cdot\mathbf{B}) - (\mathbf{S}_j\cdot\mathbf{B}) - (\mathbf{S}_j\cdot\mathbf{r}_j)(\mathbf{r}_{kj}\cdot\mathbf{B})]$	$\alpha^3 a_0^2 e$	$2\beta\frac{e^2}{mc^2}$
4.5	Spin–other-orbit Zeeman gauge correction	$\sum_{j,k}{}' \frac{1}{2}\frac{1}{r_{jk}^3}[(\mathbf{r}_{jk}\cdot\mathbf{r}_k)(\mathbf{S}_j\cdot\mathbf{B}) - (\mathbf{S}_j\cdot\mathbf{r}_k)(\mathbf{r}_{jk}\cdot\mathbf{B})]$	$\alpha^3 a_0^2 e$	$2\beta\frac{e^2}{mc^2}$
(Nuclear spin)				
4.6	Nuclear Zeeman	$\sum_\nu \frac{g_\nu}{2}\mathbf{I}_\nu\cdot\mathbf{B}$	$\left(\frac{m}{M_P}\right)\alpha a_0 e$	$2\beta_N$
4.7	Electronic nuclear Zeeman correction	$\sum_{j,\nu}\frac{g_\nu}{4}\frac{k_0}{r_{j\nu}^3}[(\mathbf{r}_j\cdot\mathbf{r}_{j\nu})(\mathbf{I}_\nu\cdot\mathbf{B}) - (\mathbf{r}_j\cdot\mathbf{I}_\nu)(\mathbf{r}_{j\nu}\cdot\mathbf{B})]$	$\left(\frac{m}{M_P}\right)\alpha^3 a_0^2 e$	$2\beta_N\frac{e^2}{mc^2}$

TABLE F-2

Origins and Destinations of Hamiltonian Terms

Term	Origin	Destination
0.0	$\underset{(4\text{-}30)}{\mathscr{H}_{12}\,\text{(first term)}}$	$\mathscr{H}_0$
0.1	$\underset{(2\text{-}64)}{\mathscr{H}^{(0)}_{1a}} \leftarrow \underset{\text{T2-4}}{\mathscr{H}^{(0)}_{1}} \leftarrow \underset{(2\text{-}58)}{\mathscr{H}^{(0)}}$	$\mathscr{H}_0$
0.2	$\underset{(2\text{-}82)}{\mathscr{H}^{(0)}_{2v}} \leftarrow \underset{\text{T2-4}}{\mathscr{H}^{(0)}_{2}} \leftarrow \underset{(2\text{-}58)}{\mathscr{H}^{(0)}}$	$\mathscr{H}_0$
0.3	$\underset{(4\text{-}34)}{\mathscr{H}_{12a}} \leftarrow \underset{(4\text{-}30)}{\mathscr{H}_{12}\,\text{(first term)}}$	$\mathscr{H}_0$
1.1	$\underset{(2\text{-}98)}{\mathscr{H}^{(1)}_{2a}} \leftarrow \underset{(2\text{-}79)}{\mathscr{H}^{(1)}_{2}} \leftarrow \underset{\text{T2-4}}{\mathscr{H}^{(1)}_{2}} \leftarrow \underset{(2\text{-}58)}{\mathscr{H}^{(1)}}$	Neglect
1.2	$\underset{(2\text{-}88)}{\mathscr{H}^{(1)}_{1av}} \leftarrow \underset{(2\text{-}83)}{\mathscr{H}^{(1)}_{1a}} \leftarrow \underset{\text{T2-4}}{\mathscr{H}^{(1)}_{1}} \leftarrow \underset{(2\text{-}58)}{\mathscr{H}^{(1)}}$	Neglect
	$\left[\underset{(2\text{-}88)(2\text{-}89)}{\mathscr{H}^{(1)}_{1av}} \leftarrow \underset{(2\text{-}89)}{\mathscr{H}^{(1)}_{1b}} \leftarrow \underset{\text{T2-4}}{\mathscr{H}^{(1)}_{1}} \leftarrow \underset{(2\text{-}58)}{\mathscr{H}^{(1)}}\right]$	
1.3	$\underset{(4\text{-}35)}{\mathscr{H}_{12b}} \leftarrow \underset{(4\text{-}32)}{\mathscr{H}_{12}\,\text{(second term)}}$	Neglect
1.4	$\underset{(4\text{-}33)}{\mathscr{H}_{12}\,\text{(last term)}} \leftarrow \underset{(4\text{-}4)}{B}$	Neglect
1.5	$\underset{(4\text{-}33)}{\mathscr{H}_{12}\,\text{(last term)}} \leftarrow \underset{(4\text{-}4)}{B}$	Neglect
1.6	$\underset{(4\text{-}33)}{\mathscr{H}_{12}\,\text{(last term)}} \leftarrow \underset{(4\text{-}4)}{B}$	Neglect
2.1	$\underset{(2\text{-}92)}{\mathscr{H}^{(1)}_{1cv}} \leftarrow \underset{(2\text{-}83)}{\mathscr{H}^{(1)}_{1c}} \leftarrow \underset{\text{T2-4}}{\mathscr{H}^{(1)}_{1}} \leftarrow \underset{(2\text{-}58)}{\mathscr{H}^{(1)}}$	D'', (9-17), (9-18); $\Delta g''$(SO), (9-39); $A^{v''}$(SO), (9-50)
2.2	$\underset{(4\text{-}37)}{\mathscr{H}_{12d}} \leftarrow \underset{(4\text{-}33)}{\mathscr{H}_{12}\,\text{(last)}} \leftarrow \underset{(4\text{-}4)}{B}$	D'', (9-17), (9-18); $\Delta g''$(2e1), (9-41); $A^{v''}$(2e1), (9-51)
2.3	$\underset{(4\text{-}36)}{\mathscr{H}_{12c}} \leftarrow \underset{(4\text{-}32)}{\mathscr{H}_{12}\,\text{(second term)}}$	D'', (9-17), (9-18); $\Delta g''$(2e1), (9-41); $A^{v''}$(2e1), (9-51)
2.4	$\underset{(4\text{-}39)}{\mathscr{H}_{12e}} \leftarrow \underset{(4\text{-}33)}{\mathscr{H}_{12}\text{(last)}} \leftarrow \underset{(4\text{-}4)}{B}$	D' (9-7)
2.5	$\underset{(4\text{-}40)}{\mathscr{H}_{12f}} \leftarrow \underset{(4\text{-}33)}{\mathscr{H}_{12}\,\text{(last)}} \leftarrow \underset{(4\text{-}4)}{B}$	Neglect[a]
2.6	$\underset{(4\text{-}33)}{\mathscr{H}_{12}\,\text{(last)}}$	$q^{vv'}$ (dipole), (9-53)

2.7	$\underset{(5\text{-}19)(5\text{-}20)}{\mathscr{H}^{(0)}_{2qv}} \leftarrow \underset{\text{T2-4}}{\mathscr{H}^{(0)}_{2}} \leftarrow \underset{(2\text{-}58)}{\mathscr{H}^{(0)}}$	q^{vv} (quadrupole), (9-52)
2.8	$\underset{(2\text{-}68)}{\mathscr{H}^{(0)}_{1bv}} \leftarrow \underset{(2\text{-}83)}{\mathscr{H}^{(0)}_{1b}} \leftarrow \underset{\text{T2-4}}{\mathscr{H}^{(0)}_{1}} \leftarrow \underset{(2\text{-}58)}{\mathscr{H}^{(0)}}$	$A^{v''}$ (SO), (9-50); $A^{v''}$ (2e1), (9-51); $q^{vv'}$ (orbital), (9-55)
2.9	$\underset{(2\text{-}99)}{\mathscr{H}^{(1)}_{2bv}} \leftarrow \underset{(2\text{-}97)}{\mathscr{H}^{(1)}_{2b}} \leftarrow \underset{\text{T2-4}}{\mathscr{H}^{(1)}_{2}} \leftarrow \underset{(2\text{-}58)}{\mathscr{H}^{(1)}}$	Neglect
2.10	$\underset{(2\text{-}73)}{\mathscr{H}^{(0)}_{1cvv'}} \leftarrow \underset{(2\text{-}83)}{\mathscr{H}^{(0)}_{1c}} \leftarrow \underset{\text{T2-4}}{\mathscr{H}^{(0)}_{1}} \leftarrow \underset{(2\text{-}58)}{\mathscr{H}^{(0)}}$	$q^{vv'}(A^2)$, (9-54) [neglect]
2.11	$\underset{(2\text{-}75)}{\mathscr{H}^{(0)}_{1dv}} \leftarrow \underset{(2\text{-}62)}{\mathscr{H}^{(0)}_{1d}} \leftarrow \underset{\text{T2-4}}{\mathscr{H}^{(0)}_{1}} \leftarrow \underset{(2\text{-}58)}{\mathscr{H}^{(0)}}$	$A^{v'}$ (dipole), (9-47)
2.12	$\underset{(2\text{-}96)}{\mathscr{H}^{(1)}_{1evv}} \leftarrow \underset{(2\text{-}83)}{\mathscr{H}^{(1)}_{1e}} \leftarrow \underset{\text{T2-4}}{\mathscr{H}^{(1)}_{1}} \leftarrow \underset{(2\text{-}58)}{\mathscr{H}^{(1)}}$	$A^{v'}$ (contact), (9-46); $q_0^{vv'(0)}$, (9-56), (9-57)
	$[\underset{(2\text{-}81)}{\mathscr{H}^{(0)}_{1dv'}}\ (\text{FW}) \leftarrow \underset{(2\text{-}75)}{\mathscr{H}^{(0)}_{1dv}} \leftarrow \underset{(2\text{-}62)}{\mathscr{H}^{(0)}_{1d}} \leftarrow \underset{\text{T2-4}}{\mathscr{H}^{(0)}_{1}} \leftarrow \underset{(2\text{-}58)}{\mathscr{H}^{(0)}}]$	
2.13	$\underset{(2\text{-}94)}{\mathscr{H}^{(1)}_{1evv'}} \leftarrow \underset{(2\text{-}83)}{\mathscr{H}^{(1)}_{1ev}} \leftarrow \underset{\text{T2-4}}{\mathscr{H}^{(1)}_{1}} \leftarrow \underset{(2\text{-}58)}{\mathscr{H}^{(1)}}$	$A^{v'}$ (SO correction), (9-48)
2.14	$\underset{(4\text{-}38)}{\mathscr{H}_{12dv}} \leftarrow \underset{(4\text{-}33)}{\mathscr{H}_{12}\ (\text{last})} \leftarrow \underset{(4\text{-}4)}{B}$	$A^{v'}$ (2e1 correction), (9-49)
2.15	$\underset{(4\text{-}36)}{\mathscr{H}_{12cv}} \leftarrow \underset{(4\text{-}32)}{\mathscr{H}_{12}\ (\text{second term})}$	$A^{v'}$ (2e1 correction), (9-49)
3.1	$\underset{(2\text{-}68)}{\mathscr{H}^{(0)}_{1b0}} \leftarrow \underset{(2\text{-}62)}{\mathscr{H}^{(0)}_{1b}} \leftarrow \underset{\text{T2-4}}{\mathscr{H}^{(0)}_{1}} \leftarrow \underset{(2\text{-}58)}{\mathscr{H}^{(0)}}$	$\Delta g''$ (SO), (9-39); $\Delta g''$ (2e1), (9-41); $\sigma^{v'}$ (9-45)
3.2	$\underset{(2\text{-}99)}{\mathscr{H}^{(1)}_{2bv}} \leftarrow \underset{(2\text{-}97)}{\mathscr{H}^{(1)}_{2b}} \leftarrow \underset{\text{T2-4}}{\mathscr{H}^{(1)}_{2}} \leftarrow \underset{(2\text{-}58)}{\mathscr{H}^{(1)}}$	Neglect
3.3	$\underset{(2\text{-}71)}{\mathscr{H}^{(0)}_{1c00}} \leftarrow \underset{(2\text{-}62)}{\mathscr{H}^{(0)}_{1c}} \leftarrow \underset{\text{T2-4}}{\mathscr{H}^{(0)}_{1}} \leftarrow \underset{(2\text{-}58)}{\mathscr{H}^{(0)}}$	Neglect
4.1	$\underset{(2\text{-}74)}{\mathscr{H}^{(0)}_{1d0}} \leftarrow \underset{(2\text{-}62)}{\mathscr{H}^{(0)}_{1d}} \leftarrow \underset{\text{T2-4}}{\mathscr{H}^{(0)}_{1}} \leftarrow \underset{(2\text{-}58)}{\mathscr{H}^{(0)}}$	g_e, (9-20)
4.2	$\underset{(2\text{-}100)}{\mathscr{H}^{(1)}_{2c0}} \leftarrow \underset{(2\text{-}97)}{\mathscr{H}^{(1)}_{2c}} \leftarrow \underset{\text{T2-4}}{\mathscr{H}^{(1)}_{2}} \leftarrow \underset{(2\text{-}58)}{\mathscr{H}^{(1)}}$	Δg^{KE}, (9-21)
4.3	$\underset{(2\text{-}93)}{\mathscr{H}^{(1)}_{1ev0}} \leftarrow \underset{(2\text{-}83)}{\mathscr{H}^{(1)}_{1e}} \leftarrow \underset{\text{T2-4}}{\mathscr{H}^{(1)}_{1}} \leftarrow \underset{(2\text{-}58)}{\mathscr{H}^{(1)}}$	$\Delta g'$ (SO), (9-38)
4.4	$\underset{(4\text{-}36)}{\mathscr{H}_{12c0}} \leftarrow \underset{(4\text{-}32)}{\mathscr{H}_{12}\ (\text{second term})}$	$\Delta g'$ (2e1), (9-40)
4.5	$\underset{(4\text{-}38)}{\mathscr{H}_{12d0}} \leftarrow \underset{(4\text{-}33)}{\mathscr{H}_{12}\ (\text{last})} \leftarrow \underset{(4\text{-}4)}{B}$	$\Delta g'$ (2e1), (9-40)
4.6	By analogy to 4.1	Nuclear Zeeman, (9-43)
4.7	$\underset{(2\text{-}72)}{\mathscr{H}^{(0)}_{1c0v}} \leftarrow \underset{(2\text{-}62)}{\mathscr{H}^{(0)}_{1c}} \leftarrow \underset{\text{T2-4}}{\mathscr{H}^{(0)}_{1}} \leftarrow \underset{(2\text{-}58)}{\mathscr{H}^{(0]}}$	$\sigma^{v'}$, (9-44)

[a] See Section 9.

the coefficient seems to include g, while the coefficient determined in the partitioning method includes g'. The partitioning approach is preferable, for several reasons indicated in Section 2, but the experimental value for the hyperfine interaction in ground state atomic hydrogen suggests that g rather than g' is correct. The nuclear g factors g_ν are assumed to be phenomenological parameters giving nuclear magnetic moments in units of the nuclear magneton β_N.

The fourth column of Table F-1 lists the coefficient multiplying each operator, in atomic units (see Appendix A). Each coefficient includes an appropriate power of the fine structure constant α, and may include a power of the electron–proton mass ratio m/M_P. The remaining factors in the coefficient suggest the appropriate dimensionality, but are in fact of magnitude one when atomic units are used. The constants are $\mathscr{E}_0$, the Hartree unit of energy, a_0, the Bohr radius, and e, the electronic charge. Note that $e^2/a_0 = \mathscr{E}_0$ and the atomic unit of magnetic field strength is $\alpha^{-1}e/a_0^2$.

Coefficients appropriate to the use of Gaussian units are given in column five. In addition to the fundamental quantities e, $\hbar$, m, and c, this listing uses the Bohr magneton $\beta = e\hbar/2mc$ and the nuclear magneton $\beta_N = e\hbar/2M_Pc$.

Table F-2 gives the "origin" and "destination" of each of the Hamiltonian terms. The origin refers to the sequence of operators obtained in the reduction of the Dirac and Breit equations to nonrelativistic form, with the notation of Sections 2 and 4. Numbers in parentheses are the numbers of equations giving these operators, and T2-4 refers to Table 2-4. The destination designations are spin Hamiltonian parameters. The notation is that of Section 9, and again numbers refer to appropriate equations.

Various terms are indicated as being neglected. The reason for this neglect is either that the term in question does not contribute to the energy differences observed in ordinary ESR experiments, or else that its effect is too small to be significant. Some terms which appear to be small must be retained to preserve gauge invariance. Other, parallel terms were then included also, even though their effects may later be neglected.

REFERENCES

Number(s) in parentheses at end of reference indicate page(s) on which the reference is cited.

1. A. Abragam, *The Principles of Nuclear Magnetism*. Oxford Univ. Press, London and New York, 1961. (90)
2. A. Abragam and B. Bleaney, *Electron Paramagnetic Resonance of Transition Ions*, Oxford Univ. Press (Clarendon), London and New York, 1970. (x)
3. A. T. Amos and B. L. Burrows, *Advan. Quant. Chem.* **7**, 289 (1973). (327)
4. A. T. Amos and G. G. Hall, *Proc. Roy. Soc.* (*London*) **A263**, 483 (1961). (244, 252)
5. A. T. Amos and L. C. Snyder, *J. Chem. Phys.* **41**, 1773 (1964). (252, 306)
6. L. Armstrong, Jr., *Theory of the Hyperfine Structure of Free Atoms*, Wiley, New York, 1971. (97)
7. P. S. Bagus and B. Liu, quoted by K. M. Sando [180], pp. 76, 93]. (272)
8. P. S. Bagus, B. Liu, and H. F. Schaefer III, *Phys. Rev.* **A2**, 555 (1970). (255, 272)
9. J. C. Baird, J. Brandenberger, K. I. Gondaria, and H. Metcalf, *Phys. Rev.* **A5**, 564 (1972). (72)
10. W. A. Barker and Z. V. Chraplyvy, *Phys. Rev.* **89**, 446 (1953). (40, 73)
11. W. A. Barker and F. N. Glover, *Phys. Rev.* **99**, 317 (1955). (83)
12. M. P. Barnett, "The Evaluation of Molecular Integrals by the Zeta Function Expansion," *Methods Computat. Phys.* **2**, 95 (1963). (281, 293)
13. D. R. Bates, K. Ledsham, and A. L. Stewart, *Philos. Trans. Roy. Soc.* (*London*) **246**, 215 (1953). (35, 107)
14. G. G. Belford, R. L. Belford, and J. F. Burkhalter, *J. Magn. Reson.* **11**, 251 (1973). (150, 151, 154)
15. R. L. Belford, P. H. Davis, G. G. Belford, and T. M. Lenhardt, in *Extended Interactions between Metal Ions in Transition Metal Complexes*," *A.C.S. Symposium Series*, No. 5, American Chemical Society, 1974, pp. 40–50. (150, 154)
16. K. F. Bergren and R. F. Wood, *Phys. Rev.* **130**, 198 (1963). (273)
17. H. A. Bethe and E. E. Salpeter, *Quantum Mechanics of One- and Two-Electron Atoms*, Springer-Verlag, Berlin, 1957, and Academic Press, New York, 1957. (47, 73, 78, 90)
18. W. A. Bingel and W. Kutzelnigg, "Symmetry Properties of Reduced Density Matrices and Natural p-States," *Advan. Quant. Chem.* **5**, 201 (1970). (208, 260)
19. S. M. Blinder, *J. Molecular Spectroscopy* **5**, 17 (1960). (47)
20. J. R. Bolton, *Mag. Reson. Rev.* **1**, 195 (1972). (326)
21. S. F. Boys, *Proc. Roy. Soc.* (*London*) **A200**, 542 (1950). (281)
22. G. Breit, *Phys. Rev.* **37**, 51 (1931). (47)
23. G. Breit and I. I. Rabi, *Phys. Rev.* **38**, 2082 (1931). (115)
24. E. Breitenberger, *Am. J. Phys.* **36**, 505 (1968). (82)
25. D. M. Brink and G. R. Satchler, *Angular Momentum*, 2nd ed., Oxford Univ. Press (Clarendon), 1968. (346)
26. K. M. Brubaker, Ph.D. Thesis, Univ. of Wisconsin, Madison, 1972. (12)

27. E. A. Burke, *Phys. Rev.* **130**, 1871 (1963). (273)
28. E. A. Burke, *Phys. Rev.* **135A**, 621 (1964). (273)
29. E. A. Burke and L. Cassar, *J. Chem. Phys.* **59**, 4035 (1973). (272)
30. E. A. Burke and J. F. Mulligan, *J. Chem. Phys.* **28**, 995 (1958). (272)
31. A. Carrington, *Microwave Spectroscopy of Free Radicals*, Academic Press, London and New York, 1974. (x, 102)
32. A. Carrington and A. D. McLachlan, *Introduction to Magnetic Resonance*, Harper & Row, New York, Evanston, and London, 1967. (1)
33. K. M. Case, *Phys. Rev.* **95**, 1323 (1954). (40)
34. E. S. Chang, R. T. Pu, and T. P. Das, *Phys. Rev.* **174**, 1 (1968). (273)
35. Z. V. Chraplyvy, *Phys. Rev.* **91**, 388 (1953). (83, 85)
36. Z. V. Chraplyvy, *Phys. Rev.* **92**, 1310 (1953). (83, 84, 85)
37. E. Clementi, *IBM J. Res. Devel. Suppl.* **9**, 2 (1965). (271)
38. J. P. Colpa and J. R. Bolton, *Molecular Phys.* **6**, 273 (1963). (320)
39. I. L. Cooper and R. McWeeny, *J. Chem. Phys.* **45**, 226 (1966). (267)
40. I. G. Csizmadia, M. C. Harrison, J. W. Moskowitz, and B. T. Sutcliffe, *Theor. Chim. Acta*. **6**, 191 (1966). (281)
41. C. F. Curtiss, "The Separation of Rotational Coordinates from the N-Particle Schroedinger Equation, II," University of Wisconsin, Madison, OOR-2 (unpublished), 1952. (102, 104)
42. A. Dalgarno, in *Quantum Theory, I. Elements*, D. R. Bates, Ed., Academic Press, New York and London, 1961, pp. 172–210. (126)
43. E. R. Davidson, "Natural Orbitals," *Advan. Quant. Chem.* **6**, 235 (1972). (260)
44. E. R. Davidson, *Reduced Density Matrices in Quantum Chemistry*, Academic Press, New York and London, 1976. (259, 270, 356)
45. D. W. Davies, *The Theory of Electric and Magnetic Properties of Molecules*, Wiley, London, New York, and Sidney, 1967, p. 52. (197)
46. P. A. M. Dirac, *Proc. Roy. Soc.* (*London*) **A117**, 610 (1928). (15)
47. P. A. M. Dirac, *The Principles of Quantum Mechanics*, 4th ed., Oxford Univ. Press, London and New York, 1958. (15, 16, 28, 43, 44)
48. P. A. M. Dirac, *Lectures on Quantum Field Theory*, Yeshiva University and Academic Press, New York, 1966. (71, 76)
49. A. R. Edmonds, *Angular Momentum in Quantum Mechanics*, Princeton Univ. Press, Princeton, New Jersey, 1957. (326)
50. R. R. Ernst, *Advan. Magn. Reson.* **2**, 1 (1966). (6)
51. P. G. Estabrooks, "On the Relativistic Two-Electron Problem," (unpublished), 1968. (83)
52. U. Fano and G. Racah, *Irreducible Tensorial Sets*, Academic Press, New York, San Francisco, and London, 1959. (326, 353, 364)
53. H. A. Farach and C. P. Poole, Jr., *Advan. Magn. Reson.* **5**, 229 (1971). (137)
54. R. W. Fessenden, *J. Chem. Phys.* **37**, 747 (1962). (119, 129)
55. M. E. Fisher, *Am. J. Phys.* **30**, 49 (1962). (123)
56. L. L. Foldy, *Phys. Rev.* **87**, 688 (1952). (40)
57. L. L. Foldy and S. Wouthuysen, *Phys. Rev.* **78**, 29 (1950). (40, 43)
58. J. H. Freed, "Electron Spin Resonance," in *Annual Rev. Phys. Chem.* **23**, 265 (1972). (326)
59. G. A. Gallup, *Internat. J. Quantum Chem.* **6**, 899 (1972). (267)
60. G. A. Gallup, "The Symmetric Group and Calculation of Energies of n-Electron Systems in Pure Spin States," *Adv. Quant. Chem.* **7**, 113 (1973). (239)
61. G. Giacometti, P. L. Nordio, and M. V. Pavan, *Theor, Chim. Acta* **1**, **404** (1963). (320)
62. W. A. Goddard III, *Phys. Rev.* **157**, 93 (1967). (253, 272)

63. W. A. Goddard III, *Phys. Rev.* **169**, 120 (1968). (272)
64. H. Goldstein, *Classical Mechanics*, Addison-Wesley, Reading, Massachusetts, 1950. (329, 357)
65. I. S. Gradshteyn and I. M. Ryzhik, *Table of Integrals, Series, and Products*, 4th ed., Yu. V. Geronimus and M. Yu. Tseytlin, Eds., A. Jeffrey, Transl., Academic Press, New York and London, 1965. (161, 312)
66. J. S. Griffith, *Molecular Phys.* **3**, 79 (1960). (168)
67. J. S. Griffith, *The Theory of Transition Metal Ions*, Cambridge Univ. Press, London and New York, 1961. (197)
68. H. Grotch and D. R. Yennie, *Rev. Mod. Phys.* **41**, 350 (1969). (75)
69. H. F. Hameka, *Advanced Quantum Chemistry*, Addison-Wesley, Reading, Massachusetts, 1965. (344)
70. D. L. Hardcastle, J. L. Gammal, and R. Keown, *J. Chem. Phys.* **49**, 1358 (1968). (271, 272)
71. D. L. Hardcastle and R. Keown, *J. Chem. Phys.* **51**, 598 (1969). (272)
72. A. Hardisson and J. E. Harriman, *J. Chem. Phys.* **46**, 3639 (1967). (249)
73. J. E. Harriman, *J. Chem. Phys.* **40**, 2827 (1964). (247, 248, 250)
74. J. E. Harriman, "On the Reduction of the Dirac Equation to Two-Component Form," Preprint 127, Uppsala Quantum Chemistry Group (unpublished), 1964. (37, 51)
75. J. E. Harriman, "The Use of Projection in SCF Spin Density Calculations," *La Structure Hyperfine Magnétique des Atomes et des Molécules*, (Colloques Internationaux du CNRS) **164**, 139 (1966). (252)
76. J. E. Harriman and K. M. Sando, *J. Chem. Phys.* **48**, 5138. (253, 306)
77. E. G. Harris, *A Pedestrian Approach to Quantum Field Theory*, Wiley, New York, 1972. (71)
78. F. E. Harris, "Molecular Orbital Theory," in *Adv. Quant. Chem.* **3**, 61 (1967). (230)
79. G. Herzberg, *Molecular Spectra and Molecular Structure, I. Spectra of Diatomic Molecules*, 2nd ed., Van Nostrand Reinhold, Princeton, New Jersey, 1950. (102)
80. J. O. Hirschfelder and P. R. Certain, *J. Chem. Phys.* **60**, 1118 (1974). (126, 130)
81. J. O. Hirschfelder and W. J. Meath, "The Nature of Intermolecular Forces," Section II, *Advan. Chem. Phys.*, **12**, 3 (1967). (102)
82. E. W. Hobson, *The Theory of Spherical and Ellipsoidal Harmonics*, Cambridge Univ. Press, London and New York, 1931. (297)
83. B. J. Howard and R. E. Moss, *Molecular Phys.* **19**, 433 (1970). (102)
84. B. J. Howard and R. E. Moss, *Molecular Phys.* **20**, 147 (1970). (102)
85. L. D. Huff, *Phys. Rev.* **38**, 501 (1931). (20)
86. R. P. Hurst, J. D. Gray, G. H. Brigman, and F. A. Matsen, *Molecular Phys.* **1**, 189 (1958). (272)
87. L. J. Hutchison, "The Dirac Equation for the H_2^+ Ion" (unpublished), 1969. (35)
88. D. J. E. Ingram, *Spectroscopy at Radio and Microwave Frequencies*, 2nd ed., Butterworth, London, 1967. (102)
89. T. Itoh, *Rev. Mod. Phys.* **37**, 159 (1965). (86)
90. M. H. Johnson and B. A. Lippman, *Phys. Rev.* **76**, 828 (1949). (20)
91. U. Kaldor, *J. Chem. Phys.* **48**, 835 (1968). (253, 254, 271, 272)
92. U. Kaldor and F. E. Harris, *Phys. Rev.* **183**, 1 (1969). (272)
93. M. Karplus and G. K. Fraenkel, *J. Chem. Phys.* **35**, 1312 (1961). (307)
94. I. Kazuhiro and H. Nakatsuji, *Chem. Phys. Lett.* **19**, 268 (1973). (273)
95. J. Kerwin and E. A. Burke, *J. Chem. Phys.* **36**, 2987 (1962). (272)
96. M. Klessinger and R. McWeeny, *J. Chem. Phys.* **42**, 3343 (1965). (308)
97. F. K. Kneubühl, *J. Chem. Phys.* **33**, 1074 (1965). (162)
98. H. Konishi and K. Morokuma, *Chem. Phys. Lett.* **12**, 408 (1971). (272, 273)

99. M. Kotani, A. Amemiya, E. Isiguro, and T. Kimura, *Tables of Molecular Integrals*, Mazureu Co., Tokyo, 1963. (225)
100. L. Landau and E. Lifschitz, *The Classical Theory of Fields*, Addison-Wesley, Reading, Massachusetts, 1951. (79, 330, 333)
101. S. Larsson, *Phys. Rev.* **169**, 49 (1968). (275)
102. S. Larsson and V. H. Smith, Jr., *Phys. Rev.* **178**, 137 (1969). (273)
103. S. Larsson and V. H. Smith, Jr., *Internat. J. Quant. Chem.* **6**, 1019 (1972). (275)
104. R. Lefebvre and C. Moser, Eds., *Correlation Effects in Atoms and Molecules, Advan. Chem. Phys.* **14**, Wiley (Interscience), New York, 1969. (267)
105. M. J. Levine and J. Wright, *Phys. Rev. Letters* **26**, 1351 (1971). (71)
106. P. O. Löwdin, *Phys. Rev.* **97**, 1474 (1955). (259, 266, 267, 356)
107. P. O. Löwdin, *Phys. Rev.* **97**, 1490 (1955). (248, 249)
108. P. O. Löwdin, *Phys. Rev.* **97**, 1509 (1955). (229, 246)
109. P. O. Löwdin, *Rev. Mod. Phys.* **32**, 328 (1960). (229)
110. P. O. Löwdin, *J. Appl. Phys. Suppl.* **33**, 251 (1962). (244)
111. P. O. Löwdin, *J. Molecular Spectroscopy* **14**, 131 (1964). (47, 48)
112. S. K. Luke, G. Hunter, R. P. McEachran, and M. Cohen, *J. Chem. Phys.* **50**, 1644 (1969). (35)
113. H. M. McConnell, *J. Chem. Phys.* **28**, 1188 (1958). (302)
114. H. M. McConnell and D. B. Chestnut, *J. Chem. Phys.* **27**, 984 (1957). (307)
115. H. M. McConnell and D. B. Chestnut, *J. Chem. Phys.* **28**, 107 (1958). (307)
116. H. M. McConnell and H. H. Dearman, *J. Chem. Phys.* **28**, 51 (1958). (307)
117. H. M. McConnell and J. Strathdee, *Molecular Phys.* **2**, 129 (1959). (293)
118. A. D. McLachlan, *Molecular Phys.* **3**, 233 (1960). (305)
119. A. D. McLachlan, H. H. Dearman, and R. Lefebvre, *J. Chem. Phys.* **33**, 65 (1960). (307, 308)
120. A. D. McLean and M. Yoshimine, *J. Chem. Phys.* **46**, 1812 (1967). (300)
121. R. McWeeny, *Proc. Roy. Soc.* (*London*) **A253**, 242 (1959). (308)
122. R. McWeeny, *Rev. Mod. Phys.* **32**, 335 (1960). (248, 249, 308, 356)
123. R. McWeeny, *J. Chem. Phys.* **42**, 1717 (1965). (164, 208)
124. R. McWeeny, *Spins in Chemistry*, Polytechnic Press of the Polytechnic Inst. of Brooklyn and Academic Press, New York, 1970. (208)
125. R. McWeeny and W. Kutzelnigg, *Internat. J. Quant. Chem.* **2**, 187 (1967). (260)
126. R. McWeeny and Y. Mizuno, *Proc. Roy. Soc.* (*London*) **A259**, 554 (1961). (208, 211, 215, 249, 317)
127. R. McWeeny and E. Steiner, "The Theory of Pair-Correlated Wave Functions," *Advan. Quantum Chem.* **2**, 93 (1965). (269)
128. R. McWeeny and B. T. Sutcliffe, *Proc. Roy. Soc.* (*London*) **A273**, 103 (1963). (308)
129. R. McWeeny and B. T. Sutcliffe, *Methods of Molecular Quantum Mechanics*, Academic Press, New York and London, 1969. (83, 236, 308)
130. W. Marshal, *Proc. Phys. Soc.* (*London*) **A78**, 113 (1961). (253)
131. J. B. Martin and A. W. Weiss, *J. Chem. Phys.* **39**, 1618 (1963). (273)
132. R. L. Matcha and C. W. Kern, *J. Chem. Phys.* **55**, 469 (1971). (277)
133. R. L. Matcha, C. W. Kern, and D. M. Schrader, *J. Chem. Phys.* **51**, 2152 (1969). (277, 300)
134. R. L. Matcha, D. J. Kouri, and C. W. Kern, *J. Chem. Phys.* **53**, 1052 (1970). (277, 294)
135. R. L. Matcha, G. Malli, and M. B. Milleur, *J. Chem. Phys.* **56**, 5982 (1972). (277)
136. F. A. Matsen, "Spin-Free Quantum Chemistry," *Advan. Quantum Chem.* **1**, 59 (1964). (222, 229)
137. M. T. Melchior, *J. Chem. Phys.* **50**, 511 (1969). (307, 320)

138. A. Messiah, *Quantum Mechanics*, Wiley, New York, 1962. (22, 59, 70, 346)
139. W. Meyer, *J. Chem. Phys.* **51**, 5149 (1969). (272)
140. M. B. Milleur and R. L. Matcha, *J. Chem. Phys.* **57**, 3029 (1972). (277)
141. M. Mizushima, *The Theory of Rotating Diatomic Molecules*, Wiley, New York, 1975. (102)
142. E. A. Moore and R. E. Moss, *Molecular Phys.* **30**, 1297 (1975). (90)
143. E. A. Moore and R. E. Moss, *Molecular Phys.* **30**, 1315 (1975). (51, 75, 90)
144. R. E. Moss, *Advanced Molecular Quantum Mechanics*, Chapman & Hall, London, 1973. (75)
145. L. T. Muus and P. W. Atkins, Eds., *Electron Spin Relaxation in Liquids*, Plenum, New York and London, 1972. (x)
146. R. K. Nesbet, *Phys. Rev.* **118**, 681 (1960). (271, 273)
147. R. K. Nesbet, "Bethe–Goldstone Calculations of the Magnetic Hyperfine Structure of Li(^{2}S) and N(^{4}S)," *La Structure Hyperfine Magnétique des Atomes et des Molécules*, Colloques Internationaux du CNRS) **164**, 87 (1966). (273)
148. R. K. Nesbet, "Computation of the Magnetic Hyperfine Structure of Atomic S-States," in *Quantum Theory of Atoms, Molecules and the Solid State*, P. O. Löwdin, Ed., Academic Press, New York and London, 1966, pp. 157–165. (273)
149. J. M. Norbeck and G. A. Gallup, *J. Am. Chem. Soc.* **96**, 3386 (1974). (322)
150. R. T. Pack, "Corrections to the Born–Oppenheimer Approximation," Ph.D. Thesis, Univ. of Wisconsin, Madison, WIS-TCI-197, 1966. (102, 104)
151. R. T. Pack and J. O. Hirschfelder, *J. Chem. Phys.* **49**, 4009 (1968). (102, 104)
152. W. K. H. Panofsky and M. Phillips, *Classical Electricity and Magnetism*, Addison-Wesley, Reading, Mass., 1955. (298, 330)
153. R. G. Parr, *The Quantum Theory of Molecular Electronic Structure*, Benjamin, New York and Amsterdam, 1964. (306)
154. L. Pauling and E. B. Wilson, Jr., *Introduction to Quantum Mechanics*, McGraw-Hill, New York, 1935. (35, 65)
155. R. Pauncz, *Alternant Molecular Orbital Method*, Saunders, Philadelphia and London, 1967. (223, 227, 229)
156. P. I. Pavlik and S. M. Blinder, *J. Chem. Phys.* **46**, 2749 (1967). (35)
157. D. H. Phillips and J. C. Schug, *J. Chem. Phys.* **61**, 1013 (1974). (249)
158. R. M. Pitzer, C. W. Kern, and W. Lipscomb, *J. Chem. Phys.* **37**, 267 (1962). (279, 286, 293, 300)
159. C. P. Poole, Jr., and H. A. Farach, *Relaxation in Magnetic Resonance*, Academic Press, New York and London, 1971. (x)
160. J. A. Pople and D. L. Beveridge, *Approximate Molecular Orbital Theory*, McGraw-Hill, New York, 1970. (303)
161. G. W. Pratt, Jr., *Phys. Rev.* **102**, 1303 (1956). (246)
162. R. H. Pritchard and C. W. Kern, *J. Chem. Phys.* **57**, 2590 (1972). (300, 301)
163. M. L. H. Pryce, *Proc. Roy. Soc.* (*London*) **A195**, 62 (1948). (98)
164. N. F. Ramsey, *Molecular Beams*, Oxford Univ. Press, London, 1963). (90, 96)
165. D. C. Reitz and S. I. Weissman, *J. Chem. Phys.* **33**, 700 (1960). (130)
166. P. Roman, *Theory of Elementary Particles*, 2nd ed., North-Holland Publ., Amsterdam, 1964. (332)
167. P. Roman, *Introduction to Quantum Field Theory*, Wiley, New York, 1969. (77)
168. C. C. J. Roothaan, *Rev. Mod. Phys.* **23**, 69 (1951). (254)
169. C. C. J. Roothaan, *Rev. Mod. Phys.* **32**, 179 (1960). (244, 254)
170. C. C. J. Roothaan, L. M. Sachs, and A. W. Weiss, *Rev. Mod. Phys.* **32**, 186 (1960). (271)
171. M. E. Rose, *Elementary Theory of Angular Momentum*, Wiley, New York,1957). (346)

172. M. E. Rose, *Relativistic Electron Theory*, Wiley, New York, 1961. (7, 18, 28, 32, 34, 40, 61)
173. K. Ruedenberg and R. D. Poshusta, "Matrix Elements and Density Matrices for Many-Electron Spin Eigenstates Built from Orthonormal Orbitals," *Advan. Quant. Chem.* **6**, 267 (1972). (236, 239)
174. K. Ruedenberg, C. C. J. Roothaan, and W. Jaunzenics, *J. Chem. Phys.* **24**, 201 (1956). (294)
175. M. B. Ruskai, "The Dirac Equation for H_2^+ in the Fixed-Nuclei Approximation" (unpublished), 1966. (35)
176. L. M. Sachs, *Phys. Rev.* **117**, 1504 (1960). (271, 272)
177. L. Salem, *The Molecular Orbital Theory of Conjugated Systems*, Benjamin, New York and Amsterdam, 1966. (304)
178. W. I. Salmon, "Geneological Electron Spin Eigenfunctions and Antisymmetric Many-Electron Wavefunctions Generated Directly from Young Diagrams," *Advan. Quant. Chem.* **8**, 37 (1974). (225)
179. W. I. Salmon and K. Ruedenberg, *J. Chem. Phys.* **57**, 2776 (1972). (260)
180. K. M. Sando, Ph.D. Thesis, Univ. of Wisconsin, Madison, 1968. (272, 274)
181. K. M. Sando and J. E. Harriman, *J. Chem. Phys.* **47**, 180 (1967). (249, 253)
182. F. Sasaki and K. Ohno, *J. Math. Phys.* **4**, 1140 (1963). (230)
183. T. C. Sayetta and J. D. Memory, *J. Chem. Phys.* **40**, 2748 (1964). (320)
184. D. M. Schrader, *J. Chem. Phys.* **41**, 3266 (1964). (298)
185. J. C. Schug, T. H. Brown, and M. Karplus, *J. Chem. Phys.* **35**, 1873 (1961). (322)
186. S. S. Schweber, *An Introduction to Relativistic Quantum Field Theory*, Harper & Row, New York, 1961. (71)
187. W. T. Scott, *The Physics of Electricity and Magnetism*, Wiley, New York, 1959. (337)
188. R. R. Sharma, *Phys. Rev.* **A13**, 517 (1976). (281)
189. J. N. Silverman, quoted by J. B. Martin and A. W. Weiss [131]. (272)
190. J. C. Slater, *Quantum Theory of Atomic Structure*, Vol. II, McGraw-Hill, New York, 1960. (86)
191. J. C. Slater, "Statistical Exchange-Correlation in the Self-Consistent Field," in *Advan. Quant. Chem.* **6**, 1 (1972). (269)
192. C. P. Slichter, *Principles of Magnetic Resonance*, Harper & Row, New York, Evanston, and London, 1963. (1)
193. V. H. Smith, Jr., *J. Chem. Phys.* **41**, 277 (1964). (230)
194. L. C. Snyder and A. T. Amos, *J. Chem. Phys.* **42**, 3670 (1965). (252, 306)
195. C. E. Soloman, International *J. Quant. Chem.* **5**, 319 (1971). (272)
196. E. O. Steinborn and K. Ruedenberg, "Rotation and Translation of Regular and Irregular Solid Spherical Harmonics," *Advan. Quant. Chem.* **7**, 1 (1973). (279)
197. A. J. Stone, *Proc. Roy. Soc.* (*London*) **A271**, 424 (1963). (194)
198. P. D. Sullivan, *Magn. Reson. Rev.* **2**, 35, 315 (1973). (326)
199. B. T. Sutcliffe, *J. Chem. Phys.* **45**, 235 (1966). (267)
200. B. N. Taylor, W. H. Parker, and D. N. Langenberg, *Rev. Mod. Phys.* **41**, 375 (1969). (72, 341)
201. E. C. Titchmarsh, *Proc. Roy. Soc.* (*London*) **A266**, 33 (1961). (38)
202. J. J. Tortorelli and J. E. Harriman, "Hyperfine Coupling Constants for the Hydrogen Molecular Ion," WIS-TCI-456, Univ. of Wisconsin Theoretical Chemistry Institute, Madison, (unpublished), 1971. (108)
203. J. J. Tortorelli and J. E. Harriman, "Energy-Spin Density Relationships for Gaussian-Type Families of Approximate Wavefunctions," WIS-TCI-464, University of Wisconsin Theoretical Chemistry Institute, Madison (unpublished), 1971. (256, 257)

204. H. Wahlquist, *J. Chem. Phys.* **35**, 1708 (1961). (6)
205. J. A. Weil, *J. Chem. Phys.* **55**, 4685 (1971). (157)
206. J. A. Weil and J. H. Anderson, *J. Chem. Phys.* **28**, 864 (1958). (157)
207. J. A. Weil and J. H. Anderson, *J. Chem. Phys.* **35**, 1410 (1961). (137)
208. A. W. Weiss, *Phys. Rev.* **122**, 1826 (1961). (273)
209. J. C. Wesley and A. Rich, *Phys. Rev. Letters* **24**, 1320 (1970). (72)
210. E. P. Wigner, *Group Theory and Its Applications to the Quantum Mechanics of Atomic Spectra*, J. J. Griffin, Transl., Academic Press, New York and London, 1959. (346, 353)
211. J. H. Wilkinson, *The Algebraic Eigenvalue Problem*, Oxford Univ. Press (Clarendon) New York and London, 1965. (154)
212. D. J. Wineland and N. F. Ramsey, *Phys. Rev.* **A5**, 821 (1972). (96)

INDEX

Physical Chemistry

A Series of Monographs

Editor: **Ernest M. Loebl**

Department of Chemistry

Polytechnic Institute of New York

Brooklyn, New York

1 W. Jost: Diffusion in Solids, Liquids, Gases, 1952
2 S. Mizushima: Structure of Molecules and Internal Rotation, 1954
3 H. H. G. Jellinek: Degradation of Vinyl Polymers, 1955
4 M. E. L. McBain and E. Hutchinson: Solubilization and Related Phenomena, 1955
5 C. H. Bamford, A. Elliott, and W. E. Hanby: Synthetic Polypeptides, 1956
6 George J. Janz: Thermodynamic Properties of Organic Compounds — Estimation Methods, Principles and Practice, Revised Edition, 1967
7 G. K. T. Conn and D. G. Avery: Infrared Methods, 1960
8 C. B. Monk: Electrolytic Dissociation, 1961
9 P. Leighton: Photochemistry of Air Pollution, 1961
10 P. J. Holmes: Electrochemistry of Semiconductors, 1962
11 H. Fujita: The Mathematical Theory of Sedimentation Analysis, 1962
12 K. Shinoda, T. Nakagawa, B. Tamamushi, and T. Isemura: Colloidal Surfactants, 1963
13 J. E. Wollrab: Rotational Spectra and Molecular Structure, 1967
14 A. Nelson Wright and C. A. Winkler: Active Nitrogen, 1968
15 Robert B. Anderson, ed.: Experimental Methods in Catalytic Research, Volume I, 1968; Robert B. Anderson and Peter T. Dawson, eds.: Volumes II and III, 1976
16 Milton Kerker: The Scattering of Light and Other Electromagnetic Radiation, 1969
17 Oleg V. Krylov: Catalysis by Nonmetals — Rules for Catalyst Selection, 1970
18 Alfred Clark: The Theory of Adsorption and Catalysis, 1970
19 Arnold Reisman: Phase Equilibria: Basic Principles, Applications, Experimental Techniques, 1970
20 J. J. Bikerman: Physical Surfaces, 1970
21 R. T. Sanderson: Chemical Bonds and Bond Energy, Second Edition, 1976
22 S. Petrucci, ed.: Ionic Interactions: From Dilute Solutions to Fused Salts (In Two Volumes), 1971

23 A. B. F. Duncan: Rydberg Series in Atoms and Molecules, 1971

24 J. R. Anderson: Chemisorption and Reactions on Metallic Films, 1971

25 E. A. Moelwyn-Hughes: Chemical Statics and Kinetics of Solution, 1971

26 Ivan Draganic and Zorica Draganic: The Radiation Chemistry of Water, 1971

27 M. B. Huglin: Light Scattering from Polymer Solutions, 1972

28 M. J. Blandamer: Introduction to Chemical Ultrasonics, 1973

29 A. I. Kitaigorodsky: Molecular Crystals and Molecules, 1973

30 Wendell Forst: Theory of Unimolecular Reactions, 1973

31 Jerry Goodisman: Diatomic Interaction Potential Theory. Volume 1, Fundamentals, 1973; Volume 2, Applications, 1973

32 Alfred Clark: The Chemisorptive Bond: Basic Concepts, 1974

33 Saul T. Epstein: The Variation Method in Quantum Chemistry, 1974

34 I. G. Kaplan: Symmetry of Many-Electron Systems, 1975

35 John R. Van Wazer and Ilyas Absar: Electron Densities in Molecules and Molecular Orbitals, 1975

36 Brian L. Silver: Irreducible Tensor Methods: An Introduction for Chemists, 1976

37 John E. Harriman: Theoretical Foundations of Electron Spin Resonance, 1978

A
B
C 8
D 9
E 0
F 1
G 2
H 3
I 4
J 5